Endocrinology of the Heart in Health and Disease

Endocrinology of the Heart in Health and Disease

Integrated, Cellular, and Molecular Endocrinology of the Heart

Edited by

Jonathan C. Schisler, MS, PhD
McAllister Heart Institute, Department of Pharmacology
The University of North Carolina at Chapel Hill
Chapel Hill, NC, United States

Charles H. Lang, PhD
Department of Cellular and Molecular Physiology
The Pennsylvania State University College of Medicine
Hershey, PA, United States

Monte S. Willis, MD, PhD
Heart Institute, Department of Pathology & Laboratory Medicine
The University of North Carolina at Chapel Hill
Chapel Hill, NC, United States

ELSEVIER

AMSTERDAM • BOSTON • HEIDELBERG • LONDON
NEW YORK • OXFORD • PARIS • SAN DIEGO
SAN FRANCISCO • SINGAPORE • SYDNEY • TOKYO

Academic Press is an imprint of Elsevier

Academic Press is an imprint of Elsevier
125 London Wall, London EC2Y 5AS, United Kingdom
525 B Street, Suite 1800, San Diego, CA 92101-4495, United States
50 Hampshire Street, 5th Floor, Cambridge, MA 02139, United States
The Boulevard, Langford Lane, Kidlington, Oxford OX5 1GB, United Kingdom

British Library Cataloguing-in-Publication Data
A catalogue record for this book is available from the British Library

Library of Congress Cataloging-in-Publication Data
A catalog record for this book is available from the Library of Congress

ISBN: 978-0-12-803111-7

For Information on all Academic Press publications
visit our website at https://www.elsevier.com

Publisher: Mica Haley
Acquisition Editor: Tari Broderick
Editorial Project Manager: Jeffrey Rossetti and Kathy Padilla
Production Project Manager: Lucía Pérez
Designer: Maria Inês Cruz

Typeset by MPS Limited, Chennai, India

We dedicate this book to our mentors and inspiration for our work in metabolism and cardiovascular disease: Heinrich Taegtmeyer, MD, William C. Stanley, PhD, Gary Lopaschuk, PhD, Martin Young, PhD, Michael Portman, MD, Doug Lewandowski, PhD, Chris Newgard, PhD, and Cam Patterson, MD, MBA. We hope to pass along their enthusiasm, guidance, and unwavering encouragement they were so generous to share with us.

Stacy, Matthew, Cole, & Erin...
thank you for letting me "go to school" in perpetuity

Aunt Kyle...
for never letting me forget my pledge to get my name on a book spine,
Lubert Stryer, I'm closing in
Jonathan

For Tina, Connor, and Declan...
the inspiration and distraction making this all possible
Monte

Contents

List of Contributors

F. Al-Mohanna
King Faisal Specialist Hospital and Research Centre & Alfaisal University Medical College, Riyadh, Saudi Arabia

J. Bartlett
Dalhousie Medicine New Brunswick (DMNB), Saint John, NB, Canada

F. Bortolotti
International Centre for Genetic Engineering and Biotechnology (ICGEB), Trieste, Italy

C.J. Charles
University of Otago, Christchurch, New Zealand

K. Chatha
Walsall Manor Hospital Walsall Healthcare NHS Trust, Walsall, United Kingdom

M. Ciccarelli
University of Salerno, Baronissi, SA, Italy

E. Coscioni
Azienda Ospedaliera Universitaria OO.RR. San Giovanni di Dio Ruggi d'Aragona, Salerno, Italy

W.C. De Mello
University of Puerto Rico, San Juan, PR, United States

G. Iaccarino
University of Salerno, Baronissi, SA, Italy

K. Kangawa
National Cerebral and Cardiovascular Center Research Institute, Suita, Osaka, Japan

M. Karmazyn
University of Western Ontario, London, ON, Canada

K. Kuwahara
Kyoto University Graduate School of Medicine, Kyoto, Japan

I. Kyrou
Aston University, Birmingham, United Kingdom; University Hospitals Coventry and Warwickshire (UHCW) NHS Trust, Coventry, United Kingdom; University of Warwick, Coventry, United Kingdom; Walsall Manor Hospital Walsall Healthcare NHS Trust, Walsall, United Kingdom

D. Ledee
University of Washington and Seattle Children's Research Institute, Seattle, WA, United States

A. Lymperopoulos
Nova Southeastern University College of Pharmacy, Fort Lauderdale, FL, United States

H.S. Mattu
University Hospitals Coventry and Warwickshire (UHCW) NHS Trust, Coventry, United Kingdom; University of Warwick, Coventry, United Kingdom

Y. Nakagawa
Kyoto University Graduate School of Medicine, Kyoto, Japan

K. Nakao
Kyoto University Graduate School of Medicine, Kyoto, Japan

T. Nishikimi
Kyoto University Graduate School of Medicine, Kyoto, Japan; Wakakusa-Tatsuma Rehabilitation Hospital, Osaka, Japan

T. Parry
University of North Carolina, Chapel Hill, NC, United States

C.J. Pemberton
University of Otago, Christchurch, New Zealand

M.A. Portman
University of Washington and Seattle Children's Research Institute, Seattle, WA, United States

T. Pulinilkunnil
Dalhousie Medicine New Brunswick (DMNB), Saint John, NB, Canada

H.S. Randeva
Aston University, Birmingham, United Kingdom; University Hospitals Coventry and Warwickshire (UHCW) NHS Trust, Coventry, United Kingdom; University of Warwick, Coventry, United Kingdom; Walsall Manor Hospital Walsall Healthcare NHS Trust, Walsall, United Kingdom

M.J. Ranek
The Johns Hopkins Medical Institutes, Baltimore, MD, United States

F.A. Recchia
Lewis Katz School of Medicine at Temple University, Philadelphia, PA, United States; Scuola Superiore Sant'Anna, Pisa, Italy

A.M. Richards
University of Otago, Christchurch, New Zealand

G. Ruozi
International Centre for Genetic Engineering and Biotechnology (ICGEB), Trieste, Italy

W.K. Samson
Saint Louis University School of Medicine, Saint Louis, MO, United States

G. Santulli
Columbia University Medical Center, New York, NY, United States

D. Sorriento
Institute of Biostructure and Bioimaging (IBB) of the Italian National Research Council (CNR), Naples, Italy

L.M. Stein
Saint Louis University School of Medicine, Saint Louis, MO, United States

P. Trivedi
Dalhousie Medicine New Brunswick (DMNB), Saint John, NB, Canada

A. Vu
Nova Southeastern University College of Pharmacy, Fort Lauderdale, FL, United States

M.S. Willis
University of North Carolina, Chapel Hill, NC, United States

G.L.C. Yosten
Saint Louis University School of Medicine, Saint Louis, MO, United States

Foreword

I never thought, until about two
months ago, I'd ever have to learn the
Krebs cycle. Now I realize I have to—James Watson
The New Anatomy of Cancer,
THE NEW YORK TIMES MAGAZINE
May 15, 2016

Like the dinosaurs from *Jurassic Park*, terms like metabolism, hormones, and homeostasis seem to belong to a bygone era. In today's world, terms like deep sequencing, gene editing, and gene-based therapies overshadow other established concepts, such as the flow of energy and the cross talk between the organs of the body. However, just as it is with cancer research, suddenly, cardiovascular research remembers its roots in metabolism (see James Watson above): new insights into the function of the heart are now emerging from an integral view interconnecting the heart with its biochemistry.

Endocrinology of the Heart in Health and Disease is a vivid example of the heart as a metabolic organ that is in seamless communication with its environment, both as a provider and as a target of hormonal signals. A group of world-class experts has come together to make a valiant effort and sort through many layers of complexity. The book will be a terrific resource for students, fellows, and investigators of all stripes. I value in particular the fact that cardiovascular research, long dominated by hemodynamics and coronary flow, is beginning to pay attention to the dynamic nature of the heart as a metabolic endocrine organ. Conceptually, *Endocrinology of the Heart in Health and Disease* fills a big gap. And, like *Jurassic Park*, the book also stands a good chance to go through more editions in years to come.

H. Taegtmeyer MD, DPhil
The University of Texas Health Science Center at Houston,
Houston, TX, United States

Preface

According to the World Health Organization, 12 million deaths per year are attributed to cardiovascular disease (CVD). This accounts for nearly one-half of all the deaths in the United States and other developed countries. In the United States, more than 60 million people have some form of CVD, with 2600 people dying every day from CVD. It is overall the leading cause of death worldwide. In contrast, the second most common cause of death, cancer, accounts for less than half as many deaths. The heart maintains constant contractility and demonstrates remarkable plasticity in the face of persistent hemodynamic changes. Not surprisingly, the heart is responsive to circulating endocrine factors from a variety of organ systems in addition to the autocrine and paracrine actions of peptide hormones that are synthesized by the heart and act both locally and throughout the vasculature.

We modeled this book loosely after the *Textbook of Nephro-Endocrinology* edited by Ajay K. Singh and Gordon H. Williams (Elsevier 2009) and *Endocrinology of the Heart* edited by W. Kaufmann and G. Wambach (Springer 1989). With *Endocrinology of the Heart in Health and Disease* in mind, we have developed a book that covers both the traditional concepts of cardio-endocrinology, the role of the various hormone systems both in health and disease, therapeutic implications, and other recent advances in the various fields represented. This textbook is intended for a wide audience including graduate students and post-doctoral fellows in a wide array of biomedical departments and PhD programs (e.g., Pathology, Physiology, Genetics, Pharmacology, Molecular Biology, Cell Biology) related to cardiovascular sciences curricula, as well as medical residents in pathology, laboratory medicine, internal medicine, cardiovascular surgery, and cardiology.

The endocrine function of the heart in both health and disease has to led a large body of research focusing on the heart both as an endocrine organ and endocrine target. Two broad themes divide the textbook: the first 5 chapters (see chapters: Cardiac Natriuretic Peptides, Adrenomedullin, Endothelin-1 as a Cardiac-Derived Autocrine, Paracrine and Intracrine Factor in Heart Health and Disease, The Cardiokines: An Expanding Family of the Heart Secretome, Novel Small Peptide Hormones) are devoted to the endocrine function of the heart, and the subsequent seven chapters (see chapters: Gut-Derived Hormones—Cardiac Effects of Ghrelin and Glucagon-Like Peptide-1, Fat Hormones, Adipokines, Neuronal Hormones and the Sympathetic/Parasympathetic Regulation of the Heart, Renin Angiotensin Aldosterone System and Heart Function, Nuclear Receptors and the Adaptive Response of the Heart, Adrenergic Receptors, Insulin Signaling in Cardiac Health and Disease) focus on the cardiovascular response to various endocrine signaling mechanisms.

THE HEART AS AN ENDOCRINE ORGAN

Chapter 1, Cardiac Natriuretic Peptides introduces the concept of the heart as an endocrine organ, a concept initially developed in 1971 with the discovery of atrial natriuretic factor in atrial cardiomyocytes. Chapter 1, Cardiac Natriuretic Peptides, Chapter 2, Adrenomedullin, Chapter 3, Endothelin-1 as a Cardiac-Derived Autocrine, Paracrine and Intracrine Factor in Heart Health and Disease, go on to detail the subsequent identification of other hormones produced in the heart such as the natriuretic peptide family (see chapter: Cardiac Natriuretic Peptides), adrenomedullin (see chapter: Adrenomedullin), and endothelin-1 (see chapter: Endothelin-1 as a Cardiac-Derived Autocrine, Paracrine and Intracrine

Factor in Heart Health and Disease), all of which mediate multiple and varied physiological and pathophysiological cardiovascular responses. Chapter 4, The Cardiokines: An Expanding Family of the Heart Secretome, describes the characterization and the emerging appreciation of the cardiac "secretome" from the various cell types that make up the heart, including myofibroblasts, myocytes, endothelial cells, adipocytes, and immune cells. Chapter 5, Novel Small Peptide Hormones, introduces the role of nestfatin-1 and adropin as well as peptides derived from the transcriptional processing of genes coding for G protein-coupled receptors; remarkably, these peptides control the translational/posttranslational processing and function of those receptors. We indicated the associations between cardiac hormone levels and cardiac pathologies throughout the text, including instances where targeting hormones resulted in therapeutic success.

THE HEART AS AN ENDOCRINE TARGET

The heart also responds both physiologically and pathophysiologically to a plethora of circulating hormones, reinforcing the importance of the heart as a target of a numerous endocrine systems such as the gut, in Chapter 6, Gut-Derived Hormones—Cardiac Effects of Ghrelin and Glucagon-Like Peptide-1; adipose, in Chapter 7, Fat Hormones, Adipokines; brain, in Chapter 8, Neuronal Hormones and the Sympathetic/Parasympathetic Regulation of the Heart; and renal, Chapter 9, Renin Angiotensin Aldosterone System and Heart Function. The heart also adapts to signals generated by ligands of numerous nuclear receptors, including glucocorticoid, estrogen, and thyroid receptors in addition to the various inputs that regulate the master and intrinsic circadian clock that affect cardiac function detailed in Chapter 10, Nuclear Receptors and the Adaptive Response of the Heart. Chapter 11, Adrenergic Receptors, covers one of the most common targets for treating cardiovascular diseases, the adrenergic receptors, which play significant roles in the sympathetic control of the heart. We also present the growing importance of insulin in maintaining energy balance throughout the body, including the heart. Chapter 12, Insulin Signaling in Cardiac Health and Disease, describes how perturbed insulin signals leads to cardiac dysfunction in several chronic conditions such as diabetes and ischemia.

Significant advances have come from basic, clinical, and translational research from a multiplicity of investigators with diverse backgrounds. These advances have come at such a rapid pace that it is difficult for textbooks on cardio-endocrinology disease to keep pace with the acceleration of molecular biology, biochemistry, physiology, and pathology. Therefore, we intend for this book to be updated every 3–4 years in order to keep pace with the ever-evolving field of cardiovascular medicine.

Jonathan C. Schisler
Charles H. Lang
Monte S. Willis

Acknowledgments

We wish to thank Mara Conner for the encouragement to take on the concept of endocrinology in the cardiovascular system and the support to see it through fruition, the chapter authors for their generous and invaluable contributions, Tari Broderick for her support during Mara's transition, and Jeffrey L. Rosetti for his expert assistance, guidance, and support throughout the publication process beyond his duties as Editorial Project Manager.

Jonathan C. Schisler
Charles H. Lang
Monte S. Willis

PART

I

THE HEART AS AN ENDOCRINE ORGAN

CHAPTER

CARDIAC NATRIURETIC PEPTIDES

1

C.J. Pemberton, C.J. Charles and A.M. Richards
University of Otago, Christchurch, New Zealand

HISTORICAL PERSPECTIVE

Since the 17th century, it has been known that the heart is capable of sensing the volume load it receives via the great veins and responding accordingly.[1] However, the precise mechanisms by which the heart could directly regulate circulation and total body fluid volume remained elusive until the latter 20th century. Experimental evidence supporting the role of the heart in volume regulation came in the 1950s from two separate observations: first, Henry et al.[2] noted that distension of the left atria in dogs resulted in an increase in urine flow, an effect dependent on intact innervation, as a blockade of the cervical vagi nerve conduction route with ice abolished the effect. Secondly, Kisch and Henry[2,3] independently pointed to the localization of receptors within the atrium as being sensitive to wall stretch. Kisch extended this finding by describing electron dense granules and a sophisticated Golgi network within atrial myocytes, similar to those noted for secretory cells. In the 1960s and '70s, these findings were extended by the work of Jamieson and Palade[4] who documented atrial electron dense granules as being identical to those of neuronal and endocrine polypeptide secreting cells. Marie et al.[5] reported that the density of these atrial granules was affected by experiments that altered fluid volume status in rats.

The first direct evidence for a cardiac factor directly involved in fluid regulation was provided by the seminal 1981 publication by Adolfo J. de Bold,[6] who documented a rapid and potent natriuresis and diuresis (i.e., a reduction in systemic sodium and water retention) in response to intravenous injection of atrial extracts. Rapid confirmation that atrial extracts also had repeatable vasorelaxant activity on vascular smooth muscle preparations generated intense research activity, which culminated in the purification and biochemical identification of the factor responsible.[7–10] This factor initially went under many names (atriopeptin, cardionatrin, auriculin, atrin), but the settled and permanent name was decided as atrial natriuretic peptide (ANP). As it was the first to be biochemically detailed, ANP provided a template for the subsequent discovery of the other two natriuretic peptide family members, B-type or brain natriuretic peptide (BNP) in 1988 and C-type natriuretic peptide (CNP) in 1990. Thus, within 9 years of de Bold's initial report, an entire family of cardiac natriuretic peptides was described, with multifaceted, powerful actions upon cardiovascular function and integrity. In contrast with ANP and BNP, CNP is not predominantly secreted by the heart but rather originates from the endothelium throughout the vasculature. Nevertheless, it is considered in the first part of this chapter, as the heart is a source of CNP which has important cardiovascular functions.

Endocrinology of the Heart in Health and Disease. DOI: http://dx.doi.org/10.1016/B978-0-12-803111-7.00001-4

GENE STRUCTURE OF NATRIURETIC PEPTIDES

ATRIAL NATRIURETIC PEPTIDE

All the natriuretic peptides have a similar gene structure in mammals, and consequently share a common biochemical homology across their propeptide sequences (Fig. 1.1). In humans, ANP is synthesized as preproANP(1-151) from the natriuretic peptide precursor A (*NPPA*) gene located at chromosome 1, 1p36.21. *NPPA* (GeneID 4878) is approximately 2.2 kB in length and contains 3 exons and 2 introns. The vast bulk of preproANP is encoded from Exon 2, with Exon 1 providing the 25 amino acid signal peptide and the first 16 amino acids of proANP. Exon 3 provides only the carboxyl terminus Tyr residue and the rest of the 3′ untranslated-poly (A) region. There is good conservation of mammalian preproANP translation from *NPPA* across all species studied with >90% nucleotide homology and very high (>95%) homology in the final mature ANP peptide produced. The 5′ upstream promoter region of human *NPPA* contains multiple regulatory elements such as GATA-4, GATA-6, Nkx2.5, MEF2, FOG-2, and several Tbx family recognition sites.[11] Many of these have an impact on human heart development. For example, mutations in the NPPA Nkx2.5 Response Elements at −243 and −112 bp upstream from the initiator methionine disrupt septation, conduction system development and chamber specification, which can contribute to diseases such as persistent AV block, Ebstein's anomaly, and aortic stenosis.[12,13]

The human *NPPA* gene contains a functional preproANP coding region polymorphism (rs5065, c.454T>C) which has the effect of altering the stop codon of preproANP to an arginine (p.Ter152Arg) and generates two extra carboxyl terminus arginine residues. The frequency of the rs5065 single nucleotide polymorphism (SNP) in the general population is approximately 14–20% and the minor allele has been associated with increased risk of stroke,[14] myocardial infarction (MI),[15] and increased susceptibility to acute coronary syndromes (ACS) and unfavorable prognosis in coronary artery disease

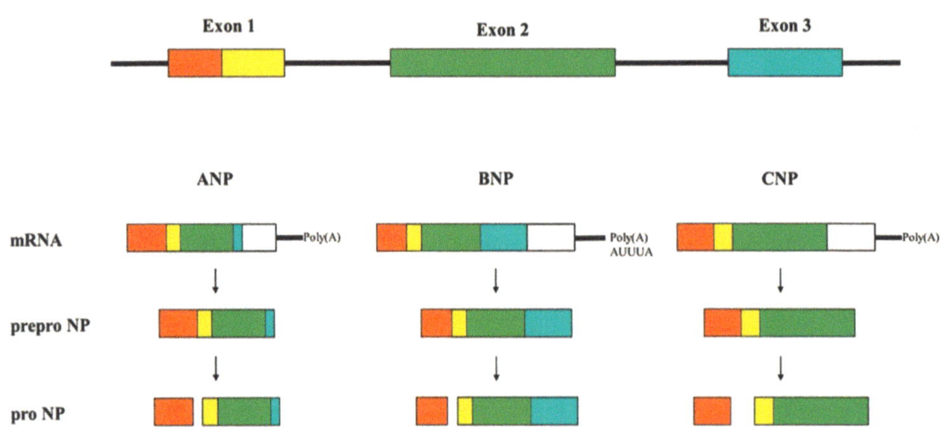

FIGURE 1.1

Generic scheme of NP gene structure. Each NP has 3 exons encoding, but translated preproCNP is devoid of exon 3, as denoted by the lack of blue shading. Individual variation in synthesis and regulation is noted in text.

(CAD).[16] Interestingly, this Arg-Arg–generating SNP is also present in mouse and rat genomes; to date, however, circulating mutant ANP with additional Arg-Arg residues at its carboxyl terminus has not been documented in human or rodent plasma. Nevertheless, in vitro experiments have shown that synthetic ANP-Arg-Arg mimicking rs5065 increases reactive oxygen species (ROS) accumulation and increases atherosclerotic gene activity in human umbilical vein endothelial cells.[17] A second polymorphism, rs5068 located in the 3′ untranslated region of NPPA (i.e., in the non-coding region), confers upon carriers of the minor allele increased circulating levels of ANP and BNP, and a concomitant lower risk of development of hypertension as evidenced by significantly lower systolic and diastolic blood pressures.[18]

BRAIN OR B-TYPE NATRIURETIC PEPTIDE

Human natriuretic peptide precursor B (*NPPB*, the gene encoding BNP, GeneID 4879) is located on the distal short arm of chromosome 1, 1p36.2 at a location only 8 kilobases 5′ upstream from *NPPA*.[19] This proximity of *NPPA* and *NPPB* suggests common regulatory elements control the expression and translation of both genes simultaneously. Like *NPPA*, *NPPB* consists of 3 exons and 2 introns,[20] but is only half the length of *NPPA*, being 0.9 kilobases.[21] The adult atrium contains 2–3 times more NPPB mRNA transcripts than the ventricle, but when chamber mass is taken into account, it is clear the bulk of cardiac NPPB synthesis resides in the cardiac ventricle.[21,22] In contrast with NPPA, human NPPB mRNA transcripts were detected in lung, thyroid, pituitary, kidney, and aorta tissues, indicating differential expression of the two hormones.[23] Like *NPPA*, the bulk of the parent product of human *NPPB* is encoded by exon 2, with the signal peptide the main product of exon 1 and a small carboxyl terminus portion encoded by exon 3. Unlike *NPPA*, across species the *NPPB* gene is not well conserved either in length, nucleotide homology, or physical location relative to *NPPA*—in fact, no two preproBNP peptides or mature forms are the same length and mature ANP and BNP forms within a single species are more homologous than mature BNP forms between species.[24]

Human *NPPB* is translated to produce preproBNP(1-134), which contains a 26-amino-acid signal peptide and the pro-peptide proBNP(1-108). Given its close proximity to *NPPA*, the 5′ promoter region of *NPPB* is also thought to be subject to regulation by AP-1, GATA-4, Nkx2.5, and MEF2 factors.[11,25–27] However, there are notable differences in the stimulated behavior of NPPB versus NPPA mRNA. First, NPPB (not NPPA) is laden with 3′ untranslated AUUUA motifs that are known to confer cellular mRNA instability (and hence lower storage levels) and must be "over-ridden" to increase translational product.[28] Related to this are the observations that phorbol esters[29] and diacylglycerol[30] increase NPPB mRNA levels, and unlike NPPA, NPPB induction does not require subsequent efficient protein synthesis.[25] Secondly, detectable increases in NPPB mRNA can occur within 1 hour of stimulation,[31] as opposed to the 8–12 hours required for NPPA. Such data are consistent with *NPPB* having the characteristics of a primary response gene. Finally, the positioning of the GATA regulatory motifs close to AP-1 and CACC box elements in the proximal 5′ promoter region of NPPB[32] is homologous to those found in products of the erythroid gene lineage (e.g., alpha and beta-globin genes) and experimental interference with these elements (e.g., deletion of the AP-1 element) reduces effective mRNA induction fourfold.[33]

Multiple SNPs are present in the coding region of human *NPPB*. Two of these give rise to silent mutations with no amino acid changes (rs35690395 and rs35628673) whereas others can yield coding sequence changes to preproBNP. The variant rs5227 (c.237C>T) confers an Arg to Leu substitution at position 25 (p.Arg25Leu), which is the penultimate amino acid prior to signal peptide cleavage at Ser26. There are other identified polymorphisms that result in coding variants within preproBNP(1-134) including p.Arg47His, p.Met93Leu, and p.Val94Phe (rs5229, rs5230, and rs35640285, respectively). It is of interest that these mutations reside in the amino terminal region of preproBNP and that no coding mutations have been reported for the mature circulating 32 amino acid form. Interestingly, a SNP in the promoter region of human NPPB (rs198389, c.-381T>C) has consistently been associated with higher circulating plasma levels of BNP forms,[34,35] but the C-allele of rs198389 is not associated with altered cardiovascular phenotype or outcomes.[35] Unsurprisingly, the above multiple polymorphisms that reside across the closely aligned *NPPA-NPPB* locus contribute to inter-individual variations in circulating ANP and BNP levels in normal health and the minor allele variants of each are associated with higher plasma natriuretic peptide, lower blood pressures, and lower risk of hypertension.[18,36] In patients with CAD it has been suggested that individual SNPs for each natriuretic peptide confers unique changes such that SNPs for ANP affect hypertension development whereas SNPs for BNP relate more to cardiac volumes.[37] These SNPs do not appear to be related to all-cause risk of mortality in the community but do associate with hospital readmission.

C-TYPE NATRIURETIC PEPTIDE

Human natriuretic peptide precursor C (*NPPC*, the gene encoding CNP, GeneID 4880) is not located near *NPPA/NPPB* but instead thought to reside on chromosome 2, 2q24-qter.[38] Defining features of *NPPC* include its extremely high conservation across all known species (greater than 90% between humans, mice, chimpanzee, dogs, and rats) and the fact that it consists of only two coding exons and one intron. A third exon in *NPPC* codes for the 3′ untranslated region only. These features have led some to speculate *NPPC* is the "prototype" natriuretic peptide gene from which *NPPA* and *NPPB* are derived.[38] PreproCNP is 126 amino acids long with exon 1 coding the 23-amino acid signal peptide and the first seven amino acids of proCNP. The remaining 96 amino acids of preproCNP are all encoded by exon 2. The mature bioactive CNP peptide is 22 amino acids long, but unlike ANP and BNP it does not have a carboxyl terminal tail, terminating at the second Cys, which completes the disulfide ring structure. Mature CNP is also 100% identical in all the above species. Originally isolated from brain,[39] the tissue distribution of NPPC mRNA has been shown to be much more equally distributed compared with NPPA/NPPB, showing high concentrations in brain and the pituitary sites, with lower amounts in kidney, bone (especially chondrocytes), blood vessels, and the heart.[40] Even though NPPC peptides are secreted by the heart,[41] these appear to originate predominantly from the general vascular endothelium as opposed to being principally synthesized by the heart, like ANP and BNP.

Factors influencing transcriptional regulation of *NPPC* have not been studied as closely as those for *NPPA/NPPB*, but the promoter of *NPPC* does possess two GC-rich regions (Sp-1 binding sites) that can be utilized by leucine zipper protein TSC22D1 and/or STK16 (a DNA-binding serine-threonine kinase) regulatory factors.[42,43] Further to this, a putative (but unverified) regulatory region containing an inverted CCAAT box, a cyclic AMP response like (CRE) box, and a TATAAA box are closely aligned in the *cis* region of the *NPPC* promoter—this feature is not present in *NPPA* or *NPPB*.[44,45] Another potential transcriptional factor implicated in *NPPC* regulation is Kruppel-like factor 2 (KLF-2). In human endothelial cells, blockade of flow-dependent up-regulated KLF-2 activity decreased the subsequent expression of NPPC,[46] which is consistent with the known experimental effects of vascular flow upon CNP production.[47]

Table 1.1 Tissue Expression, Forms, Secretion, and Metabolism of the NP

	ANP	BNP	CNP
Gene sequence homology	High	Low, species specific	Very high
Major organ of expression	Heat (atria)	Heart—atria and ventricle	Ubiquitous (brain)
Chromosomal locus	1, 1p36.21	1, 1p36.2	2, 2q24-qter
Regulatory gene motif	GATA-4, 6; Nkx2.5, MEF2, FOG-2, Tbx	AP-1, GATA-4, Nkx2.5, MEF2, AUUUA	STK16, TSC22D1, KLF-2, TATAAA
Major cardiac form	proANP	proBNP, NT-proBNP, BNP	NT-proCNP, CNP53
Cellular secretion	Regulated	Constitutive	Constitutive
Plasma forms	NT-proANP, ANP, β-ANP, cleaved ANP	NT-proBNP, proBNP, BNP?, cleaved BNP	NT-proCNP, CNP22
Cleavage enzymes	Corin, NEP, IDE	Furin, Corin?, IDE, DPP-IV	IDE, Furin, NEP
Plasma clearance	NEP, NPR-C	NEP, NPR-C	NEP, NPR-C
Bioactive receptor	NPR-A	NPR-A	NPR-B

Several polymorphisms are reported for *NPPC* within the NCBI database but the effects of these have not been well studied. A variant (G2628A) contained within the 3′ untranslated region (i.e., coded by exon 3) has been implicated with hypertension.[48] Interestingly, the minor alleles of rs11079028 and rs4796751, both of which are silent and located within the 3′ untranslated region of *NPPC*, associate with increased circulating levels of CNP peptides, but also with increased levels of BNP peptides,[37] possibly due to competition for common clearance pathways. Finally, the T allele of rs4796751 (c.*1595T>C) associates with larger cardiac volumes, suggesting a connection with cardiac dilatation.[37] Table 1.1 summaries the tissue expression, forms secreted, and metabolism of the natriuretic peptides.

TRANSLATION, PROCESSING, AND STORAGE OF CARDIAC NATRIURETIC PEPTIDES

ATRIAL NATRIURETIC PEPTIDE

ANP storage levels are 100–1000 times higher in atrial compared with ventricular myocytes. Well conserved across species, the preproANP polypeptide retains >80% homology between humans, chimpanzees, dogs, mice, and rats.[49] The 28-amino acid mature form of ANP in humans and rats differs by only one amino acid at position 12, where the human peptide contains a methionine and the rat peptide contains an isoleucine. Extra-cardiac sites of ANP production have been described but these constitute less than 1% of the capacity of the atrium.[49,50] During translocation into the lumen of the endoplasmic reticulum, the 25 amino acid signal peptide is cleaved, presumably by signal peptidase (or a similar enzyme), and the resulting proANP(1-126) peptide is transported to storage granules as the major form.[51] Aggregation of proANP into atrial secretory granules occurs via a clathrin-coated membrane system,[52] and is also mediated by calcium-binding to the amino terminus of the propeptide.[53,54] This mode of delivery is consistent with what is known for peptides that are secreted via the regulated pathway (e.g., insulin). Upon a stretch of the atrial wall caused by increased intra-cardiac volume,[55–57] or by the action of pressor hormones,[49,58] proANP(1-126) is presented to the surface of the myocyte and then cleaved by the transmembrane serine protease enzyme Corin[59] to produce proANP(1-98, NT-proANP) and the 28 amino acid, biologically active ANP(99-126, mature ANP) form, both of which appear in the circulation. The importance of Corin in ANP biochemistry is demonstrated by the fact that Corin null ($Cor^{-/-}$) mice have only proANP in their circulation and exhibit mild hypertension.[60] In turn, variations and mutations in the sequence of Corin itself result in hypertension and preeclampsia.[61–63] More recently, the generation of active Corin has been shown to be dependent upon the action of proprotein convertase PCSK6 and in PCSK6-null mice; both active Corin and proANP processing are absent.[64]

In humans there are two exceptions to this general biochemistry of proANP processing. First, failing hearts possess an antiparallel dimer of mature ANP(99-126) formed between apposing Cys bonds (known as beta-ANP) and the levels of this dimer are increased in cardiac tissue and plasma of those with severe heart failure.[65,66] Second, in the kidney an unknown enzyme is responsible for alternative, non-Corin–based processing of proANP(1-126) to generate a 32 amino acid form of ANP. This peptide, known as Urodilatin,[67] is produced exclusively in the kidney and contains four extra amino acids at its amino terminus. Urodilatin is thought to be absent (or at least undetectable) in plasma and is only observed in urine samples.[68] Synthetic urodilatin (known as Ularitide) may have potential as a vascular therapeutic agent for the treatment of acute decompensated heart failure (ADHF).[69]

BRAIN OR B-TYPE NATRIURETIC PEPTIDE

The initial discovery of BNP from porcine brain[70] was quickly updated with the observation that BNP peptide levels in the cardiac atrium are 100-fold higher than in brain tissue.[71] However, atrial and ventricular levels of BNP are much lower than ANP, and the relative ratios of the two peptides also differ between the two chambers. Thus, atrial levels of BNP are only 2–5% those of ANP, but in the ventricle they are approximately 60% those of ANP.[72–74] Extra-cardiac sites of BNP peptide are minor, with low detectable amounts only in the spinal cord, pituitary, and brain.[73,75] The length of the prepro form of BNP is highly variable across species; e.g., being 134 amino acids in humans,[76] 121 amino acids in the rat,[20] and 131 amino acids in the pig.[77] In the case of human preproBNP, signal peptidase cleavage of the 26 amino acid signal peptide forms a pro-peptide of 108 amino acids, which at some point in the Golgi-mediated transport system is glycosylated at multiple sites (Ser36, Thr37, Thr44, Thr48, Thr53, Ser58, and Thr71) in its amino terminus.[78] Unlike proANP, a portion of proBNP(1-108) is further cleaved within cardiac myocytes to form NT-proBNP(1-76) and mature BNP(77-108). Thus, cardiac myocytes contain at least three forms of immunoreactive BNP peptides, as opposed to the singular form of proANP.[79] Importantly, efficient cleavage to generate amino and carboxyl terminal BNP forms from proBNP is highly dependent upon the glycosylation status of proBNP, especially the site of Thr71.[80,81] This processing between residues 76/77 is not entirely consistent with a Corin enzyme motif, being more suggestive of a Furin (Arg-X-X-Arg) cleavage site.[78,80] Corin can process proBNP(1-108) at a site different from Furin to generate an amino terminus truncated mature form BNP(80-108).[80] However, given that proBNP is processed within cardiac granules (a location as yet unproven for Corin) it is likely that Furin is the major cardiac processing enzyme for proBNP, at least for human and rat ventricular myocytes.[81] Although some BNP colocalizes with ANP in human cardiac atrial myocyte granules, the vast majority of the peptide does not,[82,83] further underscoring the differential processing, storage, and secretion pattern of the two peptides—BNP (constitutive) versus ANP (regulated).

C-TYPE NATRIURETIC PEPTIDE

CNP is the most abundant of the natriuretic peptides in the nervous system including the pituitary and the spinal cord.[84] In the heart, CNP is not primarily expressed in the myocyte. Rather, it appears to be more prominent in cardiac fibroblasts,[85] which are presumably the main contributor, along with cardiac endothelial sources, to observed cardiac secretion.[41] Consistent with its role as a paracrine/autocrine factor, *NPPC* peptides are expressed in similar amounts to cardiac levels in noncardiac sites such as endothelial and vascular smooth muscle cells, endochondral bone, and reproductive organs.[84] *NPPC* within cells produces the 126 amino acid preproCNP, which is then further cleaved to proCNP of 103 amino acids by removal of the 23 amino acid signal peptide.[44] proCNP(1-103) is then processed intracellularly by furin to produce a 53 amino acid carboxyl terminal form (CNP53, which contains the bioactive ring structure) and the amino terminal fragment NT-proCNP.[84,86] Both CNP53 and NT-proCNP do not appear to be stored in regulated pathway secretory granules and undergo constitutive secretion in response to growth factors[87,88] and lumenal shear stress.[47]

CIRCULATING CONCENTRATIONS, FORMS, AND METABOLISM OF NATRIURETIC PEPTIDES

CIRCULATING LEVELS

All of the circulating natriuretic peptides have enriched concentrations in the cardiac coronary sinus,[41,89,90] but the level of enrichment is much more pronounced for ANP and BNP compared with CNP. For each mature peptide, average levels in the peripheral circulation in normal health approximate as follows: 20 pmol/L for ANP, 5 pmol/L for BNP, and 1 pmol/L for CNP. In comparison, NT pro forms of the natriuretic peptide circulate at 10–20 times that of the mature forms. In patients with cardiovascular disease (e.g., ADHF) circulating ANP and BNP forms are elevated up to 50-fold, depending on the severity of the disease.[91–98] This dynamic and robust profile of ANP and BNP peptides underlies their recommendation and use in the area of acute heart failure diagnosis and prognosis.[99,100] CNP peptide levels are also elevated in human[101] and experimental[102] heart failures but only modestly.

CIRCULATING FORMS AND METABOLISM

A general scheme of circulating forms of the natriuretic peptide is given in Fig. 1.2. Thus, *NPPA* and *NPPB* peptide products circulate as variable mixtures of mature ANP/BNP, NT-proANP/NT-proBNP, and proANP/proBNP forms. In the case of ANP, NT-proANP is by far the most abundant on a molar basis followed by ANP, with only a minor component of proANP. In contrast, proBNP contributes a much higher proportion of circulating NPPB forms and is much more complex due to the glycosylation status.[78] In the case of *NPPC*-related peptides, tissue CNP53 is further cleaved at secretion (via an unknown mechanism) to the 22 amino acid mature CNP form, and the circulating bioactive form is CNP22, although NT-proCNP is more abundant at a ratio of ~20:1.[41,84]

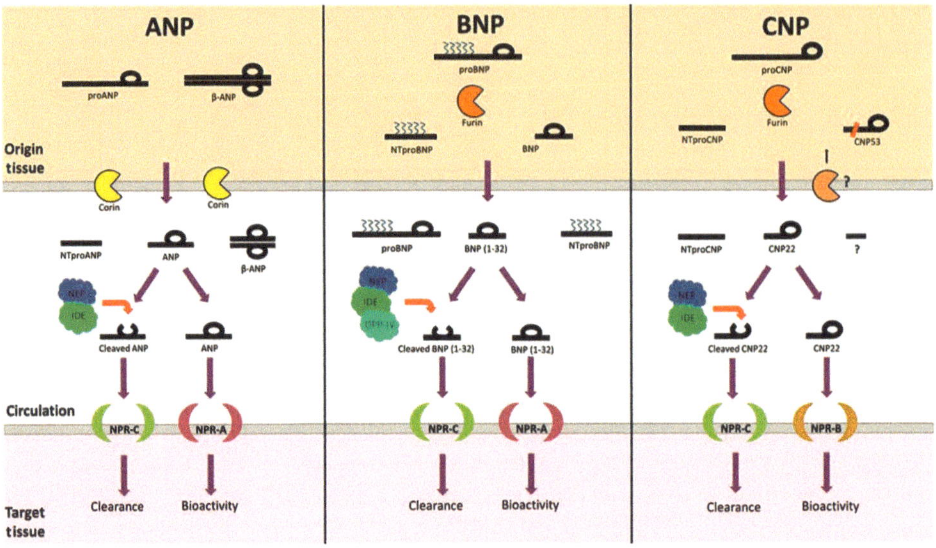

FIGURE 1.2

Tissue stored, secreted, circulating, and metabolized forms of each NP. While Corin and Furin activity for generating mature ANP and BNP, respectively, are confirmed, no such enzyme has been confirmed for CNP. proBNP and NT-proBNP are glycosylated as indicated by blue wave structures. Target tissue bioactivity and clearance receptors are as indicated in text.

However, circulating forms of natriuretic peptides are much more complex than this, as they are affected not only by what is secreted, but also by enzymatic activity and clearance mechanisms residing within the cardiovascular system. The main enzyme involved in natriuretic peptide degradation is neutral endopeptidase (also known as EC.3.4.24.11, Neprilysin, and enkephalinase A), which is highly expressed on brush border membranes in the kidney[103] but is also present in many vascular beds.[104] Neutral endopeptidase cleaves mature ANP, BNP, and CNP within the ring structure (at different sites) to produce ring open inactive metabolites,[105–107] that contribute to circulating immunoreactive forms in most assays. Cardiac coronary sinus plasma contains neutral endopeptidase cleaved mature ANP,[89] and likely cleaved mature BNP,[79] indicating that inactivation by neutral endopeptidase can occur almost at secretion, especially in patients with significant disease. Whether mature CNP suffers this same early fate via neutral endopeptidase after secretion from the heart is unknown. In contrast, the NT-pro forms of the natriuretic peptide are not thought to be affected by neutral endopeptidase metabolism.

Mature BNP [BNP(77-108)] can also be metabolized by the ubiquitous enzyme Dipeptidyl-peptidase IV (DPP-IV), which removes two amino acids from the amino terminus of the sequence (i.e., Ser-Pro) to produce BNP(79-108).[108] As well, proBNP(1-108) and NT-proBNP(1-76) also possess at their amino terminus (i.e., residues 1 and 2) the required sequence structure for DPP-IV activity and these are also both likely metabolized.[109] Whether mature forms of ANP and CNP are substrates for DPP-IV activity has not been reported, but this is unlikely as they do not possess the required sequences necessary, at least in their amino terminal regions. However, it is possible that NT-proANP or NT-proCNP may be cleaved at their amino termini as for NT-proBNP.[84]

A third enzyme that can metabolize mature forms of all three natriuretic peptides is insulin degrading enzyme. This zinc metalloprotease is ubiquitously expressed and is identified with the inactivation of insulin and amyloid-β.[110,111] Under experimental conditions, an insulin-degrading enzyme first cleaves three amino acids from the carboxyl terminus of both mature ANP and BNP,[112] with subsequent secondary cuts at the amino terminus resulting in amino and carboxyl shortened forms. Interestingly, the cleavage of mature BNP by insulin degrading enzyme is 50–100 times slower than that of ANP. In contrast, mature CNP is cleaved at its amino terminus followed by a secondary cleavage within the ring structure.[112] Whether insulin degrading enzyme plays a major role in NT-pro natriuretic peptide metabolism remains to be determined.

A fourth enzyme potentially involved in mature BNP cleavage is Meprin, but the data on this is conflicting and has yet to be adequately substantiated.[78] Instead, the other major contributing factor to circulating forms and levels of natriuretic peptides is the action of natriuretic peptide receptors, especially the clearance receptor.

NATRIURETIC PEPTIDE RECEPTORS

The bioactivity and clearance of the mature natriuretic peptides are mediated via membrane bound receptors, two of which belong to the guanylyl cyclase (GC) family. It is not known whether the amino terminal peptides of the natriuretic peptides (e.g., NT-proANP) activate these GC receptors, but there is some evidence that proANP and proBNP can activate them.[113,114] The two bioactive GC receptors (NPR-A and NPR-B) contain three domains: (1) an extracellular domain that recognizes the ring structure of the mature natriuretic peptide; (2) a transmembrane region that undergoes conformational change during natriuretic peptide binding; and (3) the intracellular region that contains the GC-element responsible for the generation of 3′,5′-guanosine cyclic monophosphate, otherwise known as cGMP, the second messenger transducing agent of the natriuretic peptide.[115]

In terms of bioactivity, NPR-A primarily mediates the actions of ANP and BNP, whereas NPR-B has a higher affinity for CNP (Fig. 1.2). However, the main receptor influencing natriuretic peptide plasma levels is NPR-C, also known as the clearance receptor. NPR-C lacks an intracellular GC-domain and is postulated to serve primarily as a removal system, binding bioactive and metabolized natriuretic peptides, internalizing them in cells, and submitting them for degradation.[84] Accordingly, NPR-C, the most widely and abundantly expressed natriuretic peptide receptor, is thought to constitute >90% of the total natriuretic peptide binding sites in endothelial cells;[116] it is highly expressed in adrenal, brain, heart, kidney, mesentery, and vascular smooth muscle tissue.[117–120] The impact of NPR-C upon circulating natriuretic peptide levels is seen in their circulating clearance. Thus, whereas the half-life of CNP[121] and ANP[122] in human plasma is around 2–3 minutes, the half-life of BNP is 10 times longer at approximately 20 minutes,[78] primarily due to the much lower affinity of BNP for NPR-C[123] and neutral endopeptidase activity.[107] Overall, the actions of neutral endopeptidase and NPR-C are thought to have equal contributions to the clearance and metabolism of the circulating mature natriuretic peptide forms.[124]

In contrast, because NT-pro forms of the natriuretic peptide are not thought to be substantially degraded by neutral endopeptidase, insulin-degrading enzyme or DPP-IV, nor cleared by NPR-C,[125] their half-lives in plasma are much longer than their mature peptide counterparts. Thus, studies in rats[126] have documented an NT-proANP half-life ~10 times longer than that of ANP (300 versus 30 seconds) whereas deconvolution analysis of endogenous NT-proBNP and BNP levels in the sheep documented a half-life of 70 minutes for NT-proBNP versus 5 minutes for mature BNP.[127]

CIRCULATING NATRIURETIC PEPTIDE SIGNAL PEPTIDES

Signal peptides have not been traditionally thought of as secreted or released products from cells that can be measured in the circulation, as it was assumed that the signal peptide was degraded after cleavage from the prepro peptide. Rather, they are well studied and documented as key components governing cellular secretion and targeting of proteins and propeptides.[128] However, it has recently been verified by immunoassay and tandem MS/MS analysis that fragments from the signal peptide regions of each of ANP, BNP, and CNP are present in human circulation.[90,129,130] The signal peptide of BNP is elevated in the plasma of patients suffering acute MI,[90] and it is also elevated with provocative testing such as dobutamine stress echocardiography.[131] MI-induced elevations in BNP signal peptide in humans occur very quickly, within 15 minutes.[132] Likewise, the signal peptide of ANP is elevated in patients after acute MI,[129] but acute MI has very little effect on plasma CNP signal peptide concentrations.[130] Instead, CNP signal peptide concentrations are acutely elevated in patients with atrial fibrillation (AF),[133] although the relevance of this finding is unclear.

An interesting biochemical feature of natriuretic peptide signal peptide fragments in the human circulation is that they are all differentially modified at their amino terminus residue. These modifications may be related to reactive species formed during oxidative stress processes in acute MI, such as glyoxal and methylglyoxal,[90] resulting in adduct formation such as formyl, methyl, and carboxyethyl groups on Leu, Ala, and Thr residues.[134] The importance of these modifications, and the presence of signal peptides in the circulation in general, remains to be determined.

ASSAYS MEASURING NATRIURETIC PEPTIDES IN THE CIRCULATION

As noted and discussed in more detail later in this chapter, measurement of the natriuretic peptides ANP and BNP are recommended by the American and European Cardiovascular guideline committees for the diagnosis and prognosis of acutely decompensated and chronic heart failure.[99,100] Of the natriuretic peptides, BNP peptides are most recommended for this purpose. Multiple providers offer clinical BNP assays for core laboratory or point of care use (e.g., Biosite, Beckmann Abbott, Siemens, Shionoria, Ortho Clinical Diagnostics), but NT-proBNP measurement is dominated by one provider, Roche Diagnostics. The benefits and drawbacks of current assays to measure these BNP forms have been comprehensively reviewed.[78] With regards to ANP peptide measurement, mature ANP is not recommended, but NT-proANP is partially indicated by one guideline.[99] An assay for mid-region NT-proANP (MR-proANP) is available on the BRAHMS/ThermoFisher Kryptor analyzer. MR-proANP has been shown to be noninferior to BNP and NT-proBNP for the diagnosis of acute heart failure,[135] and it may provide prognostic information independent to that of NT-proBNP.[136]

BIOACTIVITY

The discovery of ANP in 1981 led to the identification of a novel hormonal system sourced from the heart that is capable of affecting all tissues involved in sodium, volume, and pressure homeostasis. Most bioactivity resides within the 17 amino-acid ring of the mature peptides, with ANP and BNP actions mediated via the NPR-A. As ANP was discovered 7 years earlier than BNP, much of the work elucidating natriuretic peptide bioactivity and their physiological roles were undertaken on ANP. Subsequent studies confirmed that BNP displays a near identical array of bioactivity and both ANP and BNP are generally equipotent in inducing their respective biological actions.[137] Therefore, for the most part, the following description of biological actions for ANP apply equally to BNP. The major biological actions of ANP as reported in de Bold's initial study[6] using atrial extracts included a fall in arterial pressure and a rise in hematocrit (indicating hemoconcentration) with concomitant natriuresis and diuresis. The ensuing decade saw multiple studies further elucidating the hemodynamic, renal, and endocrine actions of the natriuretic peptides which are detailed below. Both ANP and BNP are true circulating hormones secreted by the heart. In contrast, CNP is not primarily a product of cardiac secretion and acts predominantly as a paracrine agent with a different spectrum of bioactivity and, as such, will not be reviewed in this book although it has been reviewed more broadly in *Current Pharmaceutical Design*.[138]

HEMODYNAMIC

Since the first description of ANP it has been known that natriuretic peptides lower arterial pressure,[6] and this has been subsequently shown to have a greater effect on systolic rather than diastolic pressure. Using pharmacological bolus injections of ANP in humans, it was first confirmed that the fall in arterial pressure was also associated with peripheral vasodilation.[139] Later studies employing low-dose infusions of ANP administered to man and sheep (24- and 48-hour infusions) at doses that raised circulating levels of the peptide within the physiological range showed that the reduction in arterial pressure is likely secondary to reduced filling pressures resulting in a fall in cardiac output with no evidence of direct vasodilation.[140–143] Subsequent studies infusing BNP for 4 days confirmed a similar array of hemodynamic actions in sheep.[143] Some of these effects can be attributed to a reduced plasma volume, as consistently evidenced by an increase in hematocrit associated with a movement of fluid from the vascular to extravascular space mediated by enhanced microvascular permeability of the vascular endothelium.[144] Other actions contributing to these hemodynamic effects include natriuresis and diuresis (further reducing circulating volume), inhibition of the renin-angiotensin-aldosterone system (RAAS), and inhibition of the direct vasopressor actions of angiotensin II (Ang II) and endothelin. ANP may also reduce sympathetic tone in the peripheral vasculature by a direct central inhibitory effect on sympathetic outflow.[145] Changes in heart rate are likely baroreceptor mediated in response to a fall in arterial pressure, although there are reports that heart rate rise is blunted for any given fall in blood pressure compared to that observed with agents like nitrates.[145] While the hemodynamic response to BNP in man is similar to ANP, venodilation may be more dominant than arterial vasodilation at physiological levels of the hormone.[146]

RENAL

As indicated by their name, the NPs have been known since their discovery to be natriuretic and diuretic.[6] These effects are the result of complex interactions on tubular sodium handling and reabsorption, renal hemodynamics, and a number of hormonal changes affecting renal function. The relative efficacy of natriuretic peptides as natriuretic and diuretic agents depends upon the underlying volume status and renal perfusion pressure. Short-term administration of ANP in normovolemic states induces prompt natriuresis and diuresis with smaller increases in divalent ions and phosphate excretion but no significant increase in potassium excretion.[140] These effects are in part mediated by changes in glomerular filtration rate (GFR) with dilation of renal afferent and constriction of renal efferent arterioles. Even in the absence of a change in GFR, lower doses of ANP still produce natriuresis by increasing the fractional filtration of sodium. In addition, natriuretic peptides antagonize the antinatriuretic actions of Ang II at the proximal tubule and tubular actions of arginine vasopressin and aldosterone.[147] In the setting of increased renal perfusion pressure, as occurs with volume expanded states in some forms of hypertension, the natriuretic effect of natriuretic peptides is augmented.[148] Conversely, hypotensive states exhibit clear reductions in natriuretic response. There is a good correlation between baseline blood pressure and natriuretic peptide-induced natriuresis in health.[139] In contrast, the renal response to ANP is blunted in moderate-to-severe congestive heart failure (CHF).[92] Despite CHF being a volume expanded state, cardiac output and hence renal perfusion pressure may be reduced leading to this blunted natriuretic response to ANP. Another factor that could contribute to impaired renal filtration in heart failure is an increase in venous pressure (and hence renal venous pressure), which reduces the trans-renal pressure gradient, a key determinant of filtration. There are reports that the natriuretic potency of BNP exceeds that of ANP in patients with CHF but is still blunted compared with euvolemic normal man.[149,150]

ENDOCRINE

Many of the actions of natriuretic peptides oppose those of the circulating- and tissue-based RAAS and are covered in detail in Chapter 9, Renin Angiotensin Aldosterone System and Heart Function. In humans, renin is inhibited by physiological increments in either plasma ANP or BNP, both by a direct inhibitory effect and also by enhanced delivery of sodium and chloride to the macula densa.[149,151] Aldosterone secretion is also inhibited by NPs in both sheep and man.[137,152] Small physiological increments of ANP can antagonize most secretagogues of aldosterone including potassium and adrenocorticotropin with the aldosterone stimulating effect of Ang II most affected. There is some evidence in severe heart failure that ANP inhibition of renin is attenuated,[153] but this appears not to be the case for aldosterone inhibition.[154]

INTEGRATIVE ROLE IN PHYSIOLOGY AND PATHOPHYSIOLOGY

Together, the above biological actions, along with other actions not reviewed here (including within the central nervous system), provide strong evidence for an integrative physiological role for both ANP and BNP working in tandem to maintain pressure and volume homeostasis as summarized in Fig. 1.3. This notion is also supported by numerous gene over-expression and knockout studies targeting both natriuretic peptides and their respective receptor genes.[155–159] Given the vasodilator, natriuretic/diuretic, and RAAS-inhibitory actions of the natriuretic peptides, they have long been considered to have potential benefit as therapeutic agents in the treatment of a variety of cardiovascular and pressure overload disorders.

NATRIURETIC PEPTIDE AS THERAPEUTIC AGENTS

Early studies of short-term intravenous infusions of ANP[92,160,161] and BNP[149,162] at various doses showed beneficial hemodynamic and renal effects in patients with heart failure. However, given that

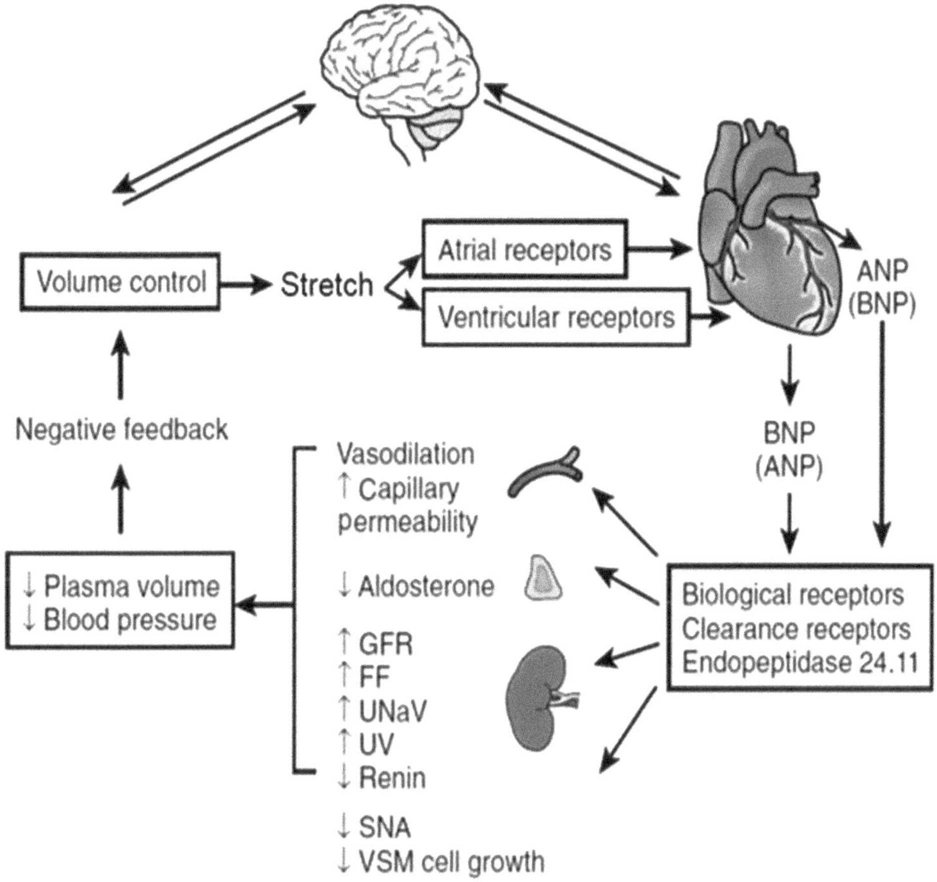

FIGURE 1.3

Schematic diagram showing the regulation and integrated actions of atrial natriuretic peptide (ANP) and B-type natriuretic peptide (BNP). GFR, glomerular filtration rate; FF, filtration fraction; UNaV, urinary sodium excretion; UV, urine volume; SNA, sympathetic nerve activity; VSM, vascular smooth muscle.

Reproduced with permission from Rademaker MT, Espiner EA. The endocrine heart. In: Becker KL, editor. Principles and practice of endocrinology and metabolism. 3rd ed. Philadelphia: Lippincott Williams & Wilkins; 2001. p. 1622–34.

the peptide nature of the natriuretic peptides necessitates intravenous infusion, this makes them only suitable as a short-term hospital or clinic-based treatment for ADHF. Based on preclinical data, ANP (marketed as carperitide) was licensed in Japan in 1995 for the treatment of ADHF. Both before and after its licensing, there has been no large-scale randomized study to confirm whether carperitide improves cardiac function, clinical symptoms, and prognosis in patients with heart failure.[163] Despite this, carperitide has been used for more than half of all heart failure patients in Japan,[164] but not used outside of that country. Evidence to date for the effect of carperitide on clinical outcomes is predominantly derived from an open-label registry and a prospective observational study with an impression that carperitide is both safe and that most patients respond, although the evidence is far from definitive, as the data are uncontrolled.[165] A recent study using a propensity score-matched analysis has reported that carperitide is associated with increased in-hospital mortality, odds ratio 2.13, compared with no carperitide, which is exacerbated in patients over 75 years old, odds ratio 2.93.[164] The authors suggest that their results strongly suggest the necessity for well-designed, randomized clinical trials of clinical safety, and efficacy of carperitide. This seems particularly relevant in light of the checkered history of the use of BNP as a therapeutic, as detailed below.

BNP (marketed as nesiritide) was approved by the FDA in 2001 for use in ADHF. As with carperitide, there were initially no large-scale clinical trials demonstrating improved mortality or demonstrating a clear advantage on outcomes such as improvements in dyspnea but rather approval was based on hemodynamic and symptomatic improvement based on studies with only mid-size cohorts, e.g., 127 patients in the Nesiritide Study Group.[166]

A number of other mid-sized studies were published in the first few years following FDA approval before red flags were raised by the publication of a metaanalysis, which reported that intravenous administration of nesiritide compared with placebo might increase serum creatinine levels indicating worsening renal function and may also increase the risk of short-term mortality.[167,168] An independent panel convened to evaluate the issue recommended that a large clinical trial be conducted to address whether nesiritide was effective and safe. The subsequent ASCEND-HF trial (over 7000 heart failure patients) compared nesiritide (72 hour intravenous infusion) to standard care on rates of self-reported dyspnea at 6 and 24 hours, rehospitalization for heart failure, all causes of death, and renal dysfunction.[169] Results showed nesiritide was not associated with either an increase or decrease in the rate of death and rehospitalization and that they had a small nonsignificant effect on dyspnea. While it was not associated with worsening renal function, nesiritide did increase rates of hypotension. On the basis of these results the authors concluded that nesiritide cannot be recommended for routine use in the broad population of patients with acute heart failure.

ENHANCING BIOACTIVITY

Due to the peptide nature of natriuretic peptides rendering IV infusion in a hospital setting as the only viable therapeutic option, for several decades researchers have sought alternative means of enhancing bioactivity of the natriuretic peptides. As stated in "Circulating Forms and Metabolism" and "Natriuretic Peptide Receptors" sections, circulating levels of natriuretic peptides are determined not only by secretion/release and excretion via the kidneys but also by two major clearance/degradation pathways. The main enzyme involved in natriuretic peptide degradation is neutral endopeptidase or neprilysin, while natriuretic peptides are also cleared via the abundant receptor NPR-C or clearance receptor. Overall, the actions of neutral endopeptidase and NPR-C are thought to contribute equally to the clearance and metabolism of the circulating mature natriuretic peptide forms both in normal physiology and in heart failure.[124,170] However, given that the agent used to block the NPR-C in those studies was also a peptide (C-$ANP_{4\text{-}23}$), there has been less emphasis on NPR-C blockade as a viable therapeutic option. Conversely, publications examining neutral endopeptidase inhibition (NEP-I) have flourished.

NEP-I

NEP-I was studied by multiple labs using a variety of different agents with the following just examples of results obtained from studies performed in normal sheep,[171] normal humans,[151] in heart-failed sheep,[172,173] and in clinical heart failure.[174] Results of these and other comparable studies showed that NEP-I consistently raised circulating levels of both ANP and BNP as well as the circulating levels of cyclic GMP. They also induced the expected array of hemodynamic, renal, and endocrine actions that reflect increased levels and activity of the natriuretic peptides. However, natriuretic peptides are not the only potential substrates for neutral endopeptidase. Ang II is also a physiologically relevant substrate for neutral endopeptidase. Low-dose stepped infusions of the Ang II administered to human volunteers on the background of 5 days dosing with the NEP-I candoxatril increased plasma Ang II levels and the pressor response with a reduction in the clearance of infused Ang II compared to placebo.[175] These results, along with other related studies,[176] suggested that there was likely to be a need to combine NEP-I with antagonism of Ang II. In preclinical studies, combined treatment with angiotensin converting enzyme inhibitors (ACE-I) and NEP-I was shown to have greater beneficial effects than treatment with either agent alone.[177]

COMBINED ACE AND NEP INHIBITORS

Given the early promise of preclinical studies with NEP-I, attention turned to the development of combined inhibitor agents that targeted both NEP-I and ACE-I in the same molecule. Subsequently, triple inhibitors, which in addition to targeting endothelin-converting enzymes, were also developed. A number of dual ACE-I/NEP-I agents, particularly the prototype Omapatrilat, showed early promise in both animal models[178] and in small cohort human heart failure studies,[179] with plasma levels of natriuretic peptides increased in association with reduction in capillary wedge and systolic arterial pressures and improvements in left ventricular and renal function. However, when Omapatrilat was taken to a large clinical trial (OVERTURE), the primary endpoint of all-cause mortality or heart failure related hospitalization did not differ significantly from ACE-I alone; however, posthoc analysis of the primary end point with the definition used in the SOLVD Treatment Trial (which included all hospitalization for heart failure) showed an 11% lower risk in patients treated with Omapatrilat.[180] Omapatrilat was also associated with significant adverse angioedema.[180] This trial in heart failure, along with the OCTAVE trial in hypertension,[181] which also showed increased risk of angioedema, essentially halted ongoing investigation of Omapatrilat and cast a shadow over NEP-I as a therapeutic mode, especially since NPs are not the only vasoactive peptides that are substrates for NEP.[175,176]

COMBINED ARB AND NEP INHIBITORS—NEW FRONTIER IN HEART FAILURE THERAPY

Despite the Omapatrilat experience, the NEP-I therapeutic story did not end. During the last decade Novartis has developed a new class of combined inhibitors based on the angiotensin type 1 receptor blocker valsartan and an NEP-I sacubitril, which they dubbed an *A*ngiotensin *R*eceptor blocker *N*eprilysin *I*nhibitor or ARN-I. Until recently their ARN-I was only known as LCZ696. The definitive trial of LCZ696 was the PARADIGM-HF trial with 8442 stable heart failure patients randomized to receive LCZ696 or enalapril in addition to recommended therapy.[182] The trial was stopped early because of an overwhelming benefit with LCZ696 compared with enalapril. The endpoints, including all-cause and cardiovascular deaths, all-cause or heart failure hospitalization and the combined primary endpoints, all showed approximately 20% reduction with LCZ696. Results from this trial first reported at major meetings in 2014 and published in September 2014 spurred fast-track approval through the US Food and Drug Administration (FDA). In July 2015, the FDA approved LCZ696, now known as Entresto, for the treatment of heart failure. This new class of drugs (ARNi) are the first new class of drugs to be approved for treatment of the general population of chronic heart failure patients in over 15 years and thus represent a "new frontier" in heart failure therapeutics.

NATRIURETIC PEPTIDES AS BIOMARKERS IN HEART FAILURE

Ideally, biomarkers reflect the pathophysiology of the condition of interest and aid clinical practice through improvements in one or more of (1) diagnosis, (2) prognosis, (3) monitoring disease progression, (4) indicating response to treatment, and (5) guiding titration of therapy.[183] The application of measurements of plasma natriuretic peptides, especially BNP and NT-proBNP, in the diagnosis of ADHF is now endorsed by all major international guidelines for the diagnosis and management of HF.[99,100] BNP and NT-proBNP are also approved as strong independent prognostic indicators in HF and are recommended as guides to titration of therapy.[100] This section of the chapter will summarize key evidence underpinning the biomarker status of NPs in HF.

NATRIURETIC PEPTIDES IN DIAGNOSIS OF ACUTE DECOMPENSATED HEART FAILURE

With the discovery of ANP and development of reliable immunoassays, it was soon clear that circulating concentrations of ANP were strongly related to the presence and severity of abnormalities of cardiac structure and function consistent with the primary role of myocardial stretch and transmural distending pressures in determining the rate of natriuretic peptide synthesis and release.[184,185] Proof of principle for plasma BNP as a diagnostic aid for discriminating ADHF from other causes of acute dyspnea was first provided in 1994 using a locally developed and validated radioimmunoassay for BNP. In a group of approximately 50 patients presenting to the emergency department with the primary complaint of recent onset breathlessness, BNP proved to have both sensitivity and negative predictive power more than 90% for ADHF.[97] Three years later Cowie et al. demonstrated similar diagnostic performance applying BNP testing in a urgent referral outpatient setting.[186] Full momentum towards adoption of BNP as a diagnostic aid for identifying ADHF among acutely symptomatic emergency department attendees came with the publication of the "Breathing Not Properly" trial conducted in seven centers in the US and western Europe, which confirmed the performance foreshadowed by the earlier New Zealand and UK studies.[187] This study recruited 1586 breathless patients (47% with ADHF) and used a commercial point of care "triage" BNP assay from Biosite (San Diego, California). A threshold value for BNP of 100pg/mL was 90% sensitive, 76% specific, had a negative predictive value (NPV) of 96% and an overall accuracy of 83% in discriminating ADHF from other causes of breathlessness. "Breathing Not Properly" also demonstrated the ability of BNP results to reduce uncertainty (measured on a scale from 1 to 100) among emergency department physicians with respect to the diagnosis of ADHF such that BNP results reduced the rates of clinically relevant uncertainty from 47% to 11%.

NT-proBNP was discovered in 1996 with proof of its presence in the human circulation and evidence of its strong association with the severity of deranged cardiac structure and function.[188,189] The diagnostic performance of this second B type natriuretic peptide in the Emergency Department was assessed first by Lainchbury et al. using an in-house radioimmunoassay and later by Januzzi et al. using a two-site commercially developed chemiluminescent immunoassay from Roche Diagnostics.[98,190] The study by Lainchbury et al. provided head-to-head comparisons of the diagnostic performance of BNP, NT-proBNP, ANP, and NT-proANP. The B type peptides performed as well as one another, comparable to earlier reports on BNP alone, and slightly better than the A type peptides.[98] While the data from the "PRIDE" study corroborated these findings with respect to the area under the receiver operating curve (area under the curve (AUC)~0.90 in both studies) for discriminating the ADHF from primary lung disease, interestingly the two studies suggested quite disparate ROC-derived optimal diagnostic threshold values.[98,190] It became apparent this reflected the strong effect of age on optimal cut-point with participants in the earlier study being older than patients in the later study. This issue was resolved by the ICON consortium which pooled data from some 1356 patients, across a wide age range, recruited in Christchurch (New Zealand), Boston (USA), Maastricht (Netherlands), and Barcelona (Spain).[191] ICON established a clinically useful common "rule-out" value (300 pg/mL) and age-adjusted "rule-in" thresholds (450 pg/mL for <50 years; >900 pg/mL for 50–75 years and >1800 pg/mL for >75 years). These cut points had excellent sensitivity and NPV and good specificity with an overall accuracy of 85% confirming similar performance to BNP as reported in the earlier reports summarized above.[191] The more recent "BACH" study conducted in 15 centers around the globe assessed test performance of BNP, NT-proBNP and mid region amino terminal proANP (MR-proANP).[192] BACH confirmed the comparability of BNP and NT-proBNP and added MR-proANP as having similar diagnostic power. Use of more than one of the three adds some additional diagnostic strength if the initial natriuretic peptide assessed gives an equivocal reading. Table 1.2 gives diagnostic test performance characteristics for BNP and NT-proBNP cut points, derived from major studies, for the detection of ADHF.

Overall diagnostic performance using the established thresholds in acutely symptomatic patients is quite reliable. Some defined patient subgroups may require additional interpretation. Elevation of B type natriuretic peptides is not specific for ADHF. Table 1.3 presents the differential diagnosis (pulmonary embolism, AF, etc.), which should be considered when elevated test results are obtained. Common confounders of B type natriuretic peptide test performance include age, the presence of reduced or preserved ejection fraction, kidney function, obesity, and AF. As for many clinical diagnostic challenges BNP/NT-proBNP levels should not to be used in isolation to determine diagnosis alone but rather as part of an integrated synthesis of history, examination, and corroboration by other tests.

Consideration of other confounding influences upon plasma natriuretic peptide concentrations is necessary for appropriate interpretation of plasma B–type natriuretic peptide results. First, as the ICON study confirmed, age is an independent determinant of natriuretic peptide levels. This does not invalidate the rule-out values of 100 pg/mL for BP and 300 pg/mL for NT-proBNP but, for values over the rule-out threshold consideration of age-adjusted limits does enhance accuracy. In younger patients (50 years of age or younger) with new onset breathlessness, an NT-proBNP level over 450 pg/mL is an almost perfect test for ADHF (AUC 0.99). Of course most HF patients are older and the AUC falls to 0.93 at 50–75 years (optimal test level 900 pg/mL) and to 0.86 for those over 75 years of age (1800 pg/mL) (Fig. 1.4). Age adjusted values are well validated for NT-proBNP but have not been established for BNP.[191]

Table 1.2 Plasma B-Type Natriuretic Peptides: Diagnostic Performance in the Emergency Department

Category of Heart Failure	Marker	Median (pg/mL)	Cut Point (pg/mL)	Sensitivity (%)	Specificity (%)	Positive Predictive Value (%)	Negative Predictive Value (%)	References
All HF								
	BNP	675	100	90	73	75	90	187
	N-BNP	4,639	300	99	60	79	89	192
HFREF								
	BNP	821	100	NR	NR	NR	NR	187
	N-BNP	6,356	300	90	89	85	93	192
HFPEF								
	BNP	413	100	86	NR	NR	96	187
	N-BNP	3,070	300	84	89	79	86	192
Non-HF								
	BNP	34						
	N-BNP	108						

The tabled values refer to the performance of the tabled cut points (BNP 100 pg/mL and NT-proBNP 300 pg/mL) in discriminating between (1) undifferentiated HF and non HF cases; (2) HFREF and non HF and (3) between HFPEF and non HF. Data are derived from the "Breathing Not Properly" and "ICON" (Refs. 187 and 192) study data sets. NR = not reported. N-BNP = NT-proBNP.

Table 1.3 Causes of Increased Plasma Cardiac Natriuretic Peptides
Cardiac
• Heart failure, acute, and chronic • Acute coronary syndromes • Atrial fibrillation • Valvular heart disease • Cardiomyopathies • Myocarditis • Cardioversion • Left ventricular hypertrophy
Noncardiac
• Age • Renal impairment • Pulmonary embolism • Pneumonia (severe) • Obstructive sleep apoea • Critical illness • Bacterial sepsis • Severe burns • Cancer chemotherapy • Toxic and metabolic insults

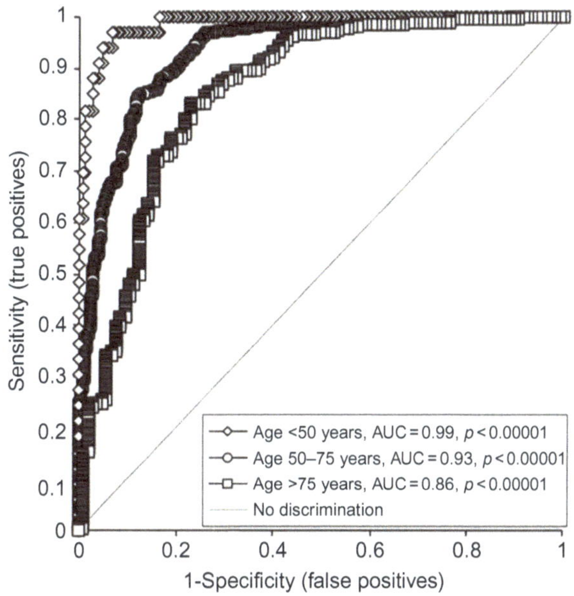

FIGURE 1.4

ROC curves for NT-proBNP-based diagnosis of acute HF across three age groups.

*Reproduced with permission from Januzzi JL, van Kimmenade R, Lainchbury J, et al. NT-proBNP testing for diagnosis and short-term prognosis in acute destabilized heart failure: an international pooled analysis of 1256 patients The International Collaborative of NT-proBNP Study. Eur Heart J 2006;**27**:330–7.*

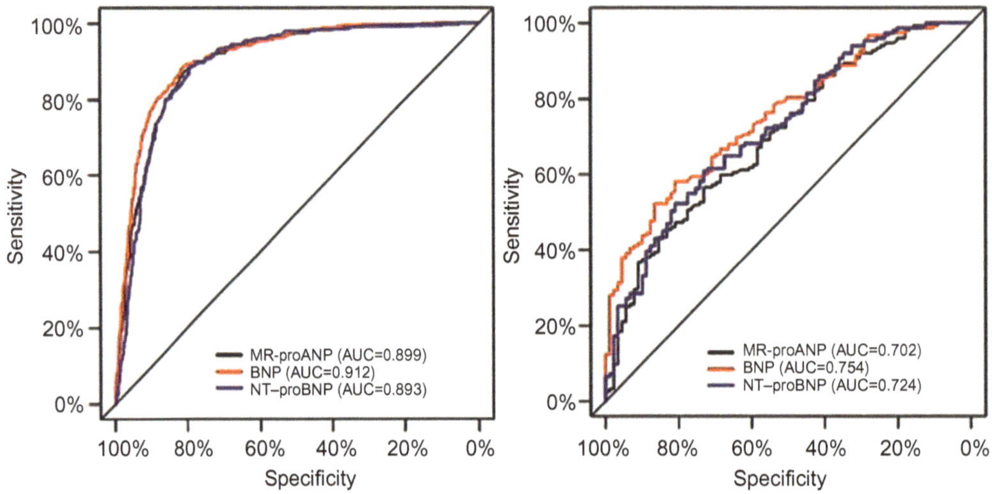

FIGURE 1.5

ROC curves for performance of NT-proBNP, BNP, and MR-proANP in the diagnosis of HF in the absence (left) and presence (right) of AF. Without AF areas under the curve (AUC) were 0.899, 0.912, and 0.893 for MR-proANP, BNP, and NTproBNP, respectively. In AF corresponding AUCs were 0.702, 0.754, and 0.724, respectively.

*Reproduced with permission from Richards AM, Di Somma S, Mueller C, Nowak R, Peacock F, Ponikowski P, Mockel M, Hogan C, Wu AHB, Clopton P, Filippatos GS, Anand I, Ng I, Daniels LB, Neath S-N, Shah K, Christenson R, Hartmann O, Anker SD, Maisel A. Atrial fibrillation impairs the diagnostic performance of cardiac natriuretic peptides in dyspneic patients: results from the biomarkers in acute heart failure (BACH) study. J Am Coll Cardiol Heart Fail 2013;***1***:192–9.*

Second, left ventricular phenotype (preserved (PEF) or reduced (REF) left ventricular ejection fraction) influences plasma B type natriuretic peptide with levels in PEF approximately half those in REF (Table 1.2) in both acute and chronic HF.[193–195] This reflects the Laplace's law through which ventricular lumenal radius, wall thickness, and intra-ventricular pressures determine individual cardiomyocyte stretch, the primary driver of natriuretic peptide synthesis and release. The "signal to noise" ratio in BNP/NT-proBNP/MR-proANP testing is so high in ADHF, characterized by extreme elevations in natriuretic peptide, their performance is only marginally reduced in PEF (Table 1.2). However, natriuretic peptide values often fall into the subdiagnostic range for those in incipient or treated HR and particularly so in HFPEF.[196,197] This emphasizes the need to apply the recommended cut-point values for acute HF in the appropriate setting; that is in patients with new onset of distressing breathlessness in whom acute HF is plausible.

AF, present in 25–40% of populations with ADHF, elevates plasma natriuretic peptide irrespective of concurrent HF.[198,199] A report from the BACH trial indicates the discriminative power of BNP/NT-proBNP for ADHF in newly dyspneic patients is clearly reduced by AF with AUCs falling from about 0.9 for those in sinus rhythm to ~0.7 in AF (Fig. 1.5).[200] As natriuretic peptide levels are raised overall by AF, sensitivity is preserved but specificity and accuracy are clearly reduced and cannot be improved by altering the cut point value despite the suggestion form some to use a higher decision level of 200 pg/mL for BNP in AF. Empirically 65–85% of dyspneic patients presenting with AF and with BNP/NT-proBNP peptide levels above 100 pg/mL and 300 pg/mL, respectively, will have HF and should therefore be treated as such until proven otherwise.[198–200]

Body mass index is inversely related to plasma natriuretic peptide concentrations in both health and HF. The underlying mechanisms are not understood.[201–203] However, in contrast to AF or renal impairment, the overall discriminative power of natriuretic peptide for ADHF is preserved in obesity with AUCs only moving from 0.9 to 0.88 between BMI<25 to >35 kg/m^2. The effect does reduce the sensitivity of BNP at 100 pg/mL and a substudy analysis from the "Breathing Not Properly" recommended reducing the BNP cut point to 50 pg/mL for BMI>30 kg/m^2.[202] Test performance of NT-proBNP is less affected by obesity.[203]

Finally, renal dysfunction elevates plasma natriuretic peptides. Plasma creatinine and estimated (e) GFR are inversely related to plasma natriuretic peptide levels.[204–206] It has been recommended that the cut point for BNP should be increased to 200 pg/mL when eGFR falls below 60 mL/min/1.73 m^2.[205] No change in cut point is generally applied to NT-proBNP values and the diagnostic performance of NT-proBNP appears less affected.[206] With kidney disease specificity and accuracy of both BNP and NT-proBNP are reduced irrespective of chosen decision thresholds.

Combined angiotensin receptor blocker/neprilysin inhibitor therapy ("ARNi") is a new potential confounder. NEP inhibitors impede metabolism of the bioactive carboxy (but not amino) terminal forms of ANP, BNP, and CNP. BNP levels are increased slightly with early dosing.[182,207] With beneficial effects upon intracardiac filling pressures and possible improved ventricular remodeling consequent to ARNi therapy, synthesis, and release of endogenous NPs will fall. In this situation NT-proBNP will reflect cardiac function better than BNP and should be the marker of choice for diagnosis of intercurrent ADHF and serial monitoring purposes when ARNI therapy is used (Fig. 1.6). This will become an increasingly common scenario as ARNis are adopted as standard therapy.

BNP AND NT-PROBNP FOR COMMUNITY SCREENING FOR CARDIAC IMPAIRMENT

In contrast to the universally recommended application of B type NPs in the diagnosis of symptomatic ADHF in the ED, the use of NPs in primary care or in community screening is not established. A single controlled trial conducted by Wright et al. provides good evidence that provision of an NT-proBNP result together with minimal tuition in its interpretation improves the accuracy of diagnosis of incipient HF among those less symptomatic patients who present to their family doctors with ankle swelling and/or progressive dyspnea on effort rather than with acute dyspnea at rest.[208] Reports from studies of community dwelling subjects, such as from the Olmstedt County, indicate NT-proBNP has good sensitivity (AUC ~0.9) for detection of asymptomatic left ventricular dysfunction.[209] An analysis of pooled data from ~5000 asymptomatic or minimally symptomatic outpatient clinic attendees indicates a sensitivity of ~90% for left ventricle ejection fraction (LVEF) <40% with thresholds markedly lower than the optimal values established for use in the ED. Optimal age-adjusted values performed as follows: sensitivity, specificity, and NPVs were: 50 years (50 pg/mL): 99.2, 57.2, and 99.7%; 50–75 years (75 pg/mL): 95.9, 51.0, and 96.8%; and >75 years (250 pg/mL): 87.9, 53.7, and 92.4%, respectively. Using only a single decision value (125 ng/L for all ages) gave sensitivities of 89.1, 91.9, and 94.3%; specificities of 84.0, 69.1, and 29.3% and NPVs of 97.7, 97.6, and 93.4%.[210] Together these results suggest NT-proBNP levels in the range 50–250 pg/mL can aid screening for incipient HF and/or significant LV dysfunction in the outpatient and community settings. Although in need of further validation, initial screening of high risk

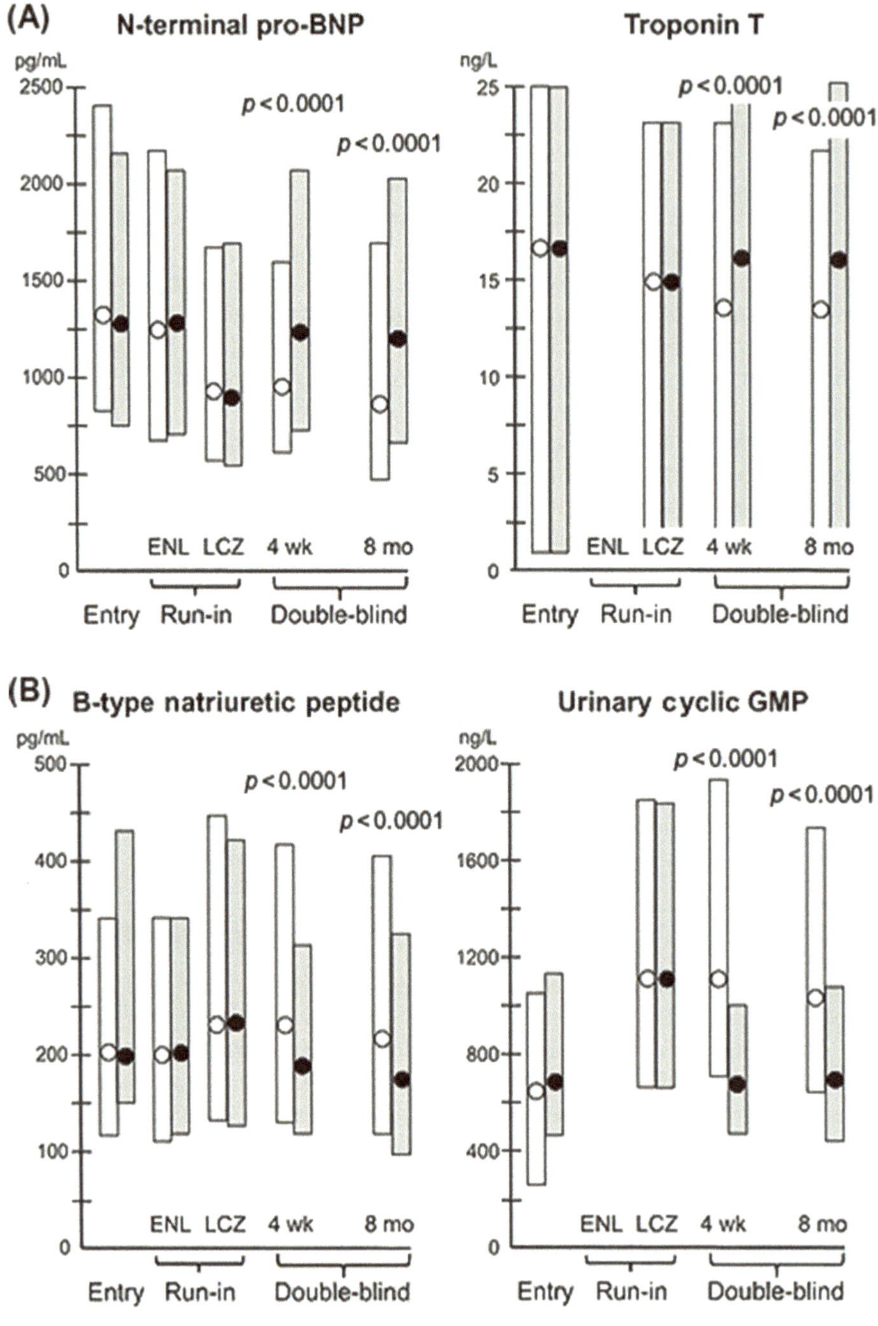

FIGURE 1.6

Median values for (A) N-terminal pro-BNP and troponin T at entry and during single-blind run-in and double-blind periods. Medians are shown in circles, and 25%/75% interquartile ranges are shown in bars, where patients in the LCZ696 group are shown in white circles and white bars and patients in the enalapril group are shown in black circles and gray bars. *p* values designate the significance of difference between the 2 groups (defined by age and cardiovascular risk and/or history) by natriuretic peptide testing progressing to cardiac imaging for those crossing the test thresholds, may offer a cost effective strategy for detection of clinically actionable asymptomatic LV dysfunction and incipient symptomatic HF in primary care.

B-TYPE NATRIURETIC PEPTIDES FOR PROGNOSIS IN HEART FAILURE

BNP and NT-proBNP are independently prognostic at all stages (A to D) of heart failure. In many analyses plasma BNP or NT-proBNP is the strongest predictor of outcomes (mortality and recurrent admission for ADHF) after multivariate analyses incorporating a comprehensive array of accepted clinical, functional, and imaging predictors. This is true for analyses in cohorts with ADHF, in chronic HF and in community-dwelling subjects with no overt heart failure. Major registry data sets (ADHERE and Get-with-the-guidelines) confirm admission BNP levels have strong predictive power for inpatient mortality in ADHF.[211,212] Bettencourt et al. demonstrated a several fold rise in risk of death or readmission at 6 months in those discharged from hospital with BNP >750 pg/mL compared with <350 pg/mL.[213]

Short- and long-term follow-up from PRIDE and ICON studies confirm the prognostic power of admission levels of NT-proBNP.[191,214] Trials of experimental therapies in chronic treated HF have provided the opportunity for biomarker substudies.[196,197] Although half of the chronic treated HFREF patients have BNP <100 pg/mL and 20% NT-proBNP<300 pg/mL, and median levels of NT-proBNP in chronic HFPEF are only ~380 pg/mL (and less than 300 pg/mL in those in normal sinus rhythm rather than AF) BNP, NT-proBNP in both HF phenotypes remain powerfully and independently prognostic for both all-cause mortality and for HF readmission. In crude unadjusted analyses the Val-Heft trial data indicate a median recruitment level plasma NT-proBNP level of ~900 pg/mL corresponded to a crude annual mortality of ~10%. In HFPEF the I-PRESERVE trial data indicate a median recruitment NT-proBNP level of ~400 pg/mL corresponded to a crude annual mortality of ~5%.

Importantly, shifts in plasma levels of B type NPs carry prognostic information. This is true in both acute and chronic settings. Bayes-Genis et al. reported higher postdischarge mortality in ADHF patients failing to reduce or increasing their NT-proBNP levels from admission to discharge compared with those in whom NT-proBNP fell by at least 30%.[215] In chronic HF the ValHeFT trial biomarker substudies demonstrated shifts in BNP between recruitment and 4 months clearly corresponding to outcomes at 23 months. Those entering the trial with BNP<100 pg/mL with similarly low levels at 4 months incurred 7.9% mortality at 23 months. Those with entry BNP >100 pg/mL which remained high

FIGURE 1.6

treatment groups. Troponin T was not measured at the end of the enalapril phase of the run-in period. (B) Median values for B-type natriuretic peptide and urinary cyclic GMP at entry and during single-blind run-in and double-blind periods. Medians are shown in circles, and 25%/75% interquartile ranges are shown in bars, where patients in the LCZ696 group are shown in white circles, and white bars and patients in the enalapril group are shown in black circles and gray bars. *p* values designate the significance of the difference between the two treatment groups. Urinary cyclic GMP was not measured at the end of the enalapril phase of the run-in period. BNP indicates B-type natriuretic peptide; ENL, end of the enalapril phase of the run-in period; and LCZ, end of the LCZ696 phase of the run-in period.

*Reproduced with permission from Packer M, McMurray JJ, Desai AS, Gong J, et al. The PARADIGM-HF investigators and coordinators. Angiotensin receptor neprilysin inhibition compared with enalapril on the risk of clinical progression in surviving patients with heart failure. Circulation 2015;**131**:54–61.*

incurred 25.4% mortality and those that changed categories reduced (12.8%) or worsened (22.7%) their risk of mortality in parallel with the shift.[216] Shifts in NT-proBNP in ValHeFT were similarly prognostic.[217] The close and consistent relationship between both baseline levels and changes in plasma B type natriuretic peptide with prognosis, together with the observed reduction in plasma concentrations of B type natriuretic peptides in parallel to a beneficial response to multiple anti-HF drug therapy and to successful device therapy, underpin the hypothesis that titration of therapy directed at lowering plasma B type natriuretic peptide levels may improve clinical outcomes.[218]

MARKER GUIDED THERAPY IN HEART FAILURE

Controlled trials of marker-guided management of chronic heart failure have been conducted in several countries since the year 2000 when the original pilot study from Troughton et al. was reported.[219] In total, more than 2000 patients have participated in trials comparing rates of key clinical outcomes with and without guidance of treatment titration by serial measurement of either BNP or NT-proBNP.[220–229] There are major variations between studies. Trial sample sizes have varied markedly with recruitment varying from under 100 to 500 participants. The average age of participants has varied from about 60 to nearly 80 years. The setting of trials has varied from specialist clinic to primary care. Target peptide levels along with the treatment algorithm used to respond to above-target BNP/NT-proBNP levels has also varied between trials. In spite of this heterogeneity, and variable neutral or positive outcomes from the individual small-to-moderate–sized trials, serial metaanalyses of summary data have consistently reported an overall benefit from the marker-guided strategy, which has reduced all-cause mortality and hospital admissions for heart failure.[230–232] This has been confirmed by a recent individual patient data metaanalysis from Troughton et al.[233] The effect of marker guidance on all-cause mortality was tested by Cox proportional hazards regression model with adjustment for study of origin, age (<75 or ≥75 years) and LVEF. Secondary endpoints included readmission for decompensated heart failure. For the endpoint of all-cause mortality, individual data from 2000 patients were available with 994 randomized to clinically guided care and 1006 to marker-guided care. Mortality was significantly reduced by guided treatment [hazard ratio = 0.62 (0.45–0.86) $p = 0.004$] with no heterogeneity between studies (Fig. 1.7). The survival benefit from guided therapy was observed over 2 years in younger (<75 years) patients [0.62 (0.45–0.85); $p = 0.004$] but not older (≥75 years) patients [0.98 (0.75–1.27); $p = 0.96$]. Hospital admissions for ADHF [0.80 (0.67–0.94); $p = 0.009$] or any cardiovascular cause [0.82 (0.67–0.99); $p = 0.048$] were reduced in the marker-guided group with no heterogeneity between studies and no interaction with age.[233]

The outcome from a larger and hopefully definitive trial, "GUIDE-IT," is awaited. This trial, implemented by Duke University, is an NHLBI collaboration (NCT01685840) planned to recruit 1100 patients with a history of clinical HF, a reduced ejection fraction (LVEF <40%) and elevated NT-proBNP to ≥2000 pg/mL within the 30 days prior to recruitment. Launched in December 2012, GUIDE-IT is at 70% recruitment and trial completion is anticipated by December 2017. The challenge faced by GUIDE-IT is ensuring adherence by multiple participating investigators to the principle of augmenting therapy if at all possible when peptide targets are not met even if conventional clinical assessment suggests "stability." The uniformity of response by clinicians to this cue will be all the more uncertain in the absence of a defined drug escalation algorithm within GUIDE-IT. The uniformity and commitment of clinical responses to persistent elevation of NT-proBNP will be critical to the trial outcome.

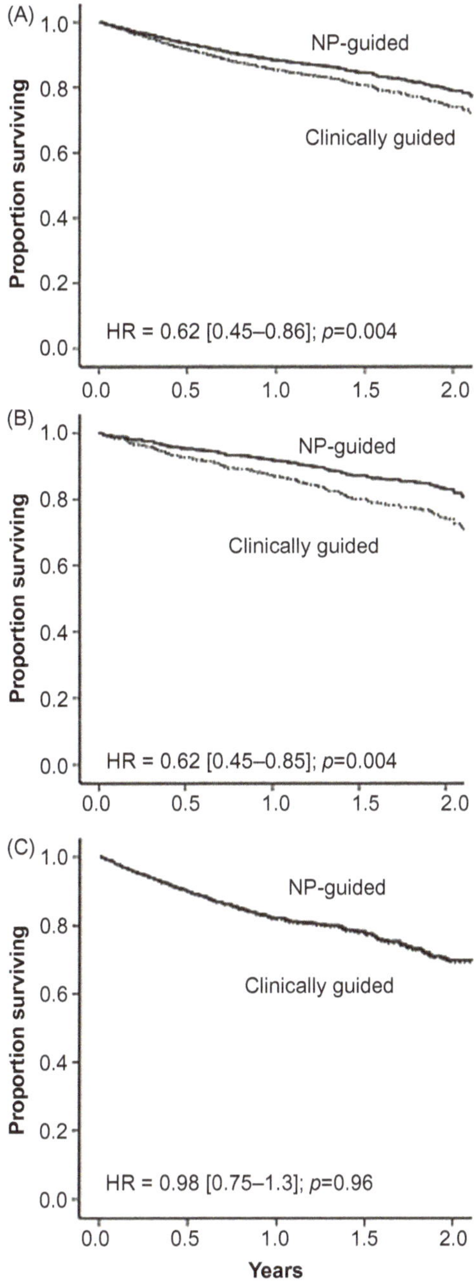

FIGURE 1.7

Kaplan–Meier survival curves for the primary endpoint, overall mortality: (A) total group, (B) below age 75 years, (C) 75 years and above.

*Reproduced with permission from Troughton RW, Frampton CM, Brunner-La Rocca H-P, Pfisterer M, Eurlings LWM, Erntell H, Persson H, O'Connor CM, Moertl D, Karlstro P, Dahlstrom U, Gaggin HK, Januzzi JL, Berger R, Richards AM, Pinto YM, Nicholls MG. Effect of B-type natriuretic peptide-guided treatment of chronic heart failure on total mortality and hospitalization: an individual patient metaanalysis. Eur Heart J 2014;***35***:1559–67.*

Should GUIDE-IT prove positive, guidelines would likely be amended to strengthen recommendations for guided treatment in HFREF. However, the role, if any, of markers in management of HFPEF will remain unclear. The only report currently available is from a substudy of 123 patients with HFPEF participating in the TIME CHF trial. In contrast to HFREF patients, no benefit from the guided strategy was observed in HFPEF cases in whom mortality and ADHF admissions were numerically higher with guided management. [234]

In the interim, current guidelines recommend use of serial marker measurements to facilitate titration of anti-HF medications to guideline mandated doses while conservatively stating whether or not such a strategy improves key clinical outcomes is yet to be confirmed.[100]

In summary, as biomarkers, the B type cardiac natriuretic peptides are established as diagnostic aids for acute heart failure and offer powerful independent prognostic information in all grades of HF. Use of serial measurements of BNP/NT-proBNP to monitor status and titrate therapy has a considerable body of supporting evidence and is cautiously recommended in some authoritative guidelines.[182] Although not yet common practice, promising epidemiological data support a role for natriuretic peptides in community screening for incipient heart failure or asymptomatic LV dysfunction.

REFERENCES

1. Harvey W. *De Motu Cordis* – the motion of the heart. Frankfurt, 1628.
2. Henry JP, Gauer OH, Reeves JL. Evidence of the atrial location of receptors influencing urine flow. *Circ Res* 1956;**4**:85–90.
3. Kisch B. Electron microscopy of the atrium of the heart. I. Guinea pig. *Exp Med Surg* 1956;**14**:99–112.
4. Jamieson JD, Palade GE. Specific granules in atrial muscle cells. *J Cell Biol* 1964;**23**:151–72.
5. Marie JP, Guillemont H, Hatt PY. Degree of granularity of the atrial cardiocytes. Morphometric study in rats subjected to different types of water and sodium load. *Pathol Biol* 1976;**24**:549–54.
6. de Bold AJ, Borenstein HB, Veress AT, Sonnenberg H. A rapid and potent natriuretic response to intravenous injection of atrial myocardial extract in rats. *Life Sci* 1981;**28**:89–94.
7. Flynn TG, de Bold ML, de Bold AJ. The amino acid sequence of an atrial peptide with potent diuretic and natriuretic properties. *Biochem Biophys Res Commun* 1983;**117**:859–65.
8. Currie MG, Geller DM, Cole BR, et al. Purification and sequence analysis of bioactive atrial peptides (atriopeptins). *Science* 1984;**223**:67–9.
9. Kangawa K, Matsuo H. Purification and complete amino acid sequence of alpha-human atrial natriuretic polypeptide (alpha-hANP). *Biochem Biophys Res Commun* 1984;**118**:131–9.
10. Atlas SA, Kleinert HD, Camargo MJ, et al. Purification, sequencing and synthesis of natriuretic and vasoactive rat atrial peptide. *Nature* 1984;**309**:717–9.
11. Hayek S, Nemer M. Cardiac natriuretic peptides: from basic discovery to clinical practice. *Cardiovasc Ther* 2011;**29**:362–76.
12. Clark KL, Yutzey KE, Benson DW. Transcription factors and congenital heart defects. *Annu Rev Physiol* 2006;**68**:97–121.
13. Schott JJ, Benson DW, Basson CT, et al. Congenital heart disease caused by mutations in the transcription factor Nkx2.5. *Science* 1998;**281**:1654–66.
14. Rubattu S, Stanzione R, Di Angelantonio E, et al. Atrial natriuretic peptide gene polymorphisms and risk of ischemic stroke in humans. *Stroke* 2004;**35**:814–8.
15. Gruchala M, Ciećwierz D, Wasag B, et al. Association of the ScaI atrial natriuretic peptide gene polymorphism with nonfatal myocardial infarction and extent of coronary artery disease. *Am Heart J* 2003;**145**:125–31.

16. Barbato E, Bartunek J, Mangiacapra F, et al. Influence of rs5065 atrial natriuretic peptide gene variant on coronary artery disease. *J Am Coll Cardiol* 2012;**59**:1763–70.
17. Scarpino S, Marchitti S, Stanzione R, et al. Reactive oxygen species-mediated effects on vascular remodeling induced by human atrial natriuretic peptide T2238C molecular variant in endothelial cells in vitro. *J Hypertens* 2009;**27**:1804–13.
18. Newton-Cheh C, Larson MG, Vasan RS, et al. Association of common variants in NPPA and NPPB with circulating natriuretic peptides and blood pressure. *Nat Genet* 2009;**41**:348–53.
19. Tamura N, Ogawa Y, Yasoda A, et al. Two cardiac natriuretic peptide genes (atrial natriuretic peptide and brain natriuretic peptide) are organized in tandem in the mouse and human genomes. *J Mol Cell Cardiol* 1996;**28**:1811–5.
20. Roy RN, Flynn TG. Organization of the gene for iso-ANP, a rat B-type natriuretic peptide. *Biochem Biophys Res Commun* 1990;**171**:416–23.
21. Hosoda K, Nakao K, Mukoyama M, et al. Expression of brain natriuretic peptide gene in human heart. Production in the ventricle. *Hypertension* 1991;**17**:1152–5.
22. Mukoyama M, Nakao K, Obata K, et al. Augmented secretion of brain natriuretic peptide in acute myocardial infarction. *Biochem Biophys Res Commun* 1991;**180**:431–6.
23. Gerbes AL, Dagnino L, Nguyen T, Nemer M. Transcription of brain natriuretic peptide and atrial natriuretic peptide genes in human tissues. *J Clin Endocrinol Metab* 1994;**78**:1307–11.
24. Rosenzweig A, Seidman CE. Atrial natriuretic factor and related peptide hormones. *Annu Rev Biochem* 1991;**60**:229–55.
25. Thuerauf DJ, Hanford DS, Glembotski CC. Regulation of rat brain natriuretic peptide transcription. A potential role for GATA-related transcription factors in myocardial cell gene expression. *J Biol Chem* 1994;**269**:17772–5.
26. Durocher D, Chen CY, Ardati A, Schwartz RJ, Nemer M. The atrial natriuretic factor promoter is a downstream target for Nkx-2.5 in the myocardium. *Mol Cell Biol* 1996;**16**:4648–55.
27. Durocher D, Charron F, Warren R, Schwartz RJ, Nemer M. The cardiac transcription factors Nkx2-5 and GATA-4 are mutual cofactors. *EMBO J* 1997;**16**:5687–96.
28. Gardner DG. Molecular biology of the natriuretic peptides. *Trends Cardiovasc Med* 1994;**4**:159–65.
29. LaPointe MC, Wu G, Garami M, Yang XP, Gardner DG. Tissue-specific expression of the human brain natriuretic peptide gene in cardiac myocytes. *Hypertension* 1996;**27**:715–22.
30. Suzuki E, Hirata Y, Kohmoto O, et al. Cellular mechanisms for synthesis and secretion of atrial natriuretic peptide and brain natriuretic peptide in cultured rat atrial cells. *Circ Res* 1992;**71**:1039–48.
31. Hanford DS, Thuerauf DJ, Murray SF, Glembotski CC. Brain natriuretic peptide is induced by alpha 1-adrenergic agonists as a primary response gene in cultured rat cardiac myocytes. *J Biol Chem* 1994;**269**:26227–33.
32. Steinhelper ME. Structure, expression, and genomic mapping of the mouse natriuretic peptide type-B gene. *Circ Res* 1993;**72**:984–92.
33. Grépin C, Dagnino L, Robitaille L, et al. A hormone-encoding gene identifies a pathway for cardiac but not skeletal muscle gene transcription. *Mol Cell Biol* 1994;**14**:3115–29.
34. Lanfear DE, Stolker JM, Marsh S, et al. Genetic variation in the B-type natriuretic peptide pathway affects BNP levels. *Cardiovasc Drugs Ther* 2007;**21**:55–62.
35. Costello-Boerrigter LC, Boerrigter G, Ameenuddin S, et al. The effect of the brain-type natriuretic peptide single-nucleotide polymorphism rs198389 on test characteristics of common assays. *Mayo Clin Proc* 2011;**86**:210–8.
36. Newton-Cheh C, Johnson T, Gateva V, et al. Genome-wide association study identifies eight loci associated with blood pressure. *Nat Genet* 2009;**41**:666–76.
37. Ellis KL, Newton-Cheh C, Wang TJ, et al. Association of genetic variation in the natriuretic peptide system with cardiovascular outcomes. *J Mol Cell Cardiol* 2011;**50**:695–701.

38. Ogawa Y, Itoh H, Yoshitake Y, et al. Molecular cloning and chromosomal assignment of the mouse C-type natriuretic peptide (CNP) gene (Nppc): comparison with the human CNP gene (NPPC). *Genomics* 1994;**24**:383–7.
39. Sudoh T, Minamino N, Kangawa K, Matsuo H. C-type natriuretic peptide: a new member of natriuretic peptide family identified in porcine brain. *Biochem Biophys Res Commun* 1990;**72**:984–92.
40. Komatsu Y, Nakao K, Suga S, et al. C-type natriuretic peptide (CNP) in rats and humans. *Endocrinology* 1991;**129**:1104–6.
41. Palmer SC, Prickett TC, Espiner EA, Yandle TG, Richards AM. Regional release and clearance of C-type natriuretic peptides in the human circulation and relation to cardiac function. *Hypertension* 2009;**54**:612–8.
42. Ohta S, Shimekake Y, Nagata K. Molecular cloning and characterization of a transcription factor for the C-type natriuretic peptide gene promoter. *Eur J Biochem* 1996;**242**:460–6.
43. Ohta S, Takeuchi M, Deguchi M, et al. A novel transcriptional factor with Ser/Thr kinase activity involved in the transforming growth factor (TGF)-beta signalling pathway. *Biochem J* 2000;**350**:395–404.
44. Tawaragi Y, Fuchimura K, Tanaka S, et al. Gene and precursor structures of human C-type natriuretic peptide. *Biochem Biophys Res Commun* 1991;**175**:645–51.
45. Ohta S, Shimekake Y, Nagata K. Cell-type-specific function of the C-type natriuretic peptide gene promoter in rat anterior pituitary-derived cultured cell lines. *Mol Cell Biol* 1993;**13**:4077–86.
46. Parmar KM, Larman HB, Dai G, et al. Integration of flow-dependent endothelial phenotypes by Kruppel-like factor 2. *J Clin Invest* 2006;**116**:49–58.
47. Chun TH, Itoh H, Ogawa Y, et al. Shear stress augments expression of C-type natriuretic peptide and adrenomedullin. *Hypertension* 1997;**29**:1296–302.
48. Ono K, Mannami T, Baba S, et al. A single-nucleotide polymorphism in C-type natriuretic peptide gene may be associated with hypertension. *Hypertens Res* 2002;**25**:727–30.
49. Ruskoaho H. Atrial natriuretic peptide: synthesis, release and metabolism. *Pharmacol Rev* 1992;**44**:479–602.
50. Vollmar AM. Atrial natriuretic peptide in peripheral organs other than the heart. *Klin Woschenschr* 1990;**68**:699–708.
51. Oikawa S, Imai M, Ueno A, et al. Cloning and sequence analysis of cDNA encoding a precursor for human atrial natriuretic polypeptide. *Nature* 1984;**309**:724–6.
52. Klein RM, Kelley KB, Merisko-Liversidge EM. A clathrin-coated vesicle-mediated pathway in atrial natriuretic peptide (ANP) secretion. *J Mol Cell Cardiol* 1993;**25**:437–52.
53. Doubell AF, Thibault G. Calcium is involved in both positive and negative modulation of the secretory system for ANP. *Am J Physiol* 1994;**266**:H1854–63.
54. Canaff L, Brechler V, Reudelhuber TL, Thibault G. Secretory granule targeting of atrial natriuretic peptide correlates with its calcium-mediated aggregation. *Proc Natl Acad Sci U S A* 1996;**93**:9483–7.
55. Bilder GE, Schofield TL, Blaine EH. Release of atrial natriuretic factor. Effects of repetitive stretch and temperature. *Am J Physiol* 1986;**251**:F817–21.
56. Edwards BS, Zimmerman RS, Schwab TR, Heublein DM, Burnett JC Jr. Atrial stretch, not pressure, is the principal determinant controlling the acute release of atrial natriuretic factor. *Circ Res* 1988;**62**:191–5.
57. Lang RE, Thölken H, Ganten D, et al. Atrial natriuretic factor--a circulating hormone stimulated by volume loading. *Nature* 1985;**314**:264–6.
58. Ruskoaho H, Vakkuri O, Arjamaa O, Vuolteenaho O, Leppäluoto J. Pressor hormones regulate atrial-stretch-induced release of atrial natriuretic peptide in the pithed rat. *Circ Res* 1989;**64**:482–92.
59. Yan W, Wu F, Morser J, Wu Q. Corin, a transmembrane cardiac serine protease, acts as a pro-atrial natriuretic peptide-converting enzyme. *Proc Natl Acad Sci U S A* 2000;**97**:8525–9.
60. Chan JC, Knudson O, Wu F, et al. Hypertension in mice lacking the proatrial natriuretic peptide convertase corin. *Proc Natl Acad Sci U S A* 2005;**102**:785–90.
61. Dries DL, Victor RG, Rame JE, et al. Corin gene minor allele defined by 2 missense mutations is common in blacks and associated with high blood pressure and hypertension. *Circulation* 2005;**112**:2403–10.

62. Wang W, Liao X, Fukuda K, et al. Corin variant associated with hypertension and cardiac hypertrophy exhibits impaired zymogen activation and natriuretic peptide processing activity. *Circ Res* 2008;**103**:502–8.
63. Cui Y, Wang W, Dong N, et al. Role of corin in trophoblast invasion and uterine spiral artery remodelling in pregnancy. *Nature* 2012;**484**:246–50.
64. Chen S, Cao P, Dong N, et al. PCSK6-mediated corin activation is essential for normal blood pressure. *Nat Med* 2015;**21**:1048–53.
65. Sugawara A, Nakao K, Morii N, et al. Synthesis of atrial natriuretic polypeptide in human failing hearts. Evidence for altered processing of atrial natriuretic polypeptide precursor and augmented synthesis of beta-human ANP. *J Clin Invest* 1988;**81**:1962–70.
66. Akimoto K, Miyata A, Kangawa K, et al. Molecular forms of atrial natriuretic peptide in the atrium of patients with cardiovascular disease. *J Clin Endocrinol Metab* 1988;**67**:93–7.
67. Schulz-Knappe P, Forssmann K, Herbst F, et al. Isolation and structural analysis of "urodilatin", a new peptide of the cardiodilatin-(ANP)-family, extracted from human urine. *Klin Wochenschr* 1988;**66**:752–9.
68. Forssmann W, Meyer M, Forssmann K. The renal urodilatin system: clinical implications. *Cardiovasc Res* 2001;**51**:450–62.
69. Anker SD, Ponikowski P, Mitrovic V, Peacock WF, Filippatos G. Ularitide for the treatment of acute decompensated heart failure: from preclinical to clinical studies. *Eur Heart J* 2015;**36**:715–23.
70. Sudoh T, Kangawa K, Minamino N, Matsuo H. A new natriuretic peptide in porcine brain. *Nature* 1988;**332**:78–81.
71. Minamino N, Aburaya M, Ueda S, Kangawa K, Matsuo H. The presence of brain natriuretic peptide of 12,000 daltons in porcine heart. *Biochem Biophys Res Commun* 1988;**155**:740–6.
72. Mukoyama M, Nakao K, Hosoda K, et al. Brain natriuretic peptide as a novel cardiac hormone in humans. Evidence for an exquisite dual natriuretic peptide system, atrial natriuretic and brain natriuretic peptide. *J Clin Invest* 1991;**87**:1402–12.
73. Ogawa Y, Nakao K, Mukoyama M, et al. Rat brain natriuretic peptide - tissue distribution and molecular form. *Endocrinology* 1990;**126**:2225–7.
74. Aburaya M, Minamino N, Kangawa K, Tanaka K, Matsuo H. Distribution and molecular forms of brain natriuretic peptide in porcine heart and blood. *Biochem Biophys Res Commun* 1989;**165**:872–9.
75. Ueda S, Minamino N, Sudoh T, Kangawa K, Matsuo H. Regional distribution of immunoreactive brain natriuretic peptide in porcine brain and spinal cord. *Biochem Biophys Res Commun* 1988;**155**:733–9.
76. Sudoh T, Maekawa K, Kojima M, et al. Cloning and sequence analysis of cDNA encoding a precursor for human brain natriuretic peptide. *Biochem Biophys Res Commun* 1989;**159**:1427–34.
77. Maekawa K, Sudoh T, Furusawa M, et al. Cloning and sequence analysis of cDNA encoding a precursor for porcine brain natriuretic peptide. *Biochem Biophys Res Commun* 1988;**157**:410–6.
78. Yandle TG, Richards AM. B-type natriuretic peptide circulating forms: analytical and bioactivity issues. *Clin Chim Acta* 2015;**448**:195–205.
79. Mahagamasekera PG, Ruygrok PN, Palmer SC, et al. B-type natriuretic peptide forms within the heart, coronary sinus, and peripheral circulation in humans: evidence for degradation before secretion. *Clin Chem* 2014;**60**:549–58.
80. Semenov AG, Tamm NN, Seferian KR, et al. Processing of pro-B-type natriuretic peptide: furin and corin as candidate convertases. *Clin Chem* 2010;**56**:1166–76.
81. Nishikimi T, Nakagawa Y, Minamino N, et al. Pro-B-type natriuretic peptide is cleaved intracellularly: impact of distance between O-glycosylation and cleavage sites. *Am J Physiol Regul Integr Comp Physiol* 2015;**309**:R639–49.
82. Nakamura S, Naruse M, Naruse K, et al. Atrial natriuretic peptide and brain natriuretic peptide coexist in the secretory granules of human cardiac myocytes. *Am J Hypertens* 1991;**4**:909–12.
83. Hasegawa K, Fujiwara H, Doyama K, et al. Ventricular expression of brain natriuretic peptide in hypertrophic cardiomyopathy. *Circulation* 1993;**88**:372–80.

84. Prickett TCR, Espiner EA. C-type natriuretic peptide (CNP) and postnatal linear growth. In: Preedy VR, editor. *Handbook of growth and growth monitoring in heath and disease*, **166**. Springer-Verlag-New York; 2012. p. 2789–809. http://dx.doi.org/10.1007/978-1-4419-1795-9.
85. Horio T, Tokudome T, Maki T, et al. Gene expression, secretion, and autocrine action of C-type natriuretic peptide in cultured adult rat cardiac fibroblasts. *Endocrinology* 2003;**144**:2279–84.
86. Wu C, Wu F, Pan J, Morser J, Wu Q. Furin-mediated processing of pro-C-type natriuretic peptide. *J Biol Chem* 2003;**278**:25847–52.
87. Suga S, Nakao K, Itoh H, et al. Endothelial production of C-type natriuretic peptide and its marked augmentation by transforming growth factor-beta. Possible existence of "vascular natriuretic peptide system". *J Clin Invest* 1992;**90**:1145–9.
88. Suga S, Itoh H, Komatsu Y, et al. Cytokine-induced C-type natriuretic peptide (CNP) secretion from vascular endothelial cells—evidence for CNP as a novel autocrine/paracrine regulator from endothelial cells. *Endocrinology* 1993;**133**:3038–41.
89. Yandle T, Crozier I, Nicholls G, et al. Amino acid sequence of atrial natriuretic peptides in human coronary sinus plasma. *Biochem Biophys Res Commun* 1987;**146**:832–9.
90. Siriwardena M, Kleffmann T, Ruygrok P, et al. B-type natriuretic peptide signal peptide circulates in human blood: evaluation as a potential biomarker of cardiac ischemia. *Circulation* 2010;**122**:255–64.
91. Burnett JC Jr, Kao PC, Hu DC, et al. Atrial natriuretic peptide elevation in congestive heart failure in the human. *Science* 1986;**231**:1145–7.
92. Cody RJ, Atlas SA, Laragh JH, et al. Atrial natriuretic factor in normal subjects and heart failure patients. Plasma levels and renal, hormonal, and hemodynamic responses to peptide infusion. *J Clin Invest* 1986;**78**:1362–74.
93. Itoh H, Nakao K, Sugawara A, et al. Gamma-atrial natriuretic polypeptide (gamma ANP)-derived peptides in human plasma: cosecretion of N-terminal gamma ANP fragment and alpha ANP. *J Clin Endocrinol Metab* 1988;**67**:429–37.
94. Sundsfjord JA, Thibault G, Larochelle P, Cantin M. Identification and plasma concentrations of the N-terminal fragment of proatrial natriuretic factor in man. *J Clin Endocrinol Metab* 1988;**66**:605–10.
95. Azizi C, Maistre G, Kalotka H, et al. Plasma levels and molecular forms of proatrial natriuretic peptides in healthy subjects and in patients with congestive heart failure. *J Endocrinol* 1996;**148**:51–7.
96. Numata Y, Dohi K, Furukawa A, et al. Immunoradiometric assay for the N-terminal fragment of proatrial natriuretic peptide in human plasma. *Clin Chem* 1998;**44**:1008–13.
97. Davis M, Espiner E, Richards G, et al. Plasma brain natriuretic peptide in assessment of acute dyspnoea. *Lancet* 1994;**343**:440–4.
98. Lainchbury JG, Campbell E, Frampton CM, et al. Brain natriuretic peptide and n-terminal brain natriuretic peptide in the diagnosis of heart failure in patients with acute shortness of breath. *J Am Coll Cardiol* 2003;**42**:728–35.
99. McMurray JJ, Adamopoulos S, Anker SD, et al. ESC guidelines for the diagnosis and treatment of acute and chronic heart failure 2012: the Task Force for the diagnosis and treatment of acute and chronic heart failure 2012 of the European Society of Cardiology. Developed in collaboration with the Heart Failure Association (HFA) of the ESC. ESC committee for practice guidelines. *Eur Heart J* 2012;**33**:1787–847.
100. Yancy CW, Jessup M, Bozkurt B, et al. 2013 ACCF/AHA guideline for the management of heart failure: executive summary: a report of the American College of Cardiology Foundation/American Heart Association Task Force on practice guidelines. *Circulation* 2013;**128**:1810–52.
101. Kalra PR, Clague JR, Bolger AP, et al. Myocardial production of C-type natriuretic peptide in chronic heart failure. *Circulation* 2003;**107**:571–3.
102. Charles CJ, Prickett TC, Espiner EA, Rademaker MT, Richards AM, Yandle TG. Regional sampling and the effects of experimental heart failure in sheep: differential responses in A, B and C-type natriuretic peptides. *Peptides* 2006;**27**:62–8.
103. Kerr MA, Kenny AJ. The purification and specificity of a neutral endopeptidase from rabbit kidney brush border. *Biochem J* 1974;**137**:477–88.

104. Turner AJ, Tanzawa K. Mammalian membrane metallopeptidases: NEP, ECE, KELL, and PEX. *FASEB J* 1997;**11**:355–64.
105. Stephenson SL, Kenny AJ. The hydrolysis of alpha-human atrial natriuretic peptide by pig kidney microvillar membranes is initiated by endopeptidase-24.11. *Biochem J* 1987;**243**:183–7.
106. Norman JA, Little D, Bolgar M, Di Donato G. Degradation of brain natriuretic peptide by neutral endopeptidase: species specific sites of proteolysis determined by mass spectrometry. *Biochem Biophys Res Commun* 1991;**175**:22–30.
107. Kenny AJ, Bourne A, Ingram J. Hydrolysis of human and pig brain natriuretic peptides, urodilatin, C-type natriuretic peptide and some C-receptor ligands by endopeptidase-24.11. *Biochem J* 1993;**291**:83–8.
108. Brandt I, Lambeir AM, Ketelslegers JM, et al. Dipeptidyl-peptidase IV converts intact B-type natriuretic peptide into its des-SerPro form. *Clin Chem* 2006;**52**:82–7.
109. Lam CS, Burnett JC Jr, Costello-Boerrigter L, Rodeheffer RJ, Redfield MM. Alternate circulating pro-B-type natriuretic peptide and B-type natriuretic peptide forms in the general population. *J Am Coll Cardiol* 2007;**49**:1193–202.
110. Duckworth WC, Garcia JV, Liepnieks JJ, et al. Drosophila insulin degrading enzyme and rat skeletal muscle insulin protease cleave insulin at similar sites. *Biochemistry* 1989;**28**:2471–7.
111. Hersh LB. The insulysin (insulin degrading enzyme) enigma. *Cell Mol Life Sci* 2006;**63**:2432–4.
112. Ralat LA, Guo Q, Ren M, et al. Insulin-degrading enzyme modulates the natriuretic peptide-mediated signaling response. *J Biol Chem* 2011;**286**:4670–9.
113. Ichiki T, Huntley BK, Sangralingham SJ, Burnett JC Jr. Pro-atrial natriuretic peptide: a novel guanylyl cyclase-A receptor activator that goes beyond atrial and B-type natriuretic peptides. *JACC Heart Fail* 2015;**3**:715–23.
114. Dickey DM, Potter LR. ProBNP(1-108) is resistant to degradation and activates guanylyl cyclase-A with reduced potency. *Clin Chem* 2011;**57**:1272–8.
115. Potter LR. Guanylyl cyclase structure, function and regulation. *Cell Signal* 2011;**23**:1921–6.
116. Leitman DC, Andresen JW, Kuno T, et al. Identification of multiple binding sites for atrial natriuretic factor by affinity cross-linking in cultured endothelial cells. *J Biol Chem* 1986;**261**:11650–5.
117. Nagase M, Katafuchi T, Hirose S, Fujita T. Tissue distribution and localization of natriuretic peptide receptor subtypes in stroke-prone spontaneously hypertensive rats. *J Hypertens* 1997;**15**:1235–43.
118. Porter JG, Arfsten A, Fuller F, et al. Isolation and functional expression of the human atrial natriuretic peptide clearance receptor cDNA. *Biochem Biophys Res Commun* 1990;**171**:796–803.
119. Suga S, Nakao K, Mukoyama M, et al. Characterization of natriuretic peptide receptors in cultured cells. *Hypertension* 1992;**19**:762–5.
120. Wilcox JN, Augustine A, Goeddel DV, Lowe DG. Differential regional expression of three natriuretic peptide receptor genes within primate tissues. *Mol Cell Biol* 1991;**11**:3454–62.
121. Hunt PJ, Richards AM, Espiner EA, Nicholls MG, Yandle TG. Bioactivity and metabolism of C-type natriuretic peptide in normal man. *J Clin Endocrinol Metab* 1994;**78**:1428–35.
122. Yandle TG, Richards AM, Nicholls MG, et al. Metabolic clearance rate and plasma half-life of alpha-human atrial natriuretic peptide in man. *Life Sci* 1986;**38**:1827–33.
123. Suga S, Nakao K, Hosoda K, et al. Receptor selectivity of natriuretic peptide family, atrial natriuretic peptide, brain natriuretic peptide, and C-type natriuretic peptide. *Endocrinology* 1992;**130**:229–39.
124. Charles CJ, Espiner EA, Nicholls MG, et al. Clearance receptors and endopeptidase 24.11: equal role in natriuretic peptide metabolism in conscious sheep. *Am J Physiol* 1996;**271**:R373–80.
125. Pemberton CJ, Yandle TG, Rademaker MT, et al. Amino-terminal proBNP in ovine plasma: evidence for enhanced secretion in response to cardiac overload. *Am J Physiol* 1998;**275**:H1200–8.
126. Thibault G, Murthy KK, Gutkowska J, et al. NH2-terminal fragment of rat pro-atrial natriuretic factor in the circulation: identification, radioimmunoassay and half-life. *Peptides* 1988;**9**:47–53.
127. Pemberton CJ, Johnson ML, Yandle TG, Espiner EA. Deconvolution analysis of cardiac natriuretic peptides during acute volume overload. *Hypertension* 2000;**36**:355–9.

128. Blobel G. Protein targeting (Nobel lecture). *Chembiochem* 2000;**1**:86–102.
129. Pemberton CJ, Siriwardena M, Kleffmann T, et al. First identification of circulating preproANP signal peptide fragments in man: initial assessment as cardiovascular biomarkers. *Clin Chem* 2012;**58**:757–67.
130. Pemberton CJ, Siriwardena M, Kleffmann T, Richards AM. CNP signal peptide fragments are present in the human circulation. *Biochem Biophys Res Commun* 2014;**449**:301–6.
131. Siriwardena M, Campbell V, Richards AM, Pemberton CJ. Cardiac biomarker responses to dobutamine stress echocardiography in healthy volunteers and patients with coronary artery disease. *Clin Chem* 2012;**58**:1492–4.
132. Liebetrau C, Gaede L, Dörr O, et al. Reference values and release kinetics of B-type natriuretic peptide signal peptide (BNPsp) in patients with acute myocardial infarction. *Clin Chem* 2015;**61**(12):1532–9. http://dx.doi.org/10.1373/clinchem.2015.244327.
133. Lee J, Than M, Aldous S, Troughton R, Richards M, Pemberton C. CNP signal peptide (CNPsp) in patients with cardiovascular disease. *Front Cardiovasc Med—Heart Fail Transpl* 2015;**2**:28. http://dx.doi.org/10.3389/fcvm.2015.00028.
134. Pemberton CJ. Signal peptides: new markers in cardiovascular disease? *Biomark Med* 2014;**8**:1013–9.
135. Maisel A, Mueller C, Nowak R, et al. Mid-region pro-hormone markers for diagnosis and prognosis in acute dyspnea: results from the BACH (Biomarkers in Acute Heart Failure) trial. *J Am Coll Cardiol* 2010;**55**:2062–76.
136. Masson S, Latini R, Carbonieri E, et al. The predictive value of stable precursor fragments of vasoactive peptides in patients with chronic heart failure: data from the GISSI-heart failure (GISSI-HF) trial. *Eur J Heart Fail* 2010;**12**:338–47.
137. Charles CJ, Espiner EA, Richards AM, Nicholls MG, Yandle TG. Comparative bioactivity of atrial, brain and C-type natriuretic peptides in conscious sheep. *Am J Physiol* 1996;**39**:R1324–31.
138. Lumsden NG, Khambata RS, Hobbs AJ. C-type natriuretic peptide (CNP): cardiovascular roles and potential as a therapeutic target. *Curr Pharm Des* 2010;**16**:4080–8.
139. Richards AM, Nicholls MG, Ikram H, et al. Renal, haemodynamic, and hormonal effects of human alpha natriuretic peptide in healthy volunteers. *Lancet* 1985;**1**:545–9.
140. Richards AM, McDonald D, Fitzpatrick MA, et al. Atrial natriuretic hormone has biological effects in man at physiological plasma concentrations. *J Clin Endocrinol Metab* 1988;**67**:1134–9.
141. Charles CJ, Espiner EA, Cameron VA, Richards AM. Hemodynamic, renal, and endocrine actions of ANF in sheep: effect of 24-h, low-dose infusions. *Am J Physiol* 1990;**258**:R1279–85.
142. Charles CJ, Espiner EA, Richards AM. Cardiovascular actions of ANF; contributions of renal, neurohumoral and hemodynamic factors in sheep. *Am J Physiol* 1993;**264**:R533–8.
143. Charles CJ, Espiner EA, Nicholls MG, Rademaker MT, Richards AM. Chronic infusions of brain natriuretic peptide in conscious sheep: bioactivity at low physiological levels. *Clin Sci* 1998;**95**:701–8.
144. Sabrane K, Kruse MN, Fabritz L, et al. Vascular endothelium is critically involved in the hypotensive and hypovolemic actions of atrial natriuretic peptides. *J Clin Invest* 2005;**115**:1666–74.
145. Floras JS. Sympathoinhibitory effects of atrial natriuretic peptide and baroreflex control of circulation. *Circulation* 1990;**81**:1860–73.
146. Houben AJ, vander Zander K, de Leeuw PW. Vascular and renal actions of brain natriuretic peptide in man: physiology and pharmacology. *Fundam Clin Pharmacol* 2005;**19**:411–9.
147. Maack T. Role of atrial natriuretic factor in volume control. *Kidney Int* 1996;**49**:1732–7.
148. Espiner EA, Richards AM. Atrial natriuretic peptide: an important factor in sodium and blood pressure regulation. *Lancet* 1989;**333**:707–10.
149. Yoshimura M, Yasue H, Morita E, et al. Hemodynamic, renal, and hormonal responses to brain natriuretic peptides in patients with congestive heart failure. *Circulation* 1991;**84**:1581–8.
150. Jensen KT, Eiskjaer H, Carstens J, Pederson EB. Renal effects of brain natriuretic peptide in patients with congestive heart failure. *Clin Sci* 1999;**96**:5–15.

151. Florkowski CM, Richards AM, Espiner EA, et al. Low-dose brain natriuretic peptide infusion in normal men and the influence of endopeptidase inhibition. *Clin Sci* 1997;**92**:255–60.
152. Hunt P, Espiner EA, Nicholls MG, et al. Differing biological effects of equimolar atrial and brain natriuretic peptide infusions in normal man. *J Clin Endocrinol Metab* 1996;**81**:3871–6.
153. Kanamori T, Wada A, Tsutamoto T, Kinoshita M. Possible regulation of renin release by ANP in dogs with heart failure. *Am J Physiol* 1995;**269**:H2281–7.
154. Rademaker MT, Charles CJ, Espiner EA, et al. Comparative bioactivity of atrial and brain natriuretic peptides in an ovine model of heart failure. *Clin Sci* 1997;**92**:159–65.
155. Barbee RW, Perry BD, Re RN, et al. Hemodynamics in transgenic mice with overexpression of atrial natriuretic factor. *Circ Res* 1994;**74**:747–51.
156. Ogawa Y, Itoh H, Tamura N, et al. Molecular cloning of the cDNA and gene that encode mouse brain natriuretic peptide gene and generation of transgenic mice that overexpress the brain natriuretic peptide gene. *J Clin Invest* 1994;**93**:1911–21.
157. Matsukawa N, Grzesik WJ, Takahashi N, et al. The natriuretic peptide clearance receptor locally modulates the physiological effects of the natriuretic peptide system. *Proc Nat Acad Sci U S A* 1999;**96**:7403–8.
158. John SW, Krege JR, Oliver PM, et al. Genetic decreases in atrial natriuretic peptides and salt-sensitive hypertension. *Science* 1995;**267**:679–81.
159. Oliver PM, John SW, Purdy KE, et al. Natriuretic peptides receptor 1 expression influences blood pressure of mice in a dose-dependent manner. *Proc Nat Acad Sci U S A* 1998;**95**:2547–51.
160. Saito Y, Nakao K, Nishimura K, et al. Clinical application of atrial natriuretic polypeptide in patients with congestive heart failure: beneficial effects on left ventricular function. *Circulation* 1987;**76**:115–24.
161. Crozier IG, Nicholls MG, Ikram H, Espiner EA, Gomez HJ, Warner NJ. Haemodynamic effects of atrial peptide infusion in heart failure. *Lancet* 1986;**2**:283–90.
162. Marcus LS, Hart D, Packer M, et al. Hemodynamic and renal excretory effects of human brain natriuretic peptide infusion in patients with congestive heart failure. *Circulation* 1996;**94**:3184–9.
163. Saito Y. Roles of atrial natriuretic peptide and its therapeutic use. *J Cardiol* 2010;**56**:262–70.
164. Matsue Y, Kagiyama N, Yoshida K, et al. Carperitide is associated with increased in-hospital mortality in acute heart failure: a propensity score-matched analysis. *J Cardiac Fail* 2015;**21**:859–64.
165. Ng TMH. Natriuretic peptides as therapy for heart failure—unfulfilled promise? *J Cardiac Fail* 2015;**21**:865–7.
166. Colucci WS, Elkayam U, Horton DP, et al. Intravenous nesiritide, a natriuretic peptide, in the treatment of decompensated congestive heart failure. Nesiritide Study Group. *N Engl J Med* 2000;**343**:246–53.
167. Sacker-Bernstein JD, Skopicki HA, Aaronson KD. Risk of worsening renal function in patients with acutely decompensated heart failure. *Circulation* 2005;**111**:1487–91.
168. Sacker-Bernstein JD, Kowalski M, Fox M, Aaronson K. Short-term risk of death after treatment with nesiritide for decompensated heart failure: a pooled analysis of randomized controlled trials. *JAMA* 2005;**293**:1900–5.
169. O'Connor CM, Starling RC, Hernandez AF, et al. Effect of nesiritide in patients with acute decompensated heart failure. *N Eng J Med* 2011;**365**:32–43.
170. Rademaker MT, Charles CJ, Kosoglou T, et al. Clearance receptors and endopeptidase: equal role in natriuretic peptide metabolism in heart failure. *Am J Physiol* 1997;**273**:H2372–9.
171. Charles CJ, Espiner EA, Cameron VA, et al. Hemodynamic and hormonal effects of neutral endopeptidase inhibitor SCH 39370 in sheep. *Hypertension* 1991;**17**:643–51.
172. Fitzpatrick MA, Rademaker MT, Charles CJ, et al. Acute hemodynamic, hormonal, and renal effects of neutral endopeptidase inhibition in ovine heart failure. *J Cardiovasc Pharmacol* 1992;**19**:635–40.
173. Rademaker MT, Charles CJ, Espiner EA, Nicholls MG, Richards AM, Kosoglou T. Neutral endopeptidase inhibition: augmented atrial and brain natriuretic peptide, haemodynamic and natriuretic responses in ovine heart failure. *Clin Sci* 1996;**91**:283–91.

174. Lainchbury JG, Richards AM, Nicholls MG, Espiner EA, Yandle TG. Brain natriuretic peptide and neutral endopeptidase inhibition in left ventricular impairment. *J Clin Endocrinol Metab* 1999;**84**:723–9.
175. Richards AM, Wittert GA, Espiner EA, Yandle TG, Ikram H, Frampton C. Effect of inhibition of endopeptidase 24.11 on responses to angiotensin II in human volunteers. *Circ Res* 1992;**71**:1501–7.
176. Richards AM, Wittert GA, Crozier IG, et al. Chronic inhibition of endopeptidase 24.11 in essential hypertension: evidence for enhanced atrial natriuretic peptide and angiotensin II. *J Hypertension* 1993;**11**:407–16.
177. Rademaker MT, Charles CJ, Espiner EA, Nicholls MG, Richards AM, Kosoglou T. Combined neutral endopeptidase and angiotensin-converting enzyme inhibition in heart failure: role of natriuretic peptides and angiotensin II. *J Cardiovasc Pharmacol* 1998;**31**:116–25.
178. Troughton RW, Rademaker MT, Powell JD, et al. Beneficial renal and hemodynamic effects of omapatrilat in mild and sever heart failure. *Hypertension* 2000;**36**:523–30.
179. McClean DR, Ikram H, Garlick AH, Richards AM, Nicholls MG, Crozier IG. The clinical, cardiac, renal, arterial and neurohormonal effects of omapatrilat, a vasopeptidase inhibitor, in patients with heart failure. *J Am Coll Cardiol* 2000;**36**:479–86.
180. Packer M, Califf RM, Konstam MA, et al. Comparison of omapatrilat and enalapril in patients with chronic heart failure. The omapatrilat versus enalapril randomized trial of utility in reducing events (OVERTURE). *Circulation* 2002;**106**:920–6.
181. Kostis JB, Packer M, Black HR, et al. Omapatrilat and enalapril in patients with hypertension: the omapatrilat cardiovascular treatment vs. enalapril (OCTAVE) trial. *Am J Hypertens* 2004;**17**:103–11.
182. McMurray JJV, Packer M, Desai AS, et al. Angiotensin-neprylisin inhibition versus enalapril in heart failure. *N Eng J Med* 2014;**371**:993–1004.
183. Richards AM. What we may expect from biomarkers in heart failure. *Heart Fail* 2009;**5**:463–70.
184. Richards AM, Cleland JGF, Tonolo G, et al. Plasma alpha natriuretic peptide in cardiac impairment. *BMJ* 1986;**293**:409–12.
185. Raine AE, Erne P, Bürgisser E, et al. Atrial natriuretic peptide and atrial pressure in patients with congestive heart failure. *N Engl J Med* 1986;**28**:533–7.
186. Cowie MR, Struthers AD, Wood DA, et al. Value of natriuretic peptides in assessment of patients with possible new heart failure in primary care. *Lancet* 1997;**350**:1349–53.
187. Maisel AS, Krishnaswamy P, Nowak RM, et al. Rapid measurement of B-type natriuretic peptide in the emergency diagnosis of heart failure. *N Engl J Med* 2002;**347**:161–7.
188. Hunt PJ, Yandle TG, Nicholls MG, Richards AM, Espiner EA. The amino-terminal portion of pro-brain natriuretic peptide (pro-BNP) circulates in human plasma. *Biochem Biophys Res Commun* 1995;**214**:1175–83.
189. Hunt PJ, Richards AM, Nicholls MG, Yandle TG, Doughty RN, Espiner EA. Immunoreactive amino-terminal pro-brain natriuretic peptide (NT-PROBNP): a new marker of cardiac impairment. *Clin Endocrinol* 1997;**47**:287–96.
190. Januzzi JL, Camargo CA, Anwaruddin S, et al. The N-terminal pro-BNP investigation of dyspnea in the emergency department (PRIDE) study. *Am J Cardiol* 2005;**95**:948–54.
191. Januzzi JL, van Kimmenade R, Lainchbury J, et al. NT-proBNP testing for diagnosis and short-term prognosis in acute destabilized heart failure: an international pooled analysis of 1256 patients The International Collaborative of NT-proBNP Study. *Eur Heart J* 2006;**27**:330–7.
192. Maisel A, Mueller C, Nowak R, et al. Mid-region prohormone ANP (MR-proANP) and procalcitonin for diagnosis of patients with acute dyspnea: primary results from the BACH (Biomarkers in ACute Heart failure) trial. *J Am Coll Cardiol* 2010;**55**:2062–76.
193. Richards AM, Januzzi Jr JL, Troughton RW. Natriuretic peptides in heart failure with preserved ejection fraction. *Heart Fail Clin* 2014;**10**:453–70.
194. O'Donoghue M, Chen A, Baggish AI, et al. The effects of ejection fraction on N-terminal proBNP and BNP levels in patients with acute CHF: analysis from the proBNP investigation of dyspnea in the emergency department (PRIDE) study. *J Cardiac Fail* 2005;**11**(Suppl. 5):S9–S14.

195. Maisel AS, McCord J, Nowak RM, et al. Bedside B-type natriuretic peptide in the emergency diagnosis of heart failure with reduced or preserved ejection fraction results from the Breathing Not Properly Multinational Study. *J Am Coll Cardiol* 2003;**41**:2010–7.
196. Masson S, Latini R, Anand IS, et al. Direct comparison of B-type natriuretic peptide (BNP) and amino-terminal proBNP in a large population of patients with chronic and symptomatic heart failure: the valsartan heart failure (Val-HeFT) data. *Clin Chem* 2006;**52**:1528–38.
197. Komajda M, Carson PE, Hetzel S, et al. Factors associated with outcome in heart failure with preserved ejection fraction findings from the irbesartan in heart failure with preserved ejection fraction study (I- PRESERVE). *Circ Heart Fail* 2011;**4**:27–35.
198. Knudsen CW, Omland T, Clopton P, et al. Impact of atrial fibrillation on the diagnostic performance of B-type natriuretic peptide concentration in dyspneic patients: an analysis from the Breathing Not Properly Multinational Study. *J Am Coll Cardiol* 2005;**46**:838–44.
199. Morello A, Lloyd-Jones DM, Chae CU, et al. Association of atrial fibrillation and amino-terminal pro–brain natriuretic peptide concentrations in dyspneic subjects with and without acute heart failure: results from the ProBNP Investigation of Dyspnea in the Emergency Department (PRIDE) study. *Am Heart J* 2007;**153**:90–7.
200. Richards AM, Di Somma S, Mueller C, et al. Atrial fibrillation impairs the diagnostic performance of cardiac natriuretic peptides in dyspneic patients: results from the Biomarkers in Acute Heart Failure (BACH) Study. *J Am Coll Cardiol Heart Fail* 2013;**1**:192–9.
201. Bayes-Genis A, Lloyd-Jones DM, Van Kimmenade RRJ, et al. The effect of body-mass index on the diagnostic and prognostic utility of plasma NT-proBNP in patients with acute dyspnea: results from the International Collaborative of NTproBNP (ICON) Study. *Arch Int Med* 2007;**167**:400–7.
202. Daniels LB, Clopton P, Bhalla V, et al. How obesity affects the cut-points for B-type natriuretic peptide in the diagnosis of acute heart failure. Results from the Breathing Not Properly Multinational Study. *Am Heart J* 2006;**151**:999–1005.
203. Bayes-Genis A, DeFilippi C, Januzzi JL. Understanding amino-terminal pro-B-type natriuretic peptide in obesity. *Am J Cardiol* 2008;**101**:89–94.
204. Richards AM, Nicholls MG, Espiner EA, et al. Comparison of B-type natriuretic peptides for assessment of cardiac function and prognosis in stable ischemic heart disease. *J Am Coll Cardiol* 2006;**47**:52–60.
205. McCullough PA, Duc P, Omland T, et al. B-type natriuretic peptide and renal function in the diagnosis of heart failure: an analysis from the Breathing Not Properly Multinational Study. *Am J Kidney Dis* 2003;**41**:571–9.
206. DeFilippi C, van Kimmenade RR, Pinto YM. Amino-terminal pro-B-type natriuretic peptide testing in renal disease. *Am J Cardiol* 2008;**101**:82–8.
207. Packer M, McMurray JJ, Desai AS, et al. Angiotensin receptor neprilysin inhibition compared with enalapril on the risk of clinical progression in surviving patients with heart failure. *Circulation* 2015;**131**:54–61.
208. Wright SP, Doughty RN, Pearl A, et al. Plasma amino-terminal brain natriuretic peptide and accuracy of heart failure diagnosis in primary care: a randomised controlled trial. *J Am Coll Cardiol* 2003;**42**: 1793–800.
209. Costello-Boerrigter LC, Boerrigter G, Redfield MM, et al. Amino-terminal pro-B-type natriuretic peptide and B-type natriuretic peptide in the general community: determinants and detection of left ventricular dysfunction. *J Am Coll Cardiol* 2006;**17**:345–53.
210. Hildebrandt P, Collinson PO, Doughty RN, et al. Age-dependent values of N-terminal pro-B-type natriuretic peptide are superior to a single cut-point for ruling out suspected systolic dysfunction in primary care. *Eur Heart J* 2010;**31**:1881–9.
211. Hsich EM, Grau-Sepulveda MV, Hernandez AF, et al. Relationship between sex, ejection fraction, and B-type natriuretic peptide levels in patients hospitalized with heart failure and associations with in hospital outcomes: findings from the Get With The Guideline-Heart Failure Registry. *Am Heart J* 2013;**166**:1063–71.

212. Fonarow GC, Peacock WF, Phillips CO, Givertz MM, Lopatin M. ADHERE Scientific Advisory Committee and Investigators Admission B-type natriuretic peptide levels and in-hospital mortality in acute decompensated heart failure. *J Am Coll Cardiol* 2007;**15**:1943–50.
213. Logeart D, Thabut G, Jourdain P, et al. Predischarge B-type natriuretic peptide assay for identifying patients at high risk of re-admission after decompensated heart failure. *J Am Coll Cardiol* 2004;**43**:635–41.
214. Chen AA, Wood MJ, Krauser DG, et al. NT-proBNP levels, echocardiographic findings, and outcomes in breathless patients: results from the ProBNP Investigation of Dyspnoea in the Emergency Department (PRIDE) echocardiographic substudy. *Eur Heart J* 2006;**27**:839–45.
215. Bettencourt P, Azevedo A, Pimenta J, Friões F, Ferreira S, Ferreira A. N-terminal-pro-brain natriuretic peptide predicts outcome after hospital discharge in heart failure patients. *Circulation* 2004;**110**:2168–74.
216. Latini R, Masson S, Wong M, et al. Incremental prognostic value of changes in B-type natriuretic peptide in heart failure. *Am J Med* 2006;**119**:e23–30.
217. Masson S, Latini R, Anand IS, et al. Prognostic value of changes in N-terminal pro-brain natriuretic peptide in Val-HeFT (Valsartan Heart Failure Trial). *J Am Coll Cardiol* 2008;**52**:997–1003.
218. Troughton RW, Richards AM, Yandle TG, Frampton CM, Nicholls MG. The effects of medications on circulating levels of cardiac natriuretic peptides. *Ann Med* 2007;**39**:242–60.
219. Troughton RW, Frampton CM, Yandle TG, Espiner EA, Nicholls MG, Richards AM. Treatment of heart failure guided by plasma aminoterminal brain natriuretic peptide(N-BNP) concentrations. *Lancet* 2000;**355**:1126–30.
220. Pfisterer M, Buser P, Rickli H, et al. BNP-guided vs symptom-guided heart failure therapy: the trial of intensified vs Standard Medical Therapy in Elderly Patients with Congestive Heart Failure (TIME-CHF) randomized trial. *JAMA* 2009;**301**:383–92.
221. Berger R, Moertl D, Peter S, et al. N-terminal pro-B-type natriuretic peptide-guided, intensive patient management in addition to multidisciplinary care in chronic heart failure: a 3-arm, prospective, randomized pilot study. *J Am Coll Cardiol* 2009;**55**:645–53.
222. Eurlings LW, van Pol PE, Kok WE, et al. Management of chronic heart failure guided by individual N-terminal pro-B-type natriuretic peptide targets: results of the PRIMA (can PRo-brain-natriuretic peptide guided therapy of chronic heart failure IMprove heart fAilure morbidity and mortality?) study. *J Am Coll Cardiol* 2010;**56**:2090–100.
223. Persson H, Erntell H, Eriksson B, Johansson G, Swedberg K, Dahlstrom U. Improved pharmacological therapy of chronic heart failure in primary care: a randomized Study of NT-proBNP Guided Management of Heart Failure - SIGNAL-HF (Swedish Intervention study - Guidelines and NT-proBNPAnaLysis in Heart Failure). *Eur J Heart Fail* 2010;**12**:1300–8.
224. Lainchbury JG, Troughton RW, Strangman KM, et al. N-terminal pro-B-type natriuretic peptide-guided treatment for chronic heart failure: results from the BATTLESCARRED (NT-proBNP-Assisted Treatment To Lessen Serial Cardiac Readmissions and Death) trial. *J Am Coll Cardiol* 2010;**55**:53–60.
225. Shah MR, Califf RM, Nohria A, et al. The STARBRITE Trial: a randomized, pilot study of B-type natriuretic peptide guided therapy in patients with advanced heart failure. *J Cardiac Fail* 2011;**17**:613–21.
226. Karlstrom P, Alehagen U, Boman K, Dahlstrom U. Brain natriuretic peptide-guided treatment does not improve morbidity and mortality in extensively treated patients with chronic heart failure: responders to treatment have a significantly better outcome. *Eur J Heart Fail* 2011;**13**:1096–103.
227. Januzzi Jr JL, Rehman SU, Mohammed AA, et al. Use of amino-terminal pro-B-type natriuretic peptide to guide outpatient therapy of patients with chronic left ventricular systolic dysfunction. *J Am Coll Cardiol* 2011;**58**:1881–9.
228. Jourdain P, Jondeau G, Funck F, Gueffet P, Le Helloco A, Donal E, et al. Plasma brain natriuretic peptide-guided therapy to improve outcome in heart failure: the STARS-BNP Multicenter Study. *J Am Coll Cardiol* 2007;**49**:1733–9.

229. Anguita M, Esteban F, Castillo JC, et al. Usefulness of brain natriuretic peptide levels, as compared with usual clinical control, for the treatment monitoring of patients with heart failure. *Med Clin* 2010;**135**:435–40.
230. Felker GM, Hasselblad V, Hernandez AF, O'Connor CM. Biomarker-guided therapy in chronic heart failure: a meta-analysis of randomized controlled trials. *Am Heart J* 2009;**158**:422–30.
231. Porapakkham P, Porapakkham P, Zimmet H, Billah B, Krum H. B-type natriuretic peptide-guided heart failure therapy: a meta-analysis. *Arch Intern Med* 2010;**170**:507–14.
232. Savarese G, Trimarco B, Dellegrottaglie S, et al. Natriuretic peptide-guided therapy in chronic heart failure: a meta-analysis of 2,686 patients in 12 randomized trials. *PLoS One* 2013;**8**:58287. http://dx.doi.org/10.1371/journal.pone.0058287.
233. Troughton RW, Frampton CM, Brunner-La Rocca H-P, et al. Effect of B-type natriuretic peptide-guided treatment of chronic heart failure on total mortality and hospitalization: an individual patient meta-analysis. *Eur Heart J* 2014;**35**:1559–67.
234. Maeder MT, Rickenbacher P, Rickli H, et al. N-terminal pro brain natriuretic peptide-guided management in patients with heart failure and preserved ejection fraction: findings from the Trial of Intensified versus standard Medical therapy in Elderly patients with Congestive Heart Failure (TIME-CHF). *Eur J Heart Fail* 2013;**15**:1148–56.

CHAPTER

2

ADRENOMEDULLIN

T. Nishikimi[1,2], K. Kuwahara[1], Y. Nakagawa[1], K. Kangawa[3] and K. Nakao[1]

[1]Kyoto University Graduate School of Medicine, Kyoto, Japan [2]Wakakusa-Tatsuma Rehabilitation Hospital, Osaka, Japan [3]National Cerebral and Cardiovascular Center Research Institute, Suita, Osaka, Japan

INTRODUCTION

Adrenomedullin (AM) was discovered in 1993 by Kitamura et al., who were monitoring cAMP activity in rat platelets from the acid extract of human pheochromocytoma tissue.[1] Human AM consists of 52 amino acids and one intramolecular disulfide bond (Fig. 2.1).[1] In addition to the adrenal gland, AM mRNA and protein are abundantly expressed in the cardiovascular system, including the ventricles, atria, lungs, kidneys, and aorta (Fig. 2.2),[2] all of which secrete AM into veins.[3,4] Adrenomedullin was initially shown to be a potent vasodilator and subsequent studies revealed that AM has diverse biological actions,[5] including the regulation other components of the cardiovascular system,[6] with the heart being both a source and a target of AM.

In this chapter, we describe the molecular forms, structures, and structure-activity relationships of AM and its receptors as well as the cardiac actions of AM, its pathophysiological function in cardiac disease, and its clinical application for the treatment of cardiac disease.

MOLECULAR FORMS, STRUCTURE, AND STRUCTURE-ACTIVITY RELATIONSHIPS OF ADRENOMEDULLIN

Adrenomedullin is produced enzymatically from a precursor molecule in two steps (Fig. 2.3). First, a signal peptide (residues 1–21) is removed from preproAM (residues 1–185) to produce proAM residues (22–185), which is subsequently cleaved by a processing enzyme into three peptides: glycine-extended AM (AM-Gly), glycine-extended proadrenomedullin N-terminal 20 peptide (also known as "PAMP", residues 22–41), and mid-regional AM (residues 45–92). Glycine-extended AM is a 53-amino-acid inactive intermediate and is converted through enzymatic amidation to active mature AM (AM-m), a 52-amino acid peptide with a C-terminal amide structure (Fig. 2.3).[5,6] Both AM-Gly and AM-m circulate in human plasma, with AM-Gly being the major molecular form; together, AM-Gly and AM-m are referred to as total AM.[4,7] Recently, mid-regional AM was identified and shown to be secreted along with total AM at equimolar levels.[8,9] However, mid-regional AM is poorly metabolized resulting in higher plasma concentrations of mid-regional AM compared to total AM. Notably, several recent studies showed that plasma levels of mid-regional AM is an important prognostic marker for heart failure,

Endocrinology of the Heart in Health and Disease. DOI: http://dx.doi.org/10.1016/B978-0-12-803111-7.00002-6

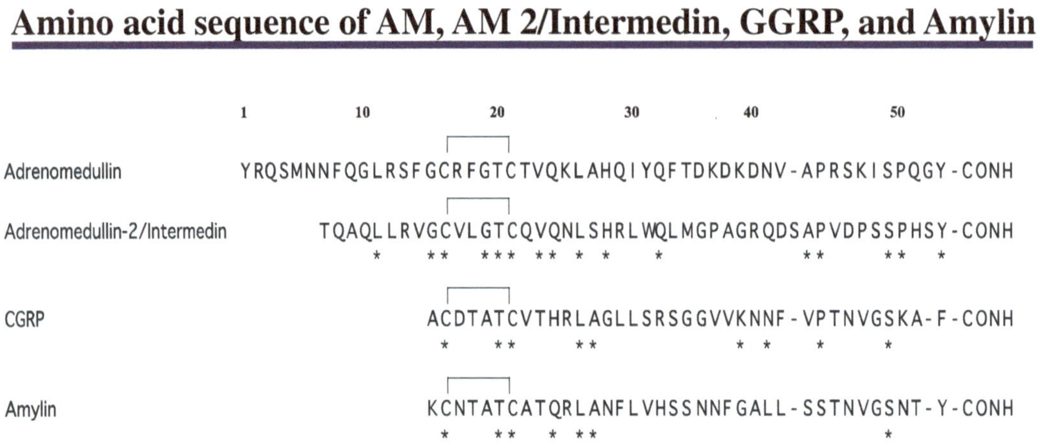

FIGURE 2.1

Comparison of the human amino acid sequences of adrenomedullin, adrenomedullin2/intermedin, calcitonin gene-related peptide (CGRP) and amylin.[5,6] Asterisk (*) indicates sequence identity with adrenomedullin.

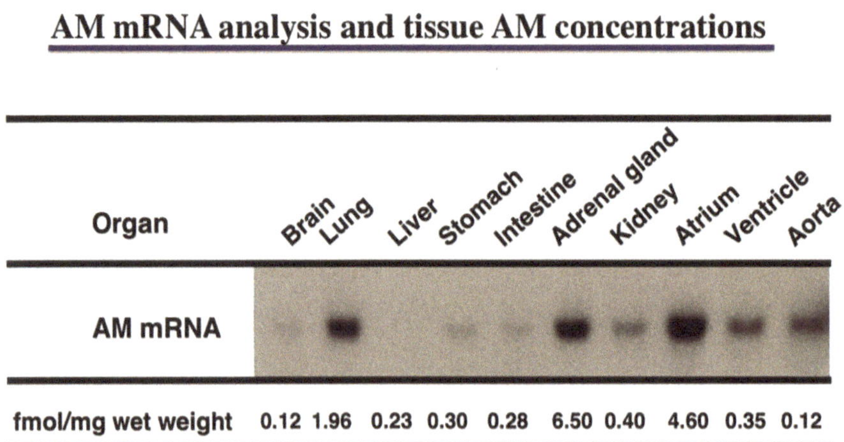

FIGURE 2.2

Adrenomedullin mRNA levels and AM concentrations determined using northern Blot analysis and radioimmunoassays, respectively, from rat tissue.[5]

myocardial infarction, atrial fibrillation, along with brain natriuretic peptide and the N-terminal fragment of brain natriuretic peptide (**for further reading on natriuretic peptides, see** chapter: Cardiac Natriuretic Peptides).[10–13]

The carboxy-terminal amino acid of AM is an amidated tyrosine (Fig. 2.1). The amidation of the peptide not only strengthens the resistance of AM to carboxypeptidase degradation, the amidation

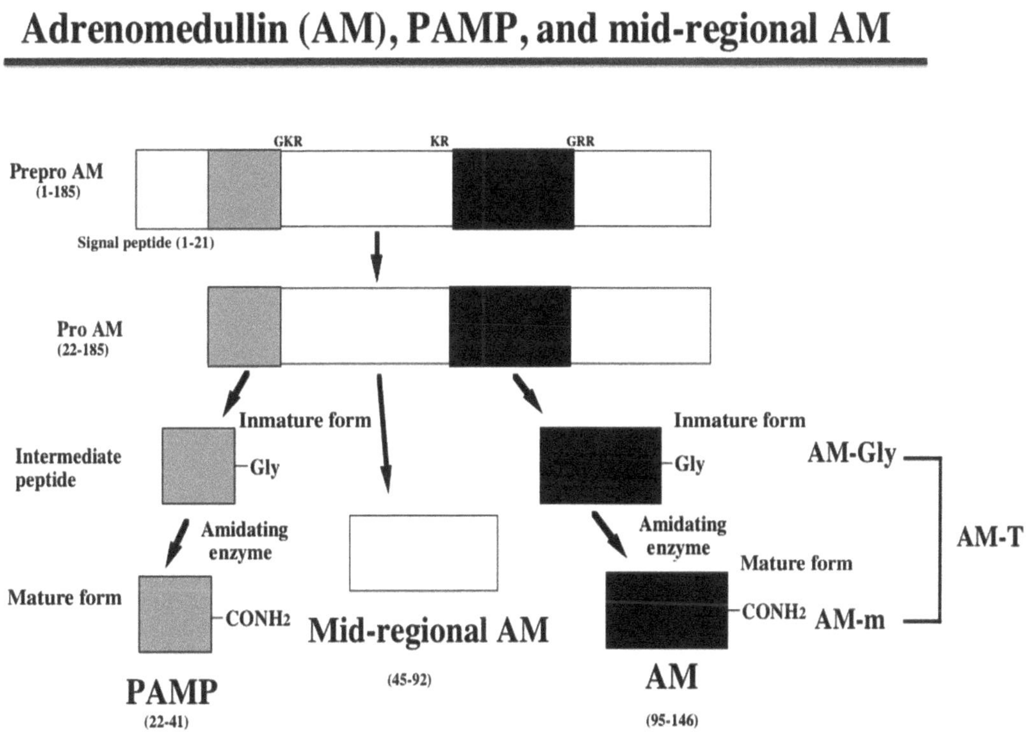

FIGURE 2.3

Schematic diagram of the biosynthesis of adrenomedullin (AM).[14] Adrenomedullin and proadrenomedullin N-terminal 20 peptide (PAMP) are cleaved from the same AM precursor (prepro AM). Prepro AM (185 amino acids) is first converted to proAM after the signal peptide is removed. ProAM is then converted to immature glycine-extended AM (AM-Gly), glycine-extended PAMP, and mid-regional AM. Finally, AM-glycine and glycine-extended PAMP are converted to active mature AM (AM-m) and PAMP with a C-terminal amide through enzymatic amidation.[6,14] AM-T = (AM-m) + (AM-Gly).

also confers biological activity to the peptide.[15] The sequence similarity of AM with human calcitonin gene-related peptide (CGRP) and amylin is not high (30%); however, this group of peptides share a carboxy-terminal amide structure and a six-residue ring structure formed by an intramolecular disulfide linkage (Fig. 2.1). Because of these structural similarities and similar pharmacological actions, AM is classified as a member of the calcitonin/CGRP family. In 2002, a new member of the AM family, adrenomedullin 2 (AM2)/intermedin, was identified separately by two groups (Fig. 2.1).[16,17] Although the sequence similarity between AM2/intermedin and AM is low (30%), the pharmacological activities of AM and AM2 are similar.

In an early study, the structure-related activities of AM were investigated using various synthetic human AM analogues. The N-terminal-truncated derivative AM-(13–52)-NH_2, which retains a cyclic structure and amidated C-terminus, exhibited a Ki and cAMP-generating activity comparable to that of intact AM-(1–52)-NH_2. By contrast, the N-terminal fragment AM-(1–10)-OH had no effect on cAMP-generating activity or receptor-binding activity, suggesting the N-terminal residues (1–12) of the AM molecule are not essential for interaction with the AM receptor.[18] In addition, removal of the C-terminal Tyr52 residue (AM-(1–51)-OH) markedly decreased the peptide's receptor binding and the cAMP response. Amidation of the C-terminal Gly51 residue (AM-(1–51)-NH_2) partially restored the receptor-binding activity and cAMP response, indicating that C-terminal amidation but not the amidated Tyr52 residue per se, is essential. Cleavage of the disulfide bond between the Cys16 and Cys21 residues (Cys(CAM)16,21 AM-NH_2) through carbamoylmethylation resulted in very weak receptor-binding activity and complete loss of the cAMP response.[18] Thus both C-terminal residue amidation and the six-residue ring structure are required for receptor binding and the cAMP response.

THE ADRENOMEDULLIN RECEPTOR

Prior to the cloning and identification of the AM receptor, binding studies identified the presence of specific AM receptors in the lung and heart as well as CGRP receptors with relatively high affinity for AM.[19] These findings suggest that AM exerts its biological effects through specific AM and/or CGRP receptors. Given the wide variety of cells and tissues with both specific CGRP and AM binding activities, it was difficult to distinguish between these two and to identify a distinct AM receptor.[20]

One component of the AM receptor complex, calcitonin receptor-like receptor (CLR), was cloned from rat hypothalamus based on homology among type B family G protein coupled receptors (GPCRs).[21] In transfection studies using several mammalian cell lines, CLR had no affinity to any known member of the calcitonin supergene family,[22] making the CLR an orphan GPCR. However, Aiyar et al. showed that when stably transfected into a cell line derived from human embryonic kidney cells (HEK-293), human CLR exhibits the pharmacology of the CGRP1 receptor,[23] suggesting HEK cells express an endogenous factor essential for the functional expression of CLR. Eventually McLatchie et al.[24] identified a cDNA encoding 148 amino-acid residues with a single transmembrane domain, which they named receptor activity modified protein 1 (RAMP1). They further showed that cotransfection of CLR and RAMP1 into COS-7 cells produced a functional CGRP1 receptor, whereas transfection of either gene alone failed to produced a functional receptor.[24] Two additional members of the RAMP family were subsequently identified through database searches and named RAMP2 and RAMP3.[24] Although the sequence similarity among the three RAMP isoforms is less than 30% within the same species, all three isoforms share conserved cysteine residues in their extracellular domain and flanking the transmembrane domain.[24] Cotransfection of CLR and RAMP2 or RAMP3 produce a functional AM receptor with high affinity for AM, but not CGRP.

Later studies confirmed that the RAMP1/CLR complex forms the CGRP receptor (Fig. 2.4, **left**), which is potently activated by CGRP. Adrenomedullin can also bind to this receptor, but with near 10-fold lower affinity than CGRP. The RAMP2/CLR complex forms an AM receptor (Fig. 2.4, **middle**), while the RAMP3/CLR complex forms an AM2 receptor (Fig. 2.4, **right**). Both the AM and AM2 receptors are potently activated by AM, whereas CGRP binds to the AM2 receptor with about 50-fold lower affinity than AM and has even less affinity for the AM receptor.[25] It is therefore now recognized that the complex of CLR with RAMP1, RAMP2, or RAMP3 produces the CGRP1, AM, or AM2 receptor, respectively (Fig. 2.4).[26] Disruption of genes encoding AM or RAMP2 is embryonically lethal in mice due to vascular defects.[27,28] On the other hand, mice with a targeted deletion of the RAMP3 gene showed no obvious vasculature changes and appear normal until old age, at which point the RAMP3 knockout mice had lower body weights than wild-type mice.[29]

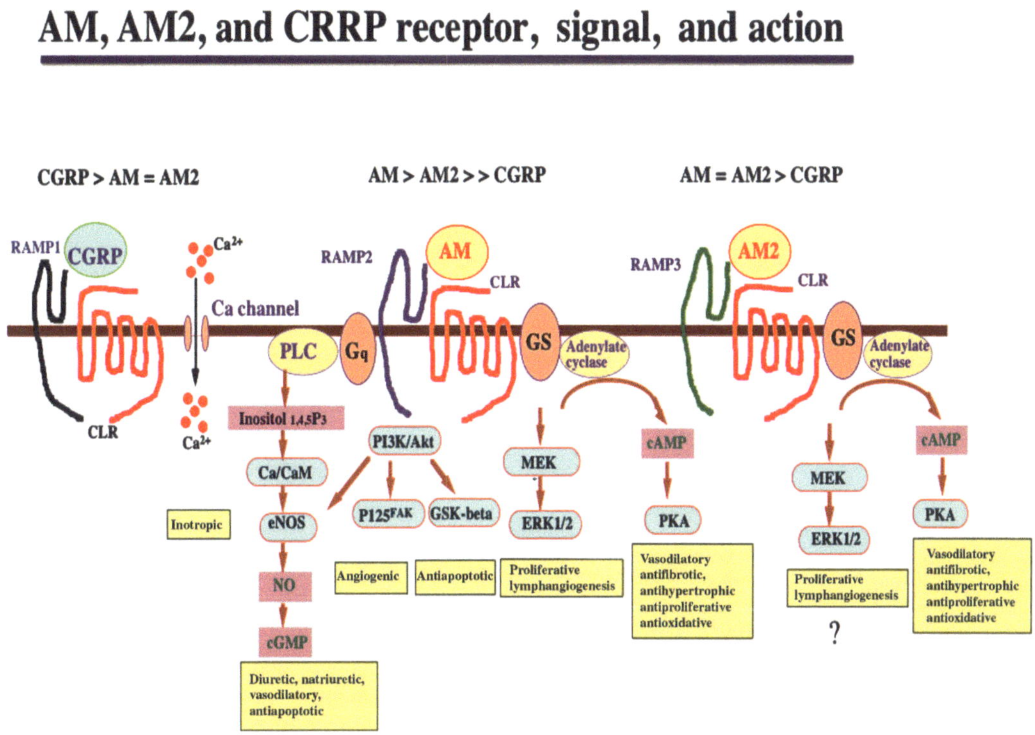

FIGURE 2.4

Adrenomedullin receptor and downstream signaling cascades. Calcitonin receptor-like receptor (CLR) and receptor activity modifying proteins (RAMPs) determine ligand selectivity for AM and calcitonin gene-related peptides (CGRP). Extracellular RAMP domains are key determinants of ligand specificity.[14,26]

CARDIAC ACTIONS OF ADRENOMEDULLIN

EFFECT OF ADRENOMEDULLIN ON CARDIAC CONTRACTILITY

In addition to its hypotensive action, AM exerts an array of cardiac effects.[5,6] Intravenous administration of AM to animals significantly increases cardiac output,[30] though it is difficult to determine whether this is a direct action or is secondary to a reduction in afterload. The first report of a direct cardiac action of AM was from Perret et al.,[31] who used a perfused rat heart model to show that AM exerts a direct negative inotropic effect. Another study showed that AM dose-dependently reduces both contractility and cytoplasmic Ca^{2+} levels in isolated rabbit cardiac myocytes via the nitric oxide/cGMP pathway.[32] Furthermore, in the presence of cytokine stimulation AM augments nitric oxide synthesis in the heart through a cAMP-dependent pathway.[33] Together, these results suggest that AM acts in the heart via a nitric oxide/cGMP pathway to suppress myocardial contractility by decreasing the availability of cytoplasmic Ca^{2+}.

By contrast, other studies demonstrated the direct inotropic effects of AM in vivo and in vitro.[34,35] Parkes and May[34] examined whether AM-induced increases in cardiac output and contractility were direct or mediated by autonomic reflexes. They examined the cardiovascular actions of AM in conscious, chronically instrumented sheep with either sympathetic, parasympathetic or autonomic ganglion blockade, to determine the role of the autonomic nervous system in mediating cardiovascular changes (**for further reading on the autonomic nervous system, see** chapter: Neuronal Hormones and the Sympathetic/Parasympathetic Regulation of the Heart). The vasodilator effects of AM on the periphery and its ability to increase cardiac output and cardiac contractility were not mediated by the autonomic nervous system but were the result of direct actions of AM on the heart and vasculature.[34] Szokodi et al.[35] reported AM-enhanced cardiac contractility via cAMP-independent mechanisms, including Ca^{2+} release from intracellular ryanodine- and thapsigargin-sensitive Ca^{2+} stores, activation of protein kinase C, and Ca^{2+} influx through L-type Ca^{2+} channels, suggesting AM is an endogenous inotropic peptide in the heart. Thereafter, the same group investigated if AM modulates blood pressure and changes in systolic and diastolic function induced by long-term administration of angiotensin II (**see** chapter: Renin Angiotensin Aldosterone System and Heart Function) or norepinephrine (**see** chapter Adrenergic Receptors) to rats.[36] They found that AM selectively inhibited the increase in blood pressure while enhancing the improvement of systolic function induced by angiotensin II. These results suggest that circulating AM primarily acts as a regulator of vascular tone and cardiac function.[36] Consistent with that idea, intravenous administration of AM enhanced left ventricular myocardial contraction and improved left ventricular relaxation without increasing myocardial oxygen consumption in patients with old myocardial infarctions and left ventricular dysfunction.[37] The discrepancies among the studies summarized above is not apparent, though they may reflect differences in the species, experimental conditions, disease models and/or age of the animals. Overall, results of in vivo animal studies are consistent with the hypothesis that AM is an endogenous inotropic peptide. This inotropic action is especially noteworthy in humans, as it may lead to the clinical application of AM in the treatment of acute heart failure.[14,38]

EFFECT OF ADRENOMEDULLIN ON CARDIAC STRUCTURE

It is now evident that AM affects cardiac structure. An early study demonstrated that AM dose-dependently increased intracellular cAMP levels in both cardiomyocytes and cardiofibroblasts.[39] In addition, AM significantly reduced angiotensin II– and fetal bovine serum–stimulated ^{14}C-phenylalanine incorporation (e.g., increased protein synthesis) into cardiomyocytes, an effect that was abolished by the AM receptor antagonist CGRP(8–37).[40] Adrenomedullin also significantly and dose-dependently reduced angiotensin II– and endothelin-1–stimulated ^{3}H-thymidine and ^{3}H-phenylalanine incorporation by cardiofibroblasts; these effects were likewise attenuated by CGRP(8–37).[41] Furthermore, AM dose-dependently suppressed DNA synthesis and collagen production in cardiofibroblasts either under basal or angiotensin II–stimulated conditions.[42] DNA and collagen synthesis by cardiofibroblasts were also suppressed by 8-bromo cAMP or the adenylate cyclase agonist forskolin and by inhibition of cAMP-specific phosphodiesterase.[42] Conversely, an AM-antisense oligo increased ^{3}H-proline incorporation and levels of collagen I and III mRNA in interleukin-1β-treated cardiofibroblasts.[43] Taken together, these results indicate that AM is an important modulator of cardiofibroblast growth that acts in an autocrine or paracrine manner, in part via cAMP signaling.

The effects of AM on cardiac hypertrophy have been studied in vivo using a rat model of pressure overload induced left ventricular hypertrophy (LVH) and heart failure using abdominal aortic banding.[44] Administration of either AM or hydralazine at the time of banding over 7 days reduced blood pressure by 10% compared to untreated rats, but only AM-treated rats showed a reduction of the left ventricular weight/body weight ratio. Left ventricular AM concentrations were 22% higher in the AM infusion group than in the untreated group, and plasma AM levels were about fivefold higher in the AM infused group. These results suggest cardiac AM exerts antifibrotic, antihypertrophic, and positive inotropic effects in the hypertrophied or failing heart.

PATHOPHYSIOLOGICAL FUNCTION OF ADRENOMEDULLIN IN CARDIAC DISEASE

CARDIAC HYPERTROPHY AND HEART FAILURE

Several clinical studies report that plasma AM levels increase in heart failure proportionally with disease severity[45–47] and that AM immunoreactivity increased in the failing heart.[46] Additionally, left ventricular AM immunoreactivity and gene expression were found to be higher in rats with heart failure compared to control rats.[48] Adrenomedullin immunoreactivity also increased in trans aortic banding–induced cardiac hypertrophy, with a strong positive correlation between levels of AM immunoreactivity and left ventricular mass.[49] Thus, cardiac AM levels are upregulated in hypertrophied and failing hearts and associated with an increase in ventricular weight and/or fetal cardiac gene expression. In human heart failure, plasma AM levels in the coronary sinus were higher than those in the aorta, suggesting cardiac AM production and secretion are increased in the failing heart.[48]

In another study, left ventricular gene expression of AM, CLR, RAMP2, and RAMP3 were increased in hypertrophied and failing hearts compared to control hearts,[50] as were cardiac levels of AM-m and AM-Gly. Moreover, the AM-m/AM-total ratio (AM-total = AM-m+ AM-Gly) was higher in the ventricles compared to plasma, and correlated with the left ventricular weight/body weight ratio.[50] These results suggest that the activity of the AM amidating enzyme as well as the AM ligand-receptor system are upregulated in hypertrophied and failing hearts (Fig. 2.5).

Whether the increased plasma and tissue levels of AM seen in hypertrophied and failing hearts have cardioprotective effects was tested using adenovirus-mediated AM gene delivery and chronic administration of AM.[51,52] Somatic gene delivery to severely hypertensive rats using an adenovirus expressing the cDNA for human AM under the control of the cytomegalovirus promoter/enhancer reduced left ventricular weight and cardiomyocyte diameter as well as decreased interstitial fibrosis and extracellular matrix formation, and a decrease in blood pressure.[51] These findings suggest that elevating AM protects against hypertension-induced cardiac remodeling.

To investigate the role of endogenous AM in the transition from LVH to heart failure, the effects of long-term AM infusion were studied in a rat model of heart failure.[52] Long-term human AM infusion decreased left ventricular end-diastolic pressure, right ventricular systolic pressure, right atrial pressure, and the left ventricular weight/body weight ratio without altering mean arterial pressure (MAP). Notably, infusion of human AM reduced endogenous plasma AM levels as well as plasma levels of renin, aldosterone, and atrial natriuretic peptide and prolonged survival.[52] A protective effect of endogenous AM against stress-induced cardiac hypertrophy was also demonstrated using heterozygous AM-null (+/−) mice.[53] Trans aortic banding led to increased heart weight/body weight ratios, left ventricular wall thickness, and perivascular fibrosis as well as the upregulation of genes encoding

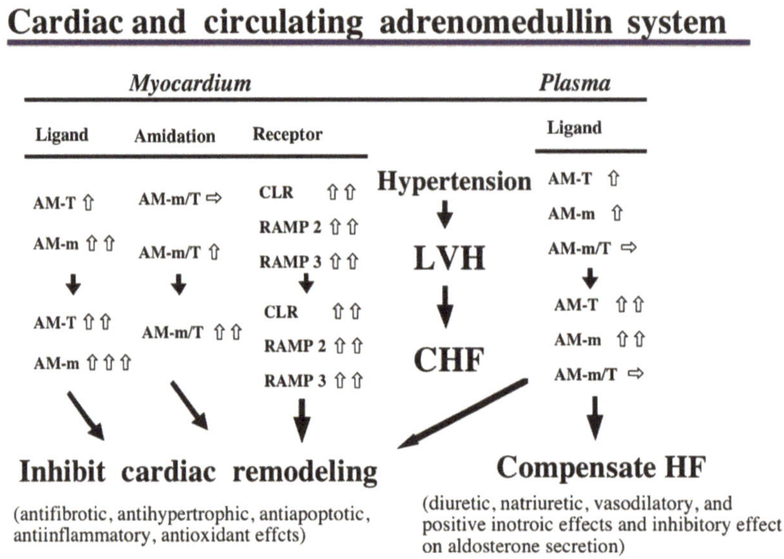

FIGURE 2.5

A working hypothesis for the function of the myocardial and circulating AM system during transition from hypertension to left ventricular hypertrophy (LVH) to heart failure.[6,50] AM-total (AM-T) = AM-mature (AM-m) + glycine-extended AM (AM-Gly).

angiotensinogen, angiotensin converting enzyme, transforming growth factor-β, collagen type I, brain natriuretic peptide, and c-fos. Across all the parameters measured, the effects were more pronounced in AM(+/−) than wild-type mice.[53] The cardioprotective effects of AM were also observed in mice overexpressing renin, a mouse model with high blood pressure, proteinuria, and cardiac hypertrophy with high levels of prorenin and active renin (see chapter: Renin Angiotensin Aldosterone System and Heart Function).[54] Interestingly, male, but not female, AM(+/−) mice with the renin transgene developed greater cardiac hypertrophy and renal damage than gender matched wild-type mice.[54] Shimosawa et al.[55] also showed that angiotensin II administration on a high-salt diet for 12 days caused marked perivascular fibrosis and intimal hyperplasia in coronary arteries in AM(+/−) mice with increased urinary excretion of 8-hydroxydeoxyguanosine and isoprostane, markers of oxidative stress. These results suggest that AM possesses a protective action against cardiovascular damage, possibly through the inhibition of oxidative stress production.[55]

Up-regulated cardiac expression of AM and its receptor appear to be an adaptive and protective response in stress-induced conditions such as cardiac hypertrophy and heart failure. This hypothesis is strongly supported by the results of recent studies using AM gene delivery, long-term AM infusion, and AM knockout mice, as described. The beneficial effects of increased AM may be associated with inhibition of the renin-angiotensin-aldosterone system (see chapter: Renin Angiotensin Aldosterone System and Heart Function) and oxidative stress, among other factors.[51–55]

Adrenomedullin and RAMP2 are highly expressed in the heart from the embryo stage through adulthood, and the genetic knockout of AM caused extreme hydrops fetalis and cardiovascular abnormalities, including overdeveloped ventricular trabeculae and underdeveloped arterial walls.[27] In addition, mice with increased AM due to a genetic modification that stabilized AM mRNA showed enlarged hearts resulting from cardiac hyperplasia during development.[56] One recent study also showed that inducible cardiac myocyte-specific RAMP2(−/−) mice exhibited cardiomyopathy-like heart failure with cardiac dilatation and myofibril disruption.[57] These studies using genetic approaches also demonstrated that AM is a powerful regulator of cardiac growth during embryogenesis, AM expression is enhanced by myocardial injury, and that AM plays a key role in the regulation of cardiac function and in the pathophysiology of heart failure.[27,56,57]

ACUTE MYOCARDIAL INFARCTION

A clinical study reported that plasma AM levels increased in patients during the early phase of acute myocardial infarction[58] In a rat model of acute myocardial infarction, expression of both AM mRNA and the peptide markedly increased in infarcted and noninfarcted regions of left ventricles.[59] Treatment with an angiotensin converting enzyme inhibitor suppressed the overproduction of AM in association with improved hemodynamics.

As described above, AM acts as an autocrine and/or paracrine factor to exert protective effects suppressing cardiac remodeling and preserving function. Consistent with that idea, Nakamura et al.[60] demonstrated that continuous administration of AM had beneficial effects on hemodynamics in a rat model of acute myocardial infarction. They also showed that AM infusion improved survival and ameliorated progression of left ventricular remodeling and heart failure with a reduction of urinary isoprostane and left ventricular mRNA levels of angiotensin converting enzyme and p22-phox, an essential component of NADPH-oxidase.[60] These results suggest that the beneficial effects of administering AM during acute myocardial infarction is due to the ability of AM to reduce left ventricular remodeling, in part by inhibiting oxidative stress and angiotensin converting enzyme expression, leading to the improvement of heart failure and reduced mortality.

To investigate whether cardiac synthesis of the mature forms of AM is accelerated in patients with acute myocardial infarction, Yasu et al.[61] used specific immunoradiometric assays to measure AM-m and AM-Gly in the aorta and coronary sinus. They found that plasma AM-m and AM-Gly levels in the aorta and coronary sinus were higher in patients with acute myocardial infarction than in normal controls. In addition, the coronary sinus-aortic step-up of AM-m, which is an index of myocardial AM-m production, was greater in patients with acute myocardial infarction than in the controls. On the other hand, there was no difference in coronary sinus-aortic step-up of AM-Gly. Patients with left ventricular dysfunction had a higher coronary sinus-aortic AM-m step-up than those without left ventricular dysfunction, and AM-m levels in the aorta and coronary sinus correlated negatively with the left ventricular ejection fraction. These results suggest that myocardial synthesis of AM-m is enhanced in patients with acute myocardial infarction, especially in patients with critical left ventricular dysfunction.[61] Thus, increased myocardial synthesis of active AM may protect against cardiac dysfunction, myocardial remodeling, or both after the onset of acute myocardial infarction in humans.

ISCHEMIA/REPERFUSION

In a rat coronary ligation ischemia/reperfusion model, AM infusion attenuated myocardial ischemia/reperfusion injury,[62] at least in part by reducing infarct size, left ventricular end-diastolic pressure, and myocardial apoptotic cell death. These beneficial effects were nearly completely abolished by pretreatment with the phosphatidylinositol 3-kinase inhibitor wortmannin, suggesting the cardioprotective effects of AM are mediated via a phosphatidylinositol 3-kinase/Akt-dependent pathway. Consistent with that idea, local AM gene transfer to the heart increased phosphorylation of Akt and glycogen synthase kinase-3β but reduced the cardiac activities of glycogen synthase kinase-3β and caspase-3. The effects of AM on glycogen synthase kinase-3β and caspase-3 activities were blocked by CGRP (residues 8–37) or by an adenovirus expressing a dominant-negative Akt.[63] Thus, AM may protect against ischemia/reperfusion-induced cardiomyocyte apoptosis via an Akt-glycogen synthase kinase-caspase signaling pathway.

The cardioprotective effect of AM against ischemia/reperfusion-induced apoptosis was confirmed using AM(+/−) mice.[64] Following 30 minutes of regional myocardial ischemia, infarct size was greater in AM(+/−) mice than in wild-type controls. Treatment with exogenous recombinant AM prior to coronary occlusion rescued the ischemia/reperfusion intolerant phenotype in AM(+/−) mice and was associated with augmented phosphorylation of Akt and endothelial nitric oxide synthase. Similarly, Nishida et al.[65] showed that treatment with AM for 10 minutes before ischemia reduced infarct size after ischemia/reperfusion. This infarct size–limiting effect of AM was abolished by a mitochondrial Ca^{2+}-activated K^+ channel blocker or by a PKA inhibitor. By contrast, AM treatment for the first 10 minutes of reperfusion reduced infarct size, and this cardioprotective effect was unchanged by the mitochondrial Ca^{2+}–activated K^+ channel blocker, but was abolished by a phosphatidylinositol 3-kinase inhibitor.[65] Thus, the cardioprotective effects of AM administered pre- and postischemia appear to be mediated by different signaling pathways.

In addition, AM reportedly induces angiogenesis and inhibits apoptosis. Three days of AM infusion plus transplantation of bone marrow–derived mononuclear cells reduced infarct size and improved cardiac function in a rat acute myocardial infarction model to a greater extent than AM alone.[66] Adrenomedullin infusion plus bone marrow–derived mononuclear cell transplantation also produced a greater increase in capillary density than AM or bone marrow–derived mononuclear cells alone, and AM markedly decreased the number of apoptotic cells among the transplanted bone marrow–derived mononuclear cells. Thus, the beneficial effects of AM infusion may reflect in part the angiogenic properties of AM itself as well as it ability to suppress apoptosis among bone marrow–derived mononuclear cells.

More recently, evidence of the mechanism by which AM exerts its beneficial effects in ischemia/reperfusion models was reported.[67] It was observed that AM stimulated nitric oxide synthesis, as indicated by increased NO_2- efflux in coronary effluent throughout reperfusion. In addition, the ability of AM to limit infarct size was associated with a 2.45-fold increase in myocardial cGMP levels 10 minutes after reperfusion, and the soluble guanylate cyclase inhibitor ODQ abolished the infarct-limiting effect of AM. Adrenomedullin appears to increase nitric oxide bioavailability in the intact myocardium, and the cytoprotective action of AM against ischemia/reperfusion injury is likely mediated via a nitric oxide/soluble guanylyl cyclase/cGMP pathway.

CLINICAL APPLICATIONS OF ADRENOMEDULLIN TO CARDIAC DISEASE

EFFECT OF ADRENOMEDULLIN ADMINISTRATION IN PATIENTS WITH HEART FAILURE

The beneficial effects of AM on experimental heart failure in animals suggest that AM administration could be effective in the treatment of human heart failure.[52,68–70] The acute effects of intravenous AM infusion (0.05 mg/kg/min) for 30 minutes on hemodynamic, renal, and hormonal responses were studied in patients with heart failure and healthy controls.[71] Adrenomedullin infusion increased the cardiac index (CI) while decreasing pulmonary capillary wedge pressure in both heart failure patients and healthy subjects. Adrenomedullin also decreased the mean pulmonary arterial pressure in heart failure patients and increased urine volume and urinary sodium excretion in both groups. Plasma aldosterone fell only during and after AM infusion in these patients with heart failure. These findings indicate that acute intravenous infusion of AM has beneficial hemodynamic, renal, and endocrine effects in patients with heart failure.[71] The effects of AM infusion in human heart failure were also studied by the Christchurch group,[72] who found that AM decreased MAP and left ventricular end-systolic volume and increased cardiac output. Despite the large drop in mean blood pressure, urine volume, urinary sodium excretion, and creatinine clearance were unchanged. Thus, short-term AM infusion appears to improve the condition of heart failure patients.

It was also tested whether long-term administration of AM (0.02 mg/kg/min) in the presence human atrial natriuretic peptide (0.05 mg/kg/min) could be an effective therapy in patients with acute decompensated heart failure in a clinical setting.[73] Seven acute decompensated heart failure patients with dyspnea and pulmonary congestion were studied. AM and recombinant human atrial natriuretic peptide were infused for 12 hours, after which human atrial natriuretic peptide was infused alone for an additional 12 hours. During the infusions hemodynamic, renal, hormonal, and oxidative stress responses were evaluated. AM plus human atrial natriuretic peptide reduced mean blood pressure, pulmonary arterial pressure, and systemic and pulmonary vascular resistance without changing heart rate, and increased cardiac output above baseline at most time-points (Fig. 2.6). In addition, AM plus human atrial natriuretic peptide reduced aldosterone, brain natriuretic peptide, and reactive oxygen species as compared to baseline measures, and increased urine volume and urinary sodium excretion. After switching to human atrial natriuretic peptide monotherapy, mean blood pressure and systemic vascular resistance increased while the CI decreased; however, urine volume or urinary excretion of sodium did not change.[73] Although this was a small pilot trial, it appears AM plus human atrial natriuretic peptide therapy is beneficial given the hemodynamic and hormonal effects in patients with acute decompensated heart failure. That said, these data are preliminary and require confirmation in a larger clinical study.

CLINICAL APPLICATION OF ADRENOMEDULLIN IN ACUTE MYOCARDIAL INFARCTION

As described above, AM appears able to reduce infarct size, inhibit myocyte apoptosis, and suppress production of reactive oxygen species, suggesting AM could potentially be useful in the treatment of acute myocardial infarction. In the first clinical pilot study of intravenous AM administration to patients with acute myocardial infarction, AM was infused at 0.0125–0.025 μg/kg/min for 12 hours.[74] During the infusion, hemodynamics remained stable in eight of the 10 patients. At 3 months postacute myocardial infarction, the wall motion index in the infarcted area was improved compared to baseline, and infarct size evaluated using cardiac magnetic resonance was decreased. These findings suggest that intravenous administration of AM could serve as an adjunct to percutaneous coronary intervention. However, these data are preliminary and require confirmation in future studies.

CLINICAL TRIALS WITH ADRENOMEDULLIN

Based on these basic and clinical results, several clinical trials were performed. Biomarkers in acute heart failure trial (http://ClinicalTrials.gov Identifier: NCT00537628) was a prospective, 15-center,

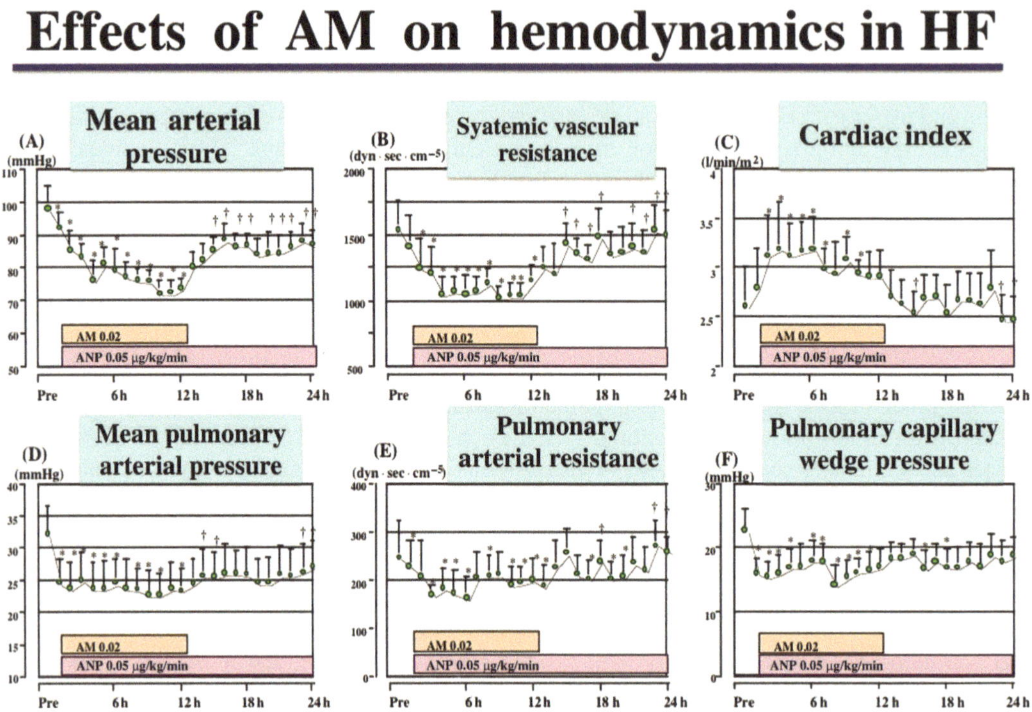

FIGURE 2.6

Effects of long-term AM administration on hemodynamics in patients with decompensated heart failure are shown. Effects of AM+ hANP (0–12h) and hANP monotherapy (12–24h) on mean arterial pressure (MAP; A), systemic vascular resistance (SVR; B), cardiac index (CI; C), mean pulmonary arterial pressure (mPAP; D), pulmonary arterial resistance (PAR; E), and pulmonary capillary wedge pressure (PCWP; F) in patients with decompensated heart failure.[73] $*p<0.05$ versus time 0.

international study of 1641 patients presenting to the emergency department with dyspnea. A superiority test of mid-regional proAM versus brain natriuretic peptide for 90-day survival and a noninferiority test of mid-regional-pro-atrial natriuretic peptide versus brain natriuretic peptide for diagnosis of acute heart failure were conducted.[10,75] Using cut-off values from receiver-operating characteristic analysis, the accuracy to predict 90-day survival of heart failure patients was 73% for mid-regional proAM and 62% for brain natriuretic peptide (difference $p<0.001$). In adjusted multivariable Cox regression, mid-regional proAM, but not brain natriuretic peptide, carried independent prognostic value ($p<0.001$). In addition, compared with brain natriuretic peptide or troponin, mid-regional proAM was superior for predicting 90-day all-cause mortality in patients presenting with acute dyspnea ($p<0.0001$). Furthermore, mid-regional proAM added significantly to all clinical variables (all adjusted hazard ratios: >3.28), and it was also superior to all other biomarkers. From these results, it was concluded that mid-regional proAM identified patients with high, 90-day mortality suggesting that brain natriuretic peptides have prognostic value in patients presenting with acute shortness of breath.

The clinical trial titled "The Role of AM on the Outcome of Severe Heart Failure: A Clinical Randomized Study" was initiated in 2010 (http://ClinicalTrials.gov Identifier: NCT01154504).[76] The study hypothesis was that the decrease of plasma AM concentration by ultrafiltration and isovolumetric hemofiltration in patients with acute III and IV class functional heart failure is more pronounced than a standard diuretic treatment and is related to clinical improvement. The primary outcome measure was plasma AM levels in different treatments: clinical, ultrafiltration, and isovolumetric hemofiltration in 90 days after randomization and at discharge. However, this study was suspended, and the reason for suspension was not provided.

Currently, only one agent is approved in nuclear medicine to study lung circulation: macroaggregates of albumin labeled with technetium (^{99m}Tc). Macroaggregates of albumin labeled with ^{99m}Tc is used almost exclusively to detect large pulmonary perfusion defects caused by embolism. Since this agent is larger than small pulmonary vessels, it becomes physically trapped, enabling external detection. The potential limitations of macroaggregates of albumin labeled with ^{99m}Tc include the inability to image the small pulmonary circulation beyond the point of obstruction. The AM receptor is abundantly expressed in human alveolar capillaries and mostly distributed at the surface of the endothelium. Therefore, the lungs contain AM binding sites at a density higher than that for any other organ studied. PulmoBind is a AM derivative labeled with ^{99m}Tc for molecular imaging of the pulmonary circulation. The phase I study (http://ClinicalTrials.gov Identifier: NCT01539889) evaluated the safety, efficacy, and dosing of PulmoBind for molecular imaging of pulmonary circulation. Healthy humans were included into escalating groups of 5 mCi, 10 mCi, or 15 mCi PulmoBind.[77] There were no safety concerns at the three dosages studied. PulmoBind was well tolerated, with no clinically significant adverse event related to the study drug. The highest dose of 15 mCi provided a favorable dosimetric profile and excellent imaging. PulmoBind is safe and provides good quality lung perfusion imaging. It is concluded that the safety/efficacy of this agent can be tested in disorders of pulmonary circulation such as pulmonary arterial hypertension.[78] Phase-II Study of the "Use of PulmoBind for Molecular Imaging of Pulmonary Hypertension (PB-02)" was recently completed (http://ClinicalTrials.gov Identifier:NCT02216279).[79] The aim of this Phase II study is to evaluate the safety of PulmoBind in participants with pulmonary hypertension and its potential to detect abnormal pulmonary circulation associated within pulmonary hypertension.

In addition, the study of "AM and Outcome in Severe Sepsis and Septic Shock" (http://ClinicalTrials.gov Identifier: NCT02393781) is currently recruiting participants.[80] The aim of this prospective study is to assess the prognostic value of bioactive plasma AM in 600 patients with severe sepsis or septic shock in an international multicenter study and to validate the findings concerning the association of AM concentration and the use of vasopressor therapy, organ failure, and outcome. Sepsis involves an overactive inflammatory response to severe bacterial infection that can compromise vascular integrity and cause tissue edema, organ dysfunction, and death. Adrenomedullin has attracted the interest of researchers because of its powerful physiological functions. An anti-AM antibody reduced the norepinephrine infusion rates required to achieve hemodynamic targets, increased urine flow, and improved creatinine clearance, which ultimately resulted in attenuated systemic inflammation and tissue apoptosis during resuscitated cecal ligation and puncture-induced septic shock in mice. In humans, plasma AM has been determined only in a small number of sepsis patients, and—except for one study—the assays used did not selectively measure the bioactive AM form and have been considered not reliable.[81–83] Therefore, the potential value of determining plasma AM in such patients cannot yet be ascertained, and the optimal cut off needs to be validated in future studies. Besides these studies, there are several studies that are partly associated with AM.[84]

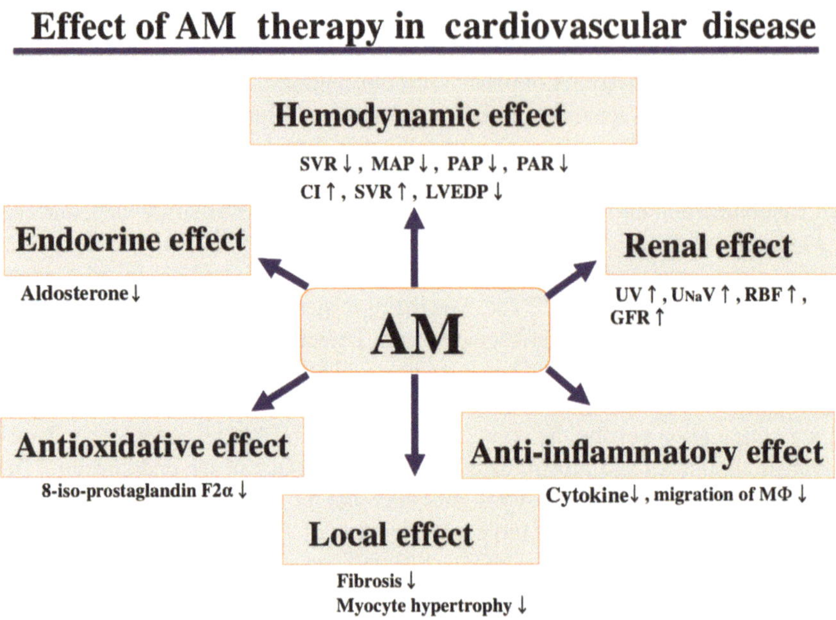

FIGURE 2.7

A working hypothesis of the mechanism of effect of AM therapy in cardiovascular disease.[14]

CONCLUSION

Over the two decades since AM was discovered, it is now known that the heart is both an important source and target of AM, with AM receptors abundantly expressed on cardiomyocytes, cardiofibroblasts, endothelial cells, and vascular smooth muscle cells. Under pathological conditions (e.g., cardiac hypertrophy, heart failure, acute myocardial infarction and ischemia/reperfusion), increased levels of AM, AM receptor, and activity of its amidating enzyme are increased. Thus, with upregulation of the cardiac AM system in common cardiac diseases, AM plays a crucial cardioprotective role, suggesting the possibility that AM may serve as an effective therapeutic agent for the treatment of various cardiovascular diseases. Consistent with this concept of AM-mediated cardioprotection, several pilot studies demonstrated the beneficial effects of AM in patients with heart failure, acute myocardial infarction, pulmonary hypertension, and ulcerative colitis.[73,74,85,86] Furthermore, clinical trials demonstrated that plasma AM levels are useful as a biomarker for heart failure, and that AM derivatives labeled with ^{99m}Tc are safe and provide quality lung perfusion imaging. A working hypothesis of the mechanism of the possible clinical use of AM in cardiovascular disease is shown in Fig. 2.7.

REFERENCES

1. Kitamura K, Kangawa K, Kawamoto M, et al. Adrenomedullin: a novel hypotensive peptide isolated from human pheochromocytoma. *Biochem Biophys Res Commun* 1993;**192**:553–60.

2. Kitamura K, Sakata J, Kangawa K, Kojima M, Matsuo H, Eto T. Cloning and characterization of cDNA encoding a precursor for humanadrenomedullin. *Biochem Biophys Res Commun* 1993;**194**:720–5.
3. Nishikimi T, Kitamura K, Saito Y, et al. Clinical studies on the sites of production and clearance of circulating adrenomedullin in human subjects. *Hypertension* 1994;**24**:600–4.
4. Nishikimi T, Matsuoka H, Shimada K, Matsuo H, Kangawa K. Production and clearance sites of two molecular forms of adrenomedullin in human plasma. *Am J Hypertens* 2000;**13**:1032–4.
5. Nishikimi T. Adrenomedullin in the kidney-renal physiological and pathophysiological roles. *Curr Med Chem* 2007;**14**:1689–99.
6. Nishikimi T, Matsuoka H. Cardiac adrenomedullin: its role in cardiac hypertrophy and heart failure. *Curr Med Chem Cardiovasc Hematol Agents* 2005;**3**:231–42.
7. Hirayama N, Kitamura K, Imamura T, et al. Molecular forms of circulating adrenomedullin in patients with congestive heart failure. *J Endocrinol* 1999;**160**:297–303.
8. Christ-Crain M, Morgenthaler NG, Struck J, Harbarth S, Bergmann A, Müller B.Mid-regional pro-adrenomedullin as a prognostic marker in sepsis: an observational study. Crit Care. 2005;9:R816-R824.
9. Dhillon OS, Khan SQ, Narayan HK, et al. Prognostic value of mid-regional pro-adrenomedullin levels taken on admission and discharge in non-ST-elevation myocardial infarction: the LAMP (Leicester Acute Myocardial Infarction Peptide) II study. *J Am Coll Cardiol* 2010;**56**:125–33.
10. Maisel A, Mueller C, Nowak R, Peacock WF, Landsberg JW, Ponikowski P, et al. Mid-region pro-hormone markers for diagnosis and prognosis in acute dyspnea: results from the BACH (Biomarkers in Acute Heart Failure) trial. *J Am Coll Cardiol* 2010;**55**:2062–76.
11. Klip IT, Voors AA, Anker SD, et al. Prognostic value of mid-regional pro-adrenomedullin in patients with heart failure after an acute myocardial infarction. *Heart* 2011;**97**:892–8.
12. Peacock WF. Novel biomarkers in acute heart failure: MR-pro-adrenomedullin. *Clin Chem Lab Med* 2014;**52**:1433–5.
13. Parwani AS, von Haehling S, Kolodziejski AI, et al. Mid-regional proadrenomedullin levels predict recurrence of atrial fibrillation after catheter ablation. *Int J Cardiol* 2015;**180**:129–33.
14. Nishikimi T, Kuwahara K, Nakagawa Y, Kangawa K, Nakao K. Adrenomedullin in cardiovascular disease: a useful biomarker, its pathological roles and therapeutic application. *Curr Protein Pept Sci* 2013;**14**:256–67.
15. Cuttitta F. Peptide amidation: signature of bioactivity. *Anat Rec* 1993;**236**:87–93.
16. Roh J, Chang CL, Bhalla A, Klein C, Hsu SY. Intermedin is a calcitonin/calcitonin gene-related peptide family peptide acting through the calcitonin receptor-like receptor/receptor activity-modifying protein receptor complexes. *J Biol Chem* 2004;**279**:7264–74.
17. Takei Y, Inoue K, Ogoshi M, Kawahara T, Bannai H, Miyano S. Identification of novel adrenomedullin in mammals: a potent cardiovascular and renal regulator. *FEBS Lett* 2004;**556**:53–8.
18. Eguchi S, Hirata Y, Iwasaki H, et al. Structure-activity relationship of adrenomedullin, a novel vasodilatory peptide, in cultured rat vascular smooth muscle cells. *Endocrinology* 1994;**135**:2454–8.
19. Owji AA, Smith DM, Coppock HA, et al. An abundant and specific binding site for the novel vasodilator adrenomedullin in the rat. *Endocrinology* 1995;**136**:2127–34.
20. Kennedy SP, Sun D, Oleynek JJ, Hoth CF, Kong J, Hill RJ. Expression of the rat adrenomedullin receptor or a putative human adrenomedullin receptor does not correlate with adrenomedullin binding or functional response. *Biochem Biophys Res Commun* 1998;**244**:832–7.
21. Njuki F, Nicholl CG, Howard A, et al. A new calcitonin-receptor-like sequence in rat pulmonary blood vessels. *Clin Sci* 1993;**85**:385–8.
22. Fluhmann B, Muff R, Hunziker W, Fischer JA, Born W. A human orphan calcitonin receptor-like structure. *Biochem Biophys Res Commun* 1995;**206**:341–7.
23. Aiyar N, Rand K, Elshourbagy NA, et al. A cDNA encoding the calcitonin gene-related peptide type 1 receptor. *J Biol Chem* 1996;**271**:11325–9.
24. McLatchie LM, Fraser NJ, Main MJ, et al. RAMPs regulate the transport and ligand specificity of the calcitonin-receptor-like receptor. *Nature* 1998;**393**:333–9.

25. Born W, Muff R, Fischer JA. Functional interaction of G protein-coupled receptors of the adrenomedullin peptide family with accessory receptor-activity-modifying proteins (RAMP). *Microsc Res Tech* 2002;**57**:14–22.
26. Hay DL, Walker CS, Poyner DR. Adrenomedullin and calcitonin gene-related peptide receptors in endocrine-related cancers: opportunities and challenges. *Endocr Relat Cancer* 2010;**18**:C1–14.
27. Caron KM, Smithies O. Extreme hydrops fetalis and cardiovascular abnormalities in mice lacking a functional Adrenomedullin gene. *Proc Natl Acad Sci USA* 2001;**98**:615–9.
28. Shindo T, Kurihara Y, Nishimatsu H, et al. Vascular abnormalities and elevated blood pressure in mice lacking adrenomedullin gene. *Circulation* 2001;**104**:1964–71.
29. Dackor R, Fritz-Six K, Smithies O, Caron K. Receptor activity-modifying proteins 2 and 3 have distinct physiological functions from embryogenesis to old age. *J Biol Chem* 2007;**282**:18094–9.
30. Ishiyama Y, Kitamura K, Ichiki Y, et al. Hemodynamic effects of a novel hypotensive peptide, humanadrenomedullin, in rats. *Eur J Pharmacol* 1993;**241**:271–3.
31. Perret M, Broussard H, LeGros T, et al. The effect of adrenomedullin on the isolated heart. *Life Sci* 1993;**53**:377–9.
32. Ikenouchi H, Kangawa K, Matsuo H, Hirata Y. Negative inotropic effect of adrenomedullin in isolated adult rabbit cardiac ventricular myocytes. *Circulation* 1997;**95**:2318–24.
33 Ikeda U, Kanbe T, Kawahara Y, Yokoyama M, Shimada K. Adrenomedullin augments inducible nitric oxide synthase expression in cytokine-stimulated cardiac myocytes. *Circulation* 1996;**94**:2560–5.
34. Parkes DG, May CN. Direct cardiac and vascular actions of adrenomedullin in conscious sheep. *Br J Pharmacol* 1997;**120**:1179–85.
35. Szokodi I, Kinnunen P, Tavi P, Weckstrom M, Toth M, Ruskoaho H. Evidence for cAMP-independent mechanisms mediating the effects of adrenomedullin, a new inotropic peptide. *Circulation* 1998;**97**:1062–70.
36. Luodonpää M, Leskinen H, Ilves M, Vuolteenaho O, Ruskoaho H. Adrenomedullin modulates hemodynamic and cardiac effects of angiotensin II in conscious rats. *Am J Physiol Regul Integr Comp Physiol* 2004;**286**:R1085–92.
37. Nagaya N, Goto Y, Satoh T, et al. Intravenous adrenomedullin in myocardial function and energy metabolism in patients after myocardial infarction. *J Cardiovasc Pharmacol* 2002;**39**:754–60.
38. Nishikimi T, Kangawa K, Nakao K. Adrenomedullin in heart failure: molecular mechanism and therapeutic implication. *Curr Hypertens Rev* 2011;**7**:273–83.
39. Nishikimi T, Horio T, Yoshihara F, Nagaya N, Matsuo H, Kangawa K. Effect of adrenomedullin on cAMP and cGMP levels in rat cardiac myocytes and nonmyocytes. *Eur J Pharmacol* 1998;**353**:337–44.
40. Tsuruda T, Kato J, Kitamura K, et al. Adrenomedullin: a possible autocrine or paracrine inhibitor of hypertrophy of cardiomyocytes. *Hypertension* 1998;**31**:505–10.
41. Tsuruda T, Kato J, Kitamura K, et al. An autocrine or a paracrine role of adrenomedullin in modulating cardiac fibroblast growth. *Cardiovasc Res* 1999;**43**:958–67.
42. Horio T, Nishikimi T, Yoshihara F, Matsuo H, Takishita S, Kangawa K. Effects of adrenomedullin on cultured rat cardiac myocytes and fibroblasts. *Eur J Pharmacol* 1999;**382**:1–9.
43. Nishikimi T, Tadokoro K, Akimoto K, et al. Response of adrenomedullin system to cytokine in cardiac fibroblasts-role of adrenomedullin as an antifibrotic factor. *Cardiovasc Res* 2005;**66**:104–13.
44. Morimoto A, Nishikimi T, Yoshihara F, et al. Ventricular adrenomedullin levels correlate with the extent of cardiac hypertrophy in rats. *Hypertension* 1999;**33**:1146–52.
45. Nishikimi T, Saito Y, Kitamura K, et al. Increased plasma levels of adrenomedullin in patients with heart failure. *J Am Coll Cardiol* 1995;**26**:1424–31.
46. Jougasaki M, Wei CM, McKinley LJ, Burnett Jr JC. Elevation of circulating and ventricular adrenomedullin in human congestive heart failure. *Circulation* 1995;**92**:286–9.
47. Kato J, Kobayashi K, Etoh T, et al. Plasma adrenomedullin concentration in patients with heart failure. *J Clin Endocrinol Metab* 1996;**81**:180–3.
48. Nishikimi T, Horio T, Sasaki T, et al. Cardiac production and secretion of adrenomedullin are increased in heart failure. *Hypertension* 1997;**30**:1369–75.

49. Yoshihara F, Nishikimi T, Horio T, et al. Ventricular adrenomedullin concentration is a sensitive biochemical marker for volume and pressure overload in rats. *Am J Physiol Heart Circ Physiol* 2000;**278**:H633–42.
50. Nishikimi T, Tadokoro K, Mori Y, et al. Ventricular adrenomedullin system in the transition from LVH to heart failure in rats. *Hypertension* 2003;**41**:512–8.
51. Dobrzynski E, Wang C, Chao J, Chao L. Adrenomedullin gene delivery attenuates hypertension, cardiac remodeling, and renal injury in deoxycorticosterone acetate-salt hypertensive rats. *Hypertension* 2000;**36**:995–1001.
52. Nishikimi T, Yoshihara F, Horinaka S, et al. Chronic administration of adrenomedullin attenuates transition from left ventricular hypertrophy to heart failure in rats. *Hypertension* 2003;**42**:1034–41.
53. Niu P, Shindo T, Iwata H, et al. Protective effects of endogenous adrenomedullin on cardiac hypertrophy, fibrosis, and renal damage. *Circulation* 2004;**109**:1789–94.
54. Caron K, Hagaman J, Nishikimi T, Kim HS, Smithies O. Adrenomedullin gene expression differences in mice do not affect blood pressure but modulate hypertension-induced pathology in males. *Proc Natl Acad Sci USA* 2007;**104**:3420–5.
55. Shimosawa T, Shibagaki Y, Ishibashi K, Kitamura K, Kangawa K, Kato S, et al. Adrenomedullin, an endogenous peptide, counteracts cardiovascular damage. *Circulation* 2002;**105**:106–11.
56. Wetzel-Strong SE, Li M, Klein KR, Nishikimi T, Caron KM. Epicardial-derived adrenomedullin drives cardiac hyperplasia during embryogenesis. *Dev Dyn* 2014;**243**:243–56.
57. Yoshizawa T, Sakurai T, Kamiyoshi A, et al. Novel regulation of cardiac metabolism and homeostasis by the adrenomedullin-receptor activity-modifying protein 2 system. *Hypertension* 2013;**61**:341–51.
58. Miyao Y, Nishikimi T, Goto Y, et al. Increased plasma adrenomedullin levels in patients with acute myocardial infarction in proportion to the clinical severity. *Heart* 1998;**79**:39–44.
59. Nagaya N, Nishikimi T, Yoshihara F, Horio T, Morimoto A, Kangawa K. Cardiac adrenomedullin gene expression and peptide accumulation after acute myocardial infarction in rats. *Am J Physiol Regul Integr Comp Physiol* 2000;**278**:R1019–26.
60. Nakamura R, Kato J, Kitamura K, et al. Adrenomedullin administration immediately after myocardial infarction ameliorates progression of heart failure in rats. *Circulation* 2004;**110**:426–31.
61. Yasu T, Nishikimi T, Kobayashi N, et al. Up-regulated synthesis of mature-type adrenomedullin in coronary circulation immediately after reperfusion in patients with anterior acute myocardial infarction. *Regul Pept* 2005;**129**:161–6.
62. Okumura H, Nagaya N, Itoh T, et al. Adrenomedullin infusion attenuates myocardial ischemia/reperfusion injury through the phosphatidylinositol 3-kinase/Akt-dependent pathway. *Circulation* 2004;**109**:242–8.
63. Yin H, Chao L, Chao J. Adrenomedullin protects against myocardial apoptosis after ischemia/reperfusion through activation of Akt-GSK signaling. *Hypertension* 2004;**43**:109–16.
64. Hamid SA, Baxter GF. A critical cytoprotective role of endogenous adrenomedullin in acute myocardial infarction. *J Mol Cell Cardiol* 2006;**41**:360–3.
65. Nishida H, Sato T, Miyazaki M, Nakaya H. Infarct size limitation by adrenomedullin: protein kinase A but not PI3-kinase is linked to mitochondrial KCa channels. *Cardiovasc Res* 2008;**77**:398–405.
66. Fujii T, Nagaya N, Iwase T, et al. Adrenomedullin enhances therapeutic potency of bone marrow transplantation for myocardial infarction in rats. *Am J Physiol Heart Circ Physiol* 2005;**288**:H1444–5.
67. Hamid SA, Totzeck M, Drexhage C, et al. Nitric oxide/cGMP signalling mediates the cardioprotective action of adrenomedullin in reperfused myocardium. *Basic Res Cardiol* 2010;**105**:257–66.
68. Nagaya N, Nishikimi T, Horio T, et al. Cardiovascular and renal effects of adrenomedullin in rats with heart failure. *Am J Physiol* 1999;**276**:R213–8.
69. Lainchbury JG, Meyer DM, Jougasaki M, Burnett Jr JC, Redfield MM. Effects of adrenomedullin on load and myocardial performance in normal and heart-failure dogs. *Am J Physiol Heart Circ Physiol* 2000;**279**:H1000–6.
70. Rademaker MT, Charles CJ, Espiner EA, Nicholls MG, Richards AM. Long-term adrenomedullin administration in experimental heart failure. *Hypertension* 2002;**40**:667–72.

71. Nagaya N, Satoh T, Nishikimi T, et al. Hemodynamic, renal, and hormonal effects of adrenomedullin infusion in patients with congestive heart failure. *Circulation* 2000;**101**:498–503.
72. Lainchbury JG, Nicholls MG, Espiner EA, Yandle TG, Lewis LK, Richards AM. Bioactivity and interactions of adrenomedullin and brain natriuretic peptide in patients with heart failure. *Hypertension* 1999;**34**:70–5.
73. Nishikimi T, Karasawa T, Inaba C, et al. Effects of long-term intravenous administration of adrenomedullin plus human atrial natriuretic peptide therapy in acute decompensated heart failure: a pilot study. *Circ J* 2009;**73**:892–8.
74. Kataoka Y, Miyazaki S, Yasuda S, et al. The first clinical pilot study of intravenous adrenomedullin administration in patients with acute myocardial infarction. *J Cardiovasc Pharmacol* 2010;**56**:413–9.
75. Maisel A, Mueller C, Nowak RM, Peacock WF, Ponikowski P, Mockel M, et al. Midregion prohormone adrenomedullin and prognosis in patients presenting with acute dyspnea: results from the BACH (Biomarkers in Acute Heart Failure) trial. *J Am Coll Cardiol* 2011;**58**:1057–67.
76. https://clinicaltrials.gov/show/NCT01154504.
77. https://clinicaltrials.gov/show/NCT01539889.
78. Harel F, Levac X, Nguyen QT, Létourneau M, Marcil S, Finnerty V, et al. Molecular imaging of the human pulmonary vascular endothelium using an adrenomedullin receptor ligand. *Mol Imaging* 2015;**14**. http://dx.doi.org/10.2310/7290.2015.00003.
79. https://clinicaltrials.gov/show/NCT02216279.
80. https://clinicaltrials.gov/show/NCT02393781.
81. Enguix-Armada A, Escobar-Conesa R, La Torre AG, De La Torre-Prados MV. Usefulness of several biomarkers in the management of septic patients: C-reactive protein, procalcitonin, presepsin and mid-regional pro-adrenomedullin. *Clin Chem Lab Med* 2016;**54**:163–8.
82. Angeletti S, Spoto S, Fogolari M, Cortigiani M, Fioravanti M, De Florio L, et al. Diagnostic and prognostic role of procalcitonin (PCT) and MR-pro-Adrenomedullin (MR-proADM) in bacterial infections. *APMIS* 2015;**123**:740–8.
83. Ohta H, Tsuji T, Asai S, Tanizaki S, Sasakura K, Teraoka H, et al. A simple immunoradiometric assay for measuring the entire molecules of adrenomedullin in human plasma. *Clin Chim Acta* 1999;**287**:131–43.
84. https://scicrunch.org/resources/data/source/nlx_154697-5/search?q=nifext_5136&l=Adrenomedullin.
85. Nagaya N, Kyotani S, Uematsu M, et al. Effects of adrenomedullin inhalation on hemodynamics and exercise capacity in patients with idiopathic pulmonary arterial hypertension. *Circulation* 2004;**109**:351–6.
86. Ashizuka S, Inatsu H, Kita T, Kitamura K. Adrenomedullin therapy in patients with refractory ulcerative colitis: a case series. *Dig Dis Sci* 2015;**61**:872–80. [Epub ahead of print].

CHAPTER

3

ENDOTHELIN-1 AS A CARDIAC-DERIVED AUTOCRINE, PARACRINE AND INTRACRINE FACTOR IN HEART HEALTH AND DISEASE

M. Karmazyn

University of Western Ontario, London, ON, Canada

INTRODUCTION

Endothelin-1 (ET-1) is a 21-amino-acid peptide initially identified by Yanagisawa and coworkers as an endothelium-derived vasoconstrictor.[1] By virtue of its ability to exert potent vasoconstrictor effects, ET-1 has attracted attention as a potential therapeutic target for the treatment of a number of cardiovascular diseases particularly with the use of endothelin receptor antagonists.[2,3] It can thus be said that the discovery of ET-1 heralded a new era in cardiovascular research. A search through PubMed using the key word "endothelin" reveals a staggering number: there have been more than 28,000 publications on this subject since 1988, the year in which ET-1 was first identified. This interest in endothelin appears to continue, with approximately 1700 publications in 2014 alone. ET-1 is actually a member of a family of endothelins, ET-1, ET-2, and ET-3, with each ET representing a distinct gene product.[4] All ETs demonstrate some degree of homogeneity in that each contains 21 amino acids as well as two disulfide bonds. Yet they demonstrate different pharmacological profiles particularly in terms of potency, which likely reflect amino acid substitutions. In fact, however, these ETs are distinguished from each other by only a few amino acid substitutions, namely two between ET-1 and ET-2, although a more substantial six amino substitutions serve to differentiate ET-3 from ET-1 (Fig. 3.1). This review will discuss primarily ET-1, as this represents not only the most abundant and potent member of the ET family, but represents the primary target for cardiovascular therapeutics.[5] Nonetheless, a potential role of ET-2 in the cardiovascular system may indeed exist although definitive evidence for this is still lacking.[6]

It is now well known that ET-1 is produced not only in the vascular endothelium but also in numerous other tissues including the heart, as will be discussed in the following section. Irrespective of its site of production, ET-1 is synthesized by the enzymatic cleavage of an amino acid precursor prepropeptide first by an endopeptidase followed by a carboxypeptidase which results in the production of the 38 amino acid pro-ET-1, also referred to as big ET-1.[7,8] The latter is then subjected to further enzymatic

Endocrinology of the Heart in Health and Disease. DOI: http://dx.doi.org/10.1016/B978-0-12-803111-7.00003-8

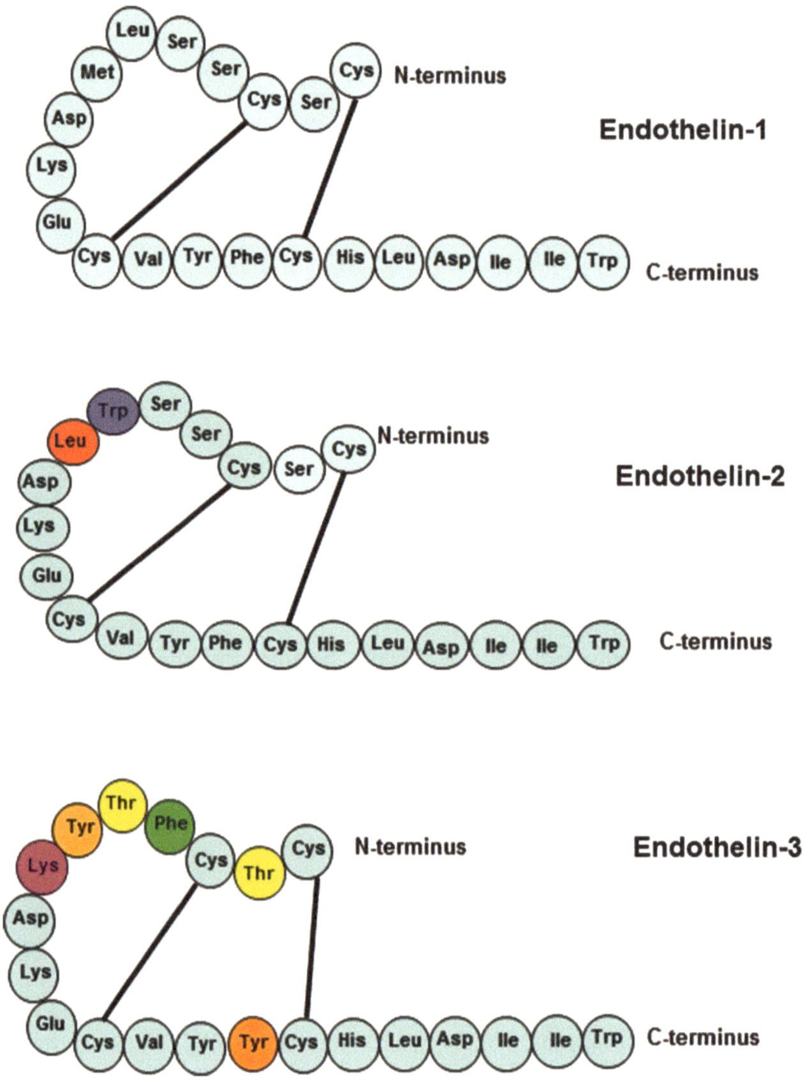

FIGURE 3.1

Amino sequences for ET-1, ET-2, and ET-3. Differences from ET-1 are shown in color. Identical disulfide bridges (Cys1-Cys15;Cys 3-Cys11) are shown for each ET.

cleavage by the phosphoramidon-sensitive endothelin converting enzyme (ECE), which results in the generation of the 21 amino acid final product (Fig. 3.2). Interestingly, ECE inhibition has been considered as a potential target for therapeutic intervention, as this would diminish the generation of ET-1 from big ET-1.[9] Thus, from a therapeutic perspective, management of ET-1–related pathologies could be potentially directed at inhibition of synthesis, i.e., ECE inhibition or targeting ET-1 receptors that

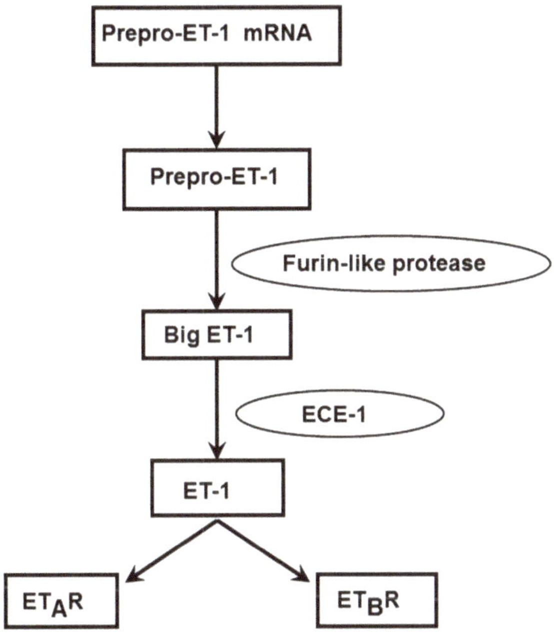

FIGURE 3.2

General scheme identifying the principal pathway of ET-1 synthesis involving the conversion of big ET-1 to ET-1 via endothelin converting enzyme-1 (ECE-1). ET-1 can exert its effect via either ETA receptor (ET_AR) or ETB receptor (ET_BR) activation.

mediate the biological effects of the peptide. However, there is evidence that big ET-1 exhibits identical vasoconstricting potencies in terms of increasing blood pressure and reducing coronary flow rate following infusion to humans,[10] which would question the validity of ECE inhibition at least with respect to attenuating vasoconstricting responses. It should be noted that there is also an alternate pathway for ET-1 synthesis from big ET-1 via the serine protease chymase,[11] although the relevance of this system to cardiac biology is uncertain.

CARDIAC PRODUCTION OF ET-1

As mentioned above, the initial site of identification of ET-1 was in the vascular endothelium and the primary effect of the peptide identified was as a potent vasoconstrictor. However, ET-1 is produced by many cell types including the cardiomyocyte, and there is now extensive and strong evidence that ET-1 functions as a paracrine, autocrine, and intracrine regulator of cardiac performance with a potential contribution to cardiac pathology. This finding should not be considered as particularly surprising, as the heart is now well known to function as an endocrine organ by virtue of its ability to produce a large number of factors particularly those acting in a paracrine or autocrine matter, as discussed throughout this volume. In the case of ET-1 there are a large number of reports documenting the ability of the heart to synthesize ET-1 as well as the ability to modulate ET-1 production under pathological conditions, in most cases by increasing ET-1 production. Indeed, these reports emerged relatively rapidly following the initial discovery of ET-1. It should be noted that the heart consists not only of cardiomyocytes but also noncardiomyocyte components such as endothelium, nerve endings, and fibroblasts, which contribute to the cardiac pathological process.[12] Thus, cardiac-derived ET-1 can originate from any of these sources. The major question that arises, and which is yet to be resolved, is what is the role of endogenously synthesized ET-1 in cardiac function or dysfunction especially under pathological conditions. As will be evident, this question is relatively difficult to address with precision since ET-1 exerts a myriad of cardiac effects which are not necessarily interrelated and in some cases diametrically opposite. Even with respect to cardiac pathology the contribution of ET-1 is not completely clear as both deleterious and beneficial effects of the peptide have been documented (see below). Nonetheless, most cardiac pathologies are associated with increased plasma levels of ET-1 although to what degree this is a reflection of increased cardiac-derived ET-1 production is not known with certainty.

Among the first demonstration that ET-1 can be produced by the cardiomyocyte was presented by Suzuki et al., who showed that cultured neonatal rat ventricular myocytes secrete ET-1 and express the enzymatic pathways for its production.[13] Moreover, the ability of myocytes to produce ET-1 was enhanced under hypoxic conditions[14] as well as mitochondrial dysfunction produced by rotenone, a mitochondrial complex 1 inhibitor,[15] thus potentially linking mitochondrial dysfunction to increased cardiac ET-1 synthesis. There appears also to be a strong stimulation to increase ET-1 synthesis and release especially during the postischemic reperfusion phase of the myocardium, a phenomenon potentially contributing to reperfusion-induced arrhythmias[16] as well as myocardial injury.[17] Thus, both ischemia and subsequent reperfusion are likely major factors dictating upregulation of ET-1 in the heart.

How cardiac ET-1 is regulated at the molecular levels is not completely understood although most studies reveal a de novo increased synthesis of the peptide under pathological conditions. There is substantial evidence from a variety of experimental models that increased ET-1 is mediated at the transcriptional level by upregulation of hypoxia-inducible factor 1.[18–20] Other factors and pathologies appear also to regulate ET-1 expression in the myocardium such as the angiotensin II AT_1 receptor since its blockade depresses cardiac ET-1 expression.[21] Diseases not directly associated with the heart such as sepsis,[22] pulmonary artery hypertension,[23] as well as obesity[24] can also increase myocardial ET-1 levels. With respect to the latter, the effect appears to be mediated by the 16 kDa satiety factor leptin (see chapter: Fat Hormones, Adipokines) whose plasma levels are increased in relation to adiposity.[25] While originally identified as a protein produced by white adipocytes, one of the so-called adipokines (see chapter: Fat Hormones, Adipokines), it is interesting that leptin is also produced by the heart including by the cardiomyocyte[26,27] thus suggesting that it could be an endogenous regulator of ET-1 synthesis at the cardiac level. In this regard it has been reported that leptin may be an important positive regulator of myocardial ET-1 expression in rats subjected to heart failure by coronary artery ligation.[28] Indeed, in that study the complete myocardial ET-1 system, including receptors, ECE, and ET-1 was upregulated in heart failure, an effect associated with abnormal expression of sarcoplasmic reticulum (SR) calcium regulatory proteins.[28]

In addition to cardiomyocytes, ET-1 is also expressed in cardiac fibroblasts where it has been proposed to contribute to fibroblast proliferation in both an autocrine and paracrine manner.[29] In addition, endocardial endothelium-derived ET-1, which may be under the control of neuropeptide Y receptors,[30] can also contribute to cardiac fibrosis and therefore play an important role in cardiac pathology.[31] Moreover, ET-1 can be produced by sympathetic neurons innervating the heart (see chapter: Adrenergic Receptors) therefore representing an additional source of cardiac-derived ET-1.[32] Interestingly, neuronally derived ET-1 is likely an important stimulator of norepinephrine release from nerve endings via ET_A receptor activation, which can contribute to pathological effects, including arrhythmogenesis and ventricular dysfunction seen with either ET-1 administration or as a consequence of endogenously released peptide.[32–35] Thus, when taken together, it is evident that cardiac-derived ET-1 can originate from multiple sources, including the cardiomyocyte, vascular endothelium, fibroblasts, and sympathetic neurons which can then influence the response to pathological stimuli (Fig. 3.3).

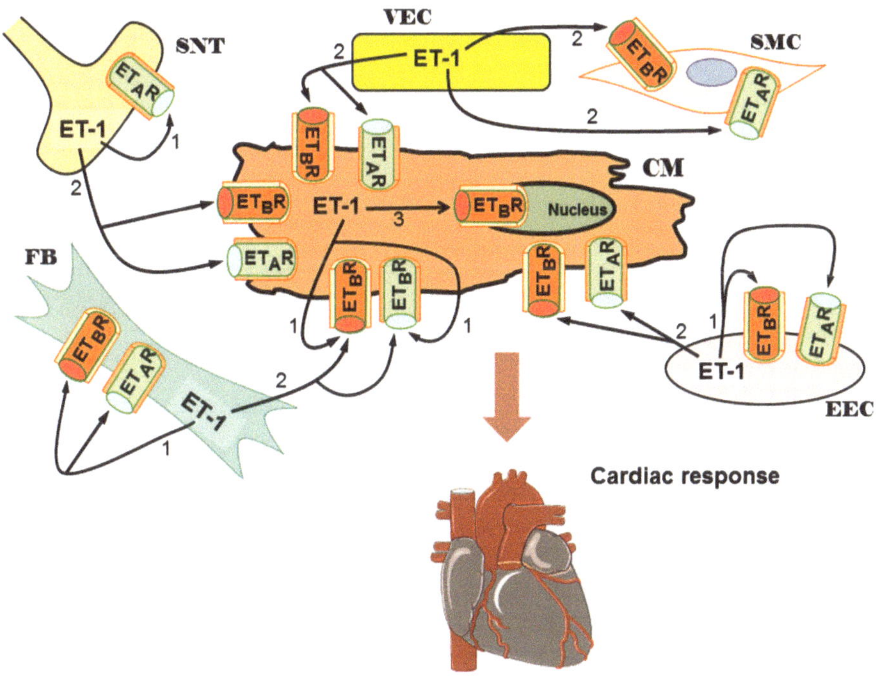

FIGURE 3.3

Interrelationship between ET-1 derived from various cellular sources within the heart. The illustration shows four different cell types capable of producing ET-1 including the cardiomyocyte (CM), vascular endothelial cell (VEC), endocardial endothelial cell (EEC) as well as the sympathetic nerve terminal (SNT). Modulation of CM function and the resultant cardiac response can be attained by ET-1 acting in an autocrine, paracrine, or intracrine manner, numbered 1, 2, and 3, respectively. For example, VEC-derived ET-1 can act directly on smooth muscle cells (SMC) to produce either vasoconstriction or vasodilatation, which is thought to occur via ET_A receptor (ET_AR) or ET_B receptor (ET_BR) activation, respectively. Paracrine roles of ET-1 (2), particularly those acting on the CM, can occur from ET-1 derived from VEC, SNT, FB, and EEC, which can directly affect the CM by activating both ET receptor subtypes expressed by CM, as discussed in the text. ET-1 produced by most of these cell types can also modulate cell behavior via an autocrine process (1). Lastly, ET-1 synthesized within the CM can also affect CM function by acting intracellularly *via* intracrine mechanisms (3) and thought to occur via targeting of nuclei primarily through ET_BR activation. See text for further discussion.

CARDIAC ET-1 PRODUCTION IN HEART DISEASE

As noted above, hypoxia and mitochondrial dysfunction result in increased cardiac production of ET-1, and the general concept of upregulation of the myocardial ET system can be applied to many cardiac disease states such as heart failure.[36] These increases in cardiac ET-1 production may be due to a number of processes and stimuli discussed in the previous section. Both animal and clinical studies show that that numerous cardiac pathologies are associated with increased circulating plasma levels of ET-1 that may originate from cardiac as well as other sources. Importantly however, increased cardiac production of ET-1 is of potential clinical relevance, as this locally produced ET-1 could represent an important autocrine, paracrine, or indeed intracrine component of cardiac regulation by this peptide. Indeed, in a rat model of renovascular hypertension, the upregulation of the cardiac ET-1 system has been implicated as an important contributor to cardiac remodeling.[37] From a clinical perspective, elevated plasma ET-1 levels have been shown to be a good indicator of poor prognosis following myocardial infarction.[38–41] ET-1 plasma levels are also elevated in patients with heart failure with plasma concentrations corresponding to heart failure severity and increasing concentrations acting as a predictor of poor outcome.[42,43] Moreover, elevated levels of ET-1 in heart failure may also contribute to increase severity of inflammation seen in these patients, thus further contributing to poor clinical outcomes.[44] As noted above, whether the heart represents a significant source of ET-1 production in heart failure is uncertain, and it is likely that numerous sources contribute to increased plasma concentrations of the peptide including the pulmonary circulation.[45] Enhanced myocardial ET-1 release has also been documented in patients with coronary heart disease undergoing angioplasty.[46]

EXPRESSION OF CARDIAC ET RECEPTORS

ET-1, and indeed all ET isoforms exert their effects via distinct membrane receptors that are linked to signaling processes through G-protein–dependent mechanisms. Three ET receptors have been identified, namely ET_A, ET_B, and ET_C although it is the ET_A and ET_B subtypes that mediate most of the biological actions of endothelins in general and ET-1 in particular. ET_C receptors have been identified in noncardiac tissue and are selectively activated by ET-3. ET receptors are generally referred to as Class A (also referred to as Class 1 or rhodopsin-like) receptors and are the most abundant of the G-protein coupled receptor (GPCR) types. Understanding the structure of ET receptors has been a critical factor for the design and development of ET receptor antagonists for cardiovascular therapeutics.[3] Activation of ET receptors initiates numerous cell signaling processes that produce diverse biological responses depending on tissue type, with responses generally prolonged, as the ligand dissociates very slowly from the ET_A receptor. The well-known vasoconstricting effect of ET-1 is an ET_A-dependent process, which results in elevations in intracellular Ca^{2+} concentrations involving both increased Ca^{2+} influx through voltage-gated Ca^{2+} channels as well as mobilization of Ca^{2+} from intracellular stores (reviewed in Ref. 47).

The heart expresses both the ET_A and ET_B receptor subtypes that have been identified both in the myocardium as well as other cell types with different receptors expressed in specific regions of the heart including vasculature and myocardium, thus demonstrating substantial heterogeneity.[48–50] As previously reviewed, both ET_A and ET_B receptors have been identified in the human heart, which indeed expresses the full complement of the ET system, including the ability to synthesize and release ET-1 thereby implicating both an autocrine and paracrine function.[7] While ET receptors appear to be heterogeneously distributed throughout the human heart, including the muscle and conduction systems,[7] there is evidence that the ET_B cell surface receptor may be more predominantly expressed in conduction fibers at least in the human heart.[49] Although the biological relevance of this is as yet unknown it may be related to a potential antiarrhythmic influence of ET_B receptor activation through diminished sympathetic nervous system stimulation especially during the early postinfarction period.[51,52] Although the issue has not been extensively explored, based on animal studies it appears that the cardiac expression levels or relative distribution of ET receptors may be determined by age with a decrease in the ET_A receptor subtype found in aged animals.[53]

INTRACELLULAR ET RECEPTORS: EVIDENCE FOR AN INTRACRINE ROLE OF ET-1 IN THE CARDIAC CELL

Although ET GPCRs are generally considered to represent cell surface receptors that initiate a cascade of intracellular signaling events, recent evidence suggests that cardiomyocyte nuclei express ET receptors that are linked to signaling pathway activation, thus providing evidence that ET-1, in addition to its role in autocrine and paracrine regulator of cardiac function, also functions as an initiator of intracrine cell signaling. As recently reviewed, these receptors expressed in nuclei could play a major role in cardiovascular regulation and contribute to cardiac pathology.[54] Interestingly, both ET_A and ET_B receptors appear to be expressed in nuclei from cardiac tissue. However, work from different laboratories suggest that the primary receptor responding to intracellular-derived ET-1 is the ET_B receptor, which mediates ET-1 induced elevations in intranuclear Ca^{2+} levels.[55,56] Thus, ET_A and ET_B receptors appear to play distinct roles in the heart via their extracellular and intracellular actions, respectively. When taken together the studies offer a potentially novel concept regarding cardiac-derived ET-1 synthesis, that includes a role for intracellularly-derived ET-1 as a regulator of cardiac function through intracrine mechanisms that have direct actions on nuclei. At present it is unknown whether other intracellular organelles express ET receptors, but this could be a possibility as various intracellular components, such as mitochondria, also express receptors for a number of biologically active ligands.

CARDIAC EFFECTS OF ET-1

ET-1 exerts a plethora of cardiac effects that can be classified as either physiological or pathophysiological. Much of what we currently know about the cardiac actions of ET-1 stems from studies in which the peptide has been added to cardiac preparations under in vitro conditions or administered in vivo. Results using the latter approach are more difficult to interpret since the cardiac response under in vivo conditions reflects direct effects of the peptide as well as secondary effects due to reflex responses, which are expected to occur following the administration of a vasopressor agent. Moreover, the cardiac effects of ET-1 will also be greatly influenced by its coronary-constricting effect even when using in vitro cardiac preparations such as perfused hearts, which are dependent on coronary artery perfusion. Indeed, a number of studies on the use of nonperfused cardiac tissues such as superfused atrial preparations, isolated myocytes, or perfused hearts have shown a positive inotropic effect of

ETs in general and ET-1 in particular.[57–60] However, these findings are not uniform, as ET-1 has also been shown to exert a direct negative inotropic effect on cardiomyocytes. The reasons for such diverse responses to ET-1 are not well understood but are unlikely to be reflective of species differences, as the negative inotropic effect of ET-1 has been documented in hearts or cardiomyocytes from different animal species.[61–63] It has been suggested that ET-1 exerts different effects on inotropic state in immature (negative inotropism) versus adult (positive inotropism) cardiomyocytes[61] although this needs to be investigated further. At the cellular level such differences in inotropic responses likely reflect the nature of Ca^{2+} responses following ET-1 administration, as discussed below.

MECHANISMS UNDERLYING INOTROPIC RESPONSES

A number of mechanisms have been proposed for the positive inotropic effect of ET-1 seen in most cardiac preparations, although as would be expected virtually all of these involve modulation of intracellular Ca^{2+} homeostasis. Among the most extensively studied is the ability of ET-1 to activate the primary Na^+-H^+ exchanger isoform (NHE-1) expressed in the heart. NHE-1 is the principal regulator of intracellular pH in the cardiac cell and its activation results in proton extrusion and therefore intracellular alkalinisation.[64] In addition, the concomitant influx of Na^+ results in elevations in intracellular Ca^{2+} either by reducing Ca^{2+} efflux via the $3Na^+$-$2Ca^{2+}$ exchanger (NCX) or producing active influx of Ca^{2+} through the reverse-mode activity of the exchanger.[65] Thus, conceptually, activation of NHE-1 could produce a positive inotropic effect either via intracellular alkalinisation thereby increasing myofilament sensitivity to Ca^{2+} or by actively increasing intracellular Ca^{2+} concentrations. It has indeed been recognized for many years that ET-1 sensitizes myofilaments to Ca^{2+}[66] and the ability of ET-1 to stimulate NHE-1 activity thus offers a logical basis for the peptide's positive inotropic effect.[67] As will be discussed later, the ability of ET-1 to activate NHE-1 also likely implicates the peptide in autocrine-paracrine regulation of contractile function as well as in cardiac pathological processes via NHE-1–dependent mechanisms. Thus, NHE-1 appears to play dual roles in response to its activation by ET-1, mediating the inotropic response as well as contributing to cardiomyocyte hypertrophy.

As noted above, in addition to increased myofilament sensitivity to Ca^{2+}, NHE-1–dependent elevations in intracellular Ca^{2+} concentrations likely also contribute to the positive inotropic effect of ET-1 as a result of increasing intracellular Ca^{2+} concentrations due to a Na^+-dependent modulation of Na^+-Ca^{2+} exchange activity, i.e., reducing efflux (normal mode) or producing influx (reverse mode) both of which result in an elevation in intracellular Ca^{2+} concentrations. With respect to ET-1, reverse mode Na^+-Ca^{2+} exchange activity may be the primary mechanism.[68] A number of studies have also shown that ET-1 can elevate intracellular Ca^{2+} through the L-type Ca^{2+} channel. This effect is thought to occur secondarily to the generation of reactive oxygen species (ROSs) including the superoxide anion derived from mitochondria and likely other intracellular sources.[60,69] A potential role for protein kinase C epsilon activation has been proposed since the ability of ET-1 to increase intracellular Ca^{2+} concentrations was absent in cardiomyocytes expressing an inactive dominant negative form of the enzyme.[70] Moreover, the ET-1 induced increased intracellular Ca^{2+} concentrations and resultant arrhythmogenesis and positive inotropic effect was abolished in atria of inositol trisphosphate receptor type 2–deficient mice (IP_3R2, the predominant IP_3R isoform in atrial myocytes), suggesting that a potential mechanism for ET-1 induced inotropy and arrhythmogenesis, at least in atria, may reflect Ca^{2+} release from SR due to IP_3R2 activation.[71] This finding may be of importance in identifying novel strategies for the treatment of atrial fibrillation. While ET-1 also increases expression of L-type Ca^{2+}

channels,[72,73] this response occurs following chronic exposure to ET-1 and is likely of more relevance to the pathological role of ET-1 such as the development of cardiac hypertrophy. In terms of the negative inotropic effect of ET-1, this effect has been attributed to reduced myofilament sensitivity to Ca^{2+} as well as a reduced Ca^{2+} transient possibly reflecting enhanced Ca^{2+}-extrusion from the myocyte via enhanced by NCX activity.[61,63]

PHYSIOLOGICAL AND PATHOPHYSIOLOGICAL ROLES OF CARDIAC-DERIVED ET-1: GENERAL CONCEPTS

While the vast majority of studies have focused on ET-1 as a factor contributing to cardiac pathology, a number of reports have also implicated this peptide as an endogenous mediator of cardiac homeostasis. Thus, the ability to identify locally produced ET-1 within the heart suggests that the peptide is likely of importance in terms of regulation of cardiac function in both health and disease. For example, endocardial endothelial-derived ET-1 may play an important role determining force-frequency relationships in the intact functioning myocardium.[74] Endogenous ET-1 production has also been related to other aspects of cardiac homeostasis including adaptation to exercise,[75] mediating the positive inotropic responses to circulating hormones including angiotensin II[76] as well as the prevention of arrhythmias during cardiac development.[77]

ET-1 AND THE AGING HEART

ET-1 may also regulate the cardiac response to aging although in this regard it is not completely clear whether it exerts a salutary or deleterious effect. It has been reported that ET-1 expression is elevated in the aged rat heart, which suggests that the peptide may play a role in the complex mechanisms underlying dysfunction of the aging heart.[78] However, a further increase in myocardial ET-1 expression was also found in these animals after exercise, suggesting a potential role in physiological adaptation.[78] Studies aimed at addressing the question of the nature of ET-1 involvement in the aging heart have been discordant. For example, in one study it was reported that mice with cardiac-specific deletion of ET-1 show an increase in cardiac susceptibility to aging particularly in terms of a deteriorating left ventricular function, increased incidence of apoptosis, and greatly reduced survival, thus implicating endogenously produced ET-1 as critical for cardiomyocyte survival during aging.[79] Therefore, this study suggests an important role for cardiac-derived ET-1 in terms of maintaining homeostasis. Conversely, it has also been proposed that cardiac ET-1 may contribute to cardiac pathology associated with aging. This was based on a comprehensive study showing that cardiac-specific deletion of the ET_A receptor attenuates aging-related hypertrophy and dysfunction possibly by favorably regulating autophagy.[80] In that study, hearts from aged mice (26–28 months) exhibited extensive myocardial dysfunction associated with hypertrophy as well as increased ROS generation, protein damage, endoplasmic reticulum stress, upregulation of a number of transcriptional factors, and downregulation of Ca^{2+} regulatory proteins as well as other changes, which were all attenuated either by ET_A receptor ablation or pharmacological antagonism whereas an ET_B receptor blocker was without effect.[80] Although the two studies involved deletion of different factors (i.e., ET-1 vs the ET_A receptor) one would assume that relatively identical phenotypes should have been evident. Moreover, evidence from another report using in vitro approaches (cultured fibroblasts), animal models, and one human subject, showed that

ET-1 is upregulated in aged fibroblasts and that this is associated with increased expression of pro-fibrosis signals.[81] In view of the importance of fibrosis to the myocardial remodeling process a potential role of ET-1 seems evident.

ASSOCIATION OF ET-1 WITH CARDIAC DISEASES

There is a large body of evidence implicating endogenous ET-1 in various cardiac pathologies that stem from studies demonstrating an upregulation of the myocardial ET system in disease states as well as direct evidence that ET-1 administration can produce deleterious effects on the heart. For example, elevated left atrial ET-1 levels are associated with increased arrhythmias and a host of other conditions in patients with structural heart disease suggesting that the peptide contributes to the genesis and maintenance of atrial fibrillation.[82] This finding agrees with an animal study referred to above demonstrating a pro-arrhythmogenic influence of ET-1 on atria, which was dependent on the presence of the IP_3R2 receptor.[71] Together, these studies suggest that targeting the ET-1 system either by preventing ET-1 synthesis or blocking ET receptors may be an effective approach in the treatment of atrial fibrillation. Other potentially deleterious roles of endogenous ET-1 have also been demonstrated, including activation of afferent sympathetic nerve fibers during myocardial ischemia[83] and contribution to infarct size expansion in a rat model of obstructive sleep apnea.[18] Moreover, based primarily on pharmacological studies utilizing either selective or nonselective ET receptor antagonists, endogenously-synthesized ET-1 has been implicated in a host of cardiac pathologies including cardiac injury as a consequence of ischemia, reperfusion, and infarction[17,84,85] possibly due to reactive oxygen stress activation.[86] Interestingly, though, the nature of the contribution of endogenous ET-1 to cardiac dysfunction under ischemic and reperfusion injury may be determined by receptor subtype as ET_B receptor antagonism appears to worsen cardiac function under these conditions.[87] Endogenous ET-1 has also been proposed as a potential contributor to cardiac dysfunction in diabetes[88] and indeed it has been shown that ET-1 expression in cardiomyocytes is upregulated under hyperglycemic conditions.[89] Additionally, ET receptor blockade prevents the cardiotoxic properties of the antineoplastic agent doxorubicin thus potentially implicating ET-1 as a mediator of the cardiotoxicity produced by this agent.[90] It would be of interest and potential importance to determine if inhibition of the cardiac ET system can reduce the cardiotoxicity of doxorubicin while maintaining its antineoplastic properties.

ET-1 IN CARDIAC HYPERTROPHY AND HEART FAILURE

Among the most widely studied aspects of ET-1 involvement in cardiovascular disease is its potential role in the development of cardiac hypertrophy and subsequent evolution to heart failure. The hypertrophic process is complex and involves an interplay between a large number of intracellular signaling factors.[91] It should also be noted that endogenous factors contributing to the hypertrophic process do not need to originate solely from the cardiomyocyte, as nonmyocytes such as endothelial cells and fibroblasts also represent a major source of diffusible factors that can contribute to hypertrophy.[12] As such, endogenously derived ET-1 meets the criteria as a potential contributor to the hypertrophic process. Furthermore, from a general perspective the ability of ET-1 to activate NHE-1 and potentially contribute to dysregulation of intracellular ion homeostasis, particularly with respect to elevations in intracellular Ca^{2+} concentrations, strongly supports this concept. Indeed, a number of studies documenting a hypertrophic effect of exogenously administered or endogenously synthesized ET-1 have implicated NHE-1 in this process.[89,92–94] Interestingly, the mechanisms underlying NHE-1 involvement in hypertrophy parallels the above-mentioned mechanisms underlying the role of NHE-1 in inotropy. Essentially, the elevations in intracellular Ca^{2+} concentrations occurring via NHE-1 activation stimulates a number of prohypertrophic pathways. Among these is the phosphatase calcineurin whose activation and the subsequent hypertrophic response appear to be a direct consequence of NHE-1 activation.[95] Calcineurin contributes to the hypertrophic response primarily by dephosphorylating the transcriptional factor nuclear factor of activated T-cells (NFAT) thus permitting its translocation into nuclei.[96] Of relevance to the hypertrophic response particularly with respect to load-induced hypertrophy and cardiac pathology, cardiomyocyte stretch has been shown to upregulate ET-1 expression which can then produce hypertrophy on its own as well as increase levels of other prohypertrophic factors such as the cytokine interleukin-18.[97,98] Moreover, it has been proposed that elevations in intracellular Na^{+} and Ca^{2+} concentrations following stretch of cardiomyocytes is dependent on NHE-1 activation, which, in turn, is dependent on the upregulation of ET-1 following stretch induction, which may be important both in terms of pathology as well as understanding the basis for the initial positive inotropic effect immediately following induction of stretch.[99]

Early activation of the cardiac ET system has been demonstrated in a canine model of tachycardia-induced heart failure,[100] and increased ET-1 production has been demonstrated in patients with chronic heart failure.[101] While the former study suggests an early activation of ET system in heart failure, this may be dependent on the experimental model. For example, in Dahl salt-sensitive hypertensive rats, ET-1 upregulation occurred during decompensated heart failure with no change during the initial compensatory period.[102] Interestingly, in that study angiotensin II upregulation occurred early during compensatory hypertrophy and preceded the increase in ET-1 synthesis. Additional evidence for ET-1 involvement in cardiac hypertrophy and heart failure originates from other studies as well from extensive evidence for a direct hypertrophic effect of the peptide, as already alluded to above with respect to NHE-1 involvement in this process. In addition to a direct hypertrophic effect of ET-1, there is substantial evidence that endogenous ET-1 mediates the hypertrophic response produced by other factors such as leptin,[103] norepinephrine,[104] and mechanical stress.[105]

In terms of mechanisms underlying the hypertrophic effect of ET-1, the potential role of NHE-1 has already been discussed. However, in addition to NHE-1 a large number of other mechanisms have been advanced as potential mediators of the direct hypertrophic effect of ET-1. These include calcineurin signaling,[106] cyclooxygenase-2 (COX-2) activation,[107] the MAPK kinase pathway,[108] inositol trisphosphate-induced Ca^{2+} release resulting in elevations in nuclear Ca^{2+} concentrations,[109] as well as the Ras homolog gene family, member A/Rho-associated, coiled-coil containing protein kinase (RhoA/ROCK pathway).[110] In this regard, it has been suggested that MAP kinase signaling, especially that involving ERK activation, predominates over RhoA/ROCK in terms of early increases in hypertrophy-associated gene expression upregulation following ET-1 administration.[111] The COX-2–dependent hypertrophic effect of ET-1 is of particular interest as these authors provided evidence that upregulation of COX-2 expression was dependent on NFAT translocation to nuclei, a calcineurin-dependent process.[107] Thus, the study suggests an ET-1-calcineurin-COX-2 axis in mediating the hypertrophic effect of ET-1. Moreover, it is possible that activation of this axis is NHE-1–dependent based on the conceptual framework discussed above implicating NHE-1 as a critical initiator of the hypertrophic process. Therefore, it is likely that many of these pathways are interrelated and act in concert to produce a hypertrophic response. Also, despite the identification of multiple pathways mediating the prohypertrophic effect of ET-1, it is possible that some pathways predominate over others as noted above for ERK activation over RhoA/ROCK signaling.[111] Nonetheless, prevention of RhoA activation abolishes the prohypertrophic effect of ET-1 implicating an important role for this pathway.[112,113] Irrespective of the exact pathway

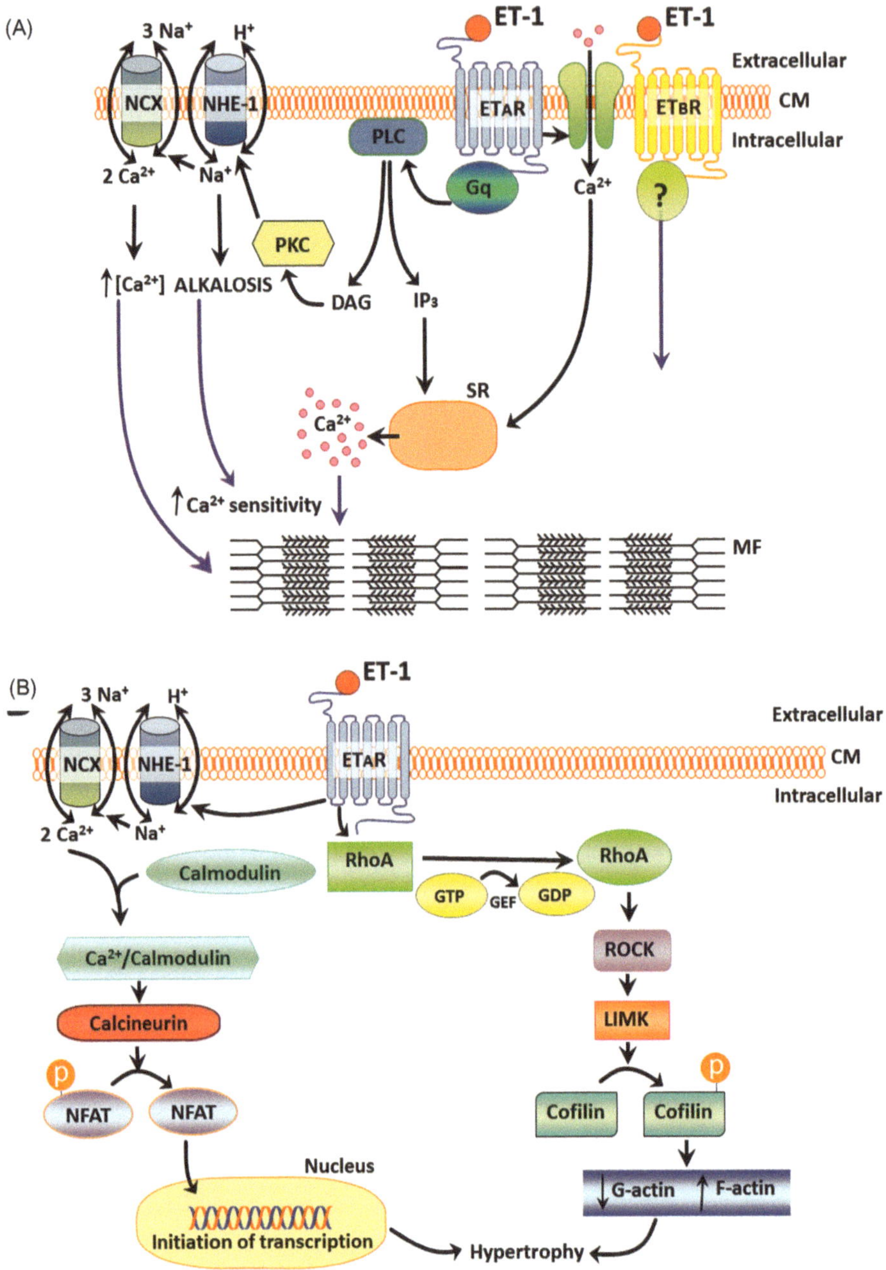

FIGURE 3.4

Cellular mechanisms underlying the inotropic (A) and hypertrophic (B) effects of ET-1 with particular emphasis on the roles of Na^+-H^+ exchange isoform 1 (NHE-1) in these processes. Panel A illustrates how activation of the ET_A (ET_AR) receptor by ET-1 activates NHE-1 activity via a Gq protein-dependent generation of diacylglycerol (DAG) leading to activation of various protein kinase C (PKC) isoforms and subsequent activation of NHE-1. The enhanced mediating the prohypertrophic effect of ET-1 the ability to induce hypertrophy may be dependent on the preservation of high mobility group box 1 (HMGB1) a multifunction nuclear DNA-binding protein whose levels are decreased in hearts of heart failure patients as well as by ET-1 treatment.[114] Interestingly, overexpression of nuclear HMG1 inhibits ET-1 induced cardiomyocyte hypertrophy.[114]

ET-1 also may exert its prohypertrophic effect by stimulating the production of intracellular factors. For example overexpression of vascular endothelial growth factor (VEGF) following ET-1 addition to cardiomyocytes has been proposed in this regard as the hypertrophic response was found to be significantly inhibited but not abolished by VEGF-neutralizing peptides.[115] Likewise, the pro-satiety factor leptin (see chapter: Fat Hormones, Adipokines) also appears to play a critical role in mediating the hypertrophic effect of ET-1 and indeed may be essential for this response since ET-1 induces intracellular leptin synthesis whereas a specific leptin receptor antagonist completely abrogates the prohypertrophic effects of ET-1.[27] A summary of the key ET-1 induced signaling mechanisms involved in cardiomyocyte inotropy and hypertrophy is shown in Fig. 3.4(A) and (B).

Although ET-1 induces hypertrophy on its own through a myriad of potential mechanisms and via mediation by many factors discussed above, there is also substantial evidence of an important role of endogenous ET-1 as a critical mediator of the hypertrophic response to many diverse factors including hyperglycemia,[89] induction of volume overload,[116] and the hypertrophic effect of angiotensin II.[117] ET-1 has also been implicated as an important player in transitioning the heart from compensatory hypertrophy to heart failure.[118] Overexpression of cardiac ET-1 in mice in the absence of other interventions leads to increased expression of pro-inflammatory cytokines and the development of heart failure and death.[119] In contrast, mice with a cardiac-specific deletion of the ET-1 are resistant to hypertrophy associated with hyperthyroidism.[120] Blocking the ET_A receptor in salt-sensitive rats with heart failure exerts a myocardial oxygen-sparing effect, suggesting that endogenously-synthesized ET-1 contributes to the maintenance of contractility at the expense of increased oxygen utilization.[121]

FIGURE 3.4 (Continued)

H^+ extrusion and generation of alkalosis results in sensitization of myofibrils (MF) to Ca^{2+} producing a positive inotropic state. In addition, NHE-1 activation and the resultant increase in intracellular Na^+ concentrations results in increased intracellular Ca^{2+} concentrations either through reducing the extrusion of Ca^{2+} via the $3Na^+$-$2Ca^{2+}$ exchanger (NCX) or by increasing influx of Ca^{2+} through reverse-mode NCX activity. Additional Ca^{2+} availability could occur by directly increasing Ca^{2+} influx through the Ca^{2+} channel in the cell membrane (CM) or by inositol trisphosphate (IP_3)-induced increased Ca^{2+} release from the sarcoplasmic reticulum (SR). Although ET-1 can also activate the ETB receptor (ETBR) in the CM, at present the function of ETBR is less well understood.
Panel B illustrates how the activation of NHE-1 and the NCX-dependent increase in intracellular Ca^{2+} concentrations induces hypertrophic cell signaling processes. The formation of a Ca^{2+}-calmodulin complex activates the phosphatase calcineurin resulting in the dephosphorylation of the transcriptional factor nuclear factor of activated T cells (NFAT) allowing nuclear import and initiation of prohypertrophic transcription. Another mechanism by which ET_AR activation could promote hypertrophy is through the activation of the Ras homolog gene family, member A/Rho-associated, coiled-coil containing protein kinase (RhoA/ROCK) pathway. The initial RhoA activation in this pathway is catalyzed by Rho guanine nucleotide exchange factors (GEF) that catalyze the exchange of GDP for GTP. Activation of ROCK leads to an increase in LIM kinase (LIMK) activity, leading to the phosphorylation and inactivation of the actin binding protein cofilin. Inactivated cofilin alters actin dynamics, demonstrated by a decreased G to F actin ratio, i.e., increased actin polymerization. This actin reorganization also contributes to the hypertrophic process.

ENDOGENOUS MODULATION OF ET-1: KEEPING ET-1 IN CHECK?

While convincing evidence supports the concept of endogenous ET-1 as a contributor to cardiac pathology the overall role of the peptide may be dictated by the presence of endogenous factors that appear to function as inhibitors of ET-1 effects. The presence of these factors may be important in cardiac pathology since reduction in their overall synthesis may exaggerate any potential deleterious effects of ET-1. Among the most recognized of these factors is nitric oxide (NO), an important vasodilator produced by the vascular endothelium but also an important regulator of cardiac function.[122] With respect to the endothelium, it is generally considered that there exists a reciprocal interaction between NO and ET-1, as these factors generally exert opposite effects on cardiovascular responses.[123] Moreover, ET-1 has been shown to stimulate NO production in the vasculature[124] as well as in the heart[125] although with respect to the latter this occurs in nuclei via ET_B receptor activation suggesting a further intracrine role of ET-1 to those discussed previously. Indirect evidence for an interplay between NO and ET-1 was shown in studies demonstrating that removal of endocardial endothelium, a major source of NO production, sensitized the myocardium to the contractile effects of ET-1.[126] Conversely, administering a NO-generating system inhibits many of the toxic effects of ET-1 on either cardiac myocytes or isolated hearts, whereas inotropic effects of the peptide are unaffected.[59] Conversely, administering an inhibitor of NO synthase unmasked cardiotoxic effects of a very low concentration of ET-1 devoid of its own effects.[59] Although NO is commonly considered as a beneficial and cardioprotective factor, there is evidence that concomitant upregulation of ET-1, such as that occurring in the postischemic reperfused heart, attenuates any potential benefit of increased NO synthesis.[127] In terms of cardiomyocyte hypertrophy, NO generation abrogates the hypertrophic effect of ET-1 through a mechanism involving inhibition of RhoA/ROCK signaling.[112]

NO also inhibits the ET system by reducing ET-1 synthesis. Thus, NO generation suppresses the upregulation of ET-1 as well as its receptors in cardiomyocytes following ischemia and reperfusion[128] and directly inhibits ET-1 secretion from endothelial cells via the activation of soluble guanylate cyclase.[129] This inverse relationship between ET-1 and NO has also been documented in humans in which administration of L-arginine, the precursor for NO synthesis, blocked the cardiovascular responses to subsequent ET-1 infusion.[130] While the inhibition of ET-1 induced effects by NO may represent physiological antagonism due to their diametrically opposite effects, there is also evidence that the antagonist effect of NO against ET-1 may involve a direct inhibition of ET-1 receptor binding in both human myocardial and vasculature tissue.[131] Thus, NO could function as an antagonist of the ET receptor, likely of the ET_A subtype.

In addition to NO, other endogenous ET-1 inhibitors may also be expressed in the heart. Among the so-called gasotransmitters such as NO, hydrogen sulfide (H_2S) has attracted substantial attention by virtue of its ability to produce a number of favorable cardiovascular responses such as vasodilation and prevention of myocardial remodeling.[132] H_2S administration was shown to inhibit the hypertrophic effect of ET, although which ET was used in the study was not mentioned.[133] Despite this limitation, it is possible that H_2S, which is produced by the heart,[134] functions as an endogenous inhibitor of ET-1 induced effects although this needs to be explored in further studies.

Another potential endogenous inhibitor of the ET system is the cardiac-derived hormone atrial natriuretic peptide (ANP) (see chapter: Cardiac Natriuretic Peptides). Although first identified as a diuretic/natriuretic and vasodilating hormone, it is now recognized that ANP exerts a plethora of cardiovascular beneficial effects.[135] One of the basis for the cardiovascular effects of ANP may lie in its ability to suppress the ET system as evidenced by its ability to attenuate ET-1 production in vascular endothelial cells.[136] In terms of cardiac pathology, a potentially important benefit of ANP is suppression of fibrosis via ET-1 downregulation in the fibroblast[137] potentially by decreasing activity of the transcriptional factor GATA-4.[29] As such, the cardiac-derived ANP may act as a suppressor of fibrosis by inhibiting ET-1 synthesis in fibroblasts in a paracrine manner. When taken together, these studies as well as those involving H_2S or NO suggest that endogenous anti-ET systems should be considered when assessing the possible role of the ET-1 in the regulation of cardiac function in both health and disease.

POTENTIAL BENEFICIAL EFFECTS OF ET-1 IN CARDIAC FUNCTION

As is evident from the preceding discussion, ET-1 is generally considered as a participant in cardiac pathology. However, this may not be the exclusive role of ET-1 in terms of regulation of heart function, as there is compelling evidence that ET-1 may also be beneficial and indeed necessary for normal cardiac performance. This has been alluded to in a preceding discussion related to aging in which ET-1 was shown to be important for cardiac homeostasis during the aging process. The concept that endogenous ET-1 may represent a cardioprotective factor has previously been reviewed and is based on the fact that ET-1 can initiate a number of pro-survival cell signaling pathways.[138] One of the benefits associated with ET-1 is the inhibition of apoptosis which has been demonstrated in a number of experimental models and with at least three different inducers of apoptosis. For example, apoptosis in cardiomyocytes induced by serum deprivation was inhibited by exogenous ET-1 likely through a tyrosine kinase pathway.[139] Interestingly, the apoptotic effect of ET-1 was not shared by angiotensin II even though both share a similar pharmacological profile and underlying GPCR-dependent cell signaling processes following activation of their respective receptors. Similar effects of ET-1 were observed in cardiomyocytes exposed to hydrogen peroxide where a calcineurin-dependent effect of ET-1 was observed.[140] As discussed, calcineurin is important for the development of hypertrophy by virtue of its ability to enhance the translocation of the transcriptional factor NFAT to the nucleus. The antiapoptotic role of calcineurin may involve the NFAT-dependent increased expression of Bcl2, a protein which inhibits the apoptotic response.[140] Induction of apoptosis by the β-adrenergic agonist isoproterenol (see chapter: Adrenergic Receptors) was also prevented by ET-1 administration.[141] Based on pharmacological interventions this was determined to be an ET_A receptor process involving a number of cell signaling pathways. Potentially related to the antiapoptotic effect of ET-1 is an earlier finding that ET-1 can reduce infarct size in isolated hearts subjected to ischemia and reperfusion through an ET_A receptor-mediated mechanism involving ATP-sensitive potassium channel activation.[142]

Although these studies suggest an antiapoptotic and cardioprotective effect of exogenous ET-1, whether endogenous ET-1 exerts similar salutary effects has not been extensively studied. As noted above, cardiac-specific ET-1 deletion enhances cardiac apoptosis in aging[79] further suggesting an antiapoptotic effect of the peptide. Vascular endothelial cell-specific deletion of ET-1 enhanced hypertrophy and left ventricular dysfunction in mice subjected to aortic coarctation further demonstrating potential benefit of endogenous ET-1 although in this model the degree of apoptosis was unaffected.[143] Using genetically modified mice expressing various levels of the ET-1 gene *Edn1* showed that a modest reduction of the gene by approximately 35% was sufficient to produce dilated cardiomyopathy and cardiac dysfunction associated with increased ventricular superoxide and matrix metalloproteinase expression which were all also associated with increased volume retention and hypertension.[144] Thus, when these studies are considered together they raise the possibility of an important role of endogenous ET-1 in cardiac homeostasis, which may affect the use of ET-1 modulators for cardiovascular therapeutics (see below).

DEVELOPMENT OF CLINICAL STRATEGIES AIMED AT TARGETING ET-1

The complexity of ET-1 and its role in heart disease renders it somewhat difficult to determine whether inhibiting ET-1-mediated effects is conducive to cardiac therapeutics particularly as it appears, based on animal studies, that ET-1 can play an important role in maintaining cardiac homeostasis in addition to participating in cardiac pathology. A number of strategies have been proposed and developed to target the ET system, the most important of which is the development of pharmacological antagonists of ET receptors in general but the ET_A receptor in particular.[145] The first such antagonist developed was bosentan, a nonspecific antagonist with relatively equal efficacy against both the ET_A and ET_B receptor, although with slightly higher affinity for the ET_A receptor subtype, which is currently in clinical use for pulmonary artery hypertension.[146] Indeed, much of the clinical progress vis á vis ET receptor blockers involves pulmonary artery hypertension, an extremely serious condition that carries a dire prognosis and for which there is no cure. The success obtained with bosentan and the superiority of bosentan over previous treatments for pulmonary artery hypertension has led to the development of newer ET receptor antagonists, the so-called "entans" with the hope of identifying better clinical outcomes. Among these antagonists are ambrisentan, which was clinically introduced in 2007 and which exhibits greater selectivity towards the ET_A receptor[147] which was followed by sitaxentan with even greater ET_A selectivity.[148] Macitentan is a more recent addition to the ET receptor antagonist family for the treatment of pulmonary artery hypertension. Although classified as a dual receptor antagonist it exhibits approximately an 800-fold greater selectivity towards the ET_A receptor.[149] Interestingly, macitentan has an additional benefit in that one of its metabolites is also biologically active adding to the efficacy of the parent compound.[150] Many other ET receptor blockers have been developed such as tezosentan, a nonselective ET_A and ET_B receptor antagonist tested in clinical trials for heart failure (see below). The development of novel potent ET receptor antagonists therefore represents an important area of research aimed at targeting the ET system for therapeutics although this has been primarily focused for the treatment of pulmonary artery hypertension. Indeed, in addition to those agents already mentioned many other ET receptor antagonists that differ in potency and selectivity have been developed by pharmaceutical companies.

As alluded to previously, targeting ECE could also serve as a potential therapeutic approach targeting the ET system although this remains primarily a theoretical concept that has not been extensively explored either experimentally or clinically for the treatment of heart disease. Moreover, as big ET-1 also exerts vasoconstricting effects[10] this could potentially negate any benefit of ET-1 inhibition.

CLINICAL EVALUATION OF ET RECEPTOR ANTAGONISTS FOR TREATING HEART DISEASE

There is extensive evidence that the ET system is upregulated in various types of heart diseases in experimental animals but also in patients with coronary heart disease as well as heart failure as exemplified by increased plasma ET-1 concentrations or concentrations of the ET-1 precursor, big ET-1, under various conditions.[43,46,151] Indeed, an elevation in plasma concentrations of the latter appears to be a better predictor of disease severity, at least with respect to heart failure than ET-1.[152,153] Moreover, the expression of the atrial ET_A receptor as well as ECE is markedly upregulated in clinical end stage heart failure whereas the ET_B receptor is decreased,[154,155] an imbalance that may contribute to the myocardial remodeling process particularly since ET_B and ET_A receptors generally tend to exert opposite effects on the cardiovascular system.[156] Interestingly, the increased cardiac ET_A expression can be reversed with a normalization of these receptors following approximately 3 months of treatment with a left ventricular assist device, likely as a consequence of cardiac unloading.[157]

The robust experimental evidence for a deleterious role of the ET system in cardiac pathology, as discussed above, coupled with clear evidence of increased ET-1 production in cardiac disease states, has provided a sound conceptual rationale for assessing the potential benefit of ET receptor blockers for the treatment of heart disease, although this has been applied primarily for the treatment of heart failure in addition to pulmonary artery hypertension. Initial short-term studies using either selective ET_A receptor blockade with the antagonist darusentan[158] or nonselective ET receptor blockade with bosentan or tezosentan[159,160] have shown a benefit in terms of improving hemodynamic properties and cardiac function in patients with heart failure. However, when administered to patients with acute heart failure, tezosentan was ineffective in terms of reducing mortality or the incidence of worsening heart failure.[161] In addition, tezosentan was also ineffective against the development of right ventricular heart failure in patients with pulmonary artery hypertension undergoing cardiac surgery.[162] Moreover large studies using long-term treatment with bosentan, a drug that produces some benefit in patients with pulmonary artery hypertension, have been disappointing because of a failure to demonstrate a benefit particularly in terms of survival. This lack of efficacy was shown in the smaller REACH-1 (Research on Endothelin Antagonism in Chronic Heart Failure) study employing 370 patients as well in the much larger international phase III ENABLE (Endothelin Antagonist Bosentan for Lowering Cardiac Events) trials.[163–165]

POTENTIAL REASONS FOR FAILED CLINICAL TRIALS

The reason for the neutral effects seen with bosentan in chronic heart failure is unknown. One possible explanation is this may be related to the use of a nonselective ET receptor antagonist, particularly since the role of the ET_B receptor in cardiac disease is not well understood. However, a selective ET_A receptor antagonist, darusentan, also failed to exert benefit in New York Heart Association (NYHA) Class 2–4 heart failure patients in the Endothelin-A Receptor Antagonist Trial in Heart Failure (EARTH) study.[166] Thus, it appears that receptor selectivity is not a determinant factor in dictating the efficacy of ET receptor blockers for the treatment of heart failure. Another issue that needs to be considered is the timing of drug administration. In this regard, in both the REACH and ENABLE trials, bosentan was administered to patients with established NYHA Stage 3 or 4 heart failure when cardiac remodeling has occurred to a large degree. It is possible that an earlier start to treatment could provide a better opportunity to blunt the remodeling process and produce a more favorable response. Indeed, it should be noted that in the EARTH study nearly 80% of patients were in NYHA Class 3 heart failure. The question then arises whether including a greater population of patients in Class 2 heart failure would produce better efficacy. Another possible explanation for the absence of clinical efficacy may lie in the observation that ET-1 produces a large amplification of the cardiac hypertrophic response by virtue of the peptide's ability, as previously alluded to, to stimulate norepinephrine release from sympathetic neurons through an ET_A receptor-dependent process.[32–35] It has therefore been suggested that concomitant use of antiadrenergic drugs in patients receiving ET receptor blockers may have precluded any potential additional benefit through ET_A receptor blockade.[35] These authors further proposed that patients with intolerance to beta receptor blockers or those with disturbed sympathetic nerve function may represent a good cohort for determining the potential benefit of ET_A receptor antagonists in heart failure. However, a recent study using sheep with pacing induced heart failure showed that while tezosentan was able to reduce cardiac sympathetic activity in control animals it had no effect on heart failure, thus suggesting that the potential benefit of tezosentan and other ET receptor antagonists, at least with respect to an anti-adrenergic effect, could be precluded in heart failure.[167] Irrespective of the underlying reasons for lack of clinical efficacy for ET receptor antagonists, the results precluded further development of these agents for cardiac therapeutics, and with respect to ET receptor antagonists, these are approved solely for the treatment of pulmonary artery hypertension. A last point needs to be reinforced, which is that endogenous ET-1 may also be beneficial in terms of maintaining cardiac homeostasis and therefore the blocking of receptors through which ET-1 exerts its effects, good or bad, may not always be desirable.

CONCLUDING COMMENTS

There is little doubt that the discovery more than 25 years ago of endothelins and ET-1 specifically was a major accomplishment in terms of furthering our understanding of the complex nature of cardiovascular homeostasis and regulation of cardiovascular function in health and disease. Among the best known effects of ET-1 is its ability to induce vasoconstriction and hence it has been implicated in many cardiovascular diseases based on this property. Although first identified in vascular endothelium, the ability of the heart, and indeed many other organs, to produce ET-1 suggests that this peptide is an important local regulator of cardiac function. Research into cardiac aspects of ET-1 has produced a wealth of information regarding the complexity of cardiac effects of this peptide and has led to the identification of receptors mediating its actions and to the development of pharmacological antagonists of ET receptors for potential cardiac therapeutics. While there has been success with ET receptor antagonists for the treatment of pulmonary artery hypertension, virtually no benefit has been found with other life-threatening conditions such as heart failure, especially in terms of survival. Improvement in therapeutic efficacy may depend on the discovery of more potent and selective ET receptor antagonists or on the development of alternate strategies to modify ET-1 function. On the other hand, it is also very possible that ablation of ET-1-mediated effects on the heart may not be entirely desirable in view of the documented beneficial role of this peptide on cardiac homeostasis. Only with continued research on this fascinating peptide can we hope to resolve this dilemma and gain greater insights into the precise role of ET-1, especially that produced with the heart, to cardiac health and disease.

ACKNOWLEDGEMENTS

Work cited from the author's laboratory has been supported by grants from the Canadian Institutes of Health Research and The Heart and Stroke Foundation of Ontario. The author holds a Canada Research Chair in Experimental Cardiology. Illustrations produced by Tracey Gan, Borna Mahmoudian and Catherine Wu and critical reading of the manuscript by Dr. Michael A Cook are gratefully acknowledged.

REFERENCES

1. Yanagisawa M, Kurihara H, Kimura S, Tomobe Y, Kobayashi M, Mitsui Y, et al. A novel potent vasoconstrictor peptide produced by vascular endothelial cells. *Nature* 1988;**332**:411–5.
2. Nasser SA, El-Mas MM. Endothelin ETA receptor antagonism in cardiovascular disease. *Eur J Pharmacol* 2014;**737**:210–3.
3. Maguire JJ, Davenport AP. Endothelin@25-new agonists, antagonists, inhibitors and emerging research frontiers: IUPHAR Review 12. *Br J Pharmacol* 2014;**171**:5555–72.
4. Inoue A, Yanagisawa M, Kimura S, Kasuya Y, Miyauchi T, Goto K, et al. The human endothelin family: three structurally and pharmacologically distinct isopeptides predicted by three separate genes. *Proc Natl Acad Sci USA* 1989;**86**:2863–7.
5. Drawnel FM, Archer CR, Roderick HL. The role of the paracrine/autocrine mediator endothelin-1 in regulation of cardiac contractility and growth. *Br J Pharmacol* 2013;**168**:296–317.
6. Ling L, Maguire JJ, Davenport AP. Endothelin-2, the forgotten isoform: emerging role in the cardiovascular system, ovarian development, immunology and cancer. *Br J Pharmacol* 2013;**168**:283–95.
7. Russell FD, Molenaar P. The human heart endothelin system: ET-1 synthesis, storage, release and effect. *Trends Pharmacol Sci* 2000;**21**:353–9.
8. Barton M, Yanagisawa M. Endothelin: 20 years from discovery to therapy. *Can J Physiol Pharmacol* 2008;**86**:485–98.
9. Turner AJ, Murphy LJ. Molecular pharmacology of endothelin converting enzymes. *Biochem Pharmacol* 1996;**26**:91–102.
10. Pernow J, Kaijser L, Lundberg JM, Ahlborg G. Comparable potent coronary constrictor effects of endothelin-1 and big endothelin-1 in humans. *Circulation* 1996;**94**:2077–82.
11. D'Orleans-Juste P, Houde M, Rae GA, Bkaily G, Carrier E, Simard E. Endothelin-1 (1–31): from chymase-dependent synthesis to cardiovascular pathologies. *Vascul Pharmacol* 2008;**49**:51–62.
12. Kamo T, Akazawa H, Komuro I. Cardiac nonmyocytes in the hub of cardiac hypertrophy. *Circ Res* 2015;**117**:89–98.
13. Suzuki T, Kumazaki T, Mitsui Y. Endothelin-1 is produced and secreted by neonatal rat cardiac myocytes in vitro. *Biochem Biophys Res Commun* 1993;**191**:823–30.
14. Kagamu H, Suzuki T, Arakawa M, Mitsui Y. Low oxygen enhances endothelin-1 (ET-1) production and responsiveness to ET-1 in cultured cardiac myocytes. *Biochem Biophys Res Commun* 1994;**202**:1612–8.
15. Yuhki KI, Miyauchi T, Kakinuma Y, Murakoshi N, Maeda S, Goto K, et al. Endothelin-1 production is enhanced by rotenone, a mitochondrial complex I inhibitor, in cultured rat cardiomyocytes. *J Cardiovasc Pharmacol* 2001;**38**:850–8.
16. Vágó H, Soós P, Zima E, Gellér L, Keltai K, Róka A, et al. Changes of endothelin-1 and big endothelin-1 levels and action potential duration during myocardial ischemia-reperfusion in dogs with and without ventricular fibrillation. *J Cardiovasc Pharmacol* 2004;**44**(Suppl. 1):S376–9.
17. Tamareille S, Terwelp M, Amirian J, Felli P, Zhang XQ, Barry WH, et al. Endothelin-1 release during the early phase of reperfusion is a mediator of myocardial reperfusion injury. *Cardiology* 2013;**125**:242–9.
18. Belaidi E, Joyeux-Faure M, Ribuot C, Launois SH, Levy P, Godin-Ribuot D. Major role for hypoxia inducible factor-1 and the endothelin system in promoting myocardial infarction and hypertension in an animal model of obstructive sleep apnea. *J Am Coll Cardiol* 2009;**53**:1309–17.
19. Yamashita K, Discher DJ, Hu J, Bishopric NH, Webster KA. Molecular regulation of the endothelin-1 gene by hypoxia. Contributions of hypoxia-inducible factor-1, activator protein-1, GATA-2, AND p300/CBP. *J Biol Chem* 2001;**276**:12645–53.
20. Kakinuma Y, Miyauchi T, Yuki K, Murakoshi N, Goto K, Yamaguchi I. Novel molecular mechanism of increased myocardial endothelin-1 expression in the failing heart involving the transcriptional factor hypoxia-inducible factor-1alpha induced for impaired myocardial energy metabolism. *Circulation* 2001;**103**:2387–94.

21. Naruse M, Tanabe A, Hara Y, Takagi S, Imaki T, Takano K. Effects of AT1 receptor antagonist and spironolactone on cardiac expression of ET-1 mRNA in SHR-SP/Izm. *J Cardiovasc Pharmacol* 2004;**44**(Suppl. 1): S1–S3.
22. Seki Y, Jesmin S, Shimojo N, Islam MM, Rahman MA, Khatun T, et al. Significant reversal of cardiac upregulated endothelin-1 system in a rat model of sepsis by landiolol hydrochloride. *Life Sci* 2014;**118**:357–63.
23. Nagendran J, Sutendra G, Paterson I, Champion HC, Webster L, Chiu B, et al. Endothelin axis is upregulated in human and rat right ventricular hypertrophy. *Circ Res* 2013;**112**:347–54. Erratum in: *Circ Res* 2014;**114**:e32.
24. Adiarto S, Emoto N, Iwasa N, Yokoyama M. Obesity-induced upregulation of myocardial endothelin-1 expression is mediated by leptin. *Biochem Biophys Res Commun* 2007;**353**:623–7.
25. Zhang Y, Proenca R, Maffei M, Barone M, Leopold L, Friedman JM. Positional cloning of the mouse obese gene and its human homologue. *Nature* 1994;**372**:425–32.
26. Purdham DM, Zou MX, Rajapurohitam V, Karmazyn M. Rat heart is a site of leptin production and action. *Am J Physiol Heart Circ Physiol* 2004;**287**:H2877–84.
27. Rajapurohitam V, Javadov S, Purdham DM, Kirshenbaum LA, Karmazyn M. An autocrine role for leptin in mediating the cardiomyocyte hypertrophic effects of angiotensin II and endothelin-1. *J Mol Cell Cardiol* 2006;**41**:265–74.
28. Na T, Dai DZ, Tang XY, Dai Y. Upregulation of leptin pathway correlates with abnormal expression of SERCA2a, phospholamban and the endothelin pathway in heart failure and reversal by CPU86017. *Naunyn Schmiedebergs Arch Pharmacol* 2007;**375**:39–49.
29. Glenn DJ, Rahmutula D, Nishimoto M, Liang F, Gardner DG. Atrial natriuretic peptide suppresses endothelin gene expression and proliferation in cardiac fibroblasts through a GATA4-dependent mechanism. *Cardiovasc Res* 2009;**84**:209–17.
30. Abdel-Samad D, Jacques D, Perreault C, Provost C. NPY regulates human endocardial endothelial cell function. *Peptides* 2007;**28**:281–7.
31. Kuruvilla L, Nair RR, Umashankar PR, Lal AV, Kartha CC. Endocardial endothelial cells stimulate proliferation and collagen synthesis of cardiac fibroblasts. *Cell Biochem Biophys* 2007;**47**:65–72.
32. Isaka M, Kudo A, Imamura M, Kawakami H, Yasuda K. Endothelin receptors, localized in sympathetic nerve terminals of the heart, modulate norepinephrine release and reperfusion arrhythmias. *Basic Res Cardiol* 2007;**102**:154–62.
33. Gottlieb SS, Harris K, Todd J, Estis J, Christenson RH, Torres V, et al. Endothelin receptors, localized in sympathetic nerve terminals of the heart, modulate norepinephrine release and reperfusion arrhythmias. *Basic Res Cardiol* 2007;**102**:154–62.
34. Lehmann LH, Stanmore DA, Backs J. The role of endothelin-1 in the sympathetic nervous system in the heart. *Life Sci* 2014;**118**(2):165–72.
35. Lehmann LH, Rostosky JS, Buss SJ, Kreusser MM, Krebs J, Mier W, et al. Essential role of sympathetic endothelin A receptors for adverse cardiac remodeling. *Proc Natl Acad Sci USA* 2014;**111**:13499–504.
36. Zolk O, Quattek J, Sitzler G, Schrader T, Nickenig G, Schnabel P, et al. Expression of endothelin-1, endothelin-converting enzyme, and endothelin receptors in chronic heart failure. *Circulation* 1999;**99**:2118–23.
37. Hocher B, George I, Rebstock J, Bauch A, Schwarz A, Neumayer HH, et al. Endothelin system-dependent cardiac remodeling in renovascular hypertension. *Hypertension* 1999;**33**:816–22.
38. Freixa X, Masotti M, Palomo M, Diaz-Ricart M, Escolar G, Guasch E, et al. Endothelin-1 levels predict endothelial progenitor cell mobilization after acute myocardial infarction. *Microvasc Res* 2011;**82**:177–81.
39. Niccoli G, Lanza GA, Shaw S, et al. Endothelin-1 and acute myocardial infarction: a no-reflow mediator after successful percutaneous myocardial revascularization. *Eur Heart J* 2006;**27**:1793–8.
40. Yip HK, Wu CJ, Chang HW, et al. Prognostic value of circulating levels of endothelin-1 in patients after acute myocardial infarction undergoing primary coronary angioplasty. *Chest* 2005;**127**:1491–7.

41. Eitel I, Nowak M, Stehl C, Adams V, Fuernau G, Hildebrand L, et al. Endothelin-1 release in acute myocardial infarction as a predictor of long-term prognosis and no-reflow assessed by contrast-enhanced magnetic resonance imaging. *Am Heart J* 2010;**159**:882–90.
42. Yin WH, Chen YH, Wei J, Jen HL, Huang WP, Young MS, et al. Associations between endothelin-1 and adiponectin in chronic heart failure. *Cardiology* 2011;**118**:207–16.
43 Kinugawa T, Kato M, Ogino K, Osaki S, Igawa O, Hisatome I, et al. Plasma endothelin-1 levels and clinical correlates in patients with chronic heart failure. *J Card Fail* 2003;**9**:318–24.
44. Gombos T, Förhécz Z, Pozsonyi Z, Wallentin S, Papassotiriou J, Kunde J, et al. Adrenomedullin and endothelin-1 are related to inflammation in chronic heart failure. *Inflamm Res* 2009;**58**:298–305.
45. von Lueder TG, Kjekshus H, Edvardsen T, ØIe E, Urheim S, Vinge LE, et al. Mechanisms of elevated plasma endothelin-1 in CHF: congestion increases pulmonary synthesis and secretion of endothelin-1. *Cardiovasc Res* 2004;**63**:41–50.
46. Taylor AJ, Bobik A, Richards M, Kaye D, Raines G, Gould P, et al. Myocardial endothelin-1 release and indices of inflammation during angioplasty for acute myocardial infarction and stable coronary artery disease. *Am Heart J* 2004;**148**:341–7.
47. Kohan DE, Rossi NF, Inscho EW, Pollock DM. Regulation of blood pressure and salt homeostasis by endothelin. *Physiol Rev* 2011;**91**:1–77.
48. Bax WA, Bruinvels AT, van Suylen RJ, Saxena PR, Hoyer D. Endothelin receptors in the human coronary artery, ventricle and atrium. A quantitative autoradiographic analysis. *Naunyn Schmiedebergs Arch Pharmacol* 1993;**348**:403–10.
49. Molenaar P, O'Reilly G, Sharkey A, Kuc RE, Harding DP, Plumpton C, et al. Characterization and localization of endothelin receptor subtypes in the human atrioventricular conducting system and myocardium. *Circ Res* 1993;**72**:526–38.
50. Godfraind T. Evidence for heterogeneity of endothelin receptor distribution in human coronary artery. *Br J Pharmacol* 1993;**110**:1201–5.
51. Oikonomidis DL, Tsalikakis DG, Baltogiannis GG, Tzallas AT, Xourgia X, Agelaki MG, et al. Endothelin-B receptors and ventricular arrhythmogenesis in the rat model of acute myocardial infarction. *Basic Res Cardiol* 2010;**105**:235–45.
52. Kolettis TM, Oikonomidis DL, Baibaki ME, Barka E, Kontonika M, Tsalikakis DG, et al. Endothelin B-receptors and sympathetic activation: impact on ventricular arrhythmogenesis during acute myocardial infarction. *Life Sci* 2014;**118**:281–7.
53. Del Ry S, Maltinti M, Giannessi D, Cavallini G, Bergamini E. Age-related changes in endothelin-1 receptor subtypes in rat heart. *Exp Aging Res* 2008;**34**:251–66.
54. Bkaily G, Al-Khoury J, Jacques D. Nuclear membranes GPCRs: implication in cardiovascular health and diseases. *Curr Vasc Pharmacol* 2014;**12**:215–22.
55. Merlen C, Farhat N, Luo X, Chatenet D, Tadevosyan A, Villeneuve LR, et al. Intracrine endothelin signaling evokes IP3-dependent increases in nucleoplasmic Ca^{2+} in adult cardiac myocytes. *J Mol Cell Cardiol* 2013;**62**:189–202.
56. Jules F, Avedanian L, Al-Khoury J, Keita R, Normand A, Bkaily G, et al. Nuclear membranes ETB receptors mediate ET-1-induced increase of nuclear calcium in human left ventricular endocardial endothelial cells. *J Cardiovasc Pharmacol* 2015;**66**:50–7.
57. Ishikawa T, Yanagisawa M, Kimura S, Goto K, Masaki T. Positive inotropic action of novel vasoconstrictor peptide endothelin on guinea pig atria. *Am J Physiol* 1988;**255**:H970–3.
58. Krämer BK, Smith TW, Kelly RA. Endothelin and increased contractility in adult rat ventricular myocytes. Role of intracellular alkalosis induced by activation of the protein kinase C-dependent Na+ -H+ exchanger. *Circ Res* 1991;**68**:269–79.

59. Ebihara Y, Haist JV, Karmazyn M. Modulation of endothelin-1 effects on rat hearts and cardiomyocytes by nitric oxide and 8-bromo cyclic GMP. *J Mol Cell Cardiol* 1996;**28**:265–77.
60. De Giusti VC, Correa MV, Villa-Abrille MC, Beltrano C, Yeves AM, de Cingolani GE, et al. The positive inotropic effect of endothelin-1 is mediated by mitochondrial reactive oxygen species. *Life Sci* 2008;**83**:264–71.
61. Kohmoto O, Ikenouchi H, Hirata Y, Momomura S, Serizawa T, Barry WH. Variable effects of endothelin-1 on [Ca2+]i transients, pHi, and contraction in ventricular myocytes. *Am J Physiol* 1993;**265**:H793–800.
62. James AF. Negative inotropic effects of endothelin-1 in mouse cardiomyocytes: evidence of a role for Na+ -Ca2+ exchange. *Br J Pharmacol* 2007;**152**:417–9.
63. Nishimaru K, Miura Y, Endoh M. Mechanisms of endothelin-1-induced decrease in contractility in adult mouse ventricular myocytes. *Br J Pharmacol* 2007;**152**:456–63.
64. Karmazyn M, Gan XT, Humphreys RA, Yoshida H, Kusumoto K. The myocardial Na+ -H+ exchange: structure, regulation, and its role in heart disease. *Circ Res* 1999;**85**:777–86.
65. Vaughan-Jones RD, Spitzer KW, Swietach P. Intracellular pH regulation in heart. *J Mol Cell Cardiol* 2009;**46**:318–31.
66. Wang JX, Paik G, Morgan JP. Endothelin 1 enhances myofilament Ca2+ responsiveness in aequorin-loaded ferret myocardium. *Circ Res* 1991;**69**:582–9.
67. Khandoudi N, Ho J, Karmazyn M. Role of Na+ -H+ exchange in mediating effects of endothelin-1 on normal and ischemic/reperfused hearts. *Circ Res* 1994;**75**:369–78.
68. Aiello EA, Villa-Abrille MC, Dulce RA, Cingolani HE, Pérez NG. Endothelin-1 stimulates the Na+ /Ca2+ exchanger reverse mode through intracellular Na+ (Na+ i)-dependent and Na+ i-independent pathways. *Hypertension* 2005;**45**:288–93.
69. Zeng Q, Zhou Q, Yao F, O'Rourke ST, Sun C. Endothelin-1 regulates cardiac L-type calcium channels via NAD(P)H oxidase-derived superoxide. *J Pharmacol Exp Ther* 2008;**326**:732–8.
70. Kang M, Chung KY. PKC-ε mediates multiple endothelin-1 actions on systolic Ca2+ and contractility in ventricular myocytes. *Biochem Biophys Res Commun* 2012;**423**:600–5.
71. Li X, Zima AV, Sheikh F, Blatter LA, Chen J. Endothelin-1-induced arrhythmogenic Ca2+ signaling is abolished in atrial myocytes of inositol-1,4,5-trisphosphate(IP3)-receptor type 2-deficient mice. *Circ Res* 2005;**96**:1274–81.
72. Yu L, Li M, She T, Shi C, Meng W, Wang B, et al. Endothelin-1 stimulates the expression of L-type Ca2+ channels in neonatal rat cardiomyocytes via the extracellular signal-regulated kinase 1/2 pathway. *J Membr Biol* 2013;**246**:343–53.
73. Puglisi JL, Yuan W, Timofeyev V, Myers RE, Chiamvimonvat N, Samarel AM, et al. Phorbol ester and endothelin-1 alter functional expression of Na+ /Ca2+ exchange, K+ , and Ca2+ currents in cultured neonatal rat myocytes. *Am J Physiol Heart Circ Physiol* 2011;**300**:H617–26.
74. Shen X, Tan Z, Zhong X, Tian Y, Wang X, Yu B, et al. Endocardial endothelium is a key determinant of force-frequency relationship in rat ventricular myocardium. *J Appl Physiol* 2013;**115**:383–93.
75. Iemitsu M, Maeda S, Otsuki T, Goto K, Miyauchi T. Time course alterations of myocardial endothelin-1 production during the formation of exercise training-induced cardiac hypertrophy. *Exp Biol Med (Maywood)* 2006;**231**:871–5.
76. Cingolani HE, Villa-Abrille MC, Cornelli M, Nolly A, Ennis IL, Garciarena C, et al. The positive inotropic effect of angiotensin II: role of endothelin-1 and reactive oxygen species. *Hypertension* 2006;**47**:727–34.
77. Karppinen S, Rapila R, Mäkikallio K, Hänninen SL, Rysä J, Vuolteenaho O, et al. Endothelin-1 signalling controls early embryonic heart rate in vitro and in vivo. *Acta Physiol (Oxf)* 2014;**210**:369–80.
78. Iemitsu M, Miyauchi T, Maeda S, Tanabe T, Irukayama-Tomobe Y, Goto K, et al. Effects of aging and subsequent exercise training on gene expression of endothelin-1 in rat heart. *Clin Sci (Lond)* 2002;**103**(Suppl. 48): 152S–7S.

79. Zhao XS, Pan W, Bekeredjian R, Shohet RV. Endogenous endothelin-1 is required for cardiomyocyte survival in vivo. *Circulation* 2006;**114**:830–7.
80. Ceylan-Isik AF, Dong M, Zhang Y, Dong F, Turdi S, Nair S, et al. Cardiomyocyte-specific deletion of endothelin receptor A rescues aging-associated cardiac hypertrophy and contractile dysfunction: role of autophagy. *Basic Res Cardiol* 2013;**108**:335.
81. Wang X, Guo Z, Ding Z, Khaidakov M, Lin J, Xu Z, et al. Endothelin-1 upregulation mediates aging-related cardiac fibrosis. *J Mol Cell Cardiol.* 2015;**80**:101–9.
82. Mayyas F, Niebauer M, Zurick A, Barnard J, Gillinov AM, Chung MK, et al. Association of left atrial endothelin-1 with atrial rhythm, size, and fibrosis in patients with structural heart disease. *Circ Arrhythm Electrophysiol* 2010;**3**:369–79.
83. Fu LW, Guo ZL, Longhurst JC. Endogenous endothelin stimulates cardiac sympathetic afferents during ischaemia. *J Physiol* 2010;**588**:2473–86.
84. Gonon AT, Bulhak A, Bröijersén A, Pernow J. Cardioprotective effect of an endothelin receptor antagonist during ischaemia/reperfusion in the severely atherosclerotic mouse heart. *Br J Pharmacol* 2005; **144**:860–6.
85. Lee TM, Chen CC, Lin MS, Chang NC. Effect of endothelin receptor antagonists on ventricular susceptibility in postinfarcted rats. *Am J Physiol Heart Circ Physiol* 2008;**294**:H1871–9.
86. Duda M, Konior A, Klemenska E, Beresewicz A. Preconditioning protects endothelium by preventing ET-1-induced activation of NADPH oxidase and xanthine oxidase in post-ischemic heart. *J Mol Cell Cardiol* 2007;**42**:400–10.
87. Yamamoto S, Matsumoto N, Kanazawa M, Fujita M, Takaoka M, Gariepy CE, et al. Different contributions of endothelin-A and endothelin-B receptors in postischemic cardiac dysfunction and norepinephrine overflow in rat hearts. *Circulation* 2005;**111**:302–9.
88. Ding Y, Zou R, Judd RL, Zhong J. Endothelin-1 receptor blockade prevented the electrophysiological dysfunction in cardiac myocytes of streptozotocin-induced diabetic rats. *Endocrine* 2006;**30**:121–7.
89. Chen S, Khan ZA, Karmazyn M, Chakrabarti S. Role of endothelin-1, sodium hydrogen exchanger-1 and mitogen activated protein kinase (MAPK) activation in glucose-induced cardiomyocyte hypertrophy. *Diabetes Metab Res Rev* 2007;**23**:356–67.
90. Schwebe M, Ameling S, Hammer E, Monzel JV, Bonitz K, Budde S, et al. Protective effects of endothelin receptor A and B inhibitors against doxorubicin-induced cardiomyopathy. *Biochem Pharmacol* 2015;**94**:109–29.
91. Tham YK, Bernardo BC, Ooi JY, Weeks KL, McMullen JR. Pathophysiology of cardiac hypertrophy and heart failure: signaling pathways and novel therapeutic targets. *Arch Toxicol* 2015;**89**:1401–38.
92. Javadov S, Rajapurohitam V, Kilić A, Zeidan A, Choi A, Karmazyn M. Anti-hypertrophic effect of NHE-1 inhibition involves GSK-3beta-dependent attenuation of mitochondrial dysfunction. *J Mol Cell Cardiol* 2009;**46**:998–1007.
93. Kilic A, Rajapurohitam V, Sandberg SM, Zeidan A, Hunter JC, Said Faruq N, et al. A novel chimeric natriuretic peptide reduces cardiomyocyte hypertrophy through the NHE-1-calcineurin pathway. *Cardiovasc Res* 2010;**88**:434–42.
94. Dulce RA, Hurtado C, Ennis IL, Garciarena CD, Alvarez MC, Caldiz C, et al. Endothelin-1 induced hypertrophic effect in neonatal rat cardiomyocytes: involvement of Na+ /H+ and Na+ /Ca2+ exchangers. *J Mol Cell Cardiol* 2006;**41**:807–15.
95. Nakamura TY, Iwata Y, Arai Y, Komamura K, Wakabayashi S. Activation of Na+ /H+ exchanger 1 is sufficient to generate Ca2+ signals that induce cardiac hypertrophy and heart failure. *Circ Res* 2008;**103**:891–9.
96. Heineke J, Ritter O. Cardiomyocyte calcineurin signaling in subcellular domains: from the sarcolemma to the nucleus and beyond. *J Mol Cell Cardiol* 2012;**52**:62–73.

97. Pikkarainen S, Tokola H, Kerkelä R, Ilves M, Mäkinen M, Orzechowski HD, et al. Inverse regulation of preproendothelin-1 and endothelin-converting enzyme-1beta genes in cardiac cells by mechanical load. *Am J Physiol Regul Integr Comp Physiol* 2006;**290**:R1639–45.
98. Naka T, Sakoda T, Doi T, Akagami T, Tsujino T, Masuyama T, et al. Mechanical stretch induced interleukin-18 (IL-18) expression through Angiotensin subtype 1 receptor (AT1R) and endothelin-1 in cardiomyocytes. *Prep Biochem Biotechnol* 2008;**38**:201–12.
99. Cingolani HE, Pérez NG, Pieske B, von Lewinski D, Camilión de Hurtado MC. Stretch-elicited Na+/H+ exchanger activation: the autocrine/paracrine loop and its mechanical counterpart. *Cardiovasc Res* 2003;**57**:953–60.
100. Motte S, van Beneden R, Mottet J, Rondelet B, Mathieu M, Havaux X, et al. Early activation of cardiac and renal endothelin systems in experimental heart failure. *Am J Physiol Heart Circ Physiol* 2003;**285**:H2482–91.
101. Parker JD, Thiessen JJ. Increased endothelin-1 production in patients with chronic heart failure. *Am J Physiol Heart Circ Physiol* 2004;**286**:H1141–5.
102. Iwanaga Y, Kihara Y, Inagaki K, Onozawa Y, Yoneda T, Kataoka K, et al. Differential effects of angiotensin II versus endothelin-1 inhibitions in hypertrophic left ventricular myocardium during transition to heart failure. *Circulation* 2001;**104**:606–12.
103. Xu FP, Chen MS, Wang YZ, Yi Q, Lin SB, Chen AF, et al. Leptin induces hypertrophy via endothelin-1-reactive oxygen species pathway in cultured neonatal rat cardiomyocytes. *Circulation* 2004;**110**:1269–75.
104. Kaddoura S, Firth JD, Boheler KR, Sugden PH, Poole-Wilson PA. Endothelin-1 is involved in norepinephrine-induced ventricular hypertrophy in vivo. Acute effects of bosentan, an orally active, mixed endothelin ETA and ETB receptor antagonist. *Circulation* 1996;**93**:2068–79.
105. Yamazaki T, Komuro I, Kudoh S, Zou Y, Shiojima I, Hiroi Y, et al. Endothelin-1 is involved in mechanical stress-induced cardiomyocyte hypertrophy. *J Biol Chem* 1996;**271**:3221–8.
106. Tongers J, Fiedler B, König D, Kempf T, Klein G, Heineke J, et al. Heme oxygenase-1 inhibition of MAP kinases, calcineurin/NFAT signaling, and hypertrophy in cardiac myocytes. *Cardiovasc Res* 2004;**63**:545–52.
107. Li H, Gao S, Ye J, Feng X, Cai Y, Liu Z, et al. COX-2 is involved in ET-1-induced hypertrophy of neonatal rat cardiomyocytes: role of NFATc3. *Mol Cell Endocrinol* 2014;**382**:998–1006.
108. Bupha-Intr T, Haizlip KM, Janssen PM. Role of endothelin in the induction of cardiac hypertrophy in vitro. *PLoS One* 2012;**7**:e43179.
109. Higazi DR, Fearnley CJ, Drawnel FM, Talasila A, Corps EM, Ritter O, et al. Endothelin-1-stimulated InsP3-induced Ca2+ release is a nexus for hypertrophic signaling in cardiac myocytes. *Mol Cell* 2009;**33**:472–82.
110. Kuwahara K, Saito Y, Nakagawa O, Kishimoto I, Harada M, Ogawa E, et al. The effects of the selective ROCK inhibitor, Y27632, on ET-1-induced hypertrophic response in neonatal rat cardiac myocytes—possible involvement of Rho/ROCK pathway in cardiac muscle cell hypertrophy. *FEBS Lett* 1999;**452**:314–8.
111. Marshall AK, Barrett OP, Cullingford TE, Shanmugasundram A, Sugden PH, Clerk A. ERK1/2 signaling dominates over RhoA signaling in regulating early changes in RNA expression induced by endothelin-1 in neonatal rat cardiomyocytes. *PLoS One* 2010;**5**:e10027.
112. Hunter JC, Zeidan A, Javadov S, Kilić A, Rajapurohitam V, Karmazyn M. Nitric oxide inhibits endothelin-1-induced neonatal cardiomyocyte hypertrophy via a RhoA-ROCK-dependent pathway. *J Mol Cell Cardiol* 2009;**47**:810–8.
113. Zeidan A, Gan XT, Thomas A, Karmazyn M. Prevention of RhoA activation and cofilin-mediated actin polymerization mediates the antihypertrophic effect of adenosine receptor agonists in angiotensin II- and endothelin-1-treated cardiomyocytes. *Mol Cell Biochem* 2014;**385**:239–48.
114. Funayama A, Shishido T, Netsu S, Narumi T, Kadowaki S, Takahashi H, et al. Cardiac nuclear high mobility group box 1 prevents the development of cardiac hypertrophy and heart failure. *Cardiovasc Res* 2013;**99**:657–64.
115. Shimojo N, Jesmin S, Zaedi S, Otsuki T, Maeda S, Yamaguchi N, et al. Contributory role of VEGF overexpression in endothelin-1-induced cardiomyocyte hypertrophy. *Am J Physiol Heart Circ Physiol* 2007;**293**(1):H474–81. Epub 2007 Mar 16.

116. Murray DB, McMillan R, Brower GL, Janicki JS. ETA selective receptor antagonism prevents ventricular remodeling in volume-overloaded rats. *Am J Physiol Heart Circ Physiol* 2009;**297**:H109–16.
117. Correa MV, Nolly MB, Caldiz CI, de Cingolani GE, Cingolani HE, Ennis IL. Endogenous endothelin 1 mediates angiotensin II-induced hypertrophy in electrically paced cardiac myocytes through EGFR transactivation, reactive oxygen species and NHE-1. *Pflugers Arch* 2014;**466**:1819–30.
118. Iwanaga Y, Kihara Y, Hasegawa K, Inagaki K, Yoneda T, Kaburagi S, et al. Cardiac endothelin-1 plays a critical role in the functional deterioration of left ventricles during the transition from compensatory hypertrophy to congestive heart failure in salt-sensitive hypertensive rats. *Circulation* 1998;**98**: 2065–73.
119. Yang LL, Gros R, Kabir MG, Sadi A, Gotlieb AI, Husain M, et al. Conditional cardiac overexpression of endothelin-1 induces inflammation and dilated cardiomyopathy in mice. *Circulation* 2004;**109**:255–61.
120. Shohet RV, Kisanuki YY, Zhao XS, Siddiquee Z, Franco F, Yanagisawa M. Mice with cardiomyocyte-specific disruption of the endothelin-1 gene are resistant to hyperthyroid cardiac hypertrophy. *Proc Natl Acad Sci USA* 2004;**101**:2088–93.
121. Noguchi T, Chen Z, Bell SP, Nyland L, LeWinter MM. Endothelin receptor blockade has an oxygen-saving effect in Dahl salt-sensitive rats with heart failure. *Am J Physiol Heart Circ Physiol* 2003;**285**:H1428–34.
122. Massion PB, Feron O, Dessy C, Balligand JL. Nitric oxide and cardiac function: ten years after, and continuing. *Circ Res* 2003;**93**:388–98.
123. Alonso D, Radomski MW. The nitric oxide-endothelin connection. *Heart Fail Rev* 2003;**8**:107–15.
124. Warner TD, Mitchell JA, de Nucci G, Vane JR. Endothelin-1 and endothelin-3 release EDRF from isolated perfused arterial vessels of the rat and rabbit. *J Cardiovasc Pharmacol* 1989;**13**(Suppl. 5):S85–8.
125. Vaniotis G, Glazkova I, Merlen C, Smith C, Villeneuve LR, Chatenet D, et al. Regulation of cardiac nitric oxide signaling by nuclear β-adrenergic and endothelin receptors. *J Mol Cell Cardiol* 2013;**62**:58–68.
126. Li K, Stewart DJ, Rouleau JL. Myocardial contractile actions of endothelin-1 in rat and rabbit papillary muscles. Role of endocardial endothelium. *Circ Res* 1991;**69**:301–12.
127. Brunner F. Interaction of nitric oxide and endothelin-1 in ischemia/reperfusion injury of rat heart. *J Mol Cell Cardiol* 1997;**29**:2363–74.
128. Gan XT, Chakrabarti S, Karmazyn M. Increased endothelin-1 and endothelin receptor expression in myocytes of ischemic and reperfused rat hearts and ventricular myocytes exposed to ischemic conditions and its inhibition by nitric oxide generation. *Can J Physiol Pharmacol* 2003;**81**:105–13.
129. Kelly LK, Wedgwood S, Steinhorn RH, Black SM. Nitric oxide decreases endothelin-1 secretion through the activation of soluble guanylate cyclase. *Am J Physiol Lung Cell Mol Physiol* 2004;**286**:L984–91.
130. Ahlborg G, Lundberg JM. Nitric oxide-endothelin-1 interaction in humans. *J Appl Physiol* 1997;**82**:1593–600.
131. Wiley KE, Davenport AP. Nitric oxide-mediated modulation of the endothelin-1 signalling pathway in the human cardiovascular system. *Br J Pharmacol* 2001;**132**:213–20.
132. Polhemus DJ, Lefer DJ. Emergence of hydrogen sulfide as an endogenous gaseous signaling molecule in cardiovascular disease. *Circ Res* 2014;**114**:730–7.
133. Yang F, Liu Z, Wang Y, Li Z, Yu H, Wang Q. Hydrogen sulfide endothelin-induced myocardial hypertrophy in rats and the mechanism involved. *Cell Biochem Biophys* 2014;**70**:1683–6.
134. Geng B, Yang J, Qi Y, Zhao J, Pang Y, Du J, et al. H2S generated by heart in rat and its effects on cardiac function. *Biochem Biophys Res Commun* 2004;**313**:362–8.
135. Song W, Wang H, Wu Q. Atrial natriuretic peptide in cardiovascular biology and disease (NPPA). *Gene* 2015;**569**:1–6.
136. Emori T, Hirata Y, Imai T, Eguchi S, Kanno K, Marumo F. Cellular mechanism of natriuretic peptides-induced inhibition of endothelin-1 biosynthesis in rat endothelial cells. *Endocrinology* 1993;**133**: 2474–80.
137. Fujisaki H, Ito H, Hirata Y, Tanaka M, Hata M, Lin M, et al. Natriuretic peptides inhibit angiotensin II-induced proliferation of rat cardiac fibroblasts by blocking endothelin-1 gene expression. *J Clin Invest* 1995;**96**:1059–61.

138. Schorlemmer A, Matter ML, Shohet RV. Cardioprotective signaling by endothelin. *Trends Cardiovasc Med* 2008;**18**:233–9.
139. Ogata Y, Takahashi M, Ueno S, Takeuchi K, Okada T, Mano H, et al. Antiapoptotic effect of endothelin-1 in rat cardiomyocytes in vitro. *Hypertension* 2003;**41**:1156–63.
140. Kakita T, Hasegawa K, Iwai-Kanai E, Adachi S, Morimoto T, Wada H, et al. Calcineurin pathway is required for endothelin-1-mediated protection against oxidant stress-induced apoptosis in cardiac myocytes. *Circ Res* 2001;**88**:1239–46.
141. Araki M, Hasegawa K, Iwai-Kanai E, Fujita M, Sawamura T, Kakita T, et al. Endothelin-1 as a protective factor against beta-adrenergic agonist-induced apoptosis in cardiac myocytes. *J Am Coll Cardiol* 2000;**36**:1411–8.
142. Bugge E, Ytrehus K. Endothelin-1 can reduce infarct size through protein kinase C and KATP channels in the isolated rat heart. *Cardiovasc Res* 1996;**32**:920–9.
143. Heiden S, Vignon-Zellweger N, Masuda S, Yagi K, Nakayama K, Yanagisawa M, et al. Vascular endothelium derived endothelin-1 is required for normal heart function after chronic pressure overload in mice. *PLoS One* 2014;**9**:e88730.
144. Hathaway CK, Grant R, Hagaman JR, Hiller S, Li F, Xu L, et al. Endothelin-1 critically influences cardiac function via superoxide-MMP9 cascade. *Proc Natl Acad Sci USA* 2015;**112**:5141–6.
145. Palmer M. Endothelin receptor antagonists: status and learning 20 years on. *Prog Med Chem* 2009;**47**:203–37.
146. Channick RN, Sitbon O, Barst RJ, Manes A, Rubin LJ. Endothelin receptor antagonists in pulmonary arterial hypertension. *J Am Coll Cardiol* 2004;**43**(12 Suppl S):62S–7S.
147. Vatter H, Seifert V. Ambrisentan, a non-peptide endothelin receptor antagonist. *Cardiovasc Drug Rev* 2006;**24**:63–76.
148. Barst RJ, Langleben D, Frost A, Horn EM, Oudiz R, Shapiro S, et al. Sitaxsentan therapy for pulmonary arterial hypertension. *Am J Respir Crit Care Med* 2004;**169**:441–7.
149. Bolli MH, Boss C, Binkert C, Buchmann S, Bur D, Hess P, et al. The discovery of N-[5-(4-bromophenyl)-6-[2-[(5-bromo-2-pyrimidinyl)oxy]ethoxy]-4-pyrimidinyl]-N′-p ropylsulfamide (Macitentan), an orally active, potent dual endothelin receptor antagonist. *J Med Chem* 2012;**55**:7849–61.
150. Sidharta PN, van Giersbergen PL, Dingemanse J. Safety, tolerability, pharmacokinetics, and pharmacodynamics of macitentan, an endothelin receptor antagonist, in an ascending multiple-dose study in healthy subjects. *J Clin Pharmacol* 2013;**54**:291–300.
151. Gottlieb SS, Harris K, Todd J, Estis J, Christenson RH, Torres V, et al. Prognostic significance of active and modified forms of endothelin 1 in patients with heart failure with reduced ejection fraction. *Clin Biochem* 2015;**48**:292–6.
152. Van Beneden R, Gurné O, Selvais PL, Ahn SA, Robert AR, Ketelslegers JM, et al. Superiority of big endothelin-1 and endothelin-1 over natriuretic peptides in predicting survival in severe congestive heart failure: a 7-year follow-up study. *J Card Fail* 2004;**10**:490–5.
153. Masson S, Latini R, Anand IS, Barlera S, Judd D, Salio M, et al. Val-HeFT investigators. The prognostic value of big endothelin-1 in more than 2,300 patients with heart failure enrolled in the Valsartan Heart Failure Trial (Val-HeFT). *J Card Fail* 2006;**12**:375–80.
154. Asano K, Bohlmeyer TJ, Westcott JY, Zisman L, Kinugawa K, Good M, et al. Altered expression of endothelin receptors in failing human left ventricles. *J Mol Cell Cardiol* 2002;**34**:833–46.
155. Morawietz H, Goettsch W, Szibor M, Barton M, Shaw S, Hakim K, et al. Increased expression of endothelin-converting enzyme-1 in failing human myocardium. *Clin Sci (Lond)* 2002;**103**(Suppl. 48):237S–240SS.
156. Schneider MP, Boesen EI, Pollock DM. Contrasting actions of endothelin ETA and ETB receptors in cardiovascular disease. *Annu Rev Pharmacol Toxicol* 2007;**47**:731–59.
157. Morawietz H, Szibor M, Goettsch W, Bartling B, Barton M, Shaw S, et al. Deloading of the left ventricle by ventricular assist device normalizes increased expression of endothelin ETA receptors but not

endothelin-converting enzyme-1 in patients with end-stage heart failure. *Circulation* 2000;**102**(Suppl. 3):III188–III193.

158. Lüscher TF, Enseleit F, Pacher R, Mitrovic V, Schulze MR, Willenbrock R, et al. Heart failure ETA receptor blockade trial. Hemodynamic and neurohumoral effects of selective endothelin A (ETA) receptor blockade in chronic heart failure: the Heart Failure ETA Receptor Blockade Trial (HEAT). *Circulation* 2002;**106**:2666–72.
159. Sütsch G, Kiowski W, Yan XW, Hunziker P, Christen S, Strobel W, et al. Short-term oral endothelin-receptor antagonist therapy in conventionally treated patients with symptomatic severe chronic heart failure. *Circulation* 1998;**98**:2262–8.
160. Torre-Amione G, Young JB, Colucci WS, Lewis BS, Pratt C, Cotter G, et al. Hemodynamic and clinical effects of tezosentan, an intravenous dual endothelin receptor antagonist, in patients hospitalized for acute decompensated heart failure. *J Am Coll Cardiol* 2003;**42**:140–7.
161. McMurray JJ, Teerlink JR, Cotter G, Bourge RC, Cleland JG, Jondeau G, et al. VERITAS Investigators. Effects of tezosentan on symptoms and clinical outcomes in patients with acute heart failure: the VERITAS randomized controlled trials. *JAMA* 2007;**298**:2009–19.
162. Denault AY, Pearl RG, Michler RE, Rao V, Tsui SS, Seitelberger R, et al. Tezosentan and right ventricular failure in patients with pulmonary hypertension undergoing cardiac surgery: the TACTICS trial. *J Cardiothorac Vasc Anesth* 2013;**27**:1212–7.
163. Packer M. Multicenter, double-blind, placebo-controlled study of long-term endothelin blockade with bosentan in chronic heart failure-results of the REACH-1 trial. *Circulation* 1998;**98**:1–3. (abstract).
164. Mylona P, Cleland JG. Update of REACH-1 and MERIT-HF clinical trials in heart failure. Cardio.net Editorial Team. *Eur J Heart Fail* 1999;**1**:197–200.
165. Coletta A, Thackray S, Nikitin N, Cleland JG. Clinical trials update: highlights of the scientific sessions of The American College of Cardiology 2002: LIFE, DANAMI 2, MADIT-2, MIRACLE-ICD, OVERTURE, OCTAVE, ENABLE 1 & 2, CHRISTMAS, AFFIRM, RACE, WIZARD, AZACS, REMATCH, BNP trial and HARDBALL. *Eur J Heart Fail* 2002;**4**:381–8.
166. Anand I, McMurray J, Cohn JN, Konstam MA, Notter T, Quitzau K, et al. EARTH investigators. Long-term effects of darusentan on left-ventricular remodelling and clinical outcomes in the Endothelin A Receptor Antagonist Trial in Heart Failure (EARTH): randomised, double-blind, placebo-controlled trial. *Lancet* 2004;**364**:347–54.
167. Abukar Y, May CN, Ramchandra R. The role of endothelin-1 in mediating changes in cardiac sympathetic nerve activity in heart failure. *Am J Physiol Regul Integr Comp Physiol* 2016; **310**:R94–9.

CHAPTER

THE CARDIOKINES: AN EXPANDING FAMILY OF THE HEART SECRETOME

4

F. Al-Mohanna

King Faisal Specialist Hospital and Research Centre & Alfaisal University Medical College, Riyadh, Saudi Arabia

INTRODUCTION

A plethora of evidence exists indicating that the heart is not just a pumping machine responsible for the delivery of nutrient and oxygen through circulating blood and its various constituents. For such a bio-machine to function successfully an intricate array of signals, including electrical, mechanical, and chemical have to be simultaneously processed to achieve the necessarily integrated response in an efficient and sustained way. The heart consists of many cell types, and understanding the basic mechanisms governing cellular behavior is key to understanding disease. Cells receive a multitude of intercellular signals simultaneously, and what determines the predominant response at any one time seems to depend on the cell type and its ability to prioritize an appropriate response. Inappropriate responses invariably lead to disease states. Cell-to-cell communication may occur in several ways including (1) direct physical contact, (2) ligand/receptor interaction, and (3) release of membrane-bound nano-vesicles containing message cargo and uptake of such vesicles by target cells. Following stimulation, an array of intracellular signals is generated. These signals are integrated in such a way that a particular stimulus will be coupled to a particular response: stimulus-response coupling. A change in intracellular signaling is interpreted differently in different cells. In addition, the resting level "set-point" of each intracellular signal may determine whether a particular ligand binding to the same receptor is altering cellular behavior in a stimulatory or inhibitory fashion. For the heart to perform its functions efficiently, its constituent cells release many signaling moieties (the secretome) in a temporally and spatially controlled manner. This chapter will briefly discuss part of the heart secretome: the cardiokines, proteins that are produced within the heart and which exert their effects within (intra-organ) and/or without (interorgan) targets.

CELLULAR COMPONENTS OF THE HEART INVOLVED IN THE CARDIAC SECRETOME

MYOFIBROBLASTS, MYOCYTES AND VASCULAR CELLS

The heart is endowed with several cell populations (Fig. 4.1) namely myofibroblasts, myocytes, and endothelial cells including those of the endocardium, myocardial capillaries, and vascular endothelial cells,[1] vascular smooth muscle cells, vascular fibroblasts, pericytes,[2,3] telocytes,[4–8] conduction

Endocrinology of the Heart in Health and Disease. DOI: http://dx.doi.org/10.1016/B978-0-12-803111-7.00004-X

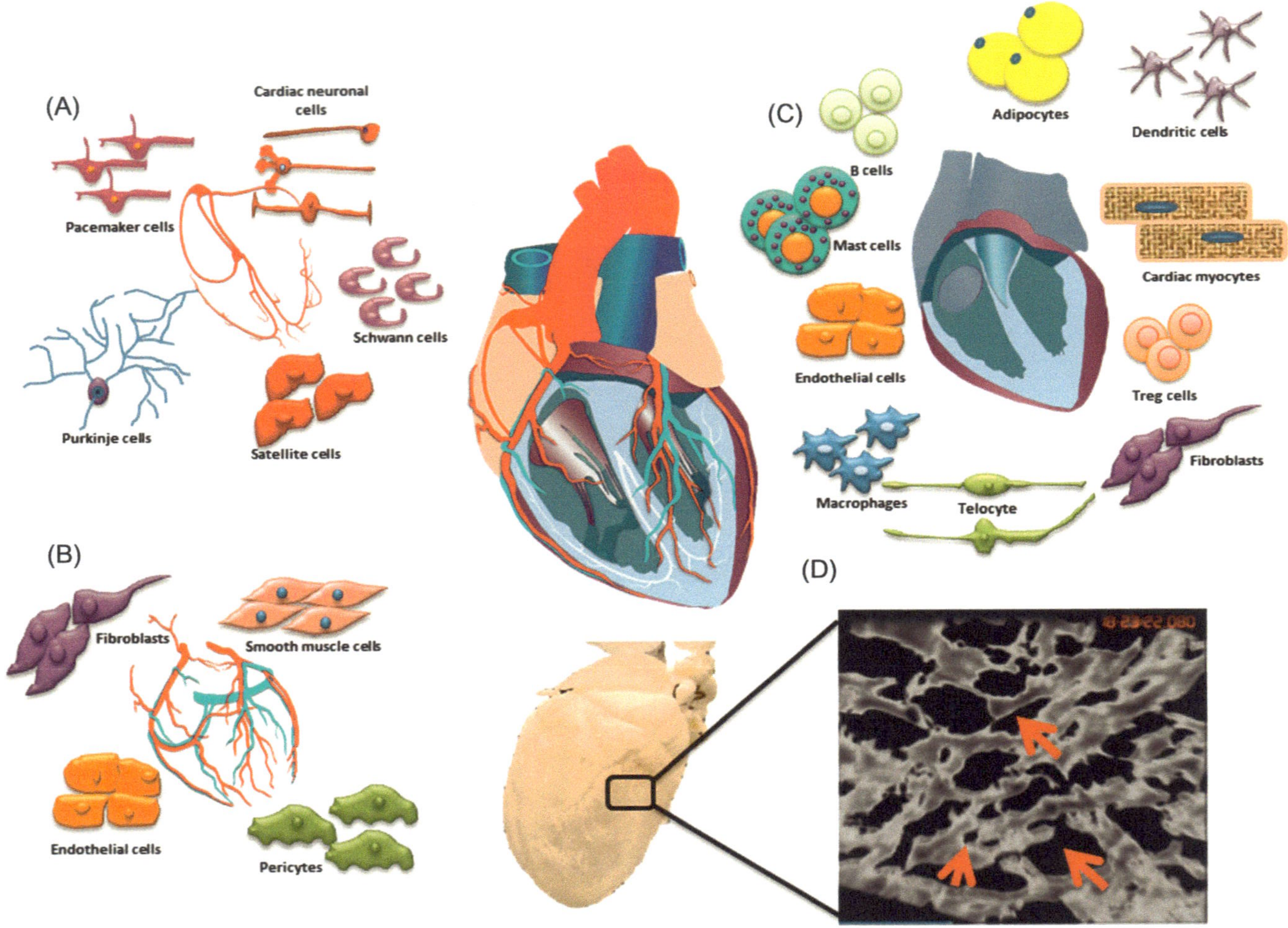

FIGURE 4.1

Simplified sketch of resident cellular components in the heart. (A) Different cell types of the conduction and neuronal cells. (B) Cell types of the heart vasculature. (C) Immune and nonimmune cell types found in the atria and ventricular components of the heart muscle. (D) Decellularized heart showing ECM within which the various cell types are embedded. The right image is a 3D reconstruction of ECM. Arrowheads show the different sized lacunae within which the cells are housed. Sketches of the heart and the various systems are modified from Human Anatomy Atlas (Visible Body), Argosy Publishing Inc.

cells, adipocytes, and immune cells.[9–11] The proportion of each is dependent upon age and species.[9–11] Myofibroblasts, like other fibroblasts, express and release a variety of growth factors and extracellular matrix (ECM) components necessary for the maintenance and repair of the heart muscle. Myofibroblasts are found throughout the heart[9] and have been implicated in cardiac remodeling following pressure and volume overload.[12,13] These cells constitute around 27% of the adult heart.[11,14] Although cardiac myocytes are generally regarded as nonregenerative (or slow), myofibroblasts, like other fibroblasts, do proliferate. Fusion between "terminally differentiated" cardiac myocytes with myofibroblasts can occur and produces hybrid cells (heterokaryons) that express markers of both cell types. The hybrid cells reenter the cell cycle and exhibit beating ability.[15–17] However, the cardiac myocyte phenotype eventually predominates.[15,16] The extent to which this fusion occurs in vivo has been demonstrated elsewhere.[15] This fusion event could provide an elegant way through which myocyte regeneration might ensue following cardiac injury. Cardiomyocytes constitute 30–50% of the heart mass, and atrial and ventricular myocytes differ in their structure and contractile function.[18,19] T-tubules are sparse in atrial myocytes, which give rise to the marked difference in calcium homeostasis and excitation contraction coupling between the atrial and ventricular myocytes.[19] In addition, the presence of atrial specific granules (ASGs) that are not seen in "normal" ventricular myocytes highlights the structural differences between the two cardiomyocytic cell types. Ventricular secretory granules, however, are seen in dilated cardiomyopathy patients.[20] ASGs are classified according to their ultrastructural phenotype into the A-, the B-, and the D-granules, and they constitute the archetypical model of cardiac endocrine system.[21] Endocardial, myocardial, and vascular endothelial cells that constitute the cardiac endothelial cells are three times the number of cardiac myocytes.[1,22] The cells express and release a number of inter- and intra-cellular signals in an auto- and paracrine fashion.[1] Endocardial and myocardial endothelial cells interact closely with the cardiomyocytes and form the "blood heart barrier" with possible role in cardiac remodeling.[1] Vascular endothelial cells, on the other hand, are part of the coronary circulation network and are not in close contact with the cardiomyocytes, functioning mainly in controlling vasomotor tone and coronary blood supply.[1] Vascular smooth muscle cells and vascular fibroblasts are part of the coronary vasculature, and like other vascular cells they interact in an auto- and paracrine fashion to regulate blood supply to the beating heart. Pericytes, found within the endomysial collagen, are the second most abundant cellular constituents of cardiac vasculature especially in the capillaries, arterioles, and postcapillary venules.[3] These cells are intimately involved in vasculogenesis/angiogenesis, coagulation, inflammation, immune responses, and blood vessel permeability.[2] The pericytes make numerous tight junctions with another cell type: the telocytes (TC). Telocytes are interstitial cells found in many organs including the heart.[5,23] The cells have long processes extending hundreds of microns (telopodes) with labyrinth interconnections between cells, generating a network that spans the various heart chambers.[23] These recently discovered cells are found in the atria and ventricles but exist in relatively higher numbers in the atria.[23] Telocytes form homocellular (TC–TC) and heterocellular junctions (TC-pericytes, TC-endothelial cells, TC-myocytes, TC-Schwann cells, and TC-immune cells) with discrete molecular structures, giving rise to an intercellular trabecular network facilitating crosstalks between the different cellular component of the working heart.[24]

CARDIAC CONDUCTION CELLS

The conduction cells of the heart are a collection of specialized excitable cells that lack the actin/myosin arrangement normally found in atrial and ventricular myocytes. These cells are considered to be specialized "modified" myocytes rather than neuronal cells. They include the pacemaker cells of the sinoatrial node (SAN), cells of the internodal pathway, cells of the atrioventricular node (AVN), cells of the bundle of His, bundle branches, and Purkinje fibers. Both adrenergic and cholinergic neuronal cells are found in the cardiac nerve plexus and cardiac ganglia. They include uni- bi- and multipolar neurons, satellite, and Schwann cells[25–28] surrounding the SAN and AVN on the surface and interatrial septum.[29]

CARDIAC ADIPOCYTES

Cardiac adipocytes are found mainly within the epicardial fat and cover around 80% of the surface of the heart.[30,31] Epicardial fat has long been neglected even though it constitutes around 20% of the human heart weight.[31] It is thought to play a protective role in healthy individuals but is associated with atrial fibrillation under pathological conditions.[32] Epicardial adipocytes are different from other adipocytes in fat depots in term of size, number per gram of tissue, and rates of fatty acid synthesis and break down.[31]

RESIDENT IMMUNE CELLS

Resident cardiac immune cells include mast cells,[33,34] macrophages,[34,35] dendritic cells,[36] T regulatory (T_{reg}) cells,[34] and B cells.[37] Out of these the cardiac macrophages are the predominant cell type. They exist in three distinct subsets: myosin heavy chain (MHC) Class II^{hi}/$CCR2^-$, and MHC Class II^{low}/$CCR2^-$ which are of embryonic origin and remain so in the adult heart.[34] These are maintained through in situ proliferation.[34,35] The third subset is $CCR2^+$ and is of monocytic origin captured and replenished from circulation.[34,35]

EXTRACELLULAR MATRIX

The ECM is the framework within which cardiac cells are embedded in lacunae of different sizes. It comprises proteoglycans for hydration and enzymatic activities and fibrous proteins, which provide the tensile strength, cross-linking elasticity, and recoil functions. ECM is a dynamic structure controlled by the matrixins (matrix metalloproteinases, MMPs) and tissue inhibitors of metalloproteinases. The expression and activities of MMPs and their inhibitors are controlled both spatially and temporally. In left ventricular remodeling, e.g., protein expression of MMP-1, -2, and -3 peaks at hypertrophy then decays to lower levels during dilatation and failure.[38] MMP-1 targets collagen I, II, and III of which the former and the later are found in the interstitium predominantly populated by fibroblasts.[39] MMP-2 on the other hand targets collagen IV, V, elastin, and proteins involved in signal transduction whereas MMP-3 targets laminin, collagen III, IV, X, and fibronectin. With more than 20 members of the matrixin family with diverse molecular targets, cardiac matrixins, and their inhibitors are considered major players in the remodeling of the heart in health and disease.

THE AUTOCRINE, PARACRINE, AND ENDOCRINE HEART: COMPONENTS OF THE CARDIAC SECRETOME

Cardiac muscle remodeling is part of the adaptive response for appropriate (physiologic) cardiac function and inappropriate (pathologic) cardiac dysfunction. The remodeling involves the many different cells found in the heart as well as the ECM within which the cells are housed. Both concentric and eccentric remodeling of the heart muscle in response to pressure- or volume-overload,[40] sterile inflammation, myocardial infarction,[41,42] or other cardiomyopathies[43] are dependent upon a number of factors released by cardiac cells through classical and nonclassical secretory pathways and also through exosomal release, in an autocrine, paracrine, and endocrine fashion. These include growth factors and inflammatory mediators necessary for cardiac cells responses to environmental stimuli, be it intrinsic or extrinsic. Many of the cell types that constitute the heart (such as the resident immune cells, myofibroblasts, endothelial cells, adipocytes, and others) are known to undergo exocytosis in response to various stimuli. Release of inflammatory mediators following myocardial infarction and in reperfusion injury has already been demonstrated.[44–47] The question as to whether cardiac myocytes per se can release inflammatory mediators and assume a pro-inflammatory phenotype has already been answered by a number of investigators,[48–50] who demonstrated the inducible release of many growth and inflammatory factors by cardiomyocytes in response to changes in homeostasis, stress, and damage. The ensuing discussion is meant to give a brief overview of a group of proteins that are collectively called cardiokines[51,52] because they are secreted by heart cells and exert their pleiotropic effects on the heart in an autocrine/paracrine and endocrine fashion. Some of these cardiokines may reach the circulation and exert additional endocrine functions. The classical endocrine secretion of atrial natriuretic peptide/brain natriuretic peptide (which are major cardiokines) from ASG, endothelin, and angiotensin/renin/aldosterone systems will not be discussed here since they are presented in detail in Chapter 1, Cardiac Natriuretic Peptides and Chapter 9, Renin Angiotensin Aldosterone System and Heart Function.

GROWTH FACTOR GENERATION IN THE HEART

TRANSFORMING GROWTH FACTOR-BETA

Transforming growth factor-beta (TGF-β) belongs to the transforming growth factor superfamily that includes bone morphogenic proteins, growth differentiation factor,[53] inhibins, activins, nodal,[54] and their associated proteins such as myostatin, and follistatin-like proteins 1 and 3 (which are known cardiokines).[52,55,56] A representative of this superfamily is TGF-β, which is a pleiotropic regulator of cellular growth and differentiation, apoptosis, migration, inflammation, fibrosis, and ECM homeostasis. It exists in different isoforms. It is synthesized as a pre-pro-polypeptide and released in a latent inactive form complexed to the mature TGF-β, latent TGF-binding protein, and latency-associated peptide[57,58] that is activated by proteolytic cleavage. The protein is ubiquitously expressed by many cell types in response to a variety of stimuli. The active TGF-β is a homodimer linked by a disulfide bond forming a cysteine knot that is characteristic of many other signaling molecules such as platelet derived growth factor (PDGF). Latent TGF-β complex is intimately associated with the ECM through latent TGF-β binding proteins (LTBPs). LTBPs are ECM components that regulate TGF-β activation and promote ECM elastogenesis. They are related to fibrillin and like TGF-β exist in multiple isoforms.[54] TGF-β association with the ECM provides the necessary positional information to keep the ECM remodeling program intact during normal physiological and pathophysiological homeostasis and illustrates the paracrine signaling mechanisms inherent within the heart muscle.[14,47] Receptors for TGF-β are widely expressed. Following binding of TGF-β to its cognate receptor type II, which is a constitutively active serine/threonine kinase, the complex dimerises with type I receptor thus bringing its GS domain to proximity for the type II receptor to activate it by serine/threonine phosphorylation. The sequentially activated type I receptor within that complex then phosphorylates SMAD-2 or -3, which releases it from SMAD anchor for receptor activation associated with type I receptor and signaling ensues through the canonical pathway.[59] SMAD, a portmanteau of homologues proteins found in *Caenorhabditis elegans* (SMA; small body size) and *Drosophila* (MAD; *mothers against decapentaplegic*), signaling continues through the binding of activated SMAD-2/3 to SMAD-4 to form a complex that translocates to the nucleus where it acts as a transcription factor in receptor-mediated gene expression responses. Other noncanonical signaling pathways, including TGF-β-activated kinase 1, mitogen-activated protein kinase (MAPK), and extracellular signal-regulated kinase (ERK), may also be deployed in response to TGF-β receptor engagement.[60]

TGF-β in its different isoforms has a profound effect on the development of the heart during embryogenesis especially in valve formation and cardiac septation.[61] In addition, necrotic myocardial cells (Fig. 4.2) release damage-associated molecular patterns (DAMPs) leading to sterile inflammation (Fig. 4.3), which, in turn, induces the release of a number of cardiokines including TGF-β.[62] Increased TGF-β levels are also seen in hypertrophic and dilated cardiomyopathies,[63,64] myocardial infarction,[65–67] cardiac injury/stress as in ischemia–reperfusion,[68] pressure overload, and others.[69,70] The cardiokine is also released by cardiac fibroblasts in response to angiotensin II stimulation.[71] The released TGF-β acts in an autocrine fashion to induce its own expression and in a paracrine fashion on the cardiomyocytes that themselves release TGF-β in response to mechanical stretch.[72] Interestingly, human cardiac fibroblasts response to mechanical stretch and TGF-β was found to be dependent on the ECM subtype.[73] Furthermore, the effect of TGF-β on cultured fibroblast is modulated by mechanical stimuli including mechanical stretch.[74] These "delicate" interactions illustrate the importance of temporal and spatial control of TGF-β autocrine/paracrine effects for the general maintenance of viable cardiac functions. The question however remains as to the contribution of the cardiac generated TGF-β to the elevated plasma levels seen after cardiac injury and hence transition from auto/paracrine to an endocrine cardiokine. Increased serum levels of TGF-β are associated with coronary artery disease in human patients.[75] Furthermore, increased serum levels precede the development of cardiac failure and correlate with cardiac fibrosis in experimental animal models.[76]

VASCULAR ENDOTHELIAL CELL GROWTH FACTOR

Vascular endothelial cell growth factor (VEGF) is a master regulator of physiologic/pathophysiologic neovascularization and vasculogenesis/angiogenesis, and an inducer of vascular endothelial cell proliferation. VEGF, also known as VEGF-A, is a member of a family of growth factors including VEGF-B, VEGF-C, VEGF-D, and the viral VEGF-E.[77] In its active form, this pleiotropic, cysteine knot cardiokine is a homodimer composed of two glycopeptides linked by disulfide bonds. In humans, alternative splicing generates more than 14 different variants (isoforms) with different activities and binding affinities.[78] The variants $VEGF_{121}$ and $VEGF_{165}$ are secreted in a soluble form whereas variants $VEGF_{189}$ and $VEGF_{206}$ are bound to ECM containing heparan sulfate glycosaminoglycans (hsGAGs) proteoglycans. Three different receptors have been identified, VEGFR1, 2, and 3 with different affinities for the different variants of VEGF. Binding of VEGF to its receptor (such as $VEGF\text{-}A_{121,145,148,165,183,189,\text{ and }206}$ to VEGFR-2)[79] causes receptor dimerization and autophosphorylation of Tyr951 and Tyr996.[79] This, in turn, binds to VEGF-associated protein followed by binding to Shc-like protein (Sck) and phospholipase C (PLC)γ activation, ultimately leading to Ras activation and ERK translocation to the nucleus where receptor-mediated gene expression ensues.[79–82] Like TGF-β, the association of VEGF with ECM demonstrates the positional information necessary for the maintenance of ECM modeling inherent in most organs including the heart. VEGF is released by vascular smooth muscle cells,[83] myofibroblasts,[84] adipocytes,[85] macrophages,[86] cardiac telocytes,[87] and cardiac myocytes.[88] It is a potent chemoattractant to

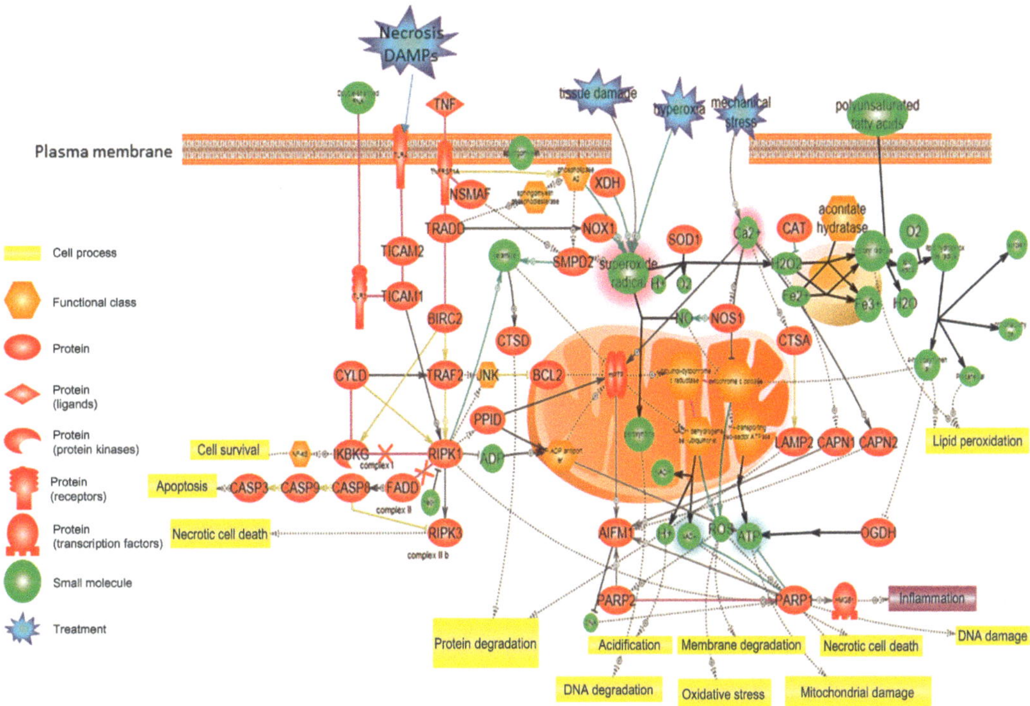

FIGURE 4.2

Cell necrosis induced by various stimuli. Abbreviations are as follows: **TNF**, tumor necrosis factor; **TLR4** Toll-like receptor 4; **TNFRSF1A** Tumor necrosis factor receptor, superfamily, member 1 A; **NSMAF** Neutral sphingomyelinase (N-SMase) activation associated factor **XDH** Xanthine dehydrogenase; **TRADD** TNFRSF1A-associated via death domain; **NOX1** NADPH oxidase 1 **SOD1** Superoxide dismutase 1, soluble; **CAT** Catalase; **TICAM2** Toll-like receptor adaptor molecule 2; **SMPD2** Sphingomyelin phosphodiesterase 2, neutral membrane (neutral sphingomyelinase); **TLR3** Toll-like receptor 3; **TICAM1** Toll-like receptor adaptor molecule 2; **BIRC2** Baculoviral IAP repeat containing 2; **CTSD** Cathepsin D; **NOS1** Nitric oxide synthase 1 (neuronal); **CTSA** Cathepsin A; **CYLD** Cylindromatosis (turban tumor syndrome); **TRAF2** TNF receptor-associated factor 2; **BCL2** B-cell CLL/lymphoma 2; **mPTP** Complex mPTP; **PPID** Peptidylprolyl isomerase D; **IKBKG** Inhibitor of kappa light polypeptide gene, nhancer in B-cells, kinase gamma; **RIPK1** Receptor (TNFRSF)-interacting serine-threonine kinase 1; **CASP3** Caspase 3, apoptosis-related cysteine peptidase; **CASP9** Caspase 9, apoptosis-related cysteine peptidase; **CASP8** Caspase 8, apoptosis-related cysteine peptidase; **FADD** Fas (TNFRSF6)-associated via death domain; **RIPK3** Receptor interacting serine-threonine kinase 3; **AIFM1** Apoptosis-inducing factor, mitochondrion-associated, 1; **PARP2** Poly (ADP-ribose) polymerase 2; **PARP1** Poly (ADP-ribose), polymerase 1; **HMGB1** High mobility group box 1; **OGDH** Oxoglutarate (alpha-ketoglutarate) dehydrogenase (lipoamide); **LAMP2** Lysosomal-associated membrane protein 2; **CAPN1** Calpain 1, (mu/I) large subunit; **CAPN2** Calpain 2, (m/II) large subunit.

The figure is generated and modified with permission from Pathway Studio®.

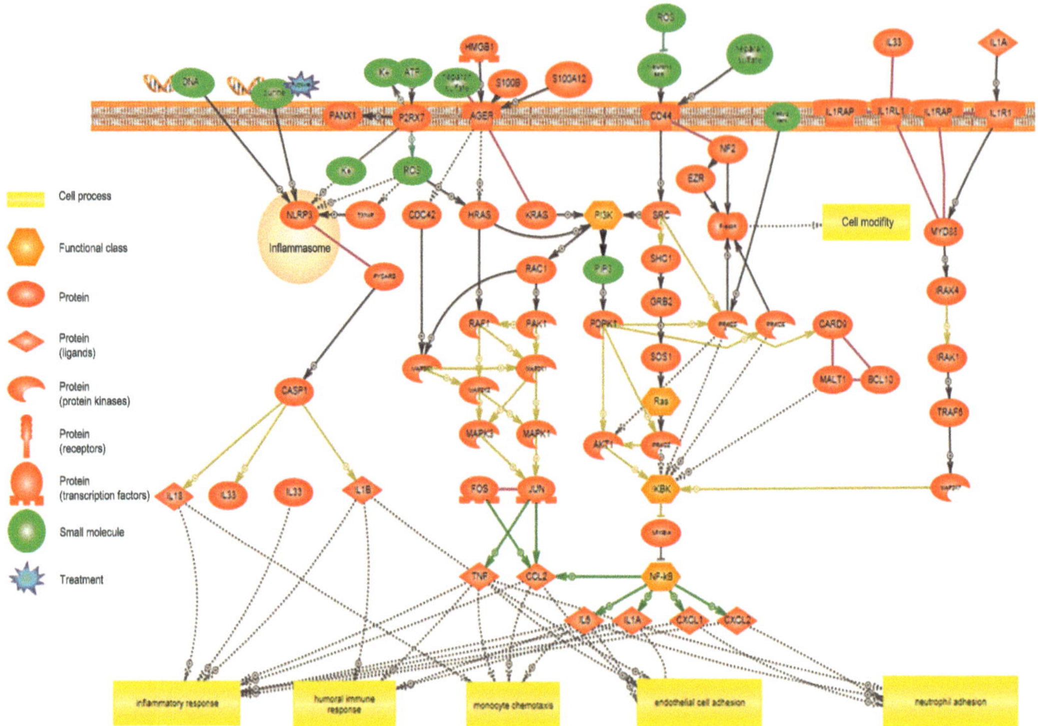

FIGURE 4.3

Sterile inflammation induced by component released from necrotic cells. Abbreviations are: **HMGB1** High mobility group box 1; **S100B** S100 calcium binding protein B; **S100A12** S100 calcium binding protein A12; **IL33** Interleukin-33; **IL1A** Interleukin-1, alpha; **PANX1** Pannexin 1; **P2RX7** Purinergic receptor P2X, ligand-gated ion channel, 7; **Ager** Advanced glycosylation end product-specific receptor; **CD44** CD44 molecule (Indian blood group); **IL1RAP** Interleukin-1 receptor accessory protein; **IL1RL1** Interleukin-1 Receptor-Like 1; **IL1R1** Interleukin-1 Receptor, Type 1; **NF2** Neurofibromin 2 (merlin); **EZR** Ezrin; **PYCARD** PYD and CARD domain containing; **NLRP3** NLR family, pyrin domain containing 3; **TXNIP** Thioredoxin interacting protein; **CDC42** Cell division cycle 42; **HRAS** Harvey rat sarcoma viral oncogene homolog; **KRAS** Kirsten rat sarcoma viral oncogene homolog; **SRC** V-src avian sarcoma (Schmidt-Ruppin A-2) viral oncogene homolog; **F-actin** Complex F-actin; **MYD88** Myoloid differentiation primary response 88; **IRAK4** Interleukin-1 receptor-associated kinase 4; **IRAK1** Interleukin-1 receptor-associated kinase; **TRAF6** TNF receptor-associated factor 6, E3 ubiquitin protein ligase; **MAP3K7** Mitogen-activated protein kinase kinase kinase 7; **RAC1** Ras-related C3 botulinum toxin substrate 1 (rho family, small GTP binding protein Rac1); **SHC1** HSC (Src homology 2 domain containing) transforming protein 1; **GRB2** Growth factor receptor-bound protein 2; **RAF1** V-raf-1 murine leukemia viral oncogene homolog 1; **PAK1** P21 protein (Cdc42/Rac)-activated kinase 1; **PDPK1** 3-phosphoinositide dependent protein; **PRKCD** Protein kinase C, delta; **PRKCE** Protein kinase C, epsilon; **CARD9** Caspase recruitment domain family, member 9; **CASP1** Caspase-1, apoptosis-related cysteine peptidase; **MAP3K1** Mitogen-activated protein kinase, kinase kinase 1, E3 ubiquitin protein ligase; **MAP2K2** Mitogen-activated protein kinase kinase 2; **MAP2K1** Mitogen-activated protein kinase kinase 1; **SOS1** Son of sevenless homolog 1 (Drosophila); **MALT1** Mucosa associated lymphoid tissue lymphoma translocation gene 1; **BCL10** B-cell CLL/lymphoma 10; **MAPK3** Mitogen-activated protein kinase 3; **MAPK1** Mitogen-activated protein kinase 1; **AKT1** c-akt murine thymoma viral oncogene; **PRKCZ** Protein kinase C, zeta; **IL18** Interleukin-18 (interferon-gamma-inducing factor); **IL33** Interleukin-33; **IL1B** Interleukin-1, beta; **FOS** FBJ murine osteosarcoma viral oncogene homolog; **JUN** Jun proto-oncogene; **NFKBIA** Nuclear factored kappa light polypeptide gene enhancer in B-cells inhibitor; **TNF** Tumor necrosis factor-α; **CCL2** Chemokine (C-C motif) ligand 2; **IL6** Interleukin-6 (interferon, beta 2); **IL1A** Interleukin-1 alpha; **CXCL1** Chemokine (C-X-C motif) ligand 1 (melanoma growth stimulating activity, alpha); **CXCL2** Chemokine (C-X-C motif) ligand 2.

The figure is generated and modified with permission from Pathway Studio®.

monocytes[89] and plays a crucial role in ECM homeostasis by inducing metalloproteinases.[90] VEGF-A, -B, -C, and -D are found in the heart.[79] Moreover, increased VEGF-A expression is found in chronic overload.[91] Expression of VEGF in its various isoforms is temporally and spatially controlled by (1) hypoxia through the hypoxia-induced factor-1α (HIF-1α) and β (HIF-1β); (2) growth factors such as TGF-β, PDGF, epidermal growth factor, and insulin-like growth factor; (3) hormones such as estrogen and testosterone; (4) cytokine/cardiokines such TNF-α, IL1-β, and interleukin-6 (IL-6) (for a comprehensive review, see Hoeben et al.)[79]; and (5) aberrant glycemic control.[92–96] Circulating VEGFs include $VEGF_{121}$ (the soluble isoform) and $VEGF_{165}$ (normally bound to cell surface and ECM). $VEGF_{145}$, $VEGF_{189}$, and $VEGF_{206}$ are only sparingly secreted and are generally bound to the ECM.[92] Changes in serum levels of VEGF are associated with cancer, pregnancy, hypoxia, and inflammation.[92] Decreased serum levels of VEGF were reported in patients with congestive heart failure.[97] In an ovine model of heart failure due to progressive increase in pressure overload, the expression of VEGF at the protein level in samples taken from the left ventricle was demonstrated to decrease during left ventricular hypertrophy and dilatation, with maximum reduction occurring at the latter. The levels were restored to control values during failure and recovery.[38] Interestingly, MMPs-1, -2, and -3 levels increase at the mRNA and protein levels with maximum change in the protein levels occurring at hypertrophy,[38] a stage in the progression to heart failure at which VEGF was reported to be low. Elevated levels have been reported in acute myocardial infarction (AMI).[98] It is, therefore, tempting to speculate that local changes in the levels of this cardiokine may underlie the serum levels, thus highlighting the transition from an auto/paracrine scenario to an endocrine scenario possibly through its exudation from the generating organ, in this case, the heart.[92] The extent of the contribution of the heart muscle to the bloodborne VEGF levels and whether such contribution induces secondary effects of VEGF elsewhere in the body is yet to be determined.

FIBROBLAST GROWTH FACTOR-2 AND FGF-16

Fibroblast growth factor-2 (FGF-2) is part of the FGF family of growth factors that includes 18 members so far, constituting a number of subclasses. These are distinct from the FGF homologous factors that do not activate FGF receptors even though they have a high degree of sequence homology with the FGF family.[99–101] FGF-2 is produced by a number of cell types including cardiac myocytes, cardiac fibroblasts, endothelial cells, and smooth muscle cells.[102] Two different isoforms arising from alternative translation of the same mRNA with different molecular weights—high molecular weight, hi-FGF-2 and low molecular weight, lo-FGF-2 isoforms—have been identified.[103] Like other members of the family, this cardiokine binds hsGAGs with high affinity. hsGAG binding is necessary for FGF-2 to engage its receptor tyrosine kinase FGFR1,[102] and signaling ensues following FGF-hsGAG-FGFR dimerization leading to the activation of protein kinase (PK)C-α and PKC- ε .[102,104] FGF-2 directly induces adult cardiac hypertrophy.[105] In a recent study of cardiac remodeling in rodents, hypertrophy, contractile dysfunction, and proIL-1β upregulation were attributed to hi-FGF-2 whereas angiogenesis and cardio-protective traits were due to lo-FGF-2.[106] In human myofibroblasts, lo-FGF-2 attenuates TGF-β-induced ECM remodeling.[107] It's been hypothesized that FGF-2 interacts with other members of the family. For instance, one study found that FGF-16 competes with FGF-2 for FGFR1 receptors.[104] Cardioprotective FGF-16 is released from the endocardium and epicardium during development and is preferentially expressed in the heart postnatally.[108,109]

INFLAMMATORY MEDIATORS GENERATED IN THE HEART

THE INFLAMMASOME

Inflammation is a normal biological response deployed by the body in order to deal with infection or damage. It is also a condition associated with common pathologies such as obesity, metabolic syndrome, dietary deficiencies, stress, and autoimmune diseases.[110–114] During inflammation, resident cells are activated, additional cells are recruited, and a number of inflammatory mediators are released both locally and globally. If successful, the inflammation subsides and normal homeostasis is restored. If not, then aberrant homeostasis persists and the unresolved inflammation continues leading ultimately to diseased state. Throughout the process an intricate balance of intercellular and interorgan mediators are maintained to ensure successful resolution. The onset of inflammation is initiated by the infecting agent or local damage, which in the absence of infection gives rise to sterile inflammation (Fig. 4.3). Central to the inflammatory response are the inflammasomes, which are supramolecular signaling complexes belonging to the pattern recognition receptor family known as the nod-like receptors (NLRs). In its simplest form the inflammasome is a tripartite complex of proteins consisting of a sensor, an adapter, and a pro-caspase. The sensor is made of a central nucleotide-binding oligomerization domain with ATPase activity (also known as NACHT), a C-terminal 20–29 amino acid long leucine-rich repeat domain with regulatory activity and a protein–protein interaction domain.[115–120] The adaptor can be an apoptosis-associated, speck-like protein with a caspase recruitment domain (ASC). ASC has two distinct domains: a protein–protein interaction domain, and caspase activation and recruitment domain (CARD). Pro-caspase typically interacts with the adaptor protein ASC through its own CARD domain.[119] The caspases involved could be caspase 1, 4, 5, and 11 depending on the species.[121] Inflammasomes are classified according to their protein–protein interaction domains, such as the pyrin domain, baculovirus inhibitor of apoptosis protein repeat (BIR) domain or CARD into NLRP, NLRC, and NAIP.[115,121] Twenty-three NLR genes have been identified in the human genome and even more in the mouse genome.[115,121,122] Fourteen human NLRPs, 7 NLRCs, and 7 NAIPs have been identified of which NLRP1, NLRP1A, NLRP1B, NLRP1C, NLRP3, NLRP4, NLRP6, NLRP7, and NLRP12 have been highlighted in different studies.[115,123,124] Pathogen-associated molecular patterns (PAMPs) and DAMPs are the two groups detected by the sensor moieties of the inflammasome. PAMPs are well characterized and are not the subject of this discussion. Five classes of endogenous DAMPs with overlapping functions have been proposed.[125,126] Class I are receptor binding DAMPs including high mobility group box 1 (HMGB1), heat shock proteins, S100 proteins including S100A8 and S100A9, β-amyloid, hyaluronan fragments generate by ECM degradation, mitochondrial formyl peptides, and mitochondrial DNA. Class II includes monosodium urate, extracellular adenosine triphosphate (ATP), reactive oxygen species (ROS), and thioredoxin interacting protein. Class III includes MHC Class I chain-related proteins A and B. Class IV includes cytoskeletal actin, nonmuscle MHC A and Class V includes unfolded/misfolded proteins involved in the unfolded protein response (UPR) associated with ER stress.[125] Exogenous DAMPs include silica and asbestos.[127]

The inflammasome NLRP3 assembly and activation in heart disease is probably the most studied. In an experimental model of sterile inflammation in the mouse heart, Mezzaroma et al.[128] demonstrated that ATP released from dying cells activates the purinergic receptor P2X7 leading to inflammasome assembly and activation. The authors demonstrated the cytoplasmic aggregation of the three component of the inflammasome at the granulation tissue and myocytes bordering the infarcted area together with the activation of caspase-1. They further demonstrated inflammasome induction in the cardiac myocytes cell line (HL-1) and showed that inhibition of inflammasome activation either pharmacologically or through silencing RNA limited the infarct size and reduced cardiac enlargement leaving compensatory hypertrophy intact.[128] The formation and activation of NLRP3 inflammasome in response to cellular necrosis (induced by pressure disruption, hypoxia, or complement-mediated injury) has also been demonstrated in other models of sterile inflammation in vitro. Moreover, mice deficient in NLRP3 and ASC were protected from renal ischemia/reperfusion (I/R) injury, suggesting the pivotal role of this inflammasome in inducing sterile inflammation.[41] A different line of evidence for the involvement of NLRP3 in myocardial dysfunction is drawn from transgenic mice, where cardiac-specific overexpression of calcineurin (CNTg) is associated with cardiac hypertrophy, ventricular dilatation, apoptosis, and inflammation.[129] In this animal model NLRP3 mRNA level is increased and is coupled to increased expression of both active caspase-1 and serum IL-1β levels. Furthermore, sustained inhibition of IL-1β by IL-1 receptor (IL-1R) antagonist reduced the pro-inflammatory response and improved fractional shortening and systolic performance.[129] Both cardiac myocytes and cardiac fibroblast have been shown to assemble and activate NLRP3 inflammasome. Supernatant from necrotic myocardial cells obtained by freeze-thawing of freshly excised mouse hearts was found to contain DAMPs including HMGB1, galectin-3, S100β, S100A8/A9, and IL-1α and induced proliferation and activation of cardiac and NIH/3T3 fibroblasts in vitro.[62] It is, therefore, possible that DAMPs may not only work in an autocrine/paracrine fashion but also in an endocrine fashion should they become blood born. In addition the same supernatant induced myocardial inflammation and fibrosis when injected locally in vivo in wildtype but not in toll-like receptor 4 (TLR4) deficient animals.[62] The question therefore arises as to the promiscuity of toll-like receptor (TLR) and to whether multiple DAMPs invoke their effect(s) synergistically or otherwise, which is yet to be answered.

Both TLRs and NLRs are differentially expressed in different tissues.[130] Different DAMPs bind to different receptors on/in the affected cells. These include but are not limited to TLR2, TLR3, TLR4, TLR9, REG-I, receptor for advanced glycation endproducts (RAGEs), cyclic guanosine monophosphate-adenosine monophosphate synthase (cGAS), CD14, CD24, CD36, CD40, and CD44.[125–127] The signaling pathways activated following receptor engagement are well reviewed, and involve I_kB kinase and MAPKs leading to (1) activation and translocation of NF-$_k$B to the nucleus; and (2) de novo synthesis of many inflammatory cytokines including proIL-1β and proIL-18. This is referred to as signal 1; signal 2 ensues via the assembly and activation of the inflammasome NLRP3. Whether a priming signal is necessary for assembly and subsequent triggering of NLRP3 induced by DAMPs is not as well-defined as that for LPS-induced NLRP3 activation, where a priming signal seems necessary and is independent of the triggering event.[131] More importantly, can inflammasomes be activated independently of plasma membrane receptor occupation? TLR or otherwise? This was partially answered by the finding that reduced cytosolic ATP levels as measured by AMP/ATP ratio, activate the NLRP1b inflammasome.[132] ATP reduction was achieved by introducing 2-deoxyglucose (2-DG) and sodium azide (NaN_3) to the cell culture medium of HT1080 human fibroblasts expressing the murine inflammasome NLRP1b. 2-DG inhibits glycolysis and NaN_3 inhibits mitochondrial respiration through blocking cytochrome c oxidase and oxidative phosphorylation[133]; both will compromise mitochondrial integrity. Arguably, two broad functions are assigned to the mitochondria: cellular metabolism and control of cell death. The mitochondria with its endosymbiont bacterial origin, has its own DAMPs (mtDAMPs) with profound effects on cellular behavior. A number of mtDAMPs are generated by dysfunctional mitochondria, these include *N*-formyl peptides (f-MIT) and mitochondrial DNA (mtDNA)[134] that may be also released to the extracellular environments and circulation from damaged cells. In fact, circulating mtDAMPs have been linked to systemic inflammatory response syndrome, similar to that induced by sepsis but without the pathogenic component.[135] Of particular interest is the f-MIT, which acts on cells, e.g., neutrophils expressing fMet-Leu-Phe receptors, leading to activation and release of many nocuous compounds including ROS and degrading enzymes existing primarily to rid the body of invading microorganisms. ROS are produced by the mitochondria through the monovalent molecular oxygen reduction pathway where superoxide in concentrations of 10–200 pM may be generated under normal homeostasis.[136] The antioxidant arsenal within the mitochondria and the cytosol are normally adequate to cope with such concentrations under normal homeostasis. However, aberrant production may overcome the "normal" homeostasis and initiate a cascade of events leading to oxidative stress with ultimate mitochondria dysfunction/destruction. Mitochondrial destruction has been clearly observed in transmission electron micrographs of heart muscle samples (left ventricular) obtained at dilatation and failure stages during progression to heart failure in an ovine model of chronic heart failure induced by pressure overload.[38] Hemodynamic stress causes mitochondrial damage,[137] and the damaged mitochondria can cause TLR9-dependent inflammation of the heart leading to myocarditis and dilated cardiomyopathy.[134,138]

Fission and fusion of mitochondria are highly regulated dynamic processes for ensuring the general "well being" of this organelle. Damaged mitochondria are removed by autophagy and both fission and fusion seem to be well-coordinated with the endoplasmic reticulum[139] at ER-mitochondria contact sites termed mitochondria-associated ER membranes (MAM). These contact sites are not membrane fusion sites but more resemble docking milieu through which exchange of "molecular information" can ensue at close proximity between the two organelles, i.e., intracellular organellar synapses.[139–142] This "molecular information" exchange includes intracellular $[Ca^{++}]_i$, ROS, and mediators of lipid metabolism[140] $[Ca^{++}]_i$ is one of most studied intracellular second messenger systems, controlling a variety of cellular behaviors including metabolic and apoptotic regulation. Bidirectional coupling of Ca^{++} between the ER and the mitochondria has been demonstrated[143] $[Ca^{++}]_i$ is stored in the ER and sequestered by mitochondria (located near the ER Ca^{++} release sites) in a well-coordinated and tightly controlled manner. At rest most cells exhibit an $[Ca^{++}]_i$ of around 100 nM (depending on the cell type). This can transiently increase to around 1 μM following stimulation with a variety of soluble and particulate stimuli, before decaying back to prestimulation levels. $[Ca^{++}]_i$ homeostasis is controlled by a myriad of coordinated actions of receptor-mediated signaling mechanisms, membrane-bound calcium channels, store and voltage-operated calcium channels, calcium release mechanisms, calcium sensor mechanisms, store replenishing mechanisms, and many more. Although high $[Ca^{++}]_i$ ($>$ 10 μM) is considered pathological, intra-ER calcium $[Ca^{++}]_{er}$ is around 1–2 mM, with varying levels of $[Ca^{++}]_{er}$ within the different regions of ER.[139,144] Intra-mitochondrial calcium $[Ca^{++}]_{mito}$ levels are 10–100 nM at rest, and escalates towards hundreds of μM upon stimulation.[142] Mitochondrial oxidative phosphorylation is controlled by $[Ca^{++}]_{mito}$ homeostasis so as to drive respiration in order to provide the necessary ATP to meet cellular energy demands.[145] An archetypical example of calcium signaling following plasma membrane receptor occupation starts with the activation of PLC, which hydrolyzes PIP_2 in a process involving heterotrimeric G proteins, producing diacylglycerol, which activate protein kinase C (PKC) and inositol 1,4,5-trisphosphate (IP_3). Binding of IP_3 to cognate receptors on the $[Ca^{++}]_i$ stores releases calcium into the cytosol. Transduction of $[Ca^{++}]_i$ to the mitochondrial intermembrane space involves the outer membrane voltage-dependent anion channel (VDAC), and its homeostasis within the mitochondrial matrix through the inner mitochondrial membrane is tightly controlled by (1) mitochondrial Ca^{++} uniporter (MCU); (2) rapid-mode uptake (RaM); (3) mitochondrial ryanodine receptor isoform (mRyR)-1 in excitable cells; and (4) the flickering of the mitochondrial permeability transition pore (mPTP), all of which are intimately linked to the mitochondrial membrane potential $\Delta\Psi_m$ through overall charge movements.[140,145] mPTP opening is associated with cytochrome C release and a burst of ROS, which exemplifies the relationship between $[Ca^{++}]_{mito}$ homeostasis and ROS production.[145] Mitochondrial ROS production activates the inflammasome NLRP3, which is normally associated with the ER. Moreover, activation of NLRP3 inflammasome leads to its accumulation in MAM together with recruitment of ASC from the cytosol.[146,147]

ER stress and Ca^{++}/ROS interplay are well investigated and reviewed.[141,142] ER stress induced by inhibition of glycoprotein synthesis, protein transfer from ER to Golgi apparatus, or emptying of the ER calcium store activates the NLRP3 inflammasome independently of the classical UPR.[148] The role of $[Ca^{++}]_i$ per se in the activation NLRP3 is somewhat controversial. A number of studies have reported the requirement of calcium for NLRP3 activation and have demonstrated that disruption of $[Ca^{++}]_i$ inhibits its activation.[149] Others have reported that K^+ efflux induces NLRP3 activation independently of $[Ca^{++}]_i$ signaling.[150] At intracellular potassium concentrations below 90 mM the NLRP3 assembly and caspase-1 recruitment occur spontaneously.[151] What transpires is that aberrant $[Ca^{++}]_i$ handling may give rise to mitochondrial/ER stress, and it is this stress that leads to NLRP3 activation. It is noteworthy, however, that both mitochondrial perturbation and ROS production have been brought to question and reported to be unnecessary for NLRP3 activation.[152] Explanations for such conflicting data are hard to reconcile. However, different cell types may activate the inflammasome differently. In addition, experimental conditions and the use of cell lines might add to the controversy thus bringing issues such as cell age (passage number) and the effect(s) of long-term cell culture on cellular behavior into the equation.

IL-1α, IL-1β, IL-18, AND IL-33

Arguably the ultimate aims of caspase-1 inflammasome activation are: (1) the proteolytic activation of proIL-1β and proIL-18 into their respective active forms IL-1β and IL-18[115,117,119,121,127]; (2) inactivation of IL-33;[153,154] and (3) induction of pyroptosis.[128] The IL-1 family of cytokines includes IL-1α and IL-1β, IL-18, IL-33, and IL-36α, β, γ together with receptor agonists IL-1Ra, IL-36Ra, IL-38, and anti-inflammatory IL-37.[155] The IL-1R family includes IL-1RI, IL-1RII, IL-1RAcP, ST2, IL-18Rα, IL-36R, IL-18Rβ, TIR8, TIGIRR-2, and TIGIRR-1.[155] IL-1α is constitutively synthesized as a precursor protein that is processed by the membrane-bound calcium-dependent cysteine protease calpain into its mature form. Both precursor and mature forms exhibit bioactivity. Necrotic cardiomyocytes release IL-1α, which, in turn, activate cardiac fibroblasts in a MAPK- and NF_kB-dependent manner.[156] The released IL-1α may act as a "danger" signal for post myocardial infarct inflammation.[156] Increased local and systemic levels of IL-1β have been demonstrated in a number of cardiovascular diseases including atherosclerosis, myocardial infarction, myocarditis, and dilated cardiomyopathy.[157] IL-1β is produced by cardiac myocytes and cardiac fibroblast in response to mechanical stretch and pressure mediated hypertrophy[158] and by cardiac macrophages.[35,159] IL-1α and IL-1β bind to the same receptor and have a similar and profound effect on local and global responses associated with left ventricular systolic dysfunction[160] IL-1β reduces cardiac contractility[160] through induction of leakage of $[Ca^{++}]_i$

from the sarcoplasmic reticulum.[119] Intra-peritoneal injection of healthy mice with recombinant IL-1β has been shown to cause a reversible left ventricular fractional shortening through modulation of the β-receptor response.[161] Like proIL-1β, proIL-18 is processed through the NLRP3 inflammasome to release the biologically active IL-18. IL-18 is known as interferon-γ-inducing factor and is elevated in patients with ischemic cardiomyopathy, and its plasma levels were higher in patients that died from heart failure.[162] Receptors for IL-18 (IL-18Rα) levels are also elevated in ischemic and dilated cardiomyopathy patients, and the levels of its endogenous inhibitor IL-18-binding protein were reduced in the failing myocardium.[162] In addition, IL-18 was found to mediate IL-1β-induced myocardium dysfunction.[160]

IL-33 is a mechanically induced cardiokine with cardio-protective functions produced by cardiac myocytes and cardiac fibroblasts.[154] The cardiokine inhibits angiotensin II- and phenylephrine-induced cardiac hypertrophy through $I_kB\alpha$ and NF_kB binding in the nucleus[154] IL-33 released by necrotic cells may serve as an alarm signal in conjunction with DAMPs.[163] Components of the IL-33 system are expressed in normal human and pressure overloaded myocardium.[163] This cardiokine is also induced by IL-1β, IFN-γ, and TNF-α[163] and is now recognized as having both pro- and anti-inflammatory activity. It is thought to facilitate the "switch" between Th1 to Th2 immune responses.[164] The receptor for IL-33 is ST2 receptor (which was an "orphan" receptor before it was discovered to bind to IL-33) with both agonist activity and nuclear binding activity.[164] Like the IL-1R antagonist, soluble ST2 "decoy" receptors are found in circulation and in the extracellular space.

INTERLEUKIN-6

IL-6, a pleiotropic cardiokine is a member of a family of cytokines that includes leukemia inhibitory factor, oncostatin M, IL-11, cardiotrophin (CT)-1, and ciliary neurotrophic factor.[78,165] It is produced by many cell types including cardiac myocytes, macrophages, fibroblasts, endothelial cells, adipocytes, and telocytes.[87] This cardiokine is produced as a precursor with different isoforms. High circulating levels have been reported in patients with congestive heart failure and were associated with myocyte hypertrophy and apoptosis.[166] In addition elevated expression of IL-6 and its receptor in donor hearts (myocytes and interstitial cells) have been associated with cardiac allograft dysfunction following transplantation.[167] The IL-6 family share a common signal transducer (gp130), which dimerizes upon receptor occupation. Intracellular signaling ensues through the janus kinase/Signal transducer and activator of transcription signaling pathway together with phosphatidylinositol-3-kinase (PI3K), Akt, MEK, and ERK.[165] The cardiokine can also bind to a soluble IL-6 receptor and the complex is sufficient to activate gp130 dimerization (IL-6 trans-signaling).[168] IL-6 expression is induced by a variety of stimuli including inflammatory mediators like IL-1β and TNF-α.[168] Moreover, neuropeptides such as urocortin (a member of corticotropin release hormone family) have been shown to induce the release of IL-6 from cardiomyocytes in a p38/MAPK/ERK- and NF_kB-dependent manner.[169]

TUMOR NECROSIS FACTOR (TNF-α) AND SOLUBLE CD40 LIGAND (SCD40L)

TNF-α is another pleiotropic cardiokine, secreted by cardiac cells in response to a variety of stimuli. Both volume and pressure overload induces TNF-α mRNA in experimental animals with higher changes in the right ventricle occurring in volume overloaded animals.[170,171] In addition, aortic banding upregulates TNF-α in C57/BL mice. This upregulation was concomitant with the development of inflammatory response, apoptosis, and cardiac hypertrophy.[172] Moreover, resident cardiac mast cells have been demonstrated to release TNF-α in response to I/R.[33] TNF-α evokes its biological activity through binding to type 1 receptor (TNFR1) and/or type 2 receptor (TNFR2). This has led to the hypothesis that binding of TNFR1 is associated with the cytotoxic effect, whereas binding to TNFR2 is more cardio-protective. It is noteworthy that the transition from auto/paracrine effect to an endocrine effect may depend on (1) the released cardiokine and whether it reaches circulation in high enough concentration[165]; (2) the expression of the appropriate receptors on target cells; (3) presence of the "decoy" receptor antagonist; and (4) cardiokine stability. The realization that heart failure is associated with high circulating levels of TNF-α prompted many studies into the use of TNF-α antagonist in patients with AMI.[173] TNF-α antagonist-based therapy has failed to confer any therapeutic benefits to AMI patients, echoing previous clinical trials where targeted therapy failed to be of any benefit clinically.[173,174]

CD40L is a trimeric transmembrane member of the TNF family expressed in many cell types including mast cells, macrophages, monocytes, B cells, T cells, endothelial cells, fibroblasts, myofibroblasts, and platelets.[175–177] A soluble form of the protein (sCD40L) is shed by activated platelets through interactions with MMP-2 and integrin $\alpha_{II}\beta_3$.[176] Elevated levels of this pro-coagulant and pro-inflammatory protein have been reported in acute coronary syndrome (ACS)[175] atherosclerosis and atherothrombosis,[178] left ventricular dysfunction, and chronic heart failure.[179] High levels of sCD40L have been demonstrated in biopsies from dilated left ventricle (LVD) in an ovine model of pressure overload. The levels returned to "control" values upon recovery.[38] The source of sCD40L was not determined in that study and thus the contribution of platelets could not be ruled out. However, since the heart contains many cell types known to express CD40L/CD40 system especially mast cells macrophages and B cells (see above), the possibility exists that the source of sCD40L measured in LVD samples may be resident cardiac cells in addition to activated platelets.

MESENCEPHALIC ASTROCYTE-DERIVED NEUROTROPHIC FACTOR (MANF), SECRETED FRIZZLED RELATED PROTEIN (SFRP)-2, AND PROTEASE INHIBITOR 16 (PI-16)

Mesencephalic astrocyte-derived neurotrophic factor is an ER/SR stress protein released upon ER/SR-calcium store depletion.[180] The cardiokine is induced in cardiomyocytes and other cardiac cells after MI.[52] The protein is antihypertrophic and its systemic administration in mice protects the heart from I/R damage.[52,180] Secreted Frizzled Related Protein is another stress-inducible, antifibrotic cardiokine released mainly by cardiac fibroblasts. Protease inhibitor 16 is an antihypertrophic cardiokine that is upregulated in the failing myocardium.[52]

HIGH MOBILITY GROUP BOX 1 PROTEIN

The HMGB1 protein, also known as amphoterin, is one of the most conserved nucleosomal proteins with 99% amino acid homology between rodent and human.[181] The protein is a member of the high mobility group proteins that are ubiquitous and highly abundant chromosomal proteins involved in many nuclear activities including transcription, replication, and DNA repair. They are broadly grouped into High Mobility Group containing AT-hook domain (HMGA), HMGB, and High Mobility Group containing Nucleosomal binding domain (HMGN).[182,183] HMGB1 is a DNA binding and bending protein localized "normally" to the nucleus but can also be seen in the cytosol[184] and the plasma membrane.[185] It is secreted by immune cells through regulated exocytosis and passively released from damaged cells as part of DAMPs.[186] In addition, viable nondamaged cells do produce and release HMGB1 is response to a variety of stimuli.[50] This nonhistone protein constitutes a danger signal alarming other cells of possible ensuing damage. It is necessary for mitochondrial integrity and is involved in regulating glycemic status since knockout mice die early after birth due to sever hypoglycemia.[187] The released HMGB1 binds to RAGEs and/or to TLR-2 and TLR-4 receptors on the plasma membranes of many cell types[188] Following binding HMGB1/receptor complexes activate a number of signaling pathways including NF-$_k$B, JAK/STAT, PI3K, and MAPK, causing the expression and release of inflammatory mediators[127,188] including TGFβ1.[189] Interestingly, HMGB1 translocation to the cytosol is induced by hypoxia[190] and by stimuli that evoke ROS production.[191] In tumor cells the translocated HMGB1 binds to mtDNA, which, in turn, leads to activation of TLR9 signaling pathway.[190] Through binding to the autophagic protein Beclin1, HMGB1 has a direct effect on cellular autophagy/apoptosis.[191,192] Exogenous HMGB1 is toxic and was demonstrated to deplete mitochondrial DNA and to induce giant mitochondria formation.[193] Increased cardiac expression of HMGB1 was demonstrated in a murine model of pressure overload. Moreover, this increased expression was accompanied by cytosolic and intercellular translocation[194] Exogenous HMGB1 has also been reported to aggravate pressure overload-induced cardiac hypertrophy and the subsequent cardiac failure.[194] Both local and systemic levels of the protein increase in patients with myocarditis.[195] Moreover, increased serum levels of HMGB1 have been demonstrated post-infarct and in LV remodeling,[196] chronic heart failure,[197] and coronary artery disease.[198] The reader is referred to Chapter 5, Novel Small Peptide Hormones where this cardiokine is discussed in detail.

MACROPHAGE MIGRATION INHIBITORY FACTOR

Macrophage migration inhibitory factor (MIF) is a pleiotropic cardiokine involved in many immune responses associated with sepsis, I/R injury, atherosclerosis,[199] and AMI.[200] The protein has chemokine-like functions and promotes the production of inflammatory mediators including TNF-α, IL-8, and IL-6.[201,202] In addition, MIF induces intercellular adhesion molecule-1-1 and vascular cell adhesion molecule-1 expression in endothelial cells thus increasing recruitment of leukocytes from circulation.[203] MIF is produced by cardiomyocytes is response to hypoxia and ROS through a PKC-dependent mechanism[199,204] and is thought to limit I/R injury through inhibition of the c-Jun N-terminal kinase signaling pathway.[205] It is also produced by immune cells, and recent data suggest that immune cell-derived MIF may exaggerate damage as appose to the cardiomyocyte-derived MIF which promotes cardiac healing.[206] A number of reports suggested that MIF may exhibit cardioprotective effect mediated by S-nitrosylation and modulation of the AMP-activated protein kinase (AMPK) following receptor engagement.[207] MIF exerts its effect through a number of receptors and coreceptors depending on the cell type. The surface receptor CD74 (otherwise known as MHC Class II chaperone invariant chain) binds to MIF and the complex recruits CD44 as a coreceptor. This leads to ERK1/2 phosphorylation before signaling ensues.[208] MIF also binds to two noncognate receptors: CXCR2 and CXCR4 chemokine receptors.[199,207]

CARDIAC EXOSOMES AND MIRNA

The exosome is a 50–100 nm lipid nanovesicle released by many cells in response to environmental inducers. The exosome content is determined by the inducer. Exosomal release of HSP 60 by adult cardiac myocyte in vitro, in response to either hypoxia/reoxygenation or alcohol, has been demonstrated.[209] Additionally, exosomes containing αvβ6 integrin isolated from cardiac endothelial cells have been shown to induce bone marrow-derived B cells to release TGF-β in an LPS/TLR4-dependent manner,[210] illustrating a true endocrine effect of the heart. Exosomes released by cardiomyocyte have been demonstrated to contain a number of DNA and miRNA (miR) cargo destined for paracrine and endocrine targets.[211] A large proportion of circulating miRs is probably exosomal.[212] Circulating miR-1, miR-133a, and urine miR-1 and miR-208 have been reported in patients with ACS and AMI, respectively.[211,213,214] In addition, histone deacetylase dependent downregulation of miR-133a is seen experimentally in pressure overloaded mice.[215] Fibroblast-derived miR-21, on the other hand, induces cardiomyocyte hypertrophy,[216] with its overexpression associated with a TGF-β regulatory mechanism in pressure overloaded mice and human patients.[217] Many of the cardiokines discussed in this chapter are affected by multiple miRs,[218] adding yet another dimension to the pathophysiological balance necessary for the "normal" function of the heart. MicroRNA signaling "mircrine"[218] is emerging as an interesting player in such pathophysiological balance both at the local auto/paracrine and distal endocrine scenarios. Moreover, cardiac specific miR208a controls liver and white adipose tissue metabolism through mediator complex subunit (MED)-13 signaling,[219–221] thereby placing the endocrine heart at the "heart" of systemic energy metabolism.

INSIGHT INTO FUTURE DIRECTIONS

Cardiovascular diseases account for more global morbidity and mortality than any other health condition. With the spiraling cost of health care, the burden of disease is set to rise at least for the foreseeable future. The search for effective and viable pharmaceutics is attracting much active research in identifying new therapeutic targets. As more cardiokines are discovered, the list of potential therapeutic targets increases. In past decades, targeting of cardiac fibrosis with anti-TGF-β therapy has given some initial success especially in animal models.[47] Anti-VEGF and anti-TNF-α therapy have also been tried with limited success.[173,222] Targeting the inflammasome, anti-IL-1β, and IL-1R antagonist have emerged as possible therapies too.[223] Recently, small molecule inhibitors of inflammasomes are hailed as possible therapeutic targets with great potential.[224,225] Unfortunately many promising targeted therapies yielded less than the expected success in human probably due to the pleiotropic nature of the cardiokines and their involvement in multiple signaling pathways (Fig. 4.4).[47,226] This apparent signaling "redundancy" is further complicated by the fact that a number of cardiokines are associated with the ECM. The association may create "positional information" directing the "normal" wear and tear of the heart muscle and ensuring "proper" physiological maintenance. In the disease state, however, positional information may be disrupted thus giving rise to inappropriate remodeling of the heart. The fact that MMPs can also proteolytically activate cardiokines such as TGF-β, IL-1β, pro-TNF, and FGFR1[227,228] suggests that any future cardiokine targeted therapy should also include the MMPs and their inhibitors.

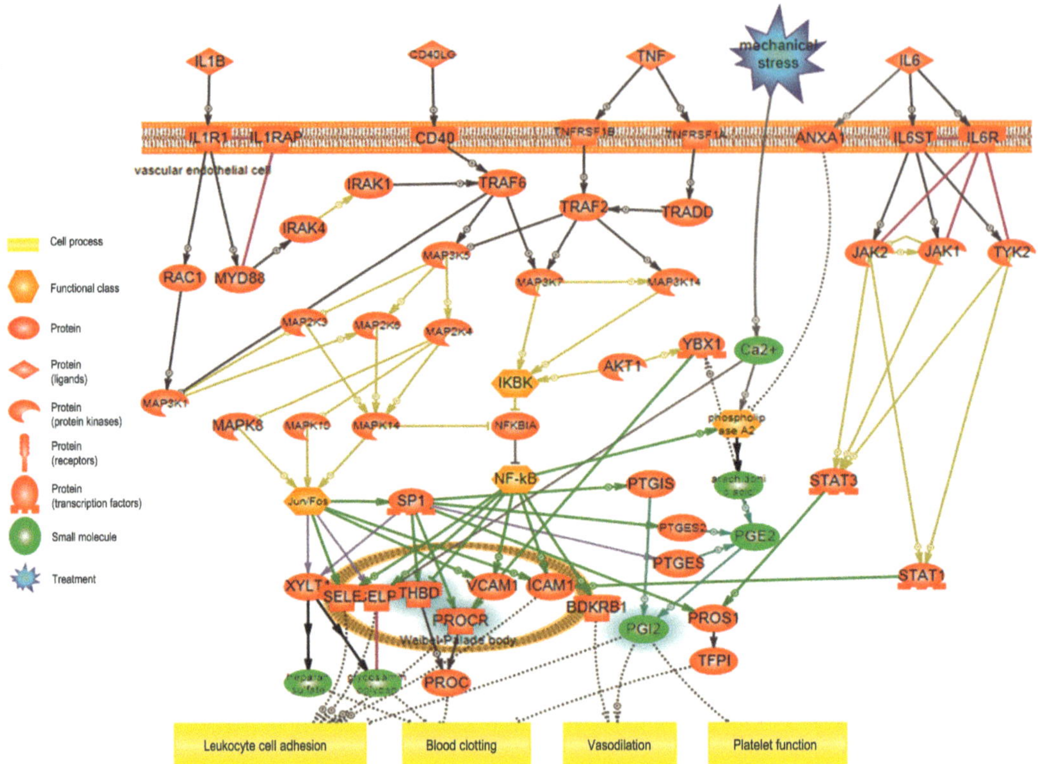

FIGURE 4.4

Cell activation due to sterile inflammation. Exemplified activation of endothelial cells by mediators released during sterile inflammation or mechanical stress. **IL1B** Interleukin-1, beta; **CD40LG** CD40 ligand; **TNF** Tumor necrosis factor-α; **IL6** Interleukin-6 (interferon, beta 2); **IL1R1** Interleukin-1 receptor, type 1; **IL1RAP** Interleukin-1 receptor accessory protein; **CD40** CD40 molecule, TNF receptor superfamily; **TNFRSF1B** Tumor necrosis factor receptor superfamily, member 1A; **ANXA1** Annexin A1; **IL6ST** Interleukin-6 signal transducer (gp130, oncostatin M receptor); **IL6R** Interleukin-6 receptor; **MYD88** Myeloid differentiation primary response 88; **IRAK4** Interleukin-1 receptor-associated kinase 4; **IRAK1** Interleukin-1 receptor-associated kinase 1; **TRAF6** TNF receptor-associated factor 6, E3 ubiquitin protein ligase; **TRAF2** TNF receptor-associated factor 2; **TRADD** TNFRSF1A-associated via death domain; **RAC1** Ras-related C3 botulinum toxin substrate 1 (rho family, small GTP binding protein Rac1); **MAP3K5** Mitogen-activated protein kinase kinase kinase 5; **MAP3K7** Mitogen-activated protein kinase kinase kinase 7; **MAP3K14** Mitogen-activated protein kinase kinase kinase 14; **MAP2K3** Mitogen-activated protein kinase kinase kinase 3; **MAP2K6** Mitogen-activated protein kinase kinase kinase 6; **MAP2K4** Mitogen-activated protein kinase kinase kinase 4; **AKT1** v-act murine thymoma viral oncogene homolog 1; **YBX1** Y box binding protein 1; **MAP3K1** Mitogen-activated protein kinase kinase kinase 1, E3 ubiquitin protein ligase; **MAPK8** Mitogen-activated protein kinase 8; **MAPK10** Mitogen-activated protein kinase 10; **MAPK14** Mitogen-activated protein kinase 14; **NFKBIA** Nuclear factor of kappa light polypeptide gene enhancer in B-cells inhibitor, alpha; **SP1** Sp1 transcription factor; **PTGIS** Prostaglandin I2 (prostacyclin) synthase; **PTGES2** Prostaglandin E synthase 2, **JAK2** Janus kinase 2; **JAK1** Janus kinase 1; **TYK2** Tyrosine kinase 2; **STAT3** Signal transducer and activator of transcription 3 (acute-phase response factor); **STAT1** Signal transducer and activator of transcription 1, 91 kDa; **PTGES** Prostaglandin E synthase; **PROS1** Protein S (alpha); **TFPI** Tissue factor pathway inhibitor (lipoprotein-associated coagulation inhibitor); **XYLT1** Xylosyltransferase 1; **SELE** Selectin E, **SELP** Selectin P (granule membrane protein 140 kDa, antigen CD62); **THBD** Thrombomodulin; **PROCR** Protein C receptor, endothelial; **VCAM1** Vascular cell adhesion molecule 1; **ICAM1** Intercellular adhesion molecule 1; **BDKRB1** Bradykinin receptor B1; **PROC** Protein C (inactivator of coagulation factors Va and VIIIa).

The figure is generated and modified with permission from Pathway Studio®.

ACKNOWLEDGEMENT

The author is indebted to Drs. KS Collison, RS Parhar, W. Conca, MA Quttainah, P Kvietys, MZ Deniro and MB Al-Joufan for their valuable discussions. My gratitude to Ms. CA Touzinte for help in processing this manuscript and Mr. M. Velasco for constructing Fig. 4.1.

REFERENCES

1. Brutsaert DL. Cardiac endothelial-myocardial signaling: its role in cardiac growth, contractile performance, and rhythmicity. *Physiol Rev* 2003;**83**(1):59–115.
2. Nees S, Weiss DR, Juchem G. Focus on cardiac pericytes. *Pflugers Arch* 2013;**465**(6):779–87.
3. Nees S, et al. Isolation, bulk cultivation, and characterization of coronary microvascular pericytes: the second most frequent myocardial cell type in vitro. *Am J Physiol Heart Circ Physiol* 2012;**302**(1): H69–84.
4. Tao L, Wang H, Wang X, Kong X, Li X. Cardiac telocytes. *Curr Stem Cell Res Ther* 2016;**11**(5):404–9.
5. Cretoiu D, et al. Human cardiac telocytes: 3D imaging by FIB-SEM tomography. *J Cell Mol Med* 2014;**18**(11):2157–64.
6. Bei Y, et al. Cardiac telocytes and fibroblasts in primary culture: different morphologies and immunophenotypes. *PLoS One* 2015;**10**(2):e0115991.
7. Zhou Q, et al. Cardiac telocytes are double positive for CD34/PDGFR-alpha. *J Cell Mol Med* 2015;**19**:2036–42.
8. Zhou J, et al. Distribution and characteristics of telocytes as nurse cells in the architectural organization of engineered heart tissues. *Sci China Life Sci* 2014;**57**(2):241–7.
9. Nag AC. Study of non-muscle cells of the adult mammalian heart: a fine structural analysis and distribution. *Cytobios* 1980;**28**(109):41–61.
10. Zak R. Development and proliferative capacity of cardiac muscle cells. *Circ Res* 1974;**35**(2) Suppl. II:17-26.
11. Banerjee I, et al. Determination of cell types and numbers during cardiac development in the neonatal and adult rat and mouse. *Am J Physiol Heart Circ Physiol* 2007;**293**(3):H1883–91.
12. Stewart Jr. JA, et al. Temporal alterations in cardiac fibroblast function following induction of pressure overload. *Cell Tissue Res* 2010;**340**(1):117–26.
13. Wei CC, et al. Cardiac kallikrein-kinin system is upregulated in chronic volume overload and mediates an inflammatory induced collagen loss. *PLoS One* 2012;**7**(6):e40110.
14. Shinde AV, Frangogiannis NG. Fibroblasts in myocardial infarction: a role in inflammation and repair. *J Mol Cell Cardiol* 2014;**70**:74–82.
15. Matsuura K, et al. Cardiomyocytes fuse with surrounding noncardiomyocytes and reenter the cell cycle. *J Cell Biol* 2004;**167**(2):351–63.
16. Matsuyama D, Kawahara K. Maintenance and characterization of spontaneous contraction rhythm in cultured cardiac myocytes fused with cardiac fibroblasts. *Biosystems* 2008;**92**(3):226–32.
17. Evans SM, et al. Heterokaryons of cardiac myocytes and fibroblasts reveal the lack of dominance of the cardiac muscle phenotype. *Mol Cell Biol* 1994;**14**(6):4269–79.
18. Smyrnias I, et al. Comparison of the T-tubule system in adult rat ventricular and atrial myocytes, and its role in excitation-contraction coupling and inotropic stimulation. *Cell Calcium* 2010;**47**(3):210–23.
19. Bootman MD, et al. Atrial cardiomyocyte calcium signalling. *Biochim Biophys Acta* 2011;**1813**(5):922–34.
20. Hasegawa K, et al. Ventricular expression of atrial and brain natriuretic peptides in dilated cardiomyopathy. An immunohistocytochemical study of the endomyocardial biopsy specimens using specific monoclonal antibodies. *Am J Pathol* 1993;**142**(1):107–16.

21. Navaratnam V. Atrial dpecific granules *Heart muscle: ultrastructural studies*. Cambridge, New York, New Rochelle, Melbourne, Sydney: Cambridge University Press; 1987. p. 120–38.
22. Anversa P, et al. Stereological measurement of cellular and subcellular hypertrophy and hyperplasia in the papillary muscle of adult rat. *J Mol Cell Cardiol* 1980;**12**(8):781–95.
23. Kostin S. Myocardial telocytes: a specific new cellular entity. *J Cell Mol Med* 2010;**14**(7):1917–21.
24. Gherghiceanu M, Popescu LM. Cardiac telocytes-their junctions and functional implications. *Cell Tissue Res* 2012;**348**(2):265–79.
25. Saburkina I, et al. Morphological pattern of intrinsic nerve plexus distributed on the rabbit heart and interatrial septum. *J Anat* 2014;**224**(5):583–93.
26. Rysevaite K, et al. Immunohistochemical characterization of the intrinsic cardiac neural plexus in whole-mount mouse heart preparations. *Heart Rhythm* 2011;**8**(5):731–8.
27. Baptista CA, Kirby ML. The cardiac ganglia: cellular and molecular aspects. *Kaohsiung J Med Sci* 1997;**13**(1):42–54.
28. Fregoso SP, Hoover DB. Development of cardiac parasympathetic neurons, glial cells, and regional cholinergic innervation of the mouse heart. *Neuroscience* 2012;**221**:28–36.
29. Singh S, et al. Hypertrophy of neurons within cardiac ganglia in human, canine, and rat heart failure: the potential role of nerve growth factor. *J Am Heart Assoc* 2013;**2**(4):e000210.
30. Shirani J, Berezowski K, Roberts WC. Quantitative measurement of normal and excessive (cor adiposum) subepicardial adipose tissue, its clinical significance, and its effect on electrocardiographic QRS voltage. *Am J Cardiol* 1995;**76**(5):414–8.
31. Rabkin SW. Epicardial fat: properties, function and relationship to obesity. *Obes Rev* 2007;**8**(3):253–61.
32. Samanta R, et al. Role of adipose tissue in the pathogenesis of cardiac arrhythmias. *Heart Rhythm* 2015.
33. Frangogiannis NG, et al. Resident cardiac mast cells degranulate and release preformed TNF-alpha, initiating the cytokine cascade in experimental canine myocardial ischemia/reperfusion. *Circulation* 1998;**98**(7):699–710.
34. Epelman S, Liu PP, Mann DL. Role of innate and adaptive immune mechanisms in cardiac injury and repair. *Nat Rev Immunol* 2015;**15**(2):117–29.
35. Epelman S, et al. Embryonic and adult-derived resident cardiac macrophages are maintained through distinct mechanisms at steady state and during inflammation. *Immunity* 2014;**40**(1):91–104.
36. Choi JH, et al. Identification of antigen-presenting dendritic cells in mouse aorta and cardiac valves. *J Exp Med* 2009;**206**(3):497–505.
37. Zouggari Y, et al. B lymphocytes trigger monocyte mobilization and impair heart function after acute myocardial infarction. *Nat Med* 2013;**19**(10):1273–80.
38. Quttainah M, et al. Progression of matrixin and cardiokine expression patterns in an ovine model of heart failure and recovery. *Int J Cardiol* 2015;**186**:77–89.
39. Eghbali M, et al. Localization of types I, III and IV collagen mRNAs in rat heart cells by in situ hybridization. *J Mol Cell Cardiol* 1989;**21**(1):103–13.
40. Mihl C, Dassen WR, Kuipers H. Cardiac remodelling: concentric versus eccentric hypertrophy in strength and endurance athletes. *Neth Heart J* 2008;**16**(4):129–33.
41. Iyer SS, et al. Necrotic cells trigger a sterile inflammatory response through the Nlrp3 inflammasome. *Proc Natl Acad Sci USA* 2009;**106**(48):20388–93.
42. Fang L, et al. Systemic inflammatory response following acute myocardial infarction. *J Geriatr Cardiol* 2015;**12**(3):305–12.
43. Huang ZG, et al. Myocardial remodeling in diabetic cardiomyopathy associated with cardiac mast cell activation. *PLoS One* 2013;**8**(3):e60827.
44. Clarke MS, et al. Contraction-induced cell wounding and release of fibroblast growth factor in heart. *Circ Res* 1995;**76**(6):927–34.

45. Gardner DG, et al. Endothelin increases the synthesis and secretion of atrial natriuretic peptide in neonatal rat cardiocytes. *Am J Physiol* 1991;**261**(2 Pt 1):E177–82.
46. Frangogiannis NG, Smith CW, Entman ML. The inflammatory response in myocardial infarction. *Cardiovasc Res* 2002;**53**(1):31–47.
47. Frangogiannis NG. The inflammatory response in myocardial injury, repair, and remodelling. *Nat Rev Cardiol* 2014;**11**(5):255–65.
48. Madorin WS, et al. Cardiac myocytes activated by septic plasma promote neutrophil transendothelial migration: role of platelet-activating factor and the chemokines LIX and KC. *Circ Res* 2004;**94**(7):944–51.
49. Yang M, et al. Important role of p38 MAP kinase/NF-kappaB signaling pathway in the sepsis-induced conversion of cardiac myocytes to a proinflammatory phenotype. *Am J Physiol Heart Circ Physiol* 2008;**294**(2):H994–1001.
50. Xu H, et al. The alarmin cytokine, high mobility group box 1, is produced by viable cardiomyocytes and mediates the lipopolysaccharide-induced myocardial dysfunction via a TLR4/phosphatidylinositol 3-kinase gamma pathway. *J Immunol* 2010;**184**(3):1492–8.
51. Doroudgar S, Glembotski CC. The cardiokine story unfolds: ischemic stress-induced protein secretion in the heart. *Trends Mol Med* 2011;**17**(4):207–14.
52. Shimano M, Ouchi N, Walsh K. Cardiokines: recent progress in elucidating the cardiac secretome. *Circulation* 2012;**126**(21):e327–32.
53. Kempf T, et al. The transforming growth factor-beta superfamily member growth-differentiation factor-15 protects the heart from ischemia/reperfusion injury. *Circ Res* 2006;**98**(3):351–60.
54. Horiguchi M, Ota M, Rifkin DB. Matrix control of transforming growth factor-beta function. *J Biochem* 2012;**152**(4):321–9.
55. Zhang WQ, et al. Lipopolysaccharide induced activin A-follistatin imbalance affects cardiac fibrosis. *Chin Med J (Engl)* 2012;**125**(12):2205–12.
56. Bootcov MR, et al. MIC-1, a novel macrophage inhibitory cytokine, is a divergent member of the TGF-beta superfamily. *Proc Natl Acad Sci USA* 1997;**94**(21):11514–9.
57. Nakajima Y, et al. Extracellular fibrillar structure of latent TGF beta binding protein-1: role in TGF beta-dependent endothelial-mesenchymal transformation during endocardial cushion tissue formation in mouse embryonic heart. *J Cell Biol* 1997;**136**(1):193–204.
58. Dobaczewski M, Chen W, Frangogiannis NG. Transforming growth factor (TGF)-beta signaling in cardiac remodeling. *J Mol Cell Cardiol* 2011;**51**(4):600–6.
59. Gomperts B, Kramer L, Tatham P. Signalling through receptor bound protein serine/threonine kinases *Signal transduction*. San Diego San Francisco New York Boston London Sydney Tokyo: Academic Press; 2002. p. 359–71.
60. Heldin CH, Miyazono K, ten Dijke P. TGF-beta signalling from cell membrane to nucleus through SMAD proteins. *Nature* 1997;**390**(6659):465–71.
61. Ramos-Mondragon R, Galindo CA, Avila G. Role of TGF-beta on cardiac structural and electrical remodeling. *Vasc Health Risk Manag* 2008;**4**(6):1289–300.
62. Zhang W, et al. Necrotic myocardial cells release damage-associated molecular patterns that provoke fibroblast activation in vitro and trigger myocardial inflammation and fibrosis in vivo. *J Am Heart Assoc* 2015;**4**(6):e001993.
63. Edgley AJ, Krum H, Kelly DJ. Targeting fibrosis for the treatment of heart failure: a role for transforming growth factor-beta. *Cardiovasc Ther* 2012;**30**(1):e30–40.
64. Ayca B, et al. Increased transforming growth factor-beta levels associated with cardiac adverse events in hypertrophic cardiomyopathy. *Clin Cardiol* 2015;**38**(6):371–7.
65. Bujak M, Frangogiannis NG. The role of TGF-beta signaling in myocardial infarction and cardiac remodeling. *Cardiovasc Res* 2007;**74**(2):184–95.

66. Euler G. Good and bad sides of TGFbeta-signaling in myocardial infarction. *Front Physiol* 2015;**6**:66.
67. Rainer PP, et al. Cardiomyocyte-specific transforming growth factor beta suppression blocks neutrophil infiltration, augments multiple cytoprotective cascades, and reduces early mortality after myocardial infarction. *Circ Res* 2014;**114**(8):1246–57.
68. Vivar R, et al. TGF-beta1 prevents simulated ischemia/reperfusion-induced cardiac fibroblast apoptosis by activation of both canonical and non-canonical signaling pathways. *Biochim Biophys Acta* 2013;**1832**(6):754–62.
69. Gong K, et al. Transforming growth factor-beta inhibits myocardial PPARgamma expression in pressure overload-induced cardiac fibrosis and remodeling in mice. *J Hypertens* 2011;**29**(9):1810–9.
70. Koitabashi N, et al. Pivotal role of cardiomyocyte TGF-beta signaling in the murine pathological response to sustained pressure overload. *J Clin Invest* 2011;**121**(6):2301–12.
71. Kawano H, et al. Angiotensin II has multiple profibrotic effects in human cardiac fibroblasts. *Circulation* 2000;**101**(10):1130–7.
72. van Wamel AJ, et al. Stretch-induced paracrine hypertrophic stimuli increase TGF-beta1 expression in cardiomyocytes. *Mol Cell Biochem* 2002;**236**(1-2):147–53.
73. Watson CJ, et al. Extracellular matrix sub-types and mechanical stretch impact human cardiac fibroblast responses to transforming growth factor beta. *Connect Tissue Res* 2014;**55**(3):248–56.
74. MacKenna D, Summerour SR, Villarreal FJ. Role of mechanical factors in modulating cardiac fibroblast function and extracellular matrix synthesis. *Cardiovasc Res* 2000;**46**(2):257–63.
75. Chen C, et al. Serum TGF-beta1 and SMAD3 levels are closely associated with coronary artery disease. *BMC Cardiovasc Disord* 2014;**14**:18.
76. Fedulov AV, et al. Serum TGF-beta 1 and TNF-alpha levels and cardiac fibrosis in experimental chronic renal failure. *Immunol Invest* 2005;**34**(2):143–52.
77. Holmes DI, Zachary I. The vascular endothelial growth factor (VEGF) family: angiogenic factors in health and disease. *Genome Biol* 2005;**6**(2):209.
78. Ibelgaufts H. Cytokine & cell online pathefinder encyclopedia. In: Ibelgaufts H, editor. COPE; 2012.
79. Hoeben A, et al. Vascular endothelial growth factor and angiogenesis. *Pharmacol Rev* 2004;**56**(4):549–80.
80. Wu LW, et al. VRAP is an adaptor protein that binds KDR, a receptor for vascular endothelial cell growth factor. *J Biol Chem* 2000;**275**(9):6059–62.
81. Warner AJ, et al. The Shc-related adaptor protein, Sck, forms a complex with the vascular-endothelial-growth-factor receptor KDR in transfected cells. *Biochem J* 2000;**347**(Pt 2):501–9.
82. Takahashi T, et al. A single autophosphorylation site on KDR/Flk-1 is essential for VEGF-A-dependent activation of PLC-gamma and DNA synthesis in vascular endothelial cells. *EMBO J* 2001;**20**(11):2768–78.
83. Shi X, et al. TGF-beta/Smad3 inhibit vascular smooth muscle cell apoptosis through an autocrine signaling mechanism involving VEGF-A. *Cell Death Dis* 2014;**5**:e1317.
84. Tsoporis JN, et al. S100B-RAGE dependent VEGF secretion by cardiac myocytes induces myofibroblast proliferation. *J Mol Cell Cardiol* 2012;**52**(2):464–73.
85. Sung HK, et al. Adipose vascular endothelial growth factor regulates metabolic homeostasis through angiogenesis. *Cell Metab* 2013;**17**(1):61–72.
86. Cho M, Hunt TK, Hussain MZ. Hydrogen peroxide stimulates macrophage vascular endothelial growth factor release. *Am J Physiol Heart Circ Physiol* 2001;**280**(5):H2357–63.
87. Albulescu R, et al. The secretome of myocardial telocytes modulates the activity of cardiac stem cells. *J Cell Mol Med* 2015;**19**(8):1783–94.
88. Yla-Herttuala S, et al. Vascular endothelial growth factors: biology and current status of clinical applications in cardiovascular medicine. *J Am Coll Cardiol* 2007;**49**(10):1015–26.
89. Barleon B, et al. Migration of human monocytes in response to vascular endothelial growth factor (VEGF) is mediated via the VEGF receptor flt-1. *Blood* 1996;**87**(8):3336–43.

90. Wang H, Keiser JA. Vascular endothelial growth factor upregulates the expression of matrix metalloproteinases in vascular smooth muscle cells: role of flt-1. *Circ Res* 1998;**83**(8):832–40.
91. Taimeh Z, et al. Vascular endothelial growth factor in heart failure. *Nat Rev Cardiol* 2013;**10**(9):519–30.
92. Jelkmann W. Pitfalls in the measurement of circulating vascular endothelial growth factor. *Clin Chem* 2001;**47**(4):617–23.
93. Kakizawa H, et al. The relationship between glycemic control and plasma vascular endothelial growth factor and endothelin-1 concentration in diabetic patients. *Metabolism* 2004;**53**(5):550–5.
94. Oltmanns KM, et al. Divergent effects of hyper- and hypoglycemia on circulating vascular endothelial growth factor in humans. *Metabolism* 2008;**57**(1):90–4.
95. Tilton RG, et al. Vascular dysfunction induced by elevated glucose levels in rats is mediated by vascular endothelial growth factor. *J Clin Invest* 1997;**99**(9):2192–202.
96. Wu LE, et al. Systemic VEGF-A neutralization ameliorates diet-induced metabolic dysfunction. *Diabetes* 2014;**63**(8):2656–67.
97. Arakawa H, et al. Decreased serum vascular endothelial growth factor concentrations in patients with congestive heart failure. *Heart* 2003;**89**(2):207–8.
98. Hojo Y, et al. Expression of vascular endothelial growth factor in patients with acute myocardial infarction. *J Am Coll Cardiol* 2000;**35**(4):968–73.
99. Ornitz DM, Itoh N. Fibroblast growth factors. *Genome Biol* 2001;**2**(3): REVIEWS3005.
100. Beenken A, Mohammadi M. The FGF family: biology, pathophysiology and therapy. *Nat Rev Drug Discov* 2009;**8**(3):235–53.
101. Itoh N, Ornitz DM. Evolution of the Fgf and Fgfr gene families. *Trends Genet* 2004;**20**(11):563–9.
102. Detillieux KA, et al. Biological activities of fibroblast growth factor-2 in the adult myocardium. *Cardiovasc Res* 2003;**57**(1):8–19.
103. Kardami E, et al. Fibroblast growth factor 2 isoforms and cardiac hypertrophy. *Cardiovasc Res* 2004;**63**(3):458–66.
104. Lu SY, et al. FGF-16 is released from neonatal cardiac myocytes and alters growth-related signaling: a possible role in postnatal development. *Am J Physiol Cell Physiol* 2008;**294**(5):C1242–9.
105. Kaye D, et al. Role of transiently altered sarcolemmal membrane permeability and basic fibroblast growth factor release in the hypertrophic response of adult rat ventricular myocytes to increased mechanical activity in vitro. *J Clin Invest* 1996;**97**(2):281–91.
106. Santiago JJ, et al. High molecular weight fibroblast growth factor-2 in the human heart is a potential target for prevention of cardiac remodeling. *PLoS One* 2014;**9**(5):e97281.
107. Svystonyuk DA, et al. Fibroblast growth factor-2 regulates human cardiac myofibroblast-mediated extracellular matrix remodeling. *J Transl Med* 2015;**13**:147.
108. Sontag DP, et al. FGF-2 and FGF-16 protect isolated perfused mouse hearts from acute doxorubicin-induced contractile dysfunction. *Cardiovasc Toxicol* 2013;**13**(3):244–53.
109. Wang J, Sontag D, Cattini PA. Heart-specific expression of FGF-16 and a potential role in postnatal cardioprotection. *Cytokine Growth Factor Rev* 2015;**26**(1):59–66.
110. McPhee JB, Schertzer JD. Immunometabolism of obesity and diabetes: microbiota link compartmentalized immunity in the gut to metabolic tissue inflammation. *Clin Sci (Lond)* 2015;**129**(12):1083–96.
111. Perez-Ruiz F, Becker MA. Inflammation: a possible mechanism for a causative role of hyperuricemia/gout in cardiovascular disease. *Curr Med Res Opin* 2015;**31**(Suppl. 2):9–14.
112. Cutolo M, Paolino S, Pizzorni C. Possible contribution of chronic inflammation in the induction of cancer in rheumatic diseases. *Clin Exp Rheumatol* 2014;**32**(6):839–47.
113. Bonaventura P, et al. Zinc and its role in immunity and inflammation. *Autoimmun Rev* 2015;**14**(4):277–85.
114. Rahman A, et al. Malnutrition and cachexia in heart failure. *JPEN J Parenter Enteral Nutr* 2015.
115. Garg NJ. Inflammasomes in cardiovascular diseases. *Am J Cardiovasc Dis* 2011;**1**(3):244–54.

116. Monie TP, Bryant CE, Gay NJ. Activating immunity: lessons from the TLRs and NLRs. *Trends Biochem Sci* 2009;**34**(11):553–61.
117. Kaparakis M, Philpott DJ, Ferrero RL. Mammalian NLR proteins; discriminating foe from friend. *Immunol Cell Biol* 2007;**85**(6):495–502.
118. Walsh JG, Muruve DA, Power C. Inflammasomes in the CNS. *Nat Rev Neurosci* 2014;**15**(2):84–97.
119. Butts B, et al. The importance of NLRP3 inflammasome in heart failure. *J Card Fail* 2015;**21**(7):586–93.
120. Guo H, Callaway JB, Ting JP. Inflammasomes: mechanism of action, role in disease, and therapeutics. *Nat Med* 2015;**21**(7):677–87.
121. Lu A, Wu H. Structural mechanisms of inflammasome assembly. *FEBS J* 2015;**282**(3):435–44.
122. Kanneganti TD. Central roles of NLRs and inflammasomes in viral infection. *Nat Rev Immunol* 2010;**10**(10):688–98.
123. Davis BK, Wen H, Ting JP. The inflammasome NLRs in immunity, inflammation, and associated diseases. *Annu Rev Immunol* 2011;**29**:707–35.
124. Guarda G, So A. Regulation of inflammasome activity. *Immunology* 2010;**130**(3):329–36.
125. Land WG. The role of damage-associated molecular patterns in human diseases: part I-promoting inflammation and immunity. *Sultan Qaboos Univ Med J* 2015;**15**(1):e9–e21.
126. Land WG. The role of damage-associated molecular patterns (DAMPs) in human diseases: part II: DAMPs as diagnostics, prognostics and therapeutics in clinical medicine. *Sultan Qaboos Univ Med J* 2015;**15**(2):e157–70.
127. Chen GY, Nunez G. Sterile inflammation: sensing and reacting to damage. *Nat Rev Immunol* 2010;**10**(12):826–37.
128. Mezzaroma E, et al. The inflammasome promotes adverse cardiac remodeling following acute myocardial infarction in the mouse. *Proc Natl Acad Sci U S A* 2011;**108**(49):19725–30.
129. Bracey NA, et al. The Nlrp3 inflammasome promotes myocardial dysfunction in structural cardiomyopathy through interleukin-1beta. *Exp Physiol* 2013;**98**(2):462–72.
130. Yin Y, et al. Inflammasomes are differentially expressed in cardiovascular and other tissues. *Int J Immunopathol Pharmacol* 2009;**22**(2):311–22.
131. Toldo S, et al. Independent roles of the priming and the triggering of the NLRP3 inflammasome in the heart. *Cardiovasc Res* 2015;**105**(2):203–12.
132. Liao KC, Mogridge J. Activation of the Nlrp1b inflammasome by reduction of cytosolic ATP. *Infect Immun* 2013;**81**(2):570–9.
133. Thompson JG, et al. Effect of inhibitors and uncouplers of oxidative phosphorylation during compaction and blastulation of bovine embryos cultured in vitro. *J Reprod Fertil* 2000;**118**(1):47–55.
134. Wenceslau CF, et al. Mitochondrial damage-associated molecular patterns and vascular function. *Eur Heart J* 2014;**35**(18):1172–7.
135. Zhang Q, et al. Circulating mitochondrial DAMPs cause inflammatory responses to injury. *Nature* 2010;**464**(7285):104–7.
136. Murphy MP. How mitochondria produce reactive oxygen species. *Biochem J* 2009;**417**(1):1–13.
137. Nakai A, et al. The role of autophagy in cardiomyocytes in the basal state and in response to hemodynamic stress. *Nat Med* 2007;**13**(5):619–24.
138. Oka T, et al. Mitochondrial DNA that escapes from autophagy causes inflammation and heart failure. *Nature* 2012;**485**(7397):251–5.
139. Marchi S, Patergnani S, Pinton P. The endoplasmic reticulum-mitochondria connection: one touch, multiple functions. *Biochim Biophys Acta* 2014;**1837**(4):461–9.
140. Raturi A, Simmen T. Where the endoplasmic reticulum and the mitochondrion tie the knot: the mitochondria-associated membrane (MAM). *Biochim Biophys Acta* 2013;**1833**(1):213–24.
141. Bhandary B, et al. An involvement of oxidative stress in endoplasmic reticulum stress and its associated diseases. *Int J Mol Sci* 2012;**14**(1):434–56.

142. Grimm S. The ER-mitochondria interface: the social network of cell death. *Biochim Biophys Acta* 2012;**1823**(2):327–34.
143. Kuba M, et al. Bidirectional Ca2+ coupling of mitochondria with the endoplasmic reticulum and regulation of multimodal Ca2+ entries in rat brown adipocytes. *Am J Physiol Cell Physiol* 2007;**292**(2):C896–908.
144. de la Fuente S, et al. Ca2+ homeostasis in the endoplasmic reticulum measured with a new low-Ca2+ -affinity targeted aequorin. *Cell Calcium* 2013;**54**(1):37–45.
145. Brookes PS, et al. Calcium, ATP, and ROS: a mitochondrial love-hate triangle. *Am J Physiol Cell Physiol* 2004;**287**(4):C817–33.
146. Sorbara MT, Girardin SE. Mitochondrial ROS fuel the inflammasome. *Cell Res* 2011;**21**(4):558–60.
147. Zhou R, et al. A role for mitochondria in NLRP3 inflammasome activation. *Nature* 2011;**469**(7329):221–5.
148. Menu P, et al. ER stress activates the NLRP3 inflammasome via an UPR-independent pathway. *Cell Death Dis* 2012;**3**:e261.
149. Murakami T, et al. Critical role for calcium mobilization in activation of the NLRP3 inflammasome. *Proc Natl Acad Sci U S A* 2012;**109**(28):11282–7.
150. Katsnelson MA, et al. K+ efflux agonists induce NLRP3 inflammasome activation independently of Ca2+ signaling. *J Immunol* 2015;**194**(8):3937–52.
151. Petrilli V, et al. Activation of the NALP3 inflammasome is triggered by low intracellular potassium concentration. *Cell Death Differ* 2007;**14**(9):1583–9.
152. Munoz-Planillo R, et al. K(+) efflux is the common trigger of NLRP3 inflammasome activation by bacterial toxins and particulate matter. *Immunity* 2013;**38**(6):1142–53.
153. Miller AM. Role of IL-33 in inflammation and disease. *J Inflamm (Lond)* 2011;**8**(1):22.
154. Sanada S, et al. IL-33 and ST2 comprise a critical biomechanically induced and cardioprotective signaling system. *J Clin Invest* 2007;**117**(6):1538–49.
155. Garlanda C, Dinarello CA, Mantovani A. The interleukin-1 family: back to the future. *Immunity* 2013;**39**(6):1003–18.
156. Lugrin J, et al. Cutting edge: IL-1alpha is a crucial danger signal triggering acute myocardial inflammation during myocardial infarction. *J Immunol* 2015;**194**(2):499–503.
157. Vicenova B, et al. Emerging role of interleukin-1 in cardiovascular diseases. *Physiol Res* 2009;**58**(4):481–98.
158. Honsho S, et al. Pressure-mediated hypertrophy and mechanical stretch induces IL-1 release and subsequent IGF-1 generation to maintain compensative hypertrophy by affecting Akt and JNK pathways. *Circ Res* 2009;**105**(11):1149–58.
159. Pinto AR, Godwin JW, Rosenthal NA. Macrophages in cardiac homeostasis, injury responses and progenitor cell mobilisation. *Stem Cell Res* 2014;**13**(3 Pt B):705–14.
160. Toldo S, et al. Interleukin-18 mediates interleukin-1-induced cardiac dysfunction. *Am J Physiol Heart Circ Physiol* 2014;**306**(7):H1025–31.
161. Van Tassell BW, et al. Interleukin-1beta induces a reversible cardiomyopathy in the mouse. *Inflamm Res* 2013;**62**(7):637–40.
162. Mallat Z, et al. Evidence for altered interleukin 18 (IL)-18 pathway in human heart failure. *FASEB J* 2004;**18**(14):1752–4.
163. Demyanets S, et al. Components of the interleukin-33/ST2 system are differentially expressed and regulated in human cardiac cells and in cells of the cardiac vasculature. *J Mol Cell Cardiol* 2013;**60**:16–26.
164. Kunes P, et al. Actual position of interleukin(IL)-33 in atherosclerosis and heart failure: great expectations or En attendant Godot? *Perfusion* 2015;**30**(5):356–74.
165. Hedayat M, et al. Proinflammatory cytokines in heart failure: double-edged swords. *Heart Fail Rev* 2010;**15**(6):543–62.
166. Wollert KC, Drexler H. The role of interleukin-6 in the failing heart. *Heart Fail Rev* 2001;**6**(2):95–103.
167. Plenz G, et al. The interleukin-6/interleukin-6-receptor system is activated in donor hearts. *J Am Coll Cardiol* 2002;**39**(9):1508–12.

168. Szabo-Fresnais N, et al. A new regulation of IL-6 production in adult cardiomyocytes by beta-adrenergic and IL-1 beta receptors and induction of cellular hypertrophy by IL-6 trans-signalling. *Cell Signal* 2010;**22**(7):1143–52.
169. Huang M, et al. Urocortin induces interleukin-6 release from rat cardiomyocytes through p38 MAP kinase, ERK and NF-kappaB activation. *J Mol Endocrinol* 2009;**42**(5):397–405.
170. Roncon-Albuquerque RJ, et al. Activation profile of pro-inflammatory cytokines in acute cardiac overload. *Rev Port Cardiol* 2005;**24**(11):1369–78.
171. Roncon-Albuquerque Jr. R, et al. Acute changes of biventricular gene expression in volume and right ventricular pressure overload. *Life Sci* 2006;**78**(22):2633–42.
172. Sun M, et al. Tumor necrosis factor-alpha mediates cardiac remodeling and ventricular dysfunction after pressure overload state. *Circulation* 2007;**115**(11):1398–407.
173. Padfield GJ, et al. Cardiovascular effects of tumour necrosis factor alpha antagonism in patients with acute myocardial infarction: a first in human study. *Heart* 2013;**99**(18):1330–5.
174. Mann DL, et al. Targeted anticytokine therapy in patients with chronic heart failure: results of the Randomized Etanercept Worldwide Evaluation (RENEWAL). *Circulation* 2004;**109**(13):1594–602.
175. Vishnevetsky D, Kiyanista VA, Gandhi PJ. CD40 ligand: a novel target in the fight against cardiovascular disease. *Ann Pharmacother* 2004;**38**(9):1500–8.
176. Choi WS, Jeon OH, Kim DS. CD40 ligand shedding is regulated by interaction between matrix metalloproteinase-2 and platelet integrin alpha(IIb)beta(3). *J Thromb Haemost* 2010;**8**(6):1364–71.
177. Elgueta R, et al. Molecular mechanism and function of CD40/CD40L engagement in the immune system. *Immunol Rev* 2009;**229**(1):152–72.
178. Pamukcu B, et al. The CD40-CD40L system in cardiovascular disease. *Ann Med* 2011;**43**(5):331–40.
179. Ueland T, et al. Soluble CD40 ligand in acute and chronic heart failure. *Eur Heart J* 2005;**26**(11):1101–7.
180. Glembotski CC, et al. Mesencephalic astrocyte-derived neurotrophic factor protects the heart from ischemic damage and is selectively secreted upon sarco/endoplasmic reticulum calcium depletion. *J Biol Chem* 2012;**287**(31):25893–904.
181. Li W, Sama AE, Wang H. Role of HMGB1 in cardiovascular diseases. *Curr Opin Pharmacol* 2006;**6**(2):130–5.
182. Billings PC, et al. Characterization of high mobility group protein binding to cisplatin-damaged DNA. *Biochem Biophys Res Commun* 1992;**188**(3):1286–94.
183. Reeves R. High mobility group (HMG) proteins: modulators of chromatin structure and DNA repair in mammalian cells. *DNA Repair (Amst)* 2015;**36**:122–36.
184. Li Y, et al. FIP200 is involved in murine pseudomonas infection by regulating HMGB1 intracellular translocation. *Cell Physiol Biochem* 2014;**33**(6):1733–44.
185. Huttunen HJ, Rauvala H. Amphoterin as an extracellular regulator of cell motility: from discovery to disease. *J Intern Med* 2004;**255**(3):351–66.
186. Klune JR, et al. HMGB1: endogenous danger signaling. *Mol Med* 2008;**14**(7–8):476–84.
187. Tang D, et al. High-mobility group box 1 is essential for mitochondrial quality control. *Cell Metab* 2011;**13**(6):701–11.
188. Anzai T. Post-infarction inflammation and left ventricular remodeling: a double-edged sword. *Circ J* 2013;**77**(3):580–7.
189. Li LC, et al. High-mobility group box 1 mediates epithelial-to-mesenchymal transition in pulmonary fibrosis involving transforming growth factor-beta1/Smad2/3 signaling. *J Pharmacol Exp Ther* 2015;**354**(3):302–9.
190. Liu Y, et al. Hypoxia induced HMGB1 and mitochondrial DNA interactions mediate tumor growth in hepatocellular carcinoma through toll-like receptor 9. *J Hepatol* 2015;**63**(1):114–21.
191. Tang D, et al. Endogenous HMGB1 regulates autophagy. *J Cell Biol* 2010;**190**(5):881–92.

192. Zhu X, et al. Cytosolic HMGB1 controls the cellular autophagy/apoptosis checkpoint during inflammation. *J Clin Invest* 2015;**125**(3):1098–110.
193. Gdynia G, et al. Danger signaling protein HMGB1 induces a distinct form of cell death accompanied by formation of giant mitochondria. *Cancer Res* 2010;**70**(21):8558–68.
194. Zhang L, et al. Extracellular high-mobility group box 1 mediates pressure overload-induced cardiac hypertrophy and heart failure. *J Cell Mol Med* 2015.
195. Bangert A, et al. Critical role of RAGE and HMGB1 in inflammatory heart disease. *Proc Natl Acad Sci U S A* 2015.
196. Kohno T, et al. Role of high-mobility group box 1 protein in post-infarction healing process and left ventricular remodelling. *Cardiovasc Res* 2009;**81**(3):565–73.
197. Liu T, et al. Increased serum HMGB1 level may predict the fatal outcomes in patients with chronic heart failure. *Int J Cardiol* 2015;**184**:318–20.
198. Yan XX, et al. Increased serum HMGB1 level is associated with coronary artery disease in nondiabetic and type 2 diabetic patients. *Atherosclerosis* 2009;**205**(2):544–8.
199. Zernecke A, Bernhagen J, Weber C. Macrophage migration inhibitory factor in cardiovascular disease. *Circulation* 2008;**117**(12):1594–602.
200. Takahashi M, et al. Elevation of plasma levels of macrophage migration inhibitory factor in patients with acute myocardial infarction. *Am J Cardiol* 2002;**89**(2):248–9.
201. Chuang CC, et al. Macrophage migration inhibitory factor regulates interleukin-6 production by facilitating nuclear factor-kappa B activation during *Vibrio vulnificus* infection. *BMC Immunol* 2010;**11**:50.
202. Das R, et al. Macrophage migration inhibitory factor (MIF) is a critical mediator of the innate immune response to Mycobacterium tuberculosis. *Proc Natl Acad Sci U S A* 2013;**110**(32):E2997–3006.
203. Cheng Q, et al. Macrophage migration inhibitory factor increases leukocyte-endothelial interactions in human endothelial cells via promotion of expression of adhesion molecules. *J Immunol* 2010;**185**(2):1238–47.
204. Takahashi M, et al. Macrophage migration inhibitory factor as a redox-sensitive cytokine in cardiac myocytes. *Cardiovasc Res* 2001;**52**(3):438–45.
205. Qi D, et al. Cardiac macrophage migration inhibitory factor inhibits JNK pathway activation and injury during ischemia/reperfusion. *J Clin Invest* 2009;**119**(12):3807–16.
206. White DA, et al. Differential roles of cardiac and leukocyte derived macrophage migration inhibitory factor in inflammatory responses and cardiac remodelling post myocardial infarction. *J Mol Cell Cardiol* 2014;**69**:32–42.
207. Rassaf T, Weber C, Bernhagen J. Macrophage migration inhibitory factor in myocardial ischaemia/reperfusion injury. *Cardiovasc Res* 2014;**102**(2):321–8.
208. Grieb G, et al. MIF and CD74-suitability as clinical biomarkers. *Mini Rev Med Chem* 2014;**14**(14):1125–31.
209. Malik ZA, et al. Cardiac myocyte exosomes: stability, HSP60, and proteomics. *Am J Physiol Heart Circ Physiol* 2013;**304**(7):H954–65.
210. Song J, et al. Cardiac endothelial cell-derived exosomes induce specific regulatory B cells. *Sci Rep* 2014;**4**:7583.
211. Zhao W, Zheng XL, Zhao SP. Exosome and its roles in cardiovascular diseases. *Heart Fail Rev* 2015;**20**(3):337–48.
212. Gallo A, et al. The majority of microRNAs detectable in serum and saliva is concentrated in exosomes. *PLoS One* 2012;**7**(3):e30679.
213. Kuwabara Y, et al. Increased microRNA-1 and microRNA-133a levels in serum of patients with cardiovascular disease indicate myocardial damage. *Circ Cardiovasc Genet* 2011;**4**(4):446–54.
214. Cheng Y, et al. A translational study of urine miRNAs in acute myocardial infarction. *J Mol Cell Cardiol* 2012;**53**(5):668–76.
215. Renaud L, et al. HDACs regulate miR-133a expression in pressure overload induced cardiac fibrosis. *Circ Heart Fail* 2015.

216. Bang C, et al. Cardiac fibroblast-derived microRNA passenger strand-enriched exosomes mediate cardiomyocyte hypertrophy. *J Clin Invest* 2014;**124**(5):2136–46.
217. Garcia R, et al. p-SMAD2/3 and DICER promote pre-miR-21 processing during pressure overload-associated myocardial remodeling. *Biochim Biophys Acta* 2015;**1852**(7):1520–30.
218. Viereck J, et al. Regulatory RNAs and paracrine networks in the heart. *Cardiovasc Res* 2014;**102**(2):290–301.
219. Grueter CE, et al. A cardiac microRNA governs systemic energy homeostasis by regulation of MED13. *Cell* 2012;**149**(3):671–83.
220. Baskin KK, et al. MED13-dependent signaling from the heart confers leanness by enhancing metabolism in adipose tissue and liver. *EMBO Mol Med* 2014;**6**(12):1610–21.
221. Nakamura M, Sadoshima J. Heart over mind: metabolic control of white adipose tissue and liver. *EMBO Mol Med* 2014;**6**(12):1521–4.
222. Koransky ML, Robbins RC, Blau HM. VEGF gene delivery for treatment of ischemic cardiovascular disease. *Trends Cardiovasc Med* 2002;**12**(3):108–14.
223. Frangogiannis NG. Interleukin-1 in cardiac injury, repair, and remodeling: pathophysiologic and translational concepts. *Discoveries (Craiova)* 2015;**3**:1.
224. Lu M, et al. Fluorofenidone inhibits macrophage IL-1beta production by suppressing inflammasome activity. *Int Immunopharmacol* 2015;**27**(1):148–53.
225. Youm YH, et al. The ketone metabolite beta-hydroxybutyrate blocks NLRP3 inflammasome-mediated inflammatory disease. *Nat Med* 2015;**21**(3):263–9.
226. Cauwe B, Van den Steen PE, Opdenakker G. The biochemical, biological, and pathological kaleidoscope of cell surface substrates processed by matrix metalloproteinases. *Crit Rev Biochem Mol Biol* 2007;**42**(3):113–85.
227. Detry B, et al. Matrix metalloproteinase-2 governs lymphatic vessel formation as an interstitial collagenase. *Blood* 2012;**119**(21):5048–56.
228. Kessenbrock K, Plaks V, Werb Z. Matrix metalloproteinases: regulators of the tumor microenvironment. *Cell* 2010;**141**(1):52–67.

CHAPTER

NOVEL SMALL PEPTIDE HORMONES

5

G.L.C. Yosten, L.M. Stein and W.K. Samson

Saint Louis University School of Medicine, Saint Louis, MO, United States

INTRODUCTION

The completion of the Human Genome Project and the birth of bioinformatics led to an explosive increase in the discovery of novel biologically active proteins and peptides. We now can scan the human genome for previously unrecognized sequences encoding not only hormones, but also small peptides derived from transcriptional processing of genes coding for G protein-coupled receptors that control translational and posttranslational processing as well as the biologic function of those receptors. These discoveries opened new avenues for the development of therapeutics and, just as important, provided novel insights into the regulation of multiple cell signaling pathways, the integrative basis of normal physiology, and the pathophysiology of disease. The rapid pace of discovery will certainly continue and we describe here some of the initial advances in the field of cardiovascular endocrinology.

ENDOCRINE FACTORS REGULATING BLOOD PRESSURE AND CARDIAC FUNCTION: NEURONOSTATIN AND ADROPIN

NEURONOSTATIN: DISCOVERY AND SITES OF PRODUCTION

Somatostatin is a peptide hormone that was originally described based on its ability to inhibit growth hormone secretion from the anterior pituitary.[1,2] It was later discovered that somatostatin-14 and the N-terminally extended form of somatostatin, somatostatin-28, are produced in a variety of tissues, including the gastrointestinal tract, pancreas, heart, and brain, where they exert primarily inhibitory effects on the secretion of other hormones in addition to growth hormone, such as insulin and glucagon.[3] The somatostatin prohormone is a 116 amino acid precursor that comprises somatostatin-14 and -28 (28 amino acids total), located at the C terminus, and a 24 amino acid signal peptide at the N terminus.[4] Between these two sequences is a 64 amino acid region that was hypothesized for many years to contain an additional biologically active molecule. Using bioinformatic analyses of conserved sequences, a potential peptide was identified in the prohormone, immediately following the signal peptide[5] (Fig. 5.1(A)). This conserved sequence was flanked by conserved dibasic residues, which could serve as potential cleavage sites. In addition, the conserved sequence terminated in a glycine-lysine pair at the C terminus, which is often indicative of a C-terminal amidation, a common feature of many biologically active peptides.

Endocrinology of the Heart in Health and Disease. DOI: http://dx.doi.org/10.1016/B978-0-12-803111-7.00005-1

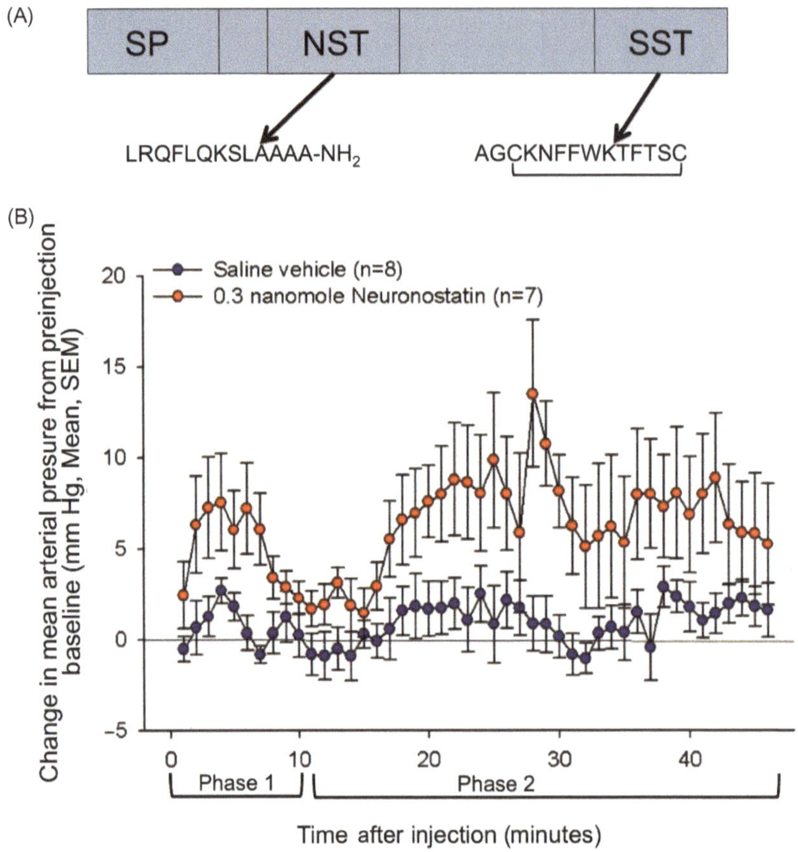

FIGURE 5.1

Neuronostatin and the central control of blood pressure. (A) Structure of the somatostatin/neuronostatin prohormone. (B) Central injection of neuronostatin increases mean arterial pressure in male rats.

*Adapted from Samson WK, Zhang JV, Avsian-Kretchmer O, et al. Neuronostatin encoded by the somatostatin gene regulates neuronal, cardiovascular, and metabolic functions. J Biol Chem 2008;***283***(46):31949–59. SP, signal peptide; NST, neuronostatin; SST, somatostatin.*

The potential peptide was synthesized and used to generate an antibody allowing the isolation of the endogenous molecule from porcine pancreas and spleen. The endogenous peptide was found to be a 13 amino acid peptide that was C-terminally amidated. The peptide was named neuronostatin given its initial identified actions on rodent cerebellar neurons ("neurono-") and its derivation from the somatostatin prohormone (-"statin").[5]

As predicted, the tissue expression profile of neuronostatin was identical to that of somatostatin in rats, with the exception that the tissue content of the two peptides differed in most tissues evaluated.[5] It was suggested that this discrepancy could be due to differential prohormone convertase expression or tissue-specific degradation of either peptide. Additionally, the peptides differ in terms of posttranslational processing—somatostatin is cyclized by the formation of disulfide bonds between cysteine residues, while neuronostatin is C-terminally amidated, which requires the presence of specific amidating enzymes. Thus, the presence or absence of amidating enzymes could determine tissue expression of neuronostatin. In addition to these differences, somatostatin and neuronostatin lack any similarity in amino acid sequence, and do not bind to the same receptors. In an in vitro assay, neuronostatin failed to activate any of the five known somatostatin receptors,[5] but appears to interact with the previously orphaned G protein-coupled receptor (GPCR), GPR107.[6] Thus, although neuronostatin is derived from the somatostatin prohormone, it appears to initiate signaling events and exert biological functions that are distinct from that of somatostatin.

NEURONOSTATIN AND THE CENTRAL CONTROL OF BLOOD PRESSURE

Although it is now known that neuronostatin exerts potent biologic action in pancreas and in other peripheral tissues including the heart, the peptide's cellular actions were initially described in brain. In particular, application of neuronostatin depolarized neurons in the paraventricular nucleus of the hypothalamus of rats.[5] Because this region of the hypothalamus is involved in blood pressure regulation, it was hypothesized that the neuronostatin acted centrally to control sympathetic nervous system activity and blood pressure (see chapter: Neuronal Hormones and the Sympathetic/Parasympathetic Regulation of the Heart). Injection of neuronostatin into the lateral cerebroventricle (icv) led to a significant, biphasic increase in mean arterial pressure (MAP) in adult, male Sprague Dawley rats.[5,7] The first phase of this response (Phase 1) was transient, and resolved within 10 minutes following injection. The second phase (Phase 2) began approximately 10–15 minutes following central infusion of neuronostatin and was maintained for ~30 minutes (Fig. 5.1(B)). Because neuronostatin depolarized both magnocellular neuroendocrine neurons, which produce vasopressin and/or oxytocin and project to the posterior pituitary and parvocellular preautonomic neurons, it was hypothesized that neuronostatin's effect on MAP was due to two separate mechanisms: activation of the sympathetic nervous system and the release of the pressor hormone, vasopressin, from the posterior pituitary. In agreement with this hypothesis, Phase 1, but not Phase 2, was blocked with peripheral pretreatment with the mixed alpha adrenergic antagonist, phentolamine (see chapter: Adrenergic Receptors), suggesting that the first, transient rise in blood pressure following neuronostatin treatment was due to activation of the sympathetic nervous system.[7] However, Phase 2, but not Phase 1, was abrogated by peripheral pretreatment with a vasopressin 1 receptor antagonist, and icv injection of neuronostatin led to a significant increase in plasma vasopressin levels in a time course consistent with the increase in MAP observed during Phase 2.[7] These data suggest that neuronostatin elevates blood pressure first through activation of the sympathetic nervous system, followed by induction of vasopressin secretion, which then acts in the systemic vasculature to increase blood pressure.

The central melanocortin system, which comprises proopiomelanocortin-producing neurons in the arcuate nucleus of the hypothalamus and nucleus of the solitary tract in the brainstem as well as melanocortin 3/4 receptor-producing neurons that are located throughout the brain, is an important neural system involved in the central regulation of blood pressure.[8] Activation of this system increased sympathetic nervous system activity and blood pressure in multiple animal models, indicating that the first phase of neuronostatin's effect on MAP could be due to an interaction with the central melanocortin system. Unexpectedly, central pretreatment with the melanocortin 3/4 receptor antagonist, SHU9119, did not affect the first phase of neuronostatin's effect; however, Phase 2 was completely abolished.[7]

Likewise, pretreatment with SHU9119 blocked the effect of neuronostatin on plasma vasopressin levels,[7] suggesting that neuronostatin's neuroendocrine effect is mediated by the central melanocortin system, while the peptide's autonomic action is due to an interaction with an alternative neural system.

NEURONOSTATIN AND CARDIAC FUNCTION

In addition to its effects in brain to modulate blood pressure, neuronostatin directly regulates cardiac function as well. In the heart, neuronostatin appears to exert primarily depressant activities. For example, neuronostatin decreased peak shortening of isolated rodent cardiomyocytes in a concentration dependent manner[9] and likewise inhibited fractional shortening and heart rate in intact hearts of C57 BL/6 mice evaluated by echocardiography.[10] In Langendorff heart preparations, neuronostatin decreased left ventricular pressure development and heart rate[9] and attenuated the endothelin-1 induced contractile response[11] (see chapter: Endothelin-1 as a Cardiac-Derived Autocrine, Paracrine and Intracrine Factor in Heart Health and Disease). Additionally, these studies revealed important information regarding the intracellular signaling mechanisms underlying neuronostatin's actions. The effect of neuronostatin on fractional shortening of isolated cardiomyocytes was blocked by application of the protein kinase A (PKA) inhibitor, H89, and the c-Jun N-terminal kinase (JNK) inhibitor, SP600125.[9] Additionally, infusion of neuronostatin-induced JNK phosphorylation and p38 MAP kinase activation in isolated perfused hearts.[11] However, neuronostatin's actions on cardiomyocytes were not altered by the protein kinase C (PKC) inhibitor, chelerythrine. Together these data suggest that neuronostatin signals via PKA- and JNK-dependent, PKC-independent mechanisms, likely via a GPCR coupled to Gαs.

ASSESSING THE PHYSIOLOGIC RELEVANCE OF NEURONOSTATIN

Attempts to establish the physiological relevance of a peptide hormone traditionally employ a compromise of production, such as the generation of knockout animals, or the use of RNA interference (i.e., siRNA, shRNA, etc.) as well as peptide overexpression studies using transgenic rodents. However, when a peptide is produced as part of a larger prohormone, like neuronostatin, generation of such model systems is challenging due to the need to maintain expression of the associated peptide (e.g., somatostatin). An alternative approach to assess physiological significance is to compromise the production of the peptide's receptor. Before this could be accomplished for neuronostatin, the neuronostatin receptor had to first be identified. Because neuronostatin signaled via PKA- and JNK-dependent mechanisms,[9,11] and because neuronostatin does not bear significant homology to any known peptides, it was hypothesized that the neuronostatin receptor was a GPCR, and in particular, one of the "orphan" GPCRs that had no known ligand.

To identify the neuronostatin receptor, a physiological approach, dubbed the "deductive ligand-receptor matching strategy" was utilized.[6] For this approach, four cell and tissue types that were known to respond to neuronostatin (and thus likely produced a neuronostatin receptor), including cardiomyocytes, hypothalamic neurons, pancreatic alpha cells, and the human gastric tumor cell line, KATOIII, were screened for the expression of orphan GPCRs using a PCR-based screening assay. Orphan GPCRs that were expressed by all four cells/tissues were considered good candidates for the neuronostatin receptor, and were subjected to further analyses. In KATOIII cells, neuronostatin enhanced cFos mRNA expression as measured by quantitative PCR (qPCR); this model system was used for further experimentation. The orphan GPCRs identified in the receptor screen were knocked down individually in KATOIII cells using siRNA; those cells were then treated with neuronostatin, and neuronostatin-induced cFos expression was evaluated. Although knockdown of GPR56 (now known to be the receptor for collagen III[12]) did not disrupt neuronostatin-induced cFos expression in KATOIII cells, knockdown of GPR107 completely inhibited neuronostatin's effect in those cells. Likewise, knockdown of GPR107 in the hypothalamus of male Sprague–Dawley rats completely blocked neuronostatin's effect on MAP, but did not alter the hypertensive action of angiotensin II. In agreement with these data, separate studies conducted using cadaveric human pancreas tissue demonstrated colocalization between neuronostatin and GPR107 on pancreatic alpha cell membranes (Fig. 5.2),[13] indicating that neuronostatin and GPR107 could physically interact.[13,14] Thus, GPR107 was considered the best candidate for the neuronostatin receptor.[6]

To evaluate the physiological significance of neuronostatin and GPR107 in the central control of blood pressure, male rats were treated with siRNA against either GPR107 or enhanced green fluorescent

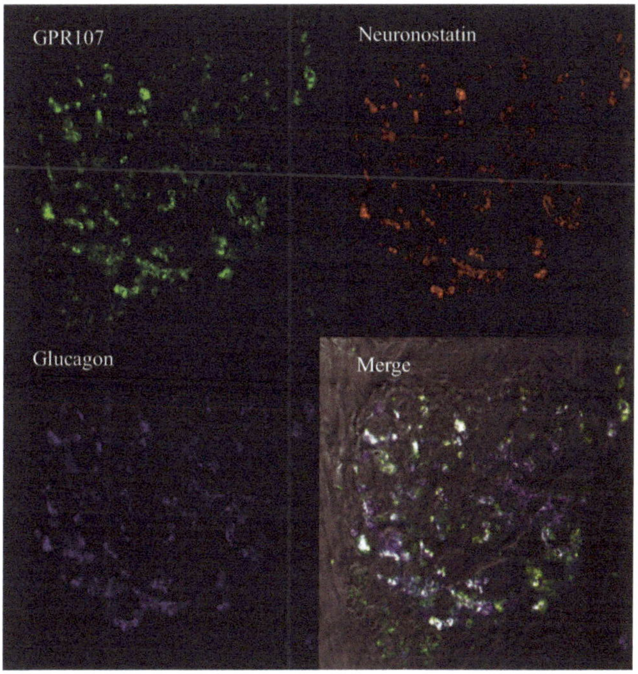

FIGURE 5.2

Colocalization of neuronostatin and GPR107 in human pancreas tissue. Human pancreas section obtained during routine autopsy at Saint Louis University Hospital were exposed to exogenous neuronostatin (30 nM), then fixed and stained using antibodies directed against GPR107 (green), neuronostatin (red), and glucagon (blue). A single islet is shown in which multiple instances of triple colocalization (white) are observed in the merged imaged (lower left panel), indicating that neuronostatin and GPR107 colocalize on alpha cell membranes.

Used with permission from Yosten GL, Elrick MM, Salvatori A, et al. Understanding peptide biology: the discovery and characterization of the novel hormone, neuronostatin. Peptides 2015; ***72****:192–5.*

protein (eGFP, siRNA control). These animals were then subjected to a baroreflex sensitivity test. Treatment with GPR107 siRNA resulted in significant knockdown of GPR107 in the hypothalamus compared to eGFP treated rats.[6] Rats with compromised GPR107 production were unable to compensate for a reduction in blood pressure with an appropriate increase in heart rate. In addition, the time between the peak change in MAP and the peak change in heart rate was significantly delayed in rats treated with GPR107 siRNA.[6] Together, these data indicate that neuronostatin and GPR107 play a physiologically relevant role in the central regulation of blood pressure, and that endogenous neuronostatin and GPR107 may act as important modulators of autonomic function under normal physiological conditions.

ADROPIN: A CARDIO-METABOLIC PEPTIDE

The recently discovered peptide hormone, adropin, is encoded by the energy homeostasis associated gene (*Enho*) and abundantly expressed in the liver and brain.[15] Adropin is a 76 amino acid peptide that exhibits complete homology among human and rodent species. Initial characterization of adropin revealed it to be an important regulator of energy homeostasis, specifically by regulating glucose and lipid metabolism as well as insulin sensitivity.[15,16] Emerging evidence also established adropin as a novel mediator of endothelial function with cardio-protective properties. Adropin is produced in the endocardium, epicardium, and myocardium[17] and constitutively expressed in human endothelial cells (EC). In addition, adropin-treated ECs exhibit enhanced proliferative and migratory abilities, indicative of a direct angiogenic effect.[18] Adropin also stimulates neovascularization in the murine model of ischemia, further suggesting an important role for adropin in endothelial function and maintenance.[18]

It is well established that vascular development and function is dependent upon activation of the vascular endothelial growth factor receptor (VEGFR2) resulting in downstream PI3K-Akt and Erk1/2 signaling cascades. In human umbilical vein EC, adropin significantly increased both VEGFR2 mRNA expression and total protein, and enhanced endothelial nitric oxide synthase (eNOS) activation via PI3K-Akt– and Erk1/2– dependent pathways (for a summary of adropin signaling, see Fig. 5.3).[18,19] Nitric oxide (NO), an endogenous vasodilator, is required for vascular homeostasis and deficiencies in NO production are thought to be at least partly responsible for the pathophysiology of atherosclerosis, diabetes, and hypertension. Therefore, adropin's involvement in NO signaling may be an important factor in endothelial maintenance, and the peptide may contribute to the pathogenesis of cardiovascular disease. It is currently not known whether adropin exerts its action centrally as a classical neuropeptide and/or exerts autocrine/paracrine effects in the periphery to regulate cardiovascular function. The identity of the adropin receptor is currently unknown and thus elucidation of the cognate receptor would allow for further characterization of the underlying mechanisms associated with adropin's cardiovascular and metabolic effects as well as identify any potential therapeutic capacity.

ADROPIN: AN INDEPENDENT RISK FACTOR FOR CARDIOVASCULAR DISEASE

Obesity-associated insulin resistance, hypertension, and dyslipidemia are significant risk factors for the development of life-threatening cardiovascular diseases.[20] As recently reviewed,[19] adropin may play important roles in the pathogenesis of these diseases. In humans, adropin has been shown to be associated with insulin resistance and negatively correlated with body mass index.[21] Normal levels of

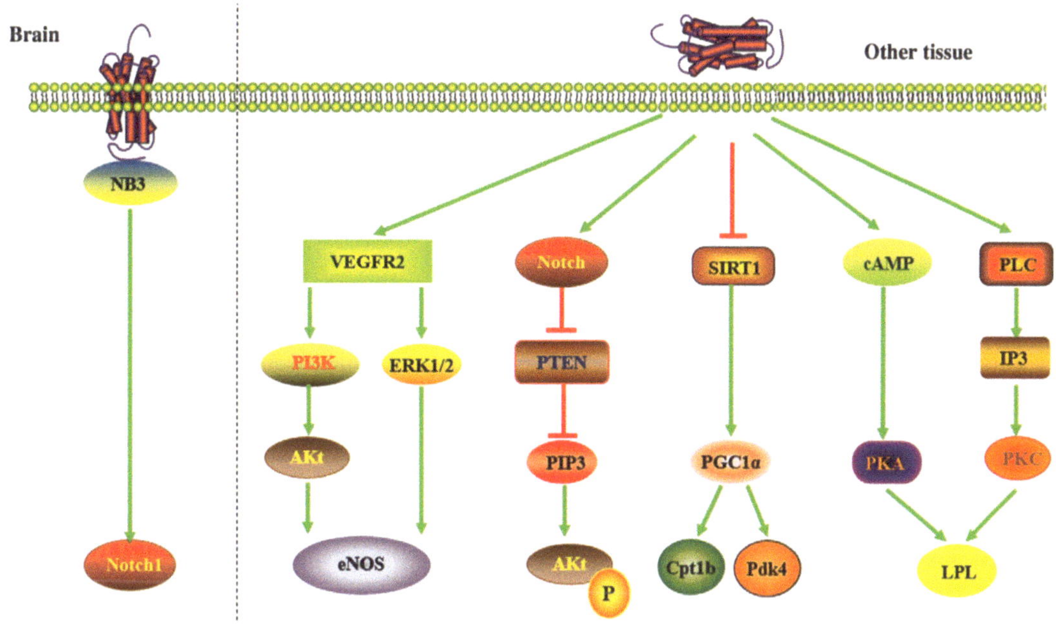

FIGURE 5.3

Schematic presentation of adropin-triggered intracellular signal transduction pathways. Adropin can regulate eNOS bioactivity and endothelial function by activating VEGFR2/PI3K/Akt and VEGFR2/ERK1/2 pathways. Adropin reduces PGC-1α through inhibition of SIRT1 and downregulation of Cpt1b and Pdk4. Adropin increases insulin-induced Akt phosphorylation by downregulating PTEN with a potential increase in the basal level of PIP3 through Notch signal pathways in muscle. Adropin stimulates LPL gene expression through activation of cAMP/PKA and PLC/IP3/PKC cascades in tilapia hepatocytes. Adropin stimulates the NB-3/Notch signaling pathway to modulate intercellular communications as a membrane-bound protein in the brain.

*Used with permission, from Li L, Xie W, Zheng XL, Yin WD, Tang CK, A novel peptide adropin in cardiovascular diseases. Clin Chim Acta 2016;***453***:107–13.*

circulating adropin concentrations vary from approximately 2–6 ng/mL,[22–24] which declines with age.[21,25] To date, several studies have investigated the potential correlation between the levels of circulating adropin and the incidence of cardiovascular disease in an attempt to identify this novel metabolic peptide as a potential cardio-pathological marker. Table 5.1 highlights recent studies assessing plasma adropin levels as a function of cardiovascular disease. There is a clear consensus among these findings that the levels of circulating adropin negatively correlate with a variety of cardiovascular diseases, leading some to speculate a cardio-protective role of adropin. This is further supported by the recent findings that aerobic exercise training, known to reduce arterial stiffness and increase cardiovascular fitness, resulted in an increases in adropin production.[23] Nonetheless, further studies are required to determine the underlying mechanism by which adropin contributes to the pathogenesis of cardiovascular disease.

Table 5.1 Association Between Circulating Adropin and Cardiovascular Disease

Cardiovascular Disease	Plasma Adropin	Reference(s)
Hypertension	Decreased	24
Atherosclerosis	Decreased	26
Coronary artery disease	Decreased	27–30
Heart failure	Increased	31
Endothelial dysfunction • Type 2 diabetes • Sleep apnea	Decreased	32,33
Cardiac syndrome X	Decreased	22

NOVEL ADIPOKINES IN THE CONTROL OF CARDIOVASCULAR FUNCTION: NESFATIN-1 AND OMENTIN

ADIPOSE TISSUE AS AN ENDOCRINE ORGAN

Although primarily a storage depot for lipids, particularly triglycerides, adipose tissue has been recognized for many years as an endocrine tissue that secretes peptide and nonpeptide hormones, angiogenic factors, and inflammatory cytokines. While the hormones secreted by adipocytes, or "adipokines," exert multiple, diverse functions, arguably one of the most important functions of adipokines is to serve as a signal of stored energy reserve (see chapter: Fat Hormones, Adipokines). For example, the production of the most widely recognized adipokine, leptin, correlates with adipocyte mass—greater adipose mass leads to higher levels of circulating leptin. Adipocyte-derived leptin acts in brain to reduce appetite; thus, leptin serves as a feedback signal so that when energy stores are adequate or excessive, leptin decreases energy intake. However, in addition to regulating appetite and energy expenditure, many anorexigenic peptides, including leptin, also enhance sympathetic nervous system activity and elevate blood pressure, which could have important implications for the development of obesity-associated hypertension. Interestingly, it appears that obese individuals develop selective resistance to adipokines such as leptin, such that they are unable to respond to the anorexigenic effect of adipokines, yet maintain sensitivity to their hypertensive effect. Since many adipokines are secreted as a function of adipocyte mass, obese individuals have high circulating levels of these proteins, suggesting that adipokines contribute to hypertension in the obese state. In recent years, multiple novel adipokines have been discovered that appear to have diverse actions with regard to the maintenance of cardiovascular function.

NESFATIN-1: DISCOVERY, PRODUCTION, AND SIGNALING

Nesfatin-1, a peptide hormone derived from the nucleobindin 2 (NUCB2) gene, was characterized initially as a DNA binding protein with calcium interacting zones due to sequence homology compared to protein domains known to exhibit these functions.[34,35] Nesfatin-1 was identified by subtraction cloning of

PPARγ-stimulated genes in the human lung tumor cell line SQ5.[34] The amino acid sequence of NUCB2 is highly conserved among humans, rats, and mice, with the human and mouse sequences exhibiting 87.4% and 95.7% homology to the rat sequence, respectively.[34] Immunohistochemical analyses revealed that nesfatin-1 was produced in rat hypothalamus, including the paraventricular nucleus and the arcuate nucleus,[34] although later studies demonstrated nesfatin-1 production by adipocytes as well.[36] Central injection of nesfatin-1 in rats led to a dose-related decrease in food intake, which, like leptin, was due to an interaction with the central melanocortin system, since the effect could be blocked by pretreatment with the melanocortin 3/4 receptor antagonist, SHU9119.[34,37] The anorexigenic effect of nesfatin-1 on food intake may be physiologically relevant, since central administration of an antisense morpholino or neutralizing antibodies directed against nesfatin-1 resulted in an exaggeration of food intake and body weight gain in rats. Interestingly, nesfatin-1 was shown to cross the blood brain barrier via a nonsaturable mechanism,[38,39] suggesting that adipocyte-derived nesfatin-1 could act in brain to exert its effects. Thus, nesfatin-1 may play a similar integrative role to that of leptin and act as an adipokine that modulates appetite and energy expenditure through activation of the sympathetic nervous system (Fig. 5.4).[40]

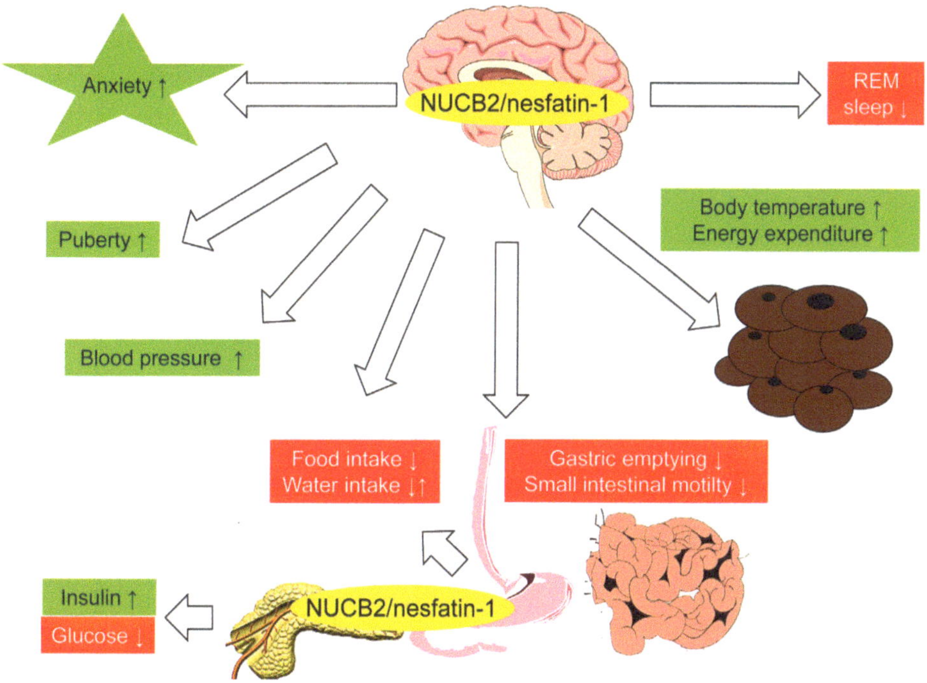

FIGURE 5.4

Pleiotropic effects of NUCB2/nesfatin-1. Stimulatory effects are indicated in green, inhibitory in red. ↑ = increase, ↓ = decrease.

*Used with permission, from Stengel A. Nesfatin-1-more than a food intake regulatory peptide. Peptides 2015;**72**:175–83.*

NESFATIN-1 AND THE CENTRAL CONTROL OF BLOOD PRESSURE

Since nesfatin-1 regulates food intake via an interaction with the central melanocortin system, which also plays critical roles in regulating cardiovascular function, nesfatin-1 was hypothesized to alter MAP. Central injection of nesfatin-1 into the lateral cerebroventricle of conscious male rats elevated MAP in a dose-related fashion.[37] The hypertensive effect of nesfatin-1 was due to an increase in sympathetic nervous system activity as peripheral pretreatment with the nonspecific alpha adrenergic antagonist, phentolamine, completely blocked nesfatin-1-induced changes in MAP.[37] Additionally, like the anorexigenic actions of the peptide, the hypertensive effect of nesfatin-1 was found to be dependent upon functional central melanocortin 3/4 receptors, since pretreatment with the melanocortin 3/4 receptor antagonist, SHU9119, inhibited the ability of nesfatin-1 to raise arterial pressure in male Sprague–Dawley rats.[37] In subsequent experiments, the downstream circuitries mediating nesfatin-1–induced increases in MAP were determined. By using antagonists against corticotrophin releasing hormone (CRH) and oxytocin receptors (Astressin2B and OVT, respectively), nesfatin-1 was shown to act via a neuronal circuit involving not only central melanocortin receptor-expressing neurons, but CRH- and oxytocin receptor-producing neurons as well.[41] Nesfatin-1 was hypothesized therefore to interact with melanocortin neurons, which synapsed either directly or indirectly with CRH-producing neurons, which in turn influenced the activity of centrally projecting oxytocin neurons. Those oxytocin neurons likely projected to brainstem autonomic centers, and upon activation, increased sympathetic nervous system activity and MAP.

If adipocyte-derived nesfatin-1 plays a role in the central regulation of blood pressure, then peripherally injected exogenous nesfatin-1 should elevate blood pressure in experimental animals. In male rats, chronic peripheral infusion of nesfatin-1 led to progressively higher blood pressures,[42] suggesting that chronic exposure to high plasma levels of nesfatin-1, such as in the setting of obesity,[43] can lead to hypertension. Nesfatin-1 antagonists therefore could prove to be effective therapy for obesity-associated hypertension; however, the nesfatin-1 receptor or receptors must first be identified.

NESFATIN-1 AND CARDIAC FUNCTION

Although the precise role of circulating or locally produced nesfatin-1 in cardiac function is not as well characterized as its contribution to the central control of blood pressure, a few key findings indicate that the peptide may be cardioprotective. For instance, nesfatin-1 has been shown to protect against cardiac dysfunction in an ischemia and reperfusion model, likely through the activation of ERK1/2 pathways.[44] Interestingly, nesfatin-1 suppresses L-type calcium channels in cardiomyocytes in a pertussis toxin-sensitive manner.[45] This effect was blocked by application of the melanocortin 4 receptor antagonist, HS024,[45] suggesting that the as yet unidentified nesfatin-1 receptor is the melanocortin 4 receptor, or that nesfatin-1 acts as an allosteric modulator of this receptor. This finding could have important implications for the regulation of the central melanocortin system and the treatment of melanocortin-dependent metabolic and cardiovascular dysfunction.

OMENTIN: DISCOVERY, EXPRESSION, AND SIGNALING

Visceral fat accumulation is associated with an increased risk for metabolic syndrome, type 2 diabetes, and cardiovascular disease. Thus, adipokines that exhibit fat depot-specific expression in omental fat could play an important role in insulin sensitivity and cardiovascular function. However, until recently, fat-specific expressed sequence tags (EST), important tools for discovery of novel peptides and proteins, were poorly catalogued in publicly available databases. Using EST analysis of human omental fat cDNA libraries, a novel 313 amino acid protein was identified and named omentin.[46] The mRNA sequence of omentin included a secretory signal sequence and a fibrinogen-related domain, and was similar to a previously identified protein called intelectin.[46] Although omentin was detected in tissues other than fat pads, including the vascular endothelium and Paneth cells of the intestine, omentin's primary site of expression appeared to be in fat.[46] Omentin was detected in the culture media of omental, but not subcutaneous, fat explants, indicating that not only was the expression of omentin fat depot-specific, but also that the protein indeed was secreted.[46] Early experiments demonstrated that omentin's intracellular effects were mediated by activation of the serine/threonine-specific protein kinase, Akt,[46] which now appears to be critical for omentin's protective effects in the blood vessels. In addition, AMP kinase has been shown to play important roles in omentin-induced vascular smooth muscle cell proliferation and neointimal formation, perhaps through ERK- and eNOS-mediated pathways (Fig. 5.5).[47]

OMENTIN AND THE VASCULATURE

One of omentin's primary sites of action appears to be in the vasculature. The protein exerts protective effects both in the vascular endothelium and in vascular smooth muscle cells. In the vascular endothelium, omentin exerts antiinflammatory activities via inhibition of tumor necrosis factor alpha (TNF alpha)-induced cyclooxygenase 2 (COX2) expression.[48] In addition, omentin promotes EC survival and differentiation. Omentin also stimulates the phosphorylation of eNOS, which plays a protective role in the vasculature through the production of NO. As expected, these effects were mediated by omentin-induced activation of Akt.[49] In a mouse model of ischemia, omentin enhanced capillary vessel formation during perfusion recovery of ischemic limbs. Omentin-induced phosphorylation of eNOS was required for this effect on revascularization.[49]

In vascular smooth muscle cells, omentin prevented platelet derived growth factor induced migration by inhibiting NOX and HSP27 pathways[50] and thus may play important antioxidant roles in these cells. Additionally, similar to its action in vascular ECs, omentin prevented TNFalpha-induced COX2 expression in smooth muscle cells.[51] In humans, high plasma levels of omentin were associated with a reduction in maximal intima media thickness of the carotid artery.[52] Thus, omentin appears to play a protective role for multiple layers of the vasculature.

THE PROTECTIVE EFFECT OF OMENTIN IN THE HEART

In humans, plasma omentin levels were negatively correlated with body mass index and waist circumference, two major risk factors for cardiovascular disease, suggesting that higher adipocyte mass leads to lower plasma levels of omentin.[52] In patients presenting with myocardial infarction, high plasma levels of omentin were associated with marked improvement of cardiac damage during recovery.[53] This effect was mirrored in mice. Omentin infusion reduced myocardial infarct size and apoptosis following ischemia and reperfusion.[53] As with omentin's protective actions in the vasculature, this effect was blocked by an Akt inhibitor as well as an inhibitor of AMP kinase, suggesting an essential role of these signaling molecules in mediating omentin-induced cardioprotection. In transgenic mice overexpression of omentin specifically in fat tissue was associated with reduced myocardial infarct size

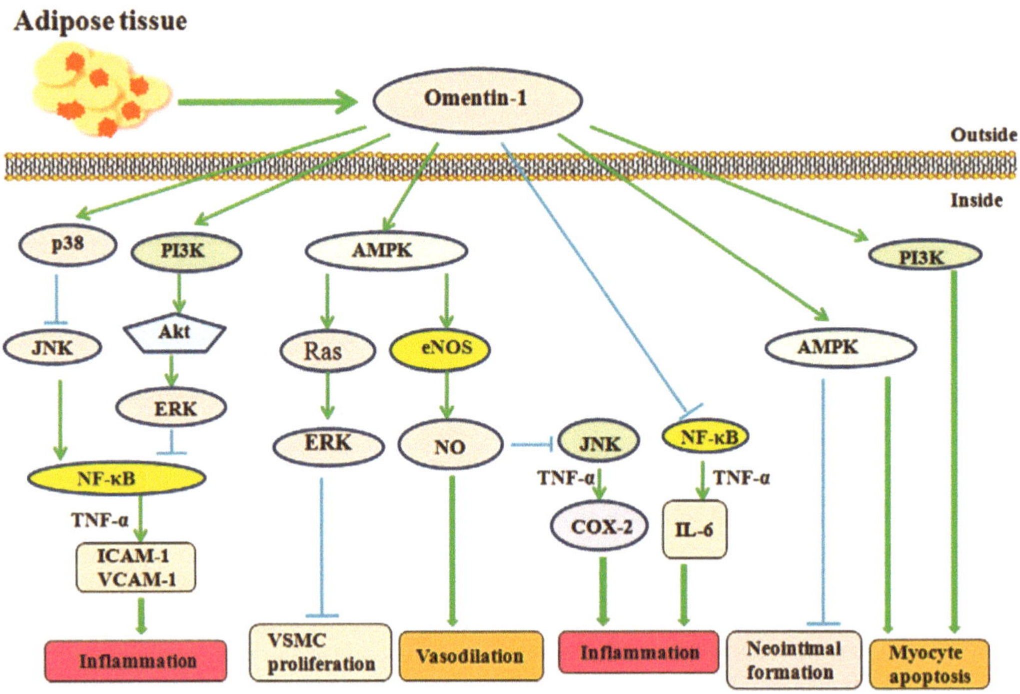

FIGURE 5.5

Schematic presentation of omentin's roles in the vasculature and intracellular signal transduction pathways. Omentin activates AMPK, which further blocks E-selection and reduces endothelial inflammation. AMPK also activates eNOS, which has vasodilation effect and blocks JNK signaling. JNK activates inflammation through TNF-α-mediated COX2 induction. Moreover, omentin inhibits the NF-κB signaling pathway and thus inhibits inflammation. Under obese state, there is a lower production of omentin, which is associated with more severe proinflammation. The antiangiogenic effect of omentin is through inhibiting Akt and NF-κB pathways and critical regulators of inflammation and angiogenesis. Omentin causes vasodilatation by increasing nitric oxide production via endothelial nitric oxide synthase. Omentin functions as an adipokine that ameliorates acute ischemic injury in the heart by suppressing myocyte apoptosis through both AMPK- and Akt-dependent mechanisms. It was also found that omentin attenuates neointimal formation after arterial injury and suppresses vascular SMC proliferation through AMPK-dependent mechanisms.

*Reproduced from Tan YL, Zheng XL, Tang CK. The protective functions of omentin in cardiovascular diseases. Clin Chim Acta 2015;***448***:98–106.*

following ischemia and reperfusion[53] and attenuation of cardiac hypertrophy and fibrosis induced by either transverse aortic constriction or infusion of angiotensin II.[54] Thus, although the physiological relevance of omentin has not been established, the protein clearly exerts beneficial actions in both the blood vessels and in the heart, and could prove to be an effective therapeutic target for the treatment of cardiovascular diseases.

ROLE OF MYOKINES IN CARDIOVASCULAR HEALTH: IRISIN

SKELETAL MUSCLE AS AN ENDOCRINE ORGAN

In addition to its role in locomotion and postural retention, skeletal muscle has long been recognized as a major contributor to whole body metabolism and glucose homeostasis.[55] Arguably the largest metabolic organ in the human body, skeletal muscle expresses high levels of the insulin receptor, and dysregulation of insulin signaling within skeletal muscle is thought to be a major contributor to insulin resistance, a hallmark feature of metabolic syndrome and type 2 diabetes. While insulin resistance is a risk factor for the development of cardiovascular disease, exercise, and in particular resistance training, has been shown to improve insulin sensitivity and reduce the incidence of cardiovascular events in individuals with metabolic syndrome. The mechanisms underlying exercise-induced cardiovascular protection are in all likelihood multifactorial; however, it was postulated for many years that a factor or factors, secreted by the skeletal muscle, played a role in the cardioprotective effect of exercise. This hypothesis was confirmed when interleukin 6 (IL-6) was identified as the first "myokine," or hormone produced and secreted by the skeletal muscle.[56] Since then, multiple myokines have been identified, thus confirming the role of the skeletal muscle as an endocrine organ, the secretory activity of which could have important implications for the regulation of cardiovascular function.

IRISIN, A NOVEL MYOKINE

PPARγ coactivator-1 α (PGC1α) is a transcription factor that plays important roles in the regulation of metabolism.[57] The expression of PGC1α is upregulated in skeletal muscle following exercise, and mild overexpression of PGC1α in muscle stimulates the browning of white subcutaneous adipose tissue, suggesting that PGC1α induces the expression of a secreted factor by the skeletal muscle which regulates adipocyte function.[57] One such gene regulated by PGC1α in the skeletal muscle is Fibronectin type III domain-containing protein 5 (Fndc5), which encodes a protein with a signal peptide, two fibronectin domains and a transmembrane domain.[57] Following proteolytic cleavage, the N-terminal domain of this protein is secreted into the extracellular space.[57] One of the major functions of this protein appears to be stimulating the browning of white adipose tissue, thus promoting thermogenesis and energy expenditure (Fig. 5.6).[57,58] Interestingly, tissue expression and plasma levels of the protein are elevated following acute exercise and exercise training,[57,59,60] and thus the cleaved protein is hypothesized to serve as an endocrine messenger between skeletal muscle and adipose tissue and may serve as the link between exercise and thermogenesis. For this reason, the protein was named irisin, after the Greek goddess Iris, the messenger of the Greek pantheon.[57]

IRISIN AND MAINTENANCE OF THE VASCULAR ENDOTHELIUM

In addition to its metabolic effects, including modulation of insulin sensitivity and white adipose tissue thermogenesis, irisin appears to act in the vascular endothelium to protect against obesity–and type 2 diabetes–associated vascular dysfunction. In cultured human ECs, irisin enhanced proliferation by promoting ERK1/2 phosphorylation, and reduced high glucose-induced EC apoptosis.[61] In addition, irisin stimulated EC migration and wound closure in an in vitro wound assay as well as stimulated tubule formation by ECs, suggesting that irisin promotes angiogenesis.[62] These effects were at least partially

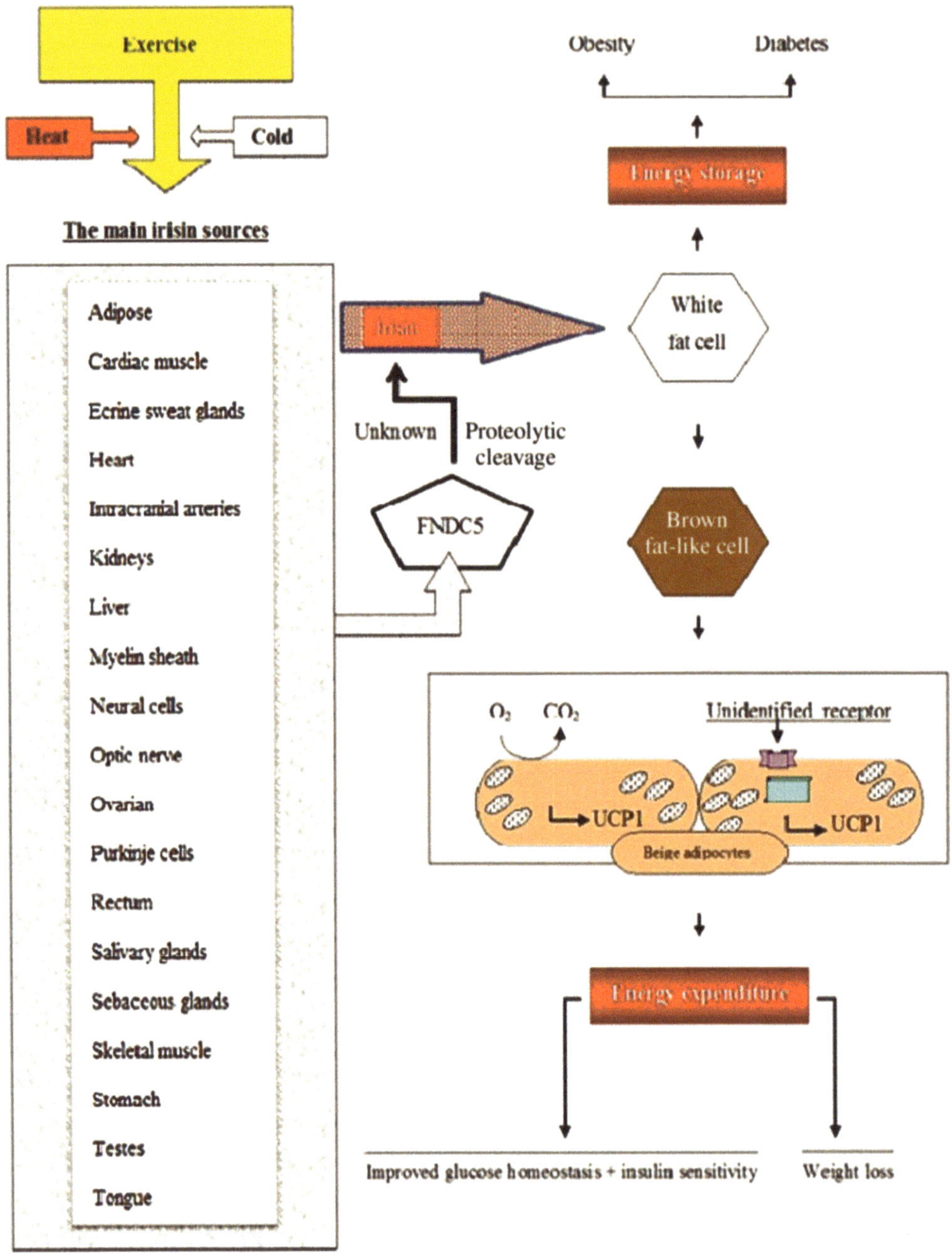

FIGURE 5.6

An overview of the major sites of irisin synthesis and the principle biochemical effects of irisin. The major sites of irisin synthesis are the heart muscle and adipose tissue. Irisin functions in the regulation of the carbohydrate mechanism.

*Used with permission from Aydin S. Three new players in energy regulation: preptin, adropin and irisin. Peptides 2014;***56***:94–110.*

reversed by treatment with an ERK inhibitor.[62] Likewise, exposure to irisin restored angiogenesis in vivo in a zebrafish model.[62] Importantly, irisin improved endothelium-dependent vasodilation in both obese[63] and type 2 diabetic[64] mice, and this effect was attenuated by treatment with an Akt or eNOS inhibitor.[63] Irisin reduced superoxide production in ex vivo aortic segments from type 2 diabetic mice, enhanced production of NO, and stimulated AMP kinase, Akt, and eNOS activation in ECs.[63,64] Irisin therefore appears to play an important role in the maintenance of the vascular endothelium, particularly in states of metabolic dysfunction.

Although the physiological significance of irisin has not been established, clinical studies revealed the potential utility of irisin as a clinical marker of cardiovascular disease. In particular, plasma and salivary irisin levels decreased in the hours following myocardial infarction.[65] This could be a reflection of the finding that cardiac muscle produces high amounts of irisin compared to skeletal muscle, even in nonexercised subjects,[66] and tissue damage following an ischemic event such as a myocardial infarction could lead to a loss of irisin-secreting cells. Treatment with irisin or irisin agonists could prove to be an effective therapeutic following a cardiovascular event or for patients with overt cardiovascular disease, since higher plasma levels of irisin were associated with a higher functional exercise capacity in patients with heart failure.[67] However, further studies are necessary to establish the importance of irisin to normal physiology and its contribution to pathological conditions. It will be important to establish the cellular mechanisms by which irisin exerts its effects (i.e., identify the irisin receptor or receptors), and to determine if and how irisin can be manipulated therapeutically for the treatment of cardiovascular diseases associated with metabolic dysfunction.

MODULATORY PEPTIDES ENCODED BY UPSTREAM SHORT OPEN READING FRAMES OF HORMONE RECEPTORS: PEP7

Genome sequencing advances enabled bioinformatics-based searches for novel signaling molecules including neuropeptides and circulating hormones. In addition, this approach has unveiled the presence of multiple translation start sites and short open reading frames (sORFs) in the 5′-leader sequences of genes encoding several G protein-coupled receptors (Fig. 5.7).[68] For example, sORFs have been identified in the genes encoding the vasopressin V1b receptor,[69] the corticotropin releasing hormone Type 1 receptor,[70] the beta 2-adrenergic receptor,[71] the retinoic acid-beta 2 receptor,[72] and the angiotensin type 1a receptor.[73] In addition to potentially controlling downstream open reading frame expression, these sORFs have been observed to control signaling initiated by ligand binding to the encoded receptor.[70,74,75]

Two alternative splice variants of the angiotensin Type 1 A (AT1aR) have been identified, each encoding the AT1aR. One variant contains exons 1, 2, and 3 with the receptor encoded in exon 3. The second variant contains only exons 1 and 3 and is the more abundant transcript. Within exon 2, a sORF encodes a seven amino acid peptide, named PEP7 (Fig. 5.8), which is highly conserved across species.[76,77] Angiotensin II signals through both G protein–dependent (phospholipase C activation) and G protein–independent (beta arrestin associated MAP kinase activation) pathways[78] (see chapter: Renin Angiotensin Aldosterone System and Heart Function). PEP7 has been demonstrated to interfere with the non-G protein–dependent signaling cascade in HEK293 cells expressing the AT1aR without interfering with angiotensin binding. This effect has physiologic relevance.

It has been recognized for some time that angiotensin II stimulation of water drinking is entirely mediated by activation of the G protein–dependent signaling cascade.[79,80] On the other hand, angiotensin

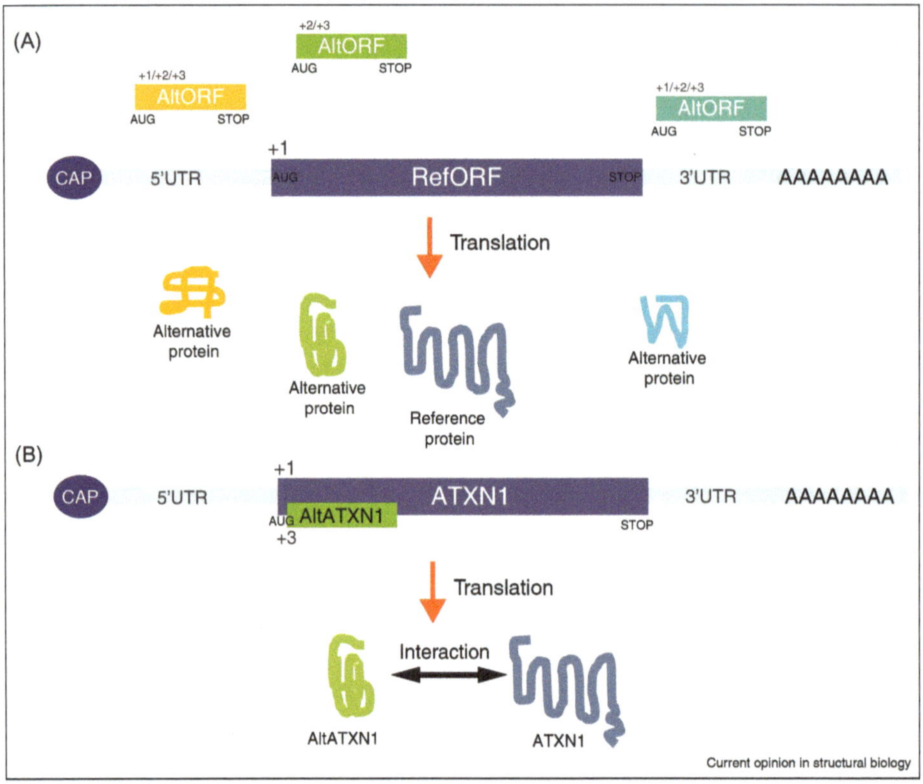

FIGURE 5.7

Alternative open reading frames (AltORFs). (A) Typical mature eukaryotic mRNA and its possible AltORFs. The reference ORF (RefORF) is defined as the coding ORF in the canonical +1 reading frame and is annotated in current nucleotide databases. An alternative ORF (AltORF) is defined as a nucleotide region comprised between a start and a stop codon (different from that of the RefORF) and is predicted to encode an alternative protein. AltORFs may be localized inside the 5′ UTR, inside the RefORF, inside the 3′ UTR. AltORFs may also partially overlap an UTR and the RefORF (not shown here for clarity purposes). In contrast to reference proteins, alternative proteins are not annotated in current protein sequence databases used in proteomics studies and therefore not searched for; (B) ATXN1 is a dual-coding transcript. The AltATXN1 coding sequence (distinct reading frame) overlaps the ATXN1 N-terminal coding sequence and interacts with the ATXN1 N-terminal domain. ATXN1 also controls the subcellular distribution of Alt-ATXN1.

*Reproduced with permission from Landry CR, Zhong X, Nielly-Thibault L, Roucou X. Found in translation: functions and evolution of a recently discovered alternative proteome. Curr Opin Struct Biol 2015;***32***:74–80.*

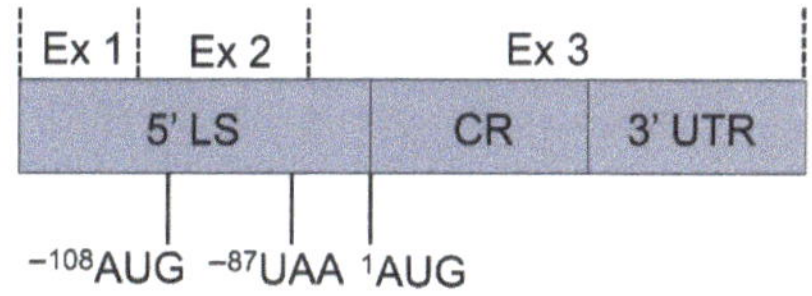

FIGURE 5.8

Angiotensin 1 receptor and PEP7. PEP7 is encoded in exon 2 between −108 and −87. Ex, exon; 5′LS, 5′ leader sequence; CR, coding region; 3′UTR, 3′ untranslated region.

II–stimulated sodium appetite is mediated by activation of the non-G protein–dependent signaling cascade.[81] As predicted by the in vitro studies, PEP7 interfered with the non-G protein–dependent action of angiotensin II in vivo, as reflected by its action to inhibit angiotensin II stimulated saline, but not water drinking in male and female rats.[77]

Thirst and sodium appetite are only two of the many actions of angiotensin II. What other actions of the hormone may be regulated by the presence of PEP7? Preliminary evidence suggests that the pressor effect of angiotensin II can be buffered by PEP7 administration.[77] The ratio of expression of the splice variant containing exons 1,2,3 (encoding in exon 2, PEP7) to that of the variant containing only exons 1 and 3 changes with aging,[77] and it has been suggested that the decrease in the expression of the longer splice variant (encoding PEP7) with aging contributes to both altered sodium sensitivity and the loss of cardio-protection with aging in human females.

The developing story of PEP7's ability to interrupt signaling of one, but not all intracellular communications activated by ligand binding may serve as a template for the development of selective receptor activity modulating compounds with potential therapeutic value. Pharmacotherapy for hypertension has depended for years upon the use of angiotensin converting enzyme inhibitors and/or angiotensin receptor blockers, compounds with frequently severe side effects and compliance issues. Will the knowledge of selective signaling modulation by an endogenously produced hormone open the door to new avenues for endocrine-based therapies? Certainly the recognition of multiple examples of sORFs encoding biologically active molecules in the upstream 5′ LS of several G protein-coupled receptors partnered with important endocrine hormones, particularly those with potent actions on cardiovascular function, promises novel insight into the mechanisms of disease and the future design of endocrine-based therapeutics.

SUMMARY AND CONCLUSIONS

Recently developed bioinformatic tools enabled the discovery of novel hormones subsequently demonstrated by pharmacologic and physiologic approaches to exert potent actions on multiple organ systems, the least of which being the cardiovascular system. In addition to providing important insight into integrative mechanisms controlling those organ systems, these discoveries open new avenues for therapeutic development. At the same time, these tools revealed previously unappreciated cellular mechanisms by which signal transduction can be manipulated, again promising future drug targets for the treatment of cardiovascular and many other diseases.

REFERENCES

1. Siler TM, VandenBerg G, Yen SS, Brazeau P, Vale W, Guillemin R. Inhibition of growth hormone release in humans by somatostatin. *J Clin Endocrinol Metabol* 1973;**37**(4):632–4.
2. Vale W, Brazeau P, Grant G, et al. Preliminary observations on the mechanism of action of somatostatin, a hypothalamic factor inhibiting the secretion of growth hormone. *C R Acad Sci Hebd Seances Acad Sci D* 1972;**275**(25):2913–6.
3. Krantic S, Goddard I, Saveanu A, et al. Novel modalities of somatostatin actions. *Eur J Endocrinol Eur Fed Endocrine Soc* 2004;**151**(6):643–55.
4. Goodman RH, Jacobs JW, Chin WW, Lund PK, Dee PC, Habener JF. Nucleotide sequence of a cloned structural gene coding for a precursor of pancreatic somatostatin. *Proc Natl Acad Sci U S A* 1980;**77**(10):5869–73.
5. Samson WK, Zhang JV, Avsian-Kretchmer O, et al. Neuronostatin encoded by the somatostatin gene regulates neuronal, cardiovascular, and metabolic functions. *J Biol Chem* 2008;**283**(46):31949–59.
6. Yosten GL, Redlinger LJ, Samson WK. Evidence for an interaction of neuronostatin with the orphan G protein-coupled receptor, GPR107. *Am J Physiol Regul Integr Comp Physiol* 2012;**303**(9):R941–9.
7. Yosten GL, Pate AT, Samson WK. Neuronostatin acts in brain to biphasically increase mean arterial pressure through sympatho-activation followed by vasopressin secretion: the role of melanocortin receptors. *Am J Physiol Regul Integr Comp Physiol* 2011;**300**(5):R1194–9.
8. Cone RD. Anatomy and regulation of the central melanocortin system. *Nat Neurosci* 2005;**8**(5):571–8.
9. Hua Y, Ma H, Samson WK, Ren J. Neuronostatin inhibits cardiac contractile function via a protein kinase A- and JNK-dependent mechanism in murine hearts. *Am J Physiol Regul Integr Comp Physiol* 2009;**297**(3):R682–9.
10. Zhu X, Hu N, Chen X, et al. Neuronostatin attenuates myocardial contractile function through inhibition of sarcoplasmic reticulum Ca2+-ATPase in murine heart. *Cell Physiol Biochem Int J Exp Cell Physiol Biochem Pharmacol* 2014;**33**(6):1921–32.
11. Vainio L, Perjes A, Ryti N, et al. Neuronostatin, a novel peptide encoded by somatostatin gene, regulates cardiac contractile function and cardiomyocyte survival. *J Biol Chem* 2012;**287**(7):4572–80.
12. Luo R, Jeong SJ, Jin Z, Strokes N, Li S, Piao X. G protein-coupled receptor 56 and collagen III, a receptor-ligand pair, regulates cortical development and lamination. *Proc Natl Acad Sci U S A* 2011;**108**(31):12925–30.
13. Yosten GL, Elrick MM, Salvatori A, et al. Understanding peptide biology: the discovery and characterization of the novel hormone, neuronostatin. *Peptides* 2015;**72**:192–5.
14. Elrick MM, Samson WK, Corbett JA, et al. Neuronostatin acts via GPR107 to increase cAMP-independent PKA phosphorylation and proglucagon mRNA accumulation in pancreatic alpha-cells. *Am J Physiol Regul Integr Comp Physiol* 2016;**310**(2):R143–55.
15. Kumar KG, Trevaskis JL, Lam DD, et al. Identification of adropin as a secreted factor linking dietary macronutrient intake with energy homeostasis and lipid metabolism. *Cell Metabol* 2008;**8**(6):468–81.
16. Ganesh Kumar K, Zhang J, Gao S, et al. Adropin deficiency is associated with increased adiposity and insulin resistance. *Obesity (Silver Spring)* 2012;**20**(7):1394–402.
17. Aydin S, Kuloglu T, Aydin S, et al. Expression of adropin in rat brain, cerebellum, kidneys, heart, liver, and pancreas in streptozotocin-induced diabetes. *Mol Cell Biochem* 2013;**380**(1–2):73–81.
18. Lovren F, Pan Y, Quan A, et al. Adropin is a novel regulator of endothelial function. *Circulation* 2010;**122** (11 Suppl):S185–92.
19. Li L, Xie W, Zheng XL, Yin WD, Tang CK. A novel peptide adropin in cardiovascular diseases. *Clin Chim Acta* 2016;**453**:107–13.
20. Reaven GM. The metabolic syndrome: time to get off the merry-go-round? *J Int Med* 2011;**269**(2):127–36.
21. Butler AA, Tam CS, Stanhope KL, et al. Low circulating adropin concentrations with obesity and aging correlate with risk factors for metabolic disease and increase after gastric bypass surgery in humans. *J Clin Endocrinol Metabol* 2012;**97**(10):3783–91.

22. Celik A, Balin M, Kobat MA, et al. Deficiency of a new protein associated with cardiac syndrome X; called adropin. *Cardiovasc Ther* 2013;**31**(3):174–8.
23. Fujie S, Hasegawa N, Sato K, et al. Aerobic exercise training-induced changes in serum adropin level are associated with reduced arterial stiffness in middle-aged and older adults. *Am J Physiol Heart Circul Physiol* 2015;**309**(10):H1642–7.
24. Gu X, Li H, Zhu X, et al. Inverse correlation between plasma adropin and ET-1 levels in essential hypertension: a cross-sectional study. *Medicine* 2015;**94**(40):e1712.
25. Nergiz S, Altinkaya SO, Kurt Omurlu I, Yuksel H, Kucuk M, Demircan Sezer S. Circulating adropin levels in patients with endometrium cancer. *Gynecol Endocrinol Off J Int Soc Gynecol Endocrinol* 2015;**31**(9):730–5.
26. Wu L, Fang J, Chen L, et al. Low serum adropin is associated with coronary atherosclerosis in type 2 diabetic and non-diabetic patients. *Clin Chem La Med* 2014;**52**(5):751–8.
27. Demircelik B, Cakmak M, Nazli Y, et al. Adropin: a new marker for predicting late saphenous vein graft disease after coronary artery bypass grafting. *Clin Invest Med Med Clin et experimentale* 2014;**37**(5):E338–44.
28. Yu HY, Zhao P, Wu MC, Liu J, Yin W. Serum adropin levels are decreased in patients with acute myocardial infarction. *Regul Pept* 2014;**190–191**:46–9.
29. Zhang C, Zhao L, Xu W, et al. Correlation of serum adropin level with coronary artery disease. *Zhonghua Yi Xue Za Zhi* 2014;**94**(16):1255–7.
30. Zhao LP, Xu WT, Wang L, et al. Serum adropin level in patients with stable coronary artery disease. *Heart Lung Circul* 2015;**24**(10):975–9.
31. Lian W, Gu X, Qin Y, Zheng X. Elevated plasma levels of adropin in heart failure patients. *Int Med (Tokyo, Japan)* 2011;**50**(15):1523–7.
32. Gozal D, Kheirandish-Gozal L, Bhattacharjee R, Molero-Ramirez H, Tan HL, Bandla HP. Circulating adropin concentrations in pediatric obstructive sleep apnea: potential relevance to endothelial function. *J Pediatr* 2013;**163**(4):1122–6.
33. Topuz M, Celik A, Aslantas T, Demir AK, Aydin S, Aydin S. Plasma adropin levels predict endothelial dysfunction like flow-mediated dilatation in patients with type 2 diabetes mellitus. *J Invest Med Off Publ Am Fed Clin Res* 2013;**61**(8):1161–4.
34. Oh IS, Shimizu H, Satoh T, et al. Identification of nesfatin-1 as a satiety molecule in the hypothalamus. *Nature* 2006;**443**(7112):709–12.
35. Barnikol-Watanabe S, Gross NA, Gotz H, et al. Human protein NEFA, a novel DNA binding/EF-hand/leucine zipper protein. Molecular cloning and sequence analysis of the cDNA, isolation and characterization of the protein. *Biol Chem Hoppe Seyler* 1994;**375**(8):497–512.
36. Ramanjaneya M, Chen J, Brown JE, et al. Identification of nesfatin-1 in human and murine adipose tissue: a novel depot-specific adipokine with increased levels in obesity. *Endocrinology* 2010;**151**(7):3169–80.
37. Yosten GL, Samson WK. Nesfatin-1 exerts cardiovascular actions in brain: possible interaction with the central melanocortin system. *Am J Physiol Regul Integr Comp Physiol* 2009;**297**(2):R330–6.
38. Pan W, Hsuchou H, Kastin AJ. Nesfatin-1 crosses the blood-brain barrier without saturation. *Peptides* 2007;**28**(11):2223–8.
39. Price TO, Samson WK, Niehoff ML, Banks WA. Permeability of the blood-brain barrier to a novel satiety molecule nesfatin-1. *Peptides* 2007;**28**(12):2372–81.
40. Stengel A. Nesfatin-1-More than a food intake regulatory peptide. *Peptides* 2015;**72**:175–83.
41. Yosten GL, Samson WK. Neural circuitry underlying the central hypertensive action of nesfatin-1: melanocortins, corticotropin-releasing hormone, and oxytocin. *Am J Physiol Regul Integr Comp Physiol* 2014;**306**(10):R722–7.
42. Ayada C, Turgut G, Turgut S, Guclu Z. The effect of chronic peripheral nesfatin-1 application on blood pressure in normal and chronic restraint stressed rats: related with circulating level of blood pressure regulators. *Gen Physiol Biophys* 2015;**34**(1):81–8.

43. Tan BK, Hallschmid M, Kern W, Lehnert H, Randeva HS. Decreased cerebrospinal fluid/plasma ratio of the novel satiety molecule, nesfatin-1/NUCB-2, in obese humans: evidence of nesfatin-1/NUCB-2 resistance and implications for obesity treatment. *J Clin Endocrinol Metabol* 2011;**96**(4):E669–73.
44. Angelone T, Filice E, Pasqua T, et al. Nesfatin-1 as a novel cardiac peptide: identification, functional characterization, and protection against ischemia/reperfusion injury. *Cell Mol Life Sci CMLS* 2013;**70**(3):495–509.
45. Ying J, Zhang Y, Gong S, et al. Nesfatin-1 suppresses cardiac L-type Ca(2)(+) channels through melanocortin type 4 receptor and the novel protein kinase C theta isoform pathway. *Cell Physiol Biochem Int J Exp Cell Physiol Biochem Pharmacol* 2015;**36**(2):555–68.
46. Yang RZ, Lee MJ, Hu H, et al. Identification of omentin as a novel depot-specific adipokine in human adipose tissue: possible role in modulating insulin action. *Am J Physiol Endocrinol Metabol* 2006;**290**(6):E1253–61.
47. Tan YL, Zheng XL, Tang CK. The protective functions of omentin in cardiovascular diseases. *Clin Chim Acta* 2015;**448**:98–106.
48. Yamawaki H, Kuramoto J, Kameshima S, Usui T, Okada M, Hara Y. Omentin, a novel adipocytokine inhibits TNF-induced vascular inflammation in human endothelial cells. *Biochem Biophys Res Commun* 2011;**408**(2):339–43.
49. Maruyama S, Shibata R, Kikuchi R, et al. Fat-derived factor omentin stimulates endothelial cell function and ischemia-induced revascularization via endothelial nitric oxide synthase-dependent mechanism. *J Biol Chem* 2012;**287**(1):408–17.
50. Kazama K, Okada M, Yamawaki H. A novel adipocytokine, omentin, inhibits platelet-derived growth factor-BB-induced vascular smooth muscle cell migration through antioxidative mechanism. *Am J Physiol Heart Circul Physiol* 2014;**306**(12):H1714–9.
51. Kazama K, Usui T, Okada M, Hara Y, Yamawaki H. Omentin plays an anti-inflammatory role through inhibition of TNF-alpha-induced superoxide production in vascular smooth muscle cells. *Eur J Pharmacol* 2012;**686**(1–3):116–23.
52. Shibata R, Takahashi R, Kataoka Y, et al. Association of a fat-derived plasma protein omentin with carotid artery intima-media thickness in apparently healthy men. *Hypertens Res Off J Jpn Soc Hyper* 2011;**34**(12):1309–12.
53. Kataoka Y, Shibata R, Ohashi K, et al. Omentin prevents myocardial ischemic injury through AMP-activated protein kinase- and Akt-dependent mechanisms. *J Am Coll Cardiol* 2014;**63**(24):2722–33.
54. Matsuo K, Shibata R, Ohashi K, et al. Omentin functions to attenuate cardiac hypertrophic response. *J Mol Cell Cardiol* 2015;**79**:195–202.
55. Iizuka K, Machida T, Hirafuji M. Skeletal muscle is an endocrine organ. *J Pharmacol Sci* 2014;**125**(2):125–31.
56. Pedersen BK, Febbraio MA. Muscles, exercise and obesity: skeletal muscle as a secretory organ. *Nat Rev Endocrinol* 2012;**8**(8):457–65.
57. Bostrom P, Wu J, Jedrychowski MP, et al. A PGC1-alpha-dependent myokine that drives brown-fat-like development of white fat and thermogenesis. *Nature* 2012;**481**(7382):463–8.
58. Aydin S. Three new players in energy regulation: preptin, adropin and irisin. *Peptides* 2014;**56**:94–110.
59. Huh JY, Mougios V, Kabasakalis A, et al. Exercise-induced irisin secretion is independent of age or fitness level and increased irisin may directly modulate muscle metabolism through AMPK activation. *J Clin Endocrinol Metabol* 2014;**99**(11):E2154–61.
60. Huh JY, Siopi A, Mougios V, Park KH, Mantzoros CS. Irisin in response to exercise in humans with and without metabolic syndrome. *J Clin Endocrinol Metabol* 2015;**100**(3):E453–7.
61. Song H, Wu F, Zhang Y, et al. Irisin promotes human umbilical vein endothelial cell proliferation through the ERK signaling pathway and partly suppresses high glucose-induced apoptosis. *PloS One* 2014;**9**(10):e110273.
62. Wu F, Song H, Zhang Y, et al. Irisin induces angiogenesis in human umbilical vein endothelial cells in vitro and in zebrafish embryos in vivo via activation of the ERK signaling pathway. *PloS One* 2015;**10**(8):e0134662.
63. Han F, Zhang S, Hou N, Wang D, Sun X. Irisin improves endothelial function in obese mice through the AMPK-eNOS pathway. *Am J Physiol Heart Circul Physiol* 2015;**309**(9):H1501–8.

64. Zhu D, Wang H, Zhang J, et al. Irisin improves endothelial function in type 2 diabetes through reducing oxidative/nitrative stresses. *J MolCell Cardiol* 2015;**87**:138–47.
65. Aydin S, Aydin S, Kobat MA, et al. Decreased saliva/serum irisin concentrations in the acute myocardial infarction promising for being a new candidate biomarker for diagnosis of this pathology. *Peptides* 2014;**56**:141–5.
66. Aydin S, Kuloglu T, Aydin S, et al. Cardiac, skeletal muscle and serum irisin responses to with or without water exercise in young and old male rats: cardiac muscle produces more irisin than skeletal muscle. *Peptides* 2014;**52**:68–73.
67. Lecker SH, Zavin A, Cao P, et al. Expression of the irisin precursor FNDC5 in skeletal muscle correlates with aerobic exercise performance in patients with heart failure. *Circul Heart Fail* 2012;**5**(6):812–8.
68. Landry CR, Zhong X, Nielly-Thibault L, Roucou X. Found in translation: functions and evolution of a recently discovered alternative proteome. *Curr Opin Struct Biol* 2015;**32**:74–80.
69. Rabadan-Diehl C, Martinez A, Volpi S, Subburaju S, Aguilera G. Inhibition of vasopressin V1b receptor translation by upstream open reading frames in the 5′-untranslated region. *J Neuroendocrinol* 2007;**19**(4):309–19.
70. Xu G, Rabadan-Diehl C, Nikodemova M, Wynn P, Spiess J, Aguilera G. Inhibition of corticotropin releasing hormone type-1 receptor translation by an upstream AUG triplet in the 5′ untranslated region. *Mol Pharmacol* 2001;**59**(3):485–92.
71. McGraw DW, Forbes SL, Kramer LA, Liggett SB. Polymorphisms of the 5′ leader cistron of the human beta2-adrenergic receptor regulate receptor expression. *J Clin Invest* 1998;**102**(11):1927–32.
72. Zimmer A, Zimmer AM, Reynolds K. Tissue specific expression of the retinoic acid receptor-beta 2: regulation by short open reading frames in the 5′-noncoding region. *J Cell Biol* 1994;**127**(4):1111–9.
73. Mori Y, Matsubara H, Murasawa S, et al. Translational regulation of angiotensin II type 1A receptor. Role of upstream AUG triplets. *Hypertension* 1996;**28**(5):810–7.
74. Wei H, Ahn S, Shenoy SK, et al. Independent beta-arrestin 2 and G protein-mediated pathways for angiotensin II activation of extracellular signal-regulated kinases 1 and 2. *Proc Natl Acad Sci U S A* 2003;**100**(19):10782–7.
75. Nomura A, Iwasaki Y, Saito M, et al. Involvement of upstream open reading frames in regulation of rat V(1b) vasopressin receptor expression. *Am J Physiol Endocrinol Metabol* 2001;**280**(5):E780–7.
76. Ji H, Zhang Y, Zheng W, Wu Z, Lee S, Sandberg K. Translational regulation of angiotensin type 1a receptor expression and signaling by upstream AUGs in the 5′ leader sequence. *J Biol Chem* 2004;**279**(44):45322–8.
77. Liu J, Yosten GL, Ji H, et al. Selective inhibition of angiotensin receptor signaling through Erk1/2 pathway by a novel peptide. *Am J Physiol Regul Integr Comp Physiol* 2014;**306**(8):R619–26.
78. Hunyady L, Catt KJ. Pleiotropic AT1 receptor signaling pathways mediating physiological and pathogenic actions of angiotensin II. *Mol Endocrinol* 2006;**20**(5):953–70.
79. Daniels D, Yee DK, Faulconbridge LF, Fluharty SJ. Divergent behavioral roles of angiotensin receptor intracellular signaling cascades. *Endocrinology* 2005;**146**(12):5552–60.
80. Daniels D, Yee DK, Fluharty SJ. Angiotensin II receptor signalling. *Exp Physiol* 2007;**92**(3):523–7.
81. Daniels D, Mietlicki EG, Nowak EL, Fluharty SJ. Angiotensin II stimulates water and NaCl intake through separate cell signalling pathways in rats. *Exp Physiol* 2009;**94**(1):130–7.

PART

II

THE HEART AS AN ENDOCRINE TARGET

CHAPTER

GUT-DERIVED HORMONES—CARDIAC EFFECTS OF GHRELIN AND GLUCAGON-LIKE PEPTIDE-1

6

G. Ruozi[1], F. Bortolotti[1] and F.A. Recchia[2,3]

[1]International Centre for Genetic Engineering and Biotechnology (ICGEB), Trieste, Italy [2]Lewis Katz School of Medicine at Temple University, Philadelphia, PA, United States [3]Scuola Superiore Sant'Anna, Pisa, Italy

GHRELIN

Peptidyl and nonpeptidyl growth hormone secretagogues (GHSs), such as growth hormone-releasing peptide 6 (GHRP-6), growth hormone-releasing peptide 2 (GHRP-2) and hexarelin have been synthesized since the early 1980s.[1,2] These peptides have different GH-releasing potency and act on the pituitary gland and on the hypothalamic arcuate nucleus through the G protein-coupled receptor GHS-receptor 1a (GHS-R1a).[3] The endogenous ligand for this receptor was later identified by Kojima and coworkers,[4] using an approach of "reverse pharmacology." Surprisingly, based on Northern blot analysis of rat tissues, ghrelin was found to be more highly expressed in the stomach than in known sites of GHS-R1a expression, namely the brain, pituitary gland or hypothalamus. This peptide was named "ghrelin," from "ghre," the Proto-Indo-European root of the word grow, and "relin" that refers to its GH-releasing activities. The purified ligand was a 28 amino acid peptide, mainly synthesized and secreted by a distinct population of endocrine cells named X/A-like cells, located predominantly in the oxyntic mucosa of the stomach.[5] Later, ghrelin mRNA was also found in many other tissues, such as the hypothalamus, pituitary gland, small intestine, adrenal gland, kidney, pancreas, liver, spleen, vein, muscle, lung, esophagus, thyroid, gall bladder, ovary, testis, breast, lymph nodes, adipose tissue, and heart, where it is expressed in atria, ventricles, and blood vessels.[6] Ghrelin protein is mainly present in the stomach, small intestine, brain, cerebellum, pituitary gland, lung, muscle, pancreas, adrenal gland, ovary, and testes.[7] Ghrelin is also produced and secreted by cardiomyocytes.[8]

Although they share common functions, there are no structural homologies between the brain-gut peptide ghrelin and the GHSs, which include GHRP-6 and hexarelin. The serine (Ser) 3 residue of ghrelin is n-octanoylated, and this modification is essential for GHS-R1a binding and for the endocrine functions of the peptide, including GH-releasing activity, stimulation of food intake, and regulation of energy homeostasis.[9] Apart from the well-described metabolic activities related to stimulation of GH-release[10] and feeding regulation,[11] it has become progressively evident that GHSs and ghrelin exert

Endocrinology of the Heart in Health and Disease. DOI: http://dx.doi.org/10.1016/B978-0-12-803111-7.00006-3

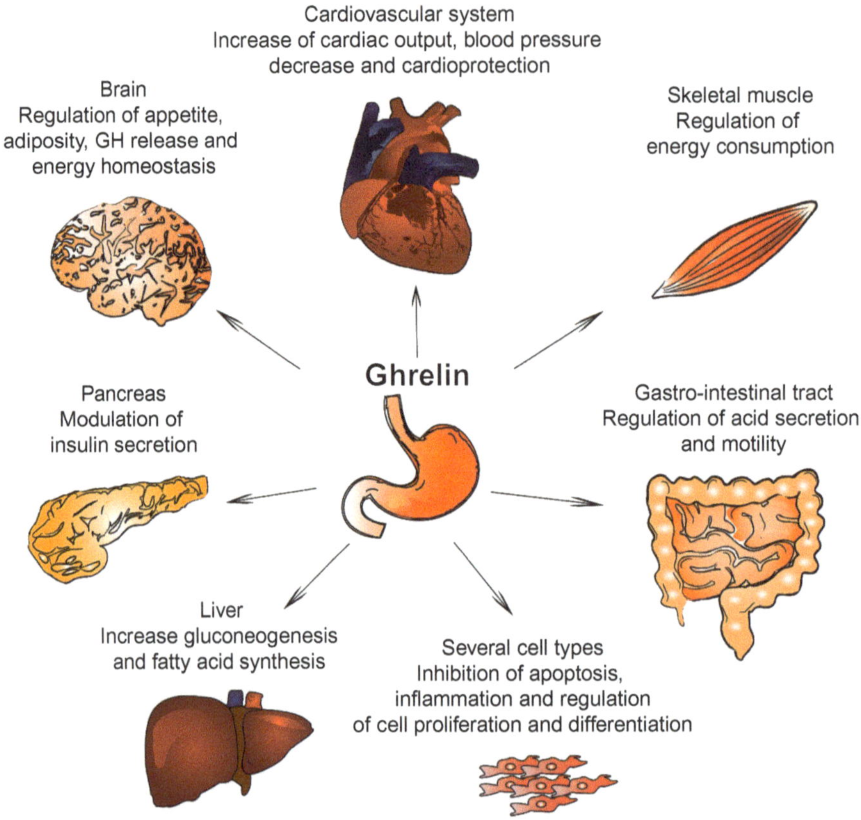

FIGURE 6.1

Main physiological functions of Ghrelin in different organs. Ghrelin exerts actions on several peripheral tissues, including pancreas, brain, heart, skeletal muscle, gastrointestinal tract and liver. Ghrelin also prevents cell death and inflammation and induces cell proliferation or differentiation of different cell types.

many other peripheral functions, including immune responses,[12] glucose and lipid metabolism,[13,14] gastrointestinal function,[15] and a wide range of cardiovascular activities[16,17] (Fig. 6.1).

GENE STRUCTURE AND DERIVED-PEPTIDES

The human ghrelin gene is located on the chromosome 3p25-26; it consists of five exons and three introns and encodes for a transcript of 511 bp, corresponding to a 117 amino acid precursor named preproghrelin (Fig. 6.2). This precursor contains a signal peptide and the proghrelin protein that yields the two mature peptides, ghrelin, and obestatin. As it enters the endoplasmic reticulum, preproghrelin is processed to proghrelin by a cleavage that removes the 23 amino acid sequence corresponding to the signal peptide sequence. Proghrelin is further processed to ghrelin by the enzyme prohormone convertase 1/3 that generates the mature 28 amino acid peptide.[18] Following proteolytic cleavage from

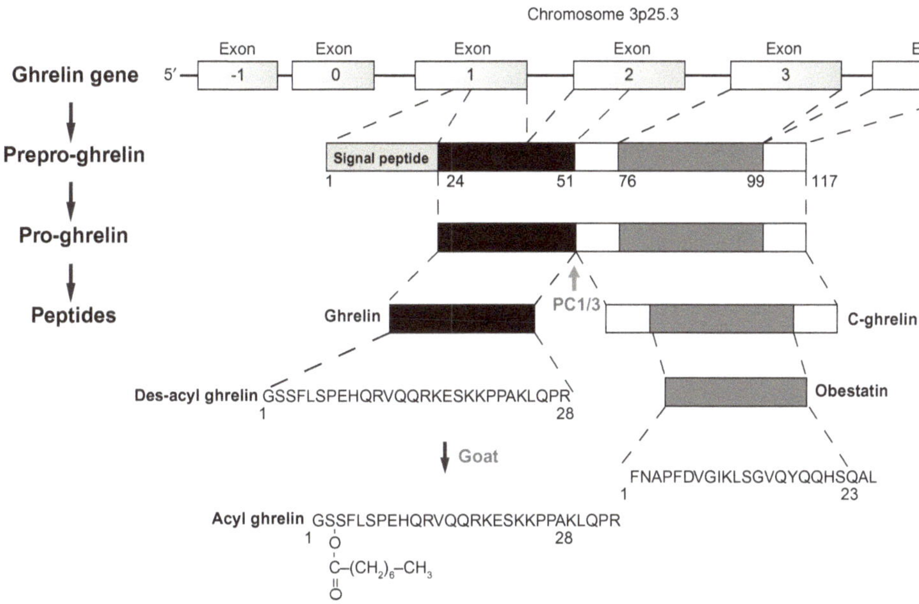

FIGURE 6.2

Structure and posttranslational processing of the ghrelin gene. Ghrelin is transcribed to yield preproghrelin, which is further processed to form the proghrelin precursor. Prohormone convertase 1/3 (PC 1/3) cleaves after arginine-28 of proghrelin, generating the mature 28 amino acid peptide. The majority of the peptide remains unacylated (des-acyl ghrelin), while a smaller portion of it undergoes a posttranslational modification, which consists of the esterification of a fatty acid on Ser3 by the enzyme GOAT to generate acyl ghrelin. In addition to ghrelin, the 23 amino acid peptide obestatin is also generated from the proghrelin precursor.

proghrelin, a posttranslational modification occurs, consisting of a fatty acid esterification, usually the n-octanoic acid (C8:0), on the third amino acidic residue, corresponding to Ser3. Only acylated-ghrelin is able to bind the GHS-R1a; therefore, this modification is essential for some ghrelin biological activities, including GH release and feeding regulation. The enzyme responsible for acylation was described in 2008 and named ghrelin-O-acyltransferase (GOAT).[19,20] GOAT is encoded by the membrane bound O-acyltransferase domain containing 4 (MBOAT4) gene and is highly conserved in vertebrates. The relative tissue distribution of GOAT mRNA matches that of ghrelin and it is highest in stomach, but, recently, low levels of GOAT expression have also been observed in other tissues, including the heart.[21]

A mechanism of alternative splicing of the ghrelin gene transcript can trigger the production of a minor active isoform of the molecule named des-Gln14-ghrelin, which is identical to the main form of the molecule, except for the deletion of glutamine in position 14. Des-Gln14-ghrelin undergoes the same process of acylation as ghrelin.[22] The presence, in much smaller amounts, of biologically active analogues of decanoylated (C10:0) or decenoylated (C10:1) ghrelin has also been reported.[23] These peptides bind the GHSR-1a receptor, but stimulate lower calcium mobilization activity and GH-release than octanoylated ghrelin.

In addition to ghrelin, another small peptide of 23 amino acids, named obestatin, is generated from the proghrelin precursor.[24,25] It was initially reported that obestatin exerted opposite effects to ghrelin on food intake, acting on a different G protein-coupled receptor (GPR39). Studies by a number of investigators failed to reproduce these data and it is now believed that GPR39 is not the cognate receptor for obestatin; hence, the effect of this peptide on feeding regulation remains controversial.[26] However, other biological functions of obestatin have been described, such as memory improvement and activation of cortical neurons.[27]

Des-acyl ghrelin, lacking O-n-octanoylation at Ser3, is also produced in the stomach and constitutes the major molecular form secreted into the circulation.[28] Plasma des-acyl/acyl ghrelin ratio ranges from 3:1 to 9:1 under different metabolic conditions.[29,30] However, des-acyl ghrelin does not bind GHS-R1a and thus does not exert the same endocrine activities as ghrelin. While des-acyl ghrelin was originally considered inactive, it has become evident this peptide exerts a number of functions, some of them common to acyl ghrelin and others different and specific, mainly in peripheral tissues, acting, for instance, on cell proliferation and metabolism. Most likely, these activities are mediated by additional, not yet identified, receptor(s) different from GHS-R1a.[31,32]

Ghrelin is highly conserved in vertebrates; rat and human sequences differ by only two residues, while the 10 amino acids in the N-terminus of the protein, containing the acylated Ser3, are identical among all mammalian ghrelins. Studies aimed at identifying the minimal sequence needed to activate GHS-R1a showed the entire sequence is not necessary for ghrelin activity: short N-terminus tetra- or penta-peptides including the first Gly-Ser-Ser(n-octanoyl)-Phe amino acids constitute the "active core" and are able to activate GHS-R1a.[33] The n-octanoyl group of ghrelin is one of the principal structural features determining its potency on GHS-R1a, which requires bulky hydrophobic groups at the side chain of Ser3.

GHRELIN RECEPTORS

Since its discovery and characterization as a GH-releasing and orexigenic factor (i.e., appetite stimulant), acyl ghrelin has been demonstrated to be a pleiotropic molecule, displaying many different functions that do not necessarily require the presence of the canonical receptor GHS-R1a. An increasing number of reports on the presence of specific binding-sites recognized by both acyl and des-acyl ghrelin[34,35] have suggested that GHS-R1a is not the only ghrelin receptor, but most likely one of the ghrelin receptor subtypes.

TYPE 1A GHS RECEPTOR (GHS-R1A)

GHS-R1a is a typical G protein-coupled receptor (GPCR) with seven transmembrane domains (7-TM). The human GHS-R gene is located on chromosome 3q26.2 and is highly conserved across species.[36] Alternative splicing of the pre-mRNA generates two transcripts encoding for GHS-R type 1a (GHS-R1a) and GHS-R type 1b (GHS-R1b).[3] The human full-length GHS-R1a is a polypeptide of 366 amino acids, which exhibits high affinity for GHSs and ghrelin. They share common binding at TM-3, while other contact points in TM sites are specific for different GHSs. In contrast, the GHS-R1b transcript is encoded by one exon and gives rise to a truncated peptide of 289 amino acids, only containing 5-TM domains with additional 24 amino acids at the C-terminus. GHS-R1b does not bind either GHSs or ghrelin and its functional activity has yet to be clearly determined. One hypothesis is that it may modulate other GPCRs, including GHS-R1a, through GPCR homo- and/or heterodimerization.[37] GHS-R1b can act as a dominant-negative regulator of GHS-R1a by reducing the cell surface expression of the receptor and, therefore, reduce its constitutive signaling.[38]

Ghrelin acts on the GHS-R1a and induces phospholipase C to give diacylglycerol and inositol-triphosphate (IP3); the resulting increase in intracellular Ca^{2+} concentration indicates that GHSR-1a is coupled with a Gq subunit. Besides the activation upon ligand-receptor interaction, GHS-R1a is constitutively highly active, signaling at approximately 50% of the ghrelin-induced activity in the absence of agonists.[39] This high level of constitutive activity may be of physiological importance as a regulator of both GH secretion and appetite control. The interaction between GHS-R1a and its ligands results in rapid desensitization and receptor internalization, mediated by clathrin-coated pits, from the cell surface to intracellular compartments. The ligand-receptor complex is therefore internalized into vesicles and then sorted into endosomes where the complex is dissociated and the receptor is finally recycled to the membrane.[40]

GHS-R1a is highly expressed in the hypothalamus and pituitary gland, consistent with its metabolic functions. However, its expression has also been reported in different areas of the CNS such as the hippocampus, substantia nigra, cortex and others, in the cervical vagal nodose ganglion and in multiple peripheral organs, such as the stomach, intestine, pancreas, thyroid, gonads, kidney, heart and vasculature, bone, and various tumors and cell lines.[6] This broad expression of the receptor is fully consistent with the rising spectrum of actions attributed to ghrelin. GHS-R1a, as its ligand ghrelin, is highly conserved among vertebrates, highlighting its important physiological functions. GHSR-1a is also able to dimerize with a number of other receptors, including the dopamine receptors 1 and 2 (D1R and D2R)[41,42] in areas associated with mood, learning and memory, and also with the melanocortin-3 receptor,[43] the serotonin 2 C receptor (5-HT2C),[44] and the somatostatin receptor subtype 5 (SSTR5) in pancreatic islets.[45] Dimerization modified the signaling pathways of the individual receptors, resulting in physiological processes not seen in the absence of dimers. Currently, heterodimers have been observed in cell lines or in hypothalamic neurons and pancreas and the interaction between GHSR-1a and GPCRs mainly involves appetite regulation, food reward, and stress. Nothing is known about heterodimerization of GHSR-1a in the heart, where the majority of the potential receptor dimerization partners are expressed; therefore, further analyses are needed to elucidate the potential influence of GHSR-1a and GPCR dimerization on ghrelin signaling in the heart.

NON TYPE 1A GHS RECEPTORS

The formation of heterodimeric receptor complexes partially accounts for the GHS-R1a alternative signaling in response to ghrelin, but there are multiple lines of evidence that other yet unidentified receptors exist (Fig. 6.3). Ghrelin also appears active in some tissues and cell lines not expressing GHS-R1a, thus supporting the hypothesis that GHS-R1a is not the only receptor for this peptide.[46–48] In addition to GPCR homologues of GHS-R1a and its splicing variant GHS-R1b, the existence of alternative receptors binding both acyl and/or des-acyl ghrelin have been reported. Moreover, an unidentified obestatin receptor must exist.

Since des-acyl ghrelin does not bind GHS-R1a, acylation at Ser3 being essential for receptor activation, the described effects induced by this peptide are likely mediated by other receptors. As indicated below, several ghrelin-sensitive tissues, including the heart, are also responsive also to des-acyl ghrelin, sometimes with different functional profiles. Both acyl and des-acyl ghrelin are able to prevent cell

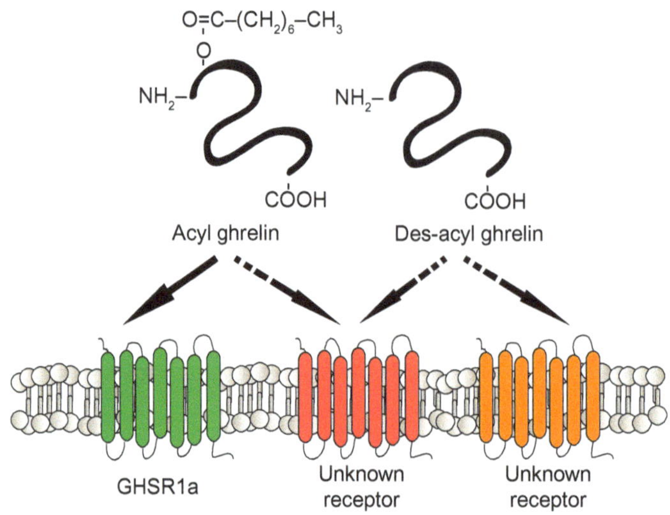

FIGURE 6.3

Acyl and des-acyl ghrelin alternative receptors. Ghrelin acylation is essential for the binding to the canonical GHS-R1a and for its endocrine functions. However, both acyl and des-acyl ghrelin, which does not bind GHS-R1a, exert several functions in tissues or cell lines not expressing GHS-R1a, supporting the hypothesis that this is not the only receptor for this peptide. Several reports have confirmed the existence of alternative receptors binding both acyl and des-acyl ghrelin as well as a specific yet unidentified receptor for the des-acyl ghrelin.

death of cultured cardiomyocytes and endothelial cells by activation of ERK1/2 and Akt pathways[31] and to improve survival and proliferation of pancreatic islet cells.[32] They also promote neurogenesis in rat fetal spinal cords,[49] increase osteoblasts proliferation,[50] and inhibit isoproterenol-induced lipolysis.[51] This evidence clearly demonstrates that at least one receptor exists, different from GHS-R1a or 1b, which is shared by the acylated and nonacylated forms of ghrelin. Moreover, the existence of receptors are able to discriminate between acyl and des-acyl ghrelin derives from the observation that, in some cells, these two peptides exert opposite functions.[13] Central administration of des-acyl ghrelin is able to stimulate food intake in GHS-R1a knockout mice, thus challenging the assumption that GHS-R1a is the only mediator of orexigenic function.[52]

Finally, there is also evidence of GHSs-specific receptors. Among these, the only one identified to date is CD36, a class B scavenger receptor expressed in many tissues such as vascular endothelium, skeletal and smooth muscle cells, monocytes, and macrophages, which is activated by hexarelin and others structurally related GHSs.[53]

GHRELIN EFFECTS ON THE CARDIOVASCULAR SYSTEM

Widespread expression of ghrelin and GHS-R1a has been found in the cardiovascular system.[6] Both GHS-R1a mRNA and protein have been detected in myocardium and aorta, even if in a much lower amount compared to the pituitary gland. Furthermore, several groups have confirmed the presence of both a putative ghrelin receptor distinct from GHS-R1a, exhibiting the same affinity for both of acyl and des-acyl ghrelin[31] as well as for a specific receptor for des-acyl ghrelin [54] in the heart. This putative receptor may be responsible for the opposing metabolic properties exhibited by acyl and des-acyl ghrelin on glucose and fatty acid uptake observed in cardiac cells.

Ghrelin can also improve energy balance, modulate the sympathetic nervous system and exert direct effects on cardiomyocyte function. Moreover, ghrelin can positively influence ventricular remodeling during pathological conditions such as myocardial infarction (MI) or chronic heart failure (CHF).[55] Acyl and des-acyl ghrelin have similar potencies in protecting the myocardium against toxic injury and cardiomyocyte depression as well in preserving endothelial cells viability.[31]

Vasoactive Function

Acyl ghrelin displays direct vasodilatory, endothelium-independent effects in humans. Intravenous injection of ghrelin peptide into healthy volunteers decreased blood pressure and increased cardiac index and stroke volume index, without changing heart rate.[56] Still in healthy humans, short-term intra-arterial infusion increased blood flow in a dose dependent manner via a GH/insulin-like growth factor (IGF)-I/nitric oxide (NO)-independent mechanism.[57] A possible mechanism explaining the ghrelin-induced vasodilation is its antagonism with the vasoconstrictor endothelin-1, observed in isolated mammary arteries.[58] The same effect was described also for des-acyl ghrelin.[59] Experiments on aortic rings harvested from GH-deficient rats demonstrated that ghrelin produces relaxation and stimulates endothelial nitric oxide synthase (eNOS).[60] eNOS activation by ghrelin was confirmed both in cultured endothelial cells and in intact vessels and depends on a ghrelin receptor/Gq protein/calcium-dependent pathway, leading to 5′-AMP activated protein kinase (AMPK) and Akt activation.[61] However, the vasodilatory effects of ghrelin and GHSs are not entirely consistent, probably due to different experimental models, routes of administration, doses and animal species. For example, it has been reported that intracoronary administration of ghrelin in pigs decreases coronary blood flow with no modification in hemodynamic parameters and plasma GH levels,[62] a response seemingly due to the inhibition of a vasodilatory β_2-adrenergic receptor-induced release of NO.

Modulation of the Sympathetic Control of Cardiovascular Function

Physiologically, acyl ghrelin is transported across the blood-brain barrier (BBB) through saturable systems that transport it from brain-to-blood and from blood-to-brain, while in mice ghrelin crosses the BBB predominantly along the brain-to-blood direction. On the contrary, des-acyl ghrelin enters the brain by nonsaturable transmembrane diffusion.[63] These transport mechanisms are essential for the peptide to target neuroendocrine networks within the central nervous system and to exert its activities on the autonomic nervous system.

Among the functions of ghrelin in the brain, an interesting mechanism that could be involved in the regulation of vascular tone is the central effect on the sympathetic system. Microinjections of acyl ghrelin in the nucleus of the tractus solitarius (NTS) suppress sympathetic activity and decrease blood pressure in rats[64] and rabbits.[65] Similarly, des-acyl ghrelin injection into the NTS reduces arterial pressure and heart rate, suggesting the desacylated form also contributes to cardiovascular regulation and that a receptor other than GHS-R1a is expressed in this bulbar nucleus.[66] The action of endogenous ghrelin on the central control of circulation has been confirmed in rats treated with [D-Lys-3]-GHRP-6, a GHS-R1a antagonist. This effect was inhibited by α- and β1-adrenoreceptor blockade, indicating it was mediated by the activation of the sympathetic nervous system.[67]

Vagal afferent terminals in the stomach and heart express ghrelin receptors, which respond to ghrelin produced in these organs sending signals to the NTS.[68,69] Blocking this system prevents the attenuation of cardiac sympathetic activity and, in turn, of arrhythmias after MI. These data therefore suggest that also peripheral ghrelin, through vagal afferent fibers, acts on the NTS to decrease peripheral sympathetic activity.[69]

Inotropic Regulation

Several studies have suggested a role of ghrelin as inotropic regulator. However, it was difficult to determine whether the observed increment of cardiac output was due to a direct effect on cardiac contractility or to reduced afterload or indirectly caused by an increased secretion of GH. Conversely, studies using isolated papillary muscles show a negative inotropic response to both of acyl and des-acyl ghrelin. This action was dependent on NO synthesis and endocardial endothelium integrity and was not mediated by GHS-R1a.[70]

Antiinflammatory Action

Ghrelin exerts potent antiinflammatory effects by inhibiting the release of cytokines such as interleukin-1 beta (IL-1β), interleukin 6 (IL-6), and tumor necrosis factor alpha (TNF-α). In addition, T lymphocytes express both ghrelin and GHS-R1a, while ghrelin secretion is increased upon T cell activation.[12] Ghrelin also displays antiinflammatory effects in endothelial cells through reducing nuclear factor (NF)-kB activation and decreasing the production of inflammatory cytokines in response to endotoxin.[71] The antiinflammatory action of ghrelin has the potential to affect several cardio-metabolic disorders associated with chronic inflammation.

Depressed cardiac contractility and endothelium-dependent vascular relaxation is also common in severe sepsis. Ghrelin levels decrease significantly during sepsis, while its administration in a rat model enhanced heart performance, attenuated the impaired endothelium-dependent vascular relaxation, and reduced organ injury by sympatho-inhibition and inflammation attenuation.[72]

Antiapoptotic Effects in Cardiac Cells

The cardioprotective effects of ghrelin can be partially explained by its inhibitory activity on molecular processes responsible for cardiomyocyte death. An antiapoptotic effect of ghrelin is detectable in primary adult and H9c2 cardiomyocytes and in endothelial cells exposed to pro-apoptotic insults, such as doxorubicin, serum withdrawal or activation by Fas ligand.[31] The proposed mechanisms involve MAPK- and PI3K/Akt-dependent pathways. Des-acyl ghrelin is similarly active, although it does not bind to and activate the ghrelin receptor. Moreover, H9c2 cardiomyocytes do not express GHS-R1a, implicating the role of another unidentified alternative ghrelin receptor. The antiapoptotic effects of acyl and des-acyl ghrelin have been confirmed in different cell types through similar signaling pathways.[8,32] In the cardiomyocyte cell line HL-1, des-acyl ghrelin binds specific sites and both acyl and des-acyl ghrelin exert antiapoptotic activities preserving cell viability and activating Akt pro-surviving pathways, despite their opposite metabolic effects on glucose and medium-length fatty acid uptake. In this regard, acyl ghrelin inhibits insulin-induced glucose uptake without influencing fatty acid uptake, whereas des-acyl ghrelin increases fatty acid uptake and glucose transporter-4 translocation to the cell membrane.[54]

Ghrelin reduced apoptosis and oxidative stress in a murine model of doxorubicin-induced cardiac injury. A number of mechanisms have been proposed to explain this cardioprotection, including the activation of antioxidant enzymes such as superoxide dismutase and catalase, the preservation of mitochondrial membrane potential and energy metabolism, and the upregulation of antiapoptotic proteins such as bcl-2. Together, these mechanisms reduce cytoplasmic cytochrome C release and prevent the activation of the NF-kB pathway.[73] Moreover, ghrelin counteracts cytokine-induced apoptosis.[74] The ability of ghrelin to reduce endoplasmic reticulum stress after ischemia-reperfusion injury is observed under both in vitro and in vivo conditions.[75] Also, des-acyl ghrelin exerts antiapoptotic effects, as shown in a rat model of isoproterenol-induced heart failure[76] and in doxorubicin-induced cardiomyopathy[77] in which it improved cardiac function. An additional pro-survival mechanism attributed to both acyl and des-acyl ghrelin is the stimulation of beneficial autophagy after MI, indeed the two peptides stimulated LC3 lipidation on autophagosome vesicles, activated the transcription of genes involved in the autophagic pathway, such as Beclin1, Atg12 and Map1LC3A and, specifically, des-acyl ghrelin triggered the removal of dysfunctional mitochondria.[78] The pro-autophagy effect of des-acyl ghrelin was confirmed in a model of diabetic cardiomyopathy.[79] Finally and importantly, ghrelin can activate cardiomyocyte AMPK,[80] a key regulator of energy homeostasis also involved in the regulation of cardiac autophagy.[81]

The more recently identified ghrelin gene-derived peptide obestatin has been reported to be protective against apoptosis in several cell types, including cardiomyocytes.[82] This antiapoptotic action appears mediated by the PKC, PI3K, and ERK1/2 pathways. Despite this evidence, to date the physiological role of obestatin is still largely unknown.

Ghrelin in the Pathophysiology of Chronic Heart Failure

Ghrelin is effective in improving cardiac performance under pathological conditions such as CHF. Rats with CHF treated with acyl ghrelin for 3 weeks displayed higher cardiac output and stroke volume compared to placebo-treated animals; furthermore, ghrelin preserved posterior wall thickness, fractional shortening and inhibited left ventricular enlargement. Ghrelin administration also increased serum GH, IGF-I levels, and body weight.[16]

Similar beneficial effects of ghrelin were observed in patients with CHF[83]: after 60 minutes of intravenous infusion, ghrelin increased mean arterial pressure without affecting heart rate. Recently, ghrelin and GHS-R1a expression have been quantified in different areas of normal and failing human hearts[84]: ghrelin was decreased in atria and ventricles of humans with CHF, while GHS-R1a was increased, possibly as a compensatory mechanism of adaptation.

Cardiac cachexia, a catabolic state characterized by weight loss and muscle wasting, occurs frequently in patients with end-stage CHF and is a negative prognostic factor. Three weeks of intravenous repeated administration of ghrelin in CHF patients improved left ventricular function, exercise capacity, decreased the plasma norepinephrine concentration, and systemic vascular resistance, and increased cardiac output.[17] Moreover, these individuals gained body weight, lean body mass, and muscle strength, which counteracted the cachectic state. Consistent with these results, ghrelin stimulates cardiac function and appetite in patients with end-stage CHF and cardiac cachexia.[85] Finally, the plasma ghrelin level is increased in cachectic patients, possibly as a compensatory mechanism in response to the anabolic-catabolic imbalance.[86,87]

One pathophysiological feature of the failing heart is a profound alteration of myocardial lipid and carbohydrate metabolism. Interestingly, the acute administration of acyl and des-acyl ghrelin enhances free fatty acid oxidation and decreases glucose oxidation, thereby partially correcting the altered energy substrate utilization observed in chronically instrumented dogs with pacing-induced heart failure.[88]

Together, vasodilatory, antiapoptotic, antiinflammatory, antioxidant, and metabolic effects may all contribute to the beneficial role of ghrelin in CHF, even if, to date, it is unknown which of these properties is the most important. No long-term clinical trials evaluating acyl and des-acyl ghrelin effects on CHF have been conducted. Should long-term administration of ghrelin prove feasible and significantly effective compared to placebo, this hormone might offer a new option for the difficult treatment of CHF.

Ghrelin in the Pathophysiology of Myocardial Infarction

Multiple lines of evidence indicate a protective effect of ghrelin on the ischemic heart. Acyl ghrelin peptide administration for 2 weeks after MI in rats mitigates sympathetic activation, improves cardiac remodeling and left ventricular function, reduces mortality and normalizes heart rate.[68,89] It is noteworthy that protective effects were also observed when ghrelin was administered less than 2 hours after MI, as it prevented malignant arrhythmias and reduced the mortality rate.[90,91] Ghrelin preserves cardiac functional parameters, reduces the post-MI scar, decreases the expression of inflammatory cytokines such as IL-1β and TNF-α and reduces matrix metalloproteinase (MMP)-2 and MMP-9 activation.[74]

In contrast, ghrelin knockout mice display an increased sympathetic activity after MI, leading to more frequent arrhythmic events, deterioration of heart function, and increased mortality. These pathological changes were efficiently reverted by ghrelin treatment.[69,92] Plasma ghrelin[93] as well as myocardial ghrelin and GHS-R1a are upregulated in isoproterenol-induced cardiac injury. As both acyl and des-acyl ghrelin proved protective against isoproterenol-induced myocardial injury and fibrosis, both peptides may function as endogenous cardioprotective factors in ischemic heart disease, acting through still unknown receptors.[76] Further support of this cardioprotective role is provided by the positive results of gene therapy with recombinant adeno–associated viral vectors carrying the ghrelin precursor gene, which preserves cardiac function by reducing the infarct size and protecting viable cardiac tissue against apoptosis, while stimulating beneficial autophagy in a murine MI model. These effects seem to be induced by both acyl and des-acyl ghrelin.[78]

Ghrelin also protects the heart against ischemia-reperfusion injury. In a Langendorff rat heart preparation subjected to ischemia-reperfusion, ghrelin improves left ventricular systolic and diastolic pressure, heart rate and coronary flow, thereby reducing ATP depletion.[94] This cardioprotection was dependent on ghrelin binding to cardiovascular receptors, which was augmented during ischemia-reperfusion.

Although further investigations are needed to establish whether the described beneficial effects of ghrelin also lead to long-term improvement of cardiac function, collectively these data suggest the potential usefulness of ghrelin as a biological therapeutic agent for the early treatment of MI.

GLUCAGON-LIKE PEPTIDE-1

Glucagon-like peptide 1 (GLP-1) is a 30 amino acid gut hormone secreted by endocrine L-cells which stimulates glucose-dependent insulin secretion in response to nutrient ingestion, resulting in reduced postprandial glycemia.

GENE STRUCTURE AND DERIVED-PEPTIDES

GLP-1 peptide was identified following cloning and characterization of the proglucagon gene on chromosome 2[95] (Fig. 6.4). In gut L-cells, proglucagon is processed to glicentin, oxyntomodulin, GLP-1 and GLP-2 by the prohormone convertase 1/3. Bioactive GLP-1 is generated from GLP-1 (1-37) and exists in two circulating forms, GLP-1 (7-37), which accounts for approximately 20% of active GLP-1, and GLP-1 (7-36) amide, the most abundant form.[96] Both GLP-1 forms are rapidly degraded by dipeptidyl peptidase (DPP)-4 to GLP-1 (9-36) amide or GLP-1 (9-37) after release. For this reason, native GLP-1 has a very short half-life (1–2 minutes) in the bloodstream; DPP-4 cleavage generates NH_2-terminally truncated metabolites that are subsequently excreted and have low affinity for the GLP-1 receptor (GLP-1R); therefore, investigating the role of intact GLP-1 in vivo requires its continuous infusion or the use of DPP-4 inhibitors.[97]

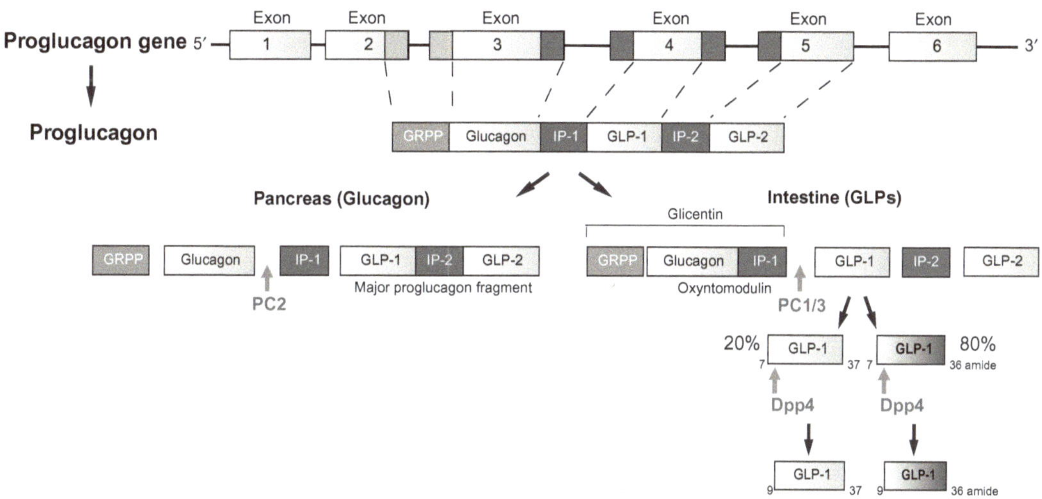

FIGURE 6.4

Structure and posttranslational processing of the proglucagon gene. Proglucagon is transcribed and cleaved by site-specific prohormone convertase 2 (PC2) and prohormone convertase 1/3 (PC 1/3) in pancreas and intestine, respectively. The precursor cleavage generates the active glucagon, glicentin-related polypeptide (GRPP), intervening peptide 1 (IP1), and the major proglucagon fragment (deriving from GLP-1, IP2, and GLP-2) in the pancreas, while in the intestine it is processed to form intervening peptide 2 (IP2), glicentin (formed by GRPP, glucagon, and IP-1), oxyntomodulin (deriving from glucagon and IP-1), GLP-1, and GLP-2. Bioactive GLP-1 is generated from GLP-1 (1-37) and exists in two circulating forms, GLP-1 (7-37), which accounts for approximately 20% of active GLP-1, and GLP-1 (7-36) amide, the most abundant one. Both GLP-1 forms are rapidly degraded by dipeptidyl peptidase (DPP)-4 to GLP-1 (9-37) or GLP-1 (9-36) amide after release in the circulation.

GLP-1 RECEPTOR

Human GLP-1R is a 463-amino acid, G protein-coupled receptor formed by eight hydrophobic domains, seven spanning the membrane plus an extracellular N-terminal domain, mainly expressed in pancreatic islets. GLP-1Rs are particularly abundant in β-cells, where they drive glucose-dependent insulin secretion, but are also present in α-cells, where they mediate the inhibition of glucagon secretion, and in the intestine, lung, kidney, heart, blood vessels, lymphocytes, and peripheral and central nervous systems.[98,99] In the cardiovascular system, GLP-1R is abundant in the vasculature, mainly in arteries and arterioles where GLP-1 exerts vasodilatory effects, whereas, in the heart, GLP-1R expression is about sixfold greater in atrial than ventricular myocytes.[100]

The GLP-1R gene is localized in chromosome 6p21 and shares sequence similarities with other receptors, such as those for the parathyroid hormone, growth hormone-releasing hormone, secretin, glucose-dependent insulinotropic polypeptide, calcitonin, vasoactive intestinal polypeptide, pituitary adenylate cyclase-activating polypeptide and glucagon.[101] GLP-1R agonists stimulate cyclic AMP formation, protein kinase A activation and cyclic AMP response element binding protein phosphorylation.[102] Moreover, GLP-1R activation is also coupled to intracellular calcium increase, inhibition of voltage-dependent K^+ currents and stimulation of ERK1/2 and phosphatidylinositol 3-kinase pathway, which is a central component of the reperfusion-injury salvage kinase pathway.[103]

In mice, GLP-1R deletion impairs glucose tolerance and alters insulin secretion after glucose ingestion, while glucagon levels, food intake, body weight, and gastric emptying are not affected.[104] GLP-1$R^{-/-}$ mice also display defects of cardiac structure and contractility, with reduced heart rate and elevated left ventricular end-diastolic pressure, supporting a role for endogenous GLP-1 in cardiovascular control.[105] The importance of GLP-1R is supported also by the observation that the GLP-1R antagonist exendin (9-39) binds the GLP-1 receptor and increases fasting time, postprandial glycemia, and plasma glucagon levels, while it reduces circulating insulin, preventing endogenous GLP-1 actions.[106] Moreover, exendin (9-39) and the metabolically inactive GLP-1 (9-36) amide can cause vascular relaxation[107] and the vasodilation induced by both of native GLP-1 and GLP-1 (9-36) persists in mice lacking the GLP-1R, indicating that the cardiovascular system likely expresses more than one GLP-1 receptor type. The specific receptor for GLP-1 (9-36) amide has not been identified yet, although this peptide not only can function as a vasodilator, but also as a beneficial modulator of cardiac function and glucose uptake under pathological conditions.[108,109]

GLP-1 RECEPTOR AGONISTS (GLP-1 RAS)

The major advantage of exogenous GLP-1 administration over conventional antidiabetic therapies, such as the sulphonylurea class of oral medications, is that its insulinotropic effects are dependent on the prevailing glucose concentration, thus reducing the risk of hypoglycemia. GLP-1 has therefore been proposed as an ideal candidate for the treatment of patients with type 2 diabetes.[110] GLP-1 also promotes the differentiation of progenitor cells derived from human pancreatic islets into β-cells, and stimulates β-cell proliferation and expansion both in healthy and diabetic rodents.[111,112] GLP-1 increases the expression of the transcription factor Pdx-1 and its binding to the insulin gene promoter, which is essential for the pro-proliferative and antiapoptotic actions of GLP-1 on β-cells.[113] Moreover, GLP-1 exerts pro-surviving effects on pancreatic cells through various mechanisms: activation of the Akt pro-surviving pathway and endoplasmic reticulum stress reduction via ERK modulation[114] plus inhibition of caspase-3 activation and nuclear fragmentation in diabetic mice.[115]

The perspective therapeutic use of GLP-1 prompted investigation of its effects on extra-pancreatic tissues (Fig. 6.5). For example, working centrally to inhibit vagal afferent nerve activity, GLP-1 inhibits gastric emptying.[116] Moreover, administration of either central or peripheral GLP-1 receptor agonists inhibits water and food intake, consistent with GLP-1 receptor localization in hypothalamic nuclei regulating satiety.[117] Finally, ghrelin binding to its receptor on L-cells "primes" them for GLP-1 secretion in response to nutrient ingestion[118] revealing a novel synergistic mechanism that involves ghrelin and GLP-1.

Given the therapeutic potential of GLP-1, a range of GLP-1 analogues and mimetics are currently being tested. Modified GLP-1 analogues are more resistant to DPP-4 degradation, exhibit longer half-lives, and are substantially more potent than native GLP-1; therefore, they are currently used for the

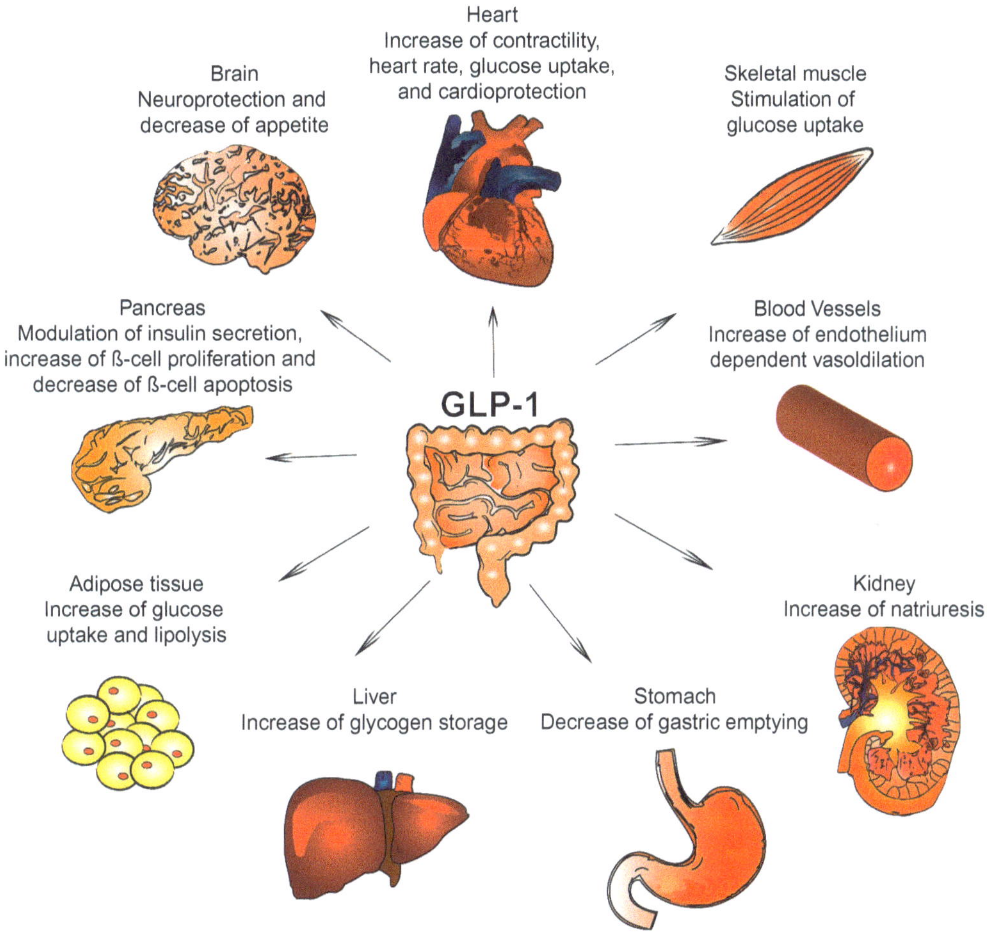

FIGURE 6.5

GLP-1 targets multiple organs. GLP-1 acts directly or indirectly on several peripheral tissues, including pancreas, brain, heart, skeletal muscle, blood vessels, kidney, stomach, liver, and adipose tissue.

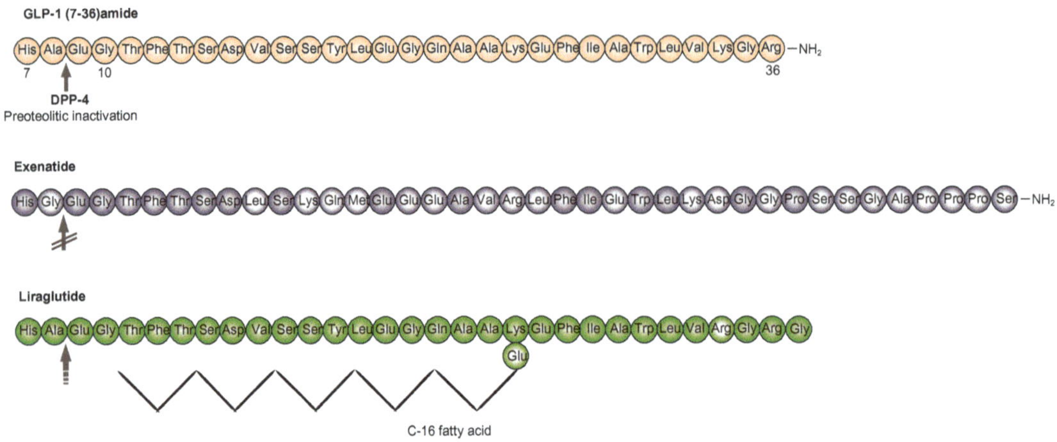

FIGURE 6.6

Structural features of GLP-1 (7-36) amide and the GLP-1 analogues exenatide and liraglutide.

Adapted from Drucker DJ, Nauck MA. The incretin system: glucagon-like peptide-1 receptor agonists and dipeptidyl peptidase-4 inhibitors in type 2 diabetes. Lancet 2006;368(9548):1696–705.

treatment of type 2 diabetic patients. Exendin-4 is a 39 amino acid GLP-1R agonist originally isolated from *Heloderma suspectum* lizard venom.[119] In mammals, the exendin-4 corresponding gene has not been identified, but the lizard protein shares 53% of amino acid sequence homology with GLP-1; hence, it represents a potent GLP-1R agonist both in vitro and in vivo. Moreover, exendin-4 contains a glycine in position 2 that confers resistance to DPP-4 cleavage and, due to higher stability, this GLP-1R agonist is a more potent glucose-lowering agent than GLP-1.

Other GLP-1 receptor agonists have been generated, such as liraglutide and exenatide (Fig. 6.6). Liraglutide is a GLP-1 analogue with 97% homology with native GLP-1, displaying only one amino acid substitution (Arg34Lys) plus a C-16 palmitic acid chain attached through a glutamyl spacer.[120] Although exenatide has about 50% homology with native GLP-1, it is identical to the exendin-4 molecule. Both exenatide and liraglutide are DPP-4 degradation resistant; the first one is a short-acting molecule, with a circulating half-life of 60–90 minutes, while liraglutide has a longer half-life of 18 hours, resulting from its noncovalent association with albumin. More recently, different peptide analogues of exendin-4 have been generated, including a long-acting version of exenatide (exenatide-LAR),[121] or others like lixisenatide, taspoglutide, and albiglutide.[122,123] Chronic treatment of type 2 diabetic patients with exenatide or liraglutide has proven effective, yielding improved glycemic control and regulation of weight and blood pressure [124,125]; these changes were paralleled by the improvement of several cardiovascular risk factors.[126–128] Long-term phase III trials, enrolling thousands of diabetic patients and analyzing cardiovascular outcomes after GLP-1 RA liraglutide (LEADER Trial) and exenatide (EXSCEL Trial) treatments, are currently ongoing.[129]

DPP-4 INHIBITORS (GLIPTINS)

A strategy complementary to the use of GLP-1R agonists is the administration of inhibitors of DPP-4, the enzyme that cleaves and inactivates GLP-1. DPP-4, also known as CD26, is a multifunctional glycoprotein protease that exists in two forms, a membrane bound form that stimulates intracellular signal pathways independent of its enzymatic activity and a circulating, soluble form, which exerts enzymatic activity and is mainly produced by lymphocytes, endothelial cells and kidney. DPP-4 is also important in glucose homeostasis, as its inactivation increases GLP-1 availability and improves glucose tolerance and insulin sensitivity.[130,131] This explains why chemical inhibitors of DPP-4, known as gliptins (e.g., sitagliptin, vildagliptin, linagliptin, saxagliptin, and alogliptin), reduce blood glucose concentration.[132] DPP-4 is a ubiquitous protease with several systemic effects: its inhibition improves endothelial function, opposes atherosclerosis and is vasoprotective, reduces the inflammatory state and influences kidney function.[133–136] The first DDP-4 inhibitor approved for the treatment of type 2 diabetes was sitagliptin, in 2006, and many others followed. They have been examined in both monotherapy and in association with metformin, glitazones, sulfonylureas, and insulin.

CARDIOVASCULAR EFFECTS OF GLP-1

As mentioned above, the beneficial effects of GLP-1 in type 2 diabetic patients are well established. Subsequent experimental and clinical investigations have also revealed the efficacy of GLP-1 in the treatment of cardiac disorders and this was not totally unexpected as GLP-1 receptors mediate important effects on the cardiovascular system. Activation of GLP-1 receptors increases systolic blood pressure and heart rate in rodents by stimulating the neural sympathetic activity.[137,138] In addition, GLP-1 has direct effects on myocardial contractility and glucose uptake in normal and postischemic myocardium. In particular, the stimulation of myocardial glucose uptake is not mediated by the classical insulin-signaling cascade involving Akt activation, but through increased NO production, p38 activation and GLUT-1 translocation.[139,140] Several studies support also direct cardioprotective roles of GLP-1 in vascular endothelium and myocardium, where GLP-1 receptors are widely expressed.[108,141] This cardioprotection is not only dependent on GLP-1-induced reduction of glycemia or on nervous control of cardiovascular function,[137] but mainly on direct cardiac effects. GLP-1R knockout mice display reduced resting heart rate, elevated left ventricular end-diastolic pressure and increased left ventricular thickness compared with wild-type mice.[105] These observations suggest a role for the GLP-1 receptor in the control of cardiac structure and function. Moreover, GLP-1 causes endothelium-independent dilation of isolated rat pulmonary artery, femoral artery and aorta.[142] In isolated cardiomyocytes, GLP-1 exerts an apparently paradoxical dual effect: while it stimulates cAMP production, this change is not associated with increased contractility, as expected, but with negative inotropism. This response is mediated by GLP-1R and completely inhibited in the presence of exendin (9–39).[143] In addition, evidence obtained from isolated heart preparations indicates that the negative inotropic effect of GLP-1 was present only when oleic acid, one of the preferential energy substrates utilized by cardiac muscle, was added to the medium and inhibited uptake and oxidation of the competing substrate glucose.[144] Such findings suggest a level of complexity that links the effects GLP-1 on cardiac contractile function to energy substrate selection. Finally, as outlined below, intravenous infusion of GLP-1 proved beneficial in various experimental models of heart failure and MI.

Diabetic Cardiomyopathy

The risk of cardiovascular disease is increased two- to fivefold in patients with type 2 diabetes compared with nondiabetic subjects; therefore, GLP-1 may represent a novel treatment strategy for diabetic patients with cardiovascular complications. In a rat model of streptozotocin (STZ)-induced type 1 diabetes, the GLP-1R agonist liraglutide reduced the typical markers of diabetic cardiomyopathy, such as myocardial steatosis, oxidative stress and apoptosis by activating the AMPK-Sirt1 pathway and independently of glucose lowering.[145] AMPK activation by GLP-1 in adult cardiomyocytes also prevents hyperglycemia-induced NADPH oxidase activation and consequent ROS production, thus reducing glucotoxicity.[146] Liraglutide also opposes the development of diabetic cardiomyopathy by inactivating the endoplasmic reticulum stress-signaling pathway in rats.[147] Moreover, chronic treatment with GLP-1 or exendin-4 restored endothelial function and vascular contraction in a STZ-induced diabetic rat model.[148] Exendin-4 has also been examined in a genetic type 2 diabetes mouse model (KKAy) and in a model of acquired type 2 diabetes induced by high-fat diet. In both cases sustained exendin-4 treatment ameliorated cardiac dysfunction, reduced left ventricular hypertrophy and reversed adverse cardiac remodeling and inflammation.[149]

In type 2 diabetes patients with stable coronary artery disease, GLP-1 treatment enhances endothelium-dependent vasodilation of the brachial artery, even though insulin resistance is not mitigated.[150] Finally, a retrospective study analyzed the cardiovascular risk in patients with type 2 diabetes treated with exenatide and concluded that these subjects are significantly less likely to exhibit cardiovascular events compared to patients treated with other glucose-lowering therapies.[151] Similar conclusions were reached by another retrospective study that analyzed the risk of major macrovascular events in type 2 diabetic patients treated with exenatide compared to insulin.[152]

Myocardial Infarction

A striking cardioprotective effect of GLP-1 and of its analogues has been found in myocardial ischemia. In isolated rat hearts, both GLP-1 and exendin-4 reduced infarct size and enhanced the recovery of contractile function after ischemia-reperfusion injury.[153] In vivo, GLP-1 infusion before ischemia protects rat hearts against myocardial injury and reduces postischemic scar size by activating pro-survival pathways. This protective effect seems to be mediated via cAMP, PI3K, or MAPK, while chemical inhibitors abolished this cardioprotection.[97] Similar results were achieved after GLP-1R agonist liraglutide pretreatment in both control and type-1 diabetic mice after infarction. Liraglutide promoted cardiomyocyte survival by activating pro-survival kinases and cytoprotective genes with a coordinate decreased incidence of cardiac rupture after MI.[141] Furthermore, the antiapoptotic effects and infarct size reduction still occurred when GLP-1 was infused at the beginning of reperfusion and not only before myocardial ischemia.[154] Moreover, exenatide treatment after ischemia reduced infarct size and improved cardiovascular parameters in a porcine model of ischemia-reperfusion injury,[155] although liraglutide did not prove efficacious in this model.[156] Finally, GLP-1 limited myocardial stunning, thus improving left ventricular regional wall motion and relaxation, after coronary occlusion and reperfusion in conscious dogs.[157]

GLP-1 effects on the heart have been confirmed in humans. In a small, nonrandomized study on patients with acute MI undergoing angioplasty, GLP-1 infusion improved left ventricular ejection fraction and global wall motion, with a consequent reduced hospitalization.[158] The benefits of this treatment persisted for months. Hemodynamic improvements were also seen in patients receiving GLP-1 before and after coronary artery bypass grafting[159,160] or after percutaneous coronary interventions.[161,162] Positive and encouraging results were obtained in a randomized trial (EXAMI Trial) evaluating the action of exenatide in patients with acute MI.[163,164]

More controversial is the outcome of DPP-4 inhibition under conditions of cardiac ischemia. It has been observed that DPP-4 genetic deficiency preserves cardiac function after MI in both normoglycemic and diabetic mice.[165] Moreover, DPP-4 inhibition, in combination with granulocyte-colony stimulating factor (G-CSF) treatment, increases cardiac regeneration and functional recovery in infarcted mice[166] and attenuates adverse cardiac remodeling in rats with chronic MI.[167] Cardioprotective effects of the DPP-4 inhibitor vildagliptin, such as the prevention of cardiac mitochondrial dysfunction, have been also reported in a porcine model of ischemia-reperfusion.[168] Clinical studies have shown that sitagliptin administration favors an improvement of left ventricular function in patients with coronary artery disease,[169] while promising results have been also obtained in a phase III randomized trial (SITAGRAMI Trial) that combined sitagliptin with G-CSF treatment in patients after acute MI.[170]

Despite evidence supporting a strategy based on DPP-4 inhibition, other studies led to an opposite conclusion. In mice, the beneficial effects of GLP-1 on cardiac functional recovery were attenuated by the DPP-4 inhibitor sitagliptin, indicating that part of the positive function of GLP-1 in the heart is possibly mediated by its breakdown product GLP-1, (9-36) not formed in the presence of DPP-4 inhibitors.[108] A recent phase IV clinical trial (SAVOR-TIMI 53), enrolling 16,492 patients, even suggested an association between the use of the DPP-4 inhibitor saxagliptin and increased hospitalization for heart failure in high-risk diabetic patients, despite improved glycemic indexes [171]; while another trial (EXAMINE) concluded that among patients with type 2 diabetes who exhibited acute coronary syndrome the rate of cardiovascular adverse events was not modified by the use of the DPP-4 inhibitor alogliptin.[172] A possible explanation for these results could be the relatively short duration of drug exposure (24 and 18 months, respectively) which may not have been sufficient to reverse the compromised condition of high-risk patients suffering from diabetes for more than 10 years.

Although more studies are warranted to draw definite conclusions, collectively the available data indicate that GLP-1 holds potential therapeutic benefit in ischemic heart disease. The exact mechanisms underlying the protective effects of GLP-1 in the ischemic heart need to be elucidated. However, it is likely that, as for other tissues, GLP-1 also activates cAMP-dependent pathways, pro-survival kinases, such as PI3K, Akt, GSK-3β, ERK1/2 and p38 MAPK, and opposes cardiomyocyte apoptosis and oxidative stress, while positively modulating myocardial metabolism.[97,143,173] During acute ischemia, cardiomyocytes switch their metabolism from fatty acid to carbohydrate utilization inducing cardiac glucose uptake.[174] In addition, it has been suggested that GLP-1 may preserve function and survival of the infarcted myocardium by limiting inflammatory cells infiltration[175] and by enhancing coronary microcirculation.[176] These effects are completely abolished by the GLP-1R antagonist exendin (9-39).[97,141] However, as mentioned above, GLP-1-induced cardioprotection is also mediated by GLP-1R-independent mechanisms, which may involve the "inactive" metabolite GLP-1 (9-36) In mice, GLP-1 (9-36) infusion improves cardiac functional recovery after ischemia-reperfusion injury.[108,177] In addition, the beneficial effects of exendin-4 or GLP-1 after ischemia-reperfusion injury are not counteracted by exendin (9-39) and persist in GLP-1R$^{-/-}$ mice,[153] thus suggesting the presence of more than one type of GLP-1 receptor in the heart.

Chronic Heart Failure

Although most of the research related to the potential applications of GLP-1 for the treatment of cardiovascular diseases has been mainly focused on cardiac ischemia, an increasing number of studies have also reported beneficial effects of GLP-1 on the failing heart. For example, continuous administration of GLP-1 for 3 months decreases cardiac apoptosis and caspase-3 activation, preserves left ventricle function and prolongs survival in spontaneously hypertensive rats with heart failure.[178] Similarly, 11 weeks of infusion of the exenatide analog AC3174 improves cardiac function, remodeling and survival in a rat model of CHF.[179] The same molecule functions as an antihypertensive agent with beneficial effects on kidneys and heart, in Dahl salt-sensitive hypertensive rats.[180,181] Consistent with results in rodents, GLP-1 administration in dogs with tachypacing-induced congestive heart failure increases cardiac output, reduces left ventricular end-diastolic pressure and improves contractility, insulin sensitivity, and myocardial glucose uptake.[182] Also the GLP-1 metabolite GLP-1 (9-36) produces similar changes,[109] thus confirming the evidence that the metabolically inactive GLP-1 (9-36) is nonetheless active on the cardiovascular system. Finally, exenatide enhances cardiac contractility and glucose uptake, with consequent reduction of brain natriuretic peptide production and prolonged survival, in a murine model of dilated cardiomyopathy.[183]

The therapeutic benefits of GLP-1 in heart failure are not documented only by experimental studies. Three days of GLP-1 infusion in a small number of type 2 diabetic patients with CHF slightly improved systolic and diastolic function.[184] In both diabetic and nondiabetic subjects with severe congestive heart failure, 5 weeks of GLP-1 $^{7-36}$ amide infusion improved left ventricular ejection fraction, myocardial oxygen consumption, functional status and quality of life.[185] These preliminary clinical studies provide encouraging data in support of the use of GLP-1 as a potential therapeutic agent for heart failure; however, further research is warranted to corroborate the positive findings, gain a deeper understanding of the underlying mechanisms and rule out long-term side effects.

REFERENCES

1. Bowers CY, Momany F, Reynolds GA, Chang D, Hong A, Chang K. Structure-activity relationships of a synthetic pentapeptide that specifically releases growth hormone in vitro. *Endocrinology* 1980;**106**(3):663–7.
2. Smith RG, Van der Ploeg LH, Howard AD, Feighner SD, Cheng K, Hickey GJ, et al. Peptidomimetic regulation of growth hormone secretion. *Endocr Rev* 1997;**18**(5):621–45.
3. Howard AD, Feighner SD, Cully DF, Arena JP, Liberator PA, Rosenblum CI, et al. A receptor in pituitary and hypothalamus that functions in growth hormone release. *Science* 1996;**273**(5277):974–7.
4. Kojima M, Hosoda H, Date Y, Nakazato M, Matsuo H, Kangawa K. Ghrelin is a growth-hormone-releasing acylated peptide from stomach. *Nature* 1999;**402**(6762):656–60.
5. Date Y, Kojima M, Hosoda H, Sawaguchi A, Mondal MS, Suganuma T, et al. Ghrelin, a novel growth hormone-releasing acylated peptide, is synthesized in a distinct endocrine cell type in the gastrointestinal tracts of rats and humans. *Endocrinology* 2000;**141**(11):4255–61.
6. Gnanapavan S, Kola B, Bustin SA, Morris DG, McGee P, Fairclough P, et al. The tissue distribution of the mRNA of ghrelin and subtypes of its receptor, GHS-R, in humans. *J Clin Endocrinol Metab* 2002;**87**(6):2988.
7. Ghelardoni S, Carnicelli V, Frascarelli S, Ronca-Testoni S, Zucchi R. Ghrelin tissue distribution: comparison between gene and protein expression. *J Endocrinol Invest* 2006;**29**(2):115–21.
8. Iglesias MJ, Pineiro R, Blanco M, Gallego R, Dieguez C, Gualillo O, et al. Growth hormone releasing peptide (ghrelin) is synthesized and secreted by cardiomyocytes. *Cardiovasc Res* 2004;**62**(3):481–8.
9. van der Lely AJ, Tschop M, Heiman ML, Ghigo E. Biological, physiological, pathophysiological, and pharmacological aspects of ghrelin. *Endocr Rev* 2004;**25**(3):426–57.
10. Malagon MM, Luque RM, Ruiz-Guerrero E, Rodriguez-Pacheco F, Garcia-Navarro S, Casanueva FF, et al. Intracellular signaling mechanisms mediating ghrelin-stimulated growth hormone release in somatotropes. *Endocrinology* 2003;**144**(12):5372–80.
11. Wren AM, Seal LJ, Cohen MA, Brynes AE, Frost GS, Murphy KG, et al. Ghrelin enhances appetite and increases food intake in humans. *J Clin Endocrinol Metab* 2001;**86**(12):5992.

12. Dixit VD, Schaffer EM, Pyle RS, Collins GD, Sakthivel SK, Palaniappan R, et al. Ghrelin inhibits leptin- and activation-induced proinflammatory cytokine expression by human monocytes and T cells. *J Clin Invest* 2004;**114**(1):57–66.
13. Gauna C, Delhanty PJ, Hofland LJ, Janssen JA, Broglio F, Ross RJ, et al. Ghrelin stimulates, whereas des-octanoyl ghrelin inhibits, glucose output by primary hepatocytes. *J Clin Endocrinol Metab* 2005;**90**(2): 1055–60.
14. Tschop M, Smiley DL, Heiman ML. Ghrelin induces adiposity in rodents. *Nature* 2000;**407**(6806):908–13.
15. Masuda Y, Tanaka T, Inomata N, Ohnuma N, Tanaka S, Itoh Z, et al. Ghrelin stimulates gastric acid secretion and motility in rats. *Biochem Biophys Res Commun* 2000;**276**(3):905–8.
16. Nagaya N, Uematsu M, Kojima M, Ikeda Y, Yoshihara F, Shimizu W, et al. Chronic administration of ghrelin improves left ventricular dysfunction and attenuates development of cardiac cachexia in rats with heart failure. *Circulation* 2001;**104**(12):1430–5.
17. Nagaya N, Moriya J, Yasumura Y, Uematsu M, Ono F, Shimizu W, et al. Effects of ghrelin administration on left ventricular function, exercise capacity, and muscle wasting in patients with chronic heart failure. *Circulation* 2004;**110**(24):3674–9.
18. Zhu X, Cao Y, Voogd K, Steiner DF. On the processing of proghrelin to ghrelin. *J Biol Chem* 2006;**281**(50):38867–70.
19. Yang J, Brown MS, Liang G, Grishin NV, Goldstein JL. Identification of the acyltransferase that octanoylates ghrelin, an appetite-stimulating peptide hormone. *Cell* 2008;**132**(3):387–96.
20. Gutierrez JA, Solenberg PJ, Perkins DR, Willency JA, Knierman MD, Jin Z, et al. Ghrelin octanoylation mediated by an orphan lipid transferase. *Proc Natl Acad Sci U S A* 2008;**105**(17):6320–5.
21. Lim CT, Kola B, Grossman A, Korbonits M. The expression of ghrelin O-acyltransferase (GOAT) in human tissues. *Endocr J* 2011;**58**(8):707–10.
22. Hosoda H, Kojima M, Matsuo H, Kangawa K. Purification and characterization of rat des-Gln14-Ghrelin, a second endogenous ligand for the growth hormone secretagogue receptor. *J Biol Chem* 2000;**275**(29):21995–2000.
23. Hosoda H, Kojima M, Mizushima T, Shimizu S, Kangawa K. Structural divergence of human ghrelin. Identification of multiple ghrelin-derived molecules produced by post-translational processing. *J Biol Chem* 2003;**278**(1):64–70.
24. Zhang JV, Ren PG, Avsian-Kretchmer O, Luo CW, Rauch R, Klein C, et al. Obestatin, a peptide encoded by the ghrelin gene, opposes ghrelin's effects on food intake. *Science* 2005;**310**(5750):996–9.
25. Chartrel N, Alvear-Perez R, Leprince J, Iturrioz X, Reaux-Le Goazigo A, Audinot V, et al. Comment on "Obestatin, a peptide encoded by the ghrelin gene, opposes ghrelin's effects on food intake". *Science* 2007;**315**(5813):766. author reply.
26. Trovato L, Gallo D, Settanni F, Gesmundo I, Ghigo E, Granata R. Obestatin: is it really doing something? *Front Horm Res* 2014;**42**:175–85.
27. Carlini VP, Schioth HB, Debarioglio SR. Obestatin improves memory performance and causes anxiolytic effects in rats. *Biochem Biophys Res Commun* 2007;**352**(4):907–12.
28. Delhanty PJ, Neggers SJ, van der Lely AJ. Should we consider des-acyl ghrelin as a separate hormone and if so, what does it do? *Front Horm Res* 2014;**42**:163–74.
29. Toshinai K, Mondal MS, Nakazato M, Date Y, Murakami N, Kojima M, et al. Upregulation of Ghrelin expression in the stomach upon fasting, insulin-induced hypoglycemia, and leptin administration. *Biochem Biophys Res Commun* 2001;**281**(5):1220–5.
30. Yoshimoto A, Mori K, Sugawara A, Mukoyama M, Yahata K, Suganami T, et al. Plasma ghrelin and desacyl ghrelin concentrations in renal failure. *J Am Soc Nephrol* 2002;**13**(11):2748–52.
31. Baldanzi G, Filigheddu N, Cutrupi S, Catapano F, Bonissoni S, Fubini A, et al. Ghrelin and des-acyl ghrelin inhibit cell death in cardiomyocytes and endothelial cells through ERK1/2 and PI 3-kinase/AKT. *J Cell Biol* 2002;**159**(6):1029–37.

32. Granata R, Settanni F, Biancone L, Trovato L, Nano R, Bertuzzi F, et al. Acylated and unacylated ghrelin promote proliferation and inhibit apoptosis of pancreatic beta-cells and human islets: involvement of 3′,5′-cyclic adenosine monophosphate/protein kinase A, extracellular signal-regulated kinase 1/2, and phosphatidyl inositol 3-Kinase/Akt signaling. *Endocrinology* 2007;**148**(2):512–29.
33. Bednarek MA, Feighner SD, Pong SS, McKee KK, Hreniuk DL, Silva MV, et al. Structure-function studies on the new growth hormone-releasing peptide, ghrelin: minimal sequence of ghrelin necessary for activation of growth hormone secretagogue receptor 1a. *J Med Chem* 2000;**43**(23):4370–6.
34. Bedendi I, Alloatti G, Marcantoni A, Malan D, Catapano F, Ghe C, et al. Cardiac effects of ghrelin and its endogenous derivatives des-octanoyl ghrelin and des-Gln14-ghrelin. *Eur J Pharmacol* 2003;**476**(1–2):87–95.
35. Muccioli G, Baragli A, Granata R, Papotti M, Ghigo E. Heterogeneity of ghrelin/growth hormone secretagogue receptors. Toward the understanding of the molecular identity of novel ghrelin/GHS receptors. *Neuroendocrinology* 2007;**86**(3):147–64.
36. Camina JP. Cell biology of the ghrelin receptor. *J Neuroendocrinol* 2006;**18**(1):65–76.
37. Chu KM, Chow KB, Leung PK, Lau PN, Chan CB, Cheng CH, et al. Over-expression of the truncated ghrelin receptor polypeptide attenuates the constitutive activation of phosphatidylinositol-specific phospholipase C by ghrelin receptors but has no effect on ghrelin-stimulated extracellular signal-regulated kinase 1/2 activity. *Int J Biochem Cell Biol* 2007;**39**(4):752–64.
38. Leung PK, Chow KB, Lau PN, Chu KM, Chan CB, Cheng CH, et al. The truncated ghrelin receptor polypeptide (GHS-R1b) acts as a dominant-negative mutant of the ghrelin receptor. *Cell Signal* 2007;**19**(5):1011–22.
39. Holst B, Holliday ND, Bach A, Elling CE, Cox HM, Schwartz TW. Common structural basis for constitutive activity of the ghrelin receptor family. *J Biol Chem* 2004;**279**(51):53806–17.
40. Camina JP, Carreira MC, El Messari S, Llorens-Cortes C, Smith RG, Casanueva FF. Desensitization and endocytosis mechanisms of ghrelin-activated growth hormone secretagogue receptor 1a. *Endocrinology* 2004;**145**(2):930–40.
41. Jiang H, Betancourt L, Smith RG. Ghrelin amplifies dopamine signaling by cross talk involving formation of growth hormone secretagogue receptor/dopamine receptor subtype 1 heterodimers. *Mol Endocrinol* 2006;**20**(8):1772–85.
42. Kern A, Albarran-Zeckler R, Walsh HE, Smith RG. Apo-ghrelin receptor forms heteromers with DRD2 in hypothalamic neurons and is essential for anorexigenic effects of DRD2 agonism. *Neuron* 2012;**73**(2):317–32.
43. Rediger A, Tarnow P, Bickenbach A, Schaefer M, Krude H, Gruters A, et al. Heterodimerization of hypothalamic G-protein-coupled receptors involved in weight regulation. *Obes Facts* 2009;**2**(2):80–6.
44. Schellekens H, van Oeffelen WE, Dinan TG, Cryan JF. Promiscuous dimerization of the growth hormone secretagogue receptor (GHS-R1a) attenuates ghrelin-mediated signaling. *J Biol Chem* 2013;**288**(1):181–91.
45. Park S, Jiang H, Zhang H, Smith RG. Modification of ghrelin receptor signaling by somatostatin receptor-5 regulates insulin release. *Proc Natl Acad Sci U S A* 2012;**109**(46):19003–8.
46. Filigheddu N, Gnocchi VF, Coscia M, Cappelli M, Porporato PE, Taulli R, et al. Ghrelin and des-acyl ghrelin promote differentiation and fusion of C2C12 skeletal muscle cells. *Mol Biol Cell* 2007;**18**(3):986–94.
47. Gauna C, Delhanty PJ, van Aken MO, Janssen JA, Themmen AP, Hofland LJ, et al. Unacylated ghrelin is active on the INS-1E rat insulinoma cell line independently of the growth hormone secretagogue receptor type 1a and the corticotropin releasing factor 2 receptor. *Mol Cell Endocrinol* 2006;**251**(1–2):103–11.
48. Thompson NM, Gill DA, Davies R, Loveridge N, Houston PA, Robinson IC, et al. Ghrelin and des-octanoyl ghrelin promote adipogenesis directly in vivo by a mechanism independent of the type 1a growth hormone secretagogue receptor. *Endocrinology* 2004;**145**(1):234–42.
49. Sato M, Nakahara K, Goto S, Kaiya H, Miyazato M, Date Y, et al. Effects of ghrelin and des-acyl ghrelin on neurogenesis of the rat fetal spinal cord. *Biochem Biophys Res Commun* 2006;**350**(3):598–603.
50. Delhanty PJ, van der Eerden BC, van der Velde M, Gauna C, Pols HA, Jahr H, et al. Ghrelin and unacylated ghrelin stimulate human osteoblast growth via mitogen-activated protein kinase (MAPK)/phosphoinositide 3-kinase (PI3K) pathways in the absence of GHS-R1a. *J Endocrinol* 2006;**188**(1):37–47.

51. Muccioli G, Pons N, Ghe C, Catapano F, Granata R, Ghigo E. Ghrelin and des-acyl ghrelin both inhibit isoproterenol-induced lipolysis in rat adipocytes via a non-type 1a growth hormone secretagogue receptor. *Eur J Pharmacol* 2004;**498**(1–3):27–35.
52. Toshinai K, Yamaguchi H, Sun Y, Smith RG, Yamanaka A, Sakurai T, et al. Des-acyl ghrelin induces food intake by a mechanism independent of the growth hormone secretagogue receptor. *Endocrinology* 2006;**147**(5):2306–14.
53. Demers A, McNicoll N, Febbraio M, Servant M, Marleau S, Silverstein R, et al. Identification of the growth hormone-releasing peptide binding site in CD36: a photoaffinity cross-linking study. *Biochem J* 2004;**382**(Pt 2):417–24.
54. Lear PV, Iglesias MJ, Feijoo-Bandin S, Rodriguez-Penas D, Mosquera-Leal A, Garcia-Rua V, et al. Des-acyl ghrelin has specific binding sites and different metabolic effects from ghrelin in cardiomyocytes. *Endocrinology* 2010;**151**(7):3286–98.
55. Granata R, Isgaard J, Alloatti G, Ghigo E. Cardiovascular actions of the ghrelin gene-derived peptides and growth hormone-releasing hormone. *Exp Biol Med (Maywood)* 2011;**236**(5):505–14.
56. Nagaya N, Kojima M, Uematsu M, Yamagishi M, Hosoda H, Oya H, et al. Hemodynamic and hormonal effects of human ghrelin in healthy volunteers. *Am J Physiol Regul Integr Comp Physiol* 2001;**280**(5):R1483–7.
57. Okumura H, Nagaya N, Enomoto M, Nakagawa E, Oya H, Kangawa K. Vasodilatory effect of ghrelin, an endogenous peptide from the stomach. *J Cardiovasc Pharmacol* 2002;**39**(6):779–83.
58. Wiley KE, Davenport AP. Comparison of vasodilators in human internal mammary artery: ghrelin is a potent physiological antagonist of endothelin-1. *Br J Pharmacol* 2002;**136**(8):1146–52.
59. Kleinz MJ, Maguire JJ, Skepper JN, Davenport AP. Functional and immunocytochemical evidence for a role of ghrelin and des-octanoyl ghrelin in the regulation of vascular tone in man. *Cardiovasc Res* 2006;**69**(1):227–35.
60. Shimizu Y, Nagaya N, Teranishi Y, Imazu M, Yamamoto H, Shokawa T, et al. Ghrelin improves endothelial dysfunction through growth hormone-independent mechanisms in rats. *Biochem Biophys Res Commun* 2003;**310**(3):830–5.
61. Xu X, Jhun BS, Ha CH, Jin ZG. Molecular mechanisms of ghrelin-mediated endothelial nitric oxide synthase activation. *Endocrinology* 2008;**149**(8):4183–92.
62. Grossini E, Molinari C, Mary DA, Ghigo E, Bona G, Vacca G. Intracoronary ghrelin infusion decreases coronary blood flow in anesthetized pigs. *Endocrinology* 2007;**148**(2):806–12.
63. Banks WA, Tschop M, Robinson SM, Heiman ML. Extent and direction of ghrelin transport across the blood-brain barrier is determined by its unique primary structure. *J Pharmacol Exp Ther* 2002;**302**(2):822–7.
64. Lin Y, Matsumura K, Fukuhara M, Kagiyama S, Fujii K, Iida M. Ghrelin acts at the nucleus of the solitary tract to decrease arterial pressure in rats. *Hypertension* 2004;**43**(5):977–82.
65. Matsumura K, Tsuchihashi T, Fujii K, Abe I, Iida M. Central ghrelin modulates sympathetic activity in conscious rabbits. *Hypertension* 2002;**40**(5):694–9.
66. Tsubota Y, Owada-Makabe K, Yukawa K, Maeda M. Hypotensive effect of des-acyl ghrelin at nucleus tractus solitarii of rat. *Neuroreport* 2005;**16**(2):163–6.
67. Vlasova MA, Jarvinen K, Herzig KH. Cardiovascular effects of ghrelin antagonist in conscious rats. *Regul Pept* 2009;**156**(1–3):72–6.
68. Soeki T, Kishimoto I, Schwenke DO, Tokudome T, Horio T, Yoshida M, et al. Ghrelin suppresses cardiac sympathetic activity and prevents early left ventricular remodeling in rats with myocardial infarction. *Am J Physiol Heart Circ Physiol* 2008;**294**(1):H426–32.
69. Mao Y, Tokudome T, Otani K, Kishimoto I, Nakanishi M, Hosoda H, et al. Ghrelin prevents incidence of malignant arrhythmia after acute myocardial infarction through vagal afferent nerves. *Endocrinology* 2012;**153**(7):3426–34.
70. Soares JB, Rocha-Sousa A, Castro-Chaves P, Henriques-Coelho T, Leite-Moreira AF. Inotropic and lusitropic effects of ghrelin and their modulation by the endocardial endothelium, NO, prostaglandins, GHS-R1a and KCa channels. *Peptides* 2006;**27**(7):1616–23.

71. Li WG, Gavrila D, Liu X, Wang L, Gunnlaugsson S, Stoll LL, et al. Ghrelin inhibits proinflammatory responses and nuclear factor-kappaB activation in human endothelial cells. *Circulation* 2004;**109**(18):2221–6.
72. Wu R, Chaung WW, Dong W, Ji Y, Barrera R, Nicastro J, et al. Ghrelin maintains the cardiovascular stability in severe sepsis. *J Surg Res* 2012;**178**(1):370–7.
73. Xu Z, Lin S, Wu W, Tan H, Wang Z, Cheng C, et al. Ghrelin prevents doxorubicin-induced cardiotoxicity through TNF-alpha/NF-kappaB pathways and mitochondrial protective mechanisms. *Toxicology* 2008;**247**(2–3):133–8.
74. Huang CX, Yuan MJ, Huang H, Wu G, Liu Y, Yu SB, et al. Ghrelin inhibits post-infarct myocardial remodeling and improves cardiac function through anti-inflammation effect. *Peptides* 2009;**30**(12):2286–91.
75. Zhang GG, Teng X, Liu Y, Cai Y, Zhou YB, Duan XH, et al. Inhibition of endoplasm reticulum stress by ghrelin protects against ischemia/reperfusion injury in rat heart. *Peptides* 2009;**30**(6):1109–16.
76. Li L, Zhang LK, Pang YZ, Pan CS, Qi YF, Chen L, et al. Cardioprotective effects of ghrelin and des-octanoyl ghrelin on myocardial injury induced by isoproterenol in rats. *Acta Pharmacol Sin* 2006;**27**(5):527–35.
77. Pei XM, Yung BY, Yip SP, Ying M, Benzie IF, Siu PM. Desacyl ghrelin prevents doxorubicin-induced myocardial fibrosis and apoptosis via the GHSR-independent pathway. *Am J Physiol Endocrinol Metab* 2014;**306**(3):E311–23.
78. Ruozi G, Bortolotti F, Falcione A, Dal Ferro M, Ukovich L, Macedo A, et al. AAV-mediated in vivo functional selection of tissue-protective factors against ischaemia. *Nat Commun* 2015;**6**:7388.
79. Pei XM, Yung BY, Yip SP, Chan LW, Wong CS, Ying M, et al. Protective effects of desacyl ghrelin on diabetic cardiomyopathy. *Acta Diabetol* 2014;**52**(2):293–306.
80. Kola B, Hubina E, Tucci SA, Kirkham TC, Garcia EA, Mitchell SE, et al. Cannabinoids and ghrelin have both central and peripheral metabolic and cardiac effects via AMP-activated protein kinase. *J Biol Chem* 2005;**280**(26):25196–201.
81. Mihaylova MM, Shaw RJ. The AMPK signalling pathway coordinates cell growth, autophagy and metabolism. *Nat Cell Biol* 2011;**13**(9):1016–23.
82. Alloatti G, Arnoletti E, Bassino E, Penna C, Perrelli MG, Ghe C, et al. Obestatin affords cardioprotection to the ischemic-reperfused isolated rat heart and inhibits apoptosis in cultures of similarly stressed cardiomyocytes. *Am J Physiol Heart Circ Physiol* 2010;**299**(2):H470–81.
83. Nagaya N, Miyatake K, Uematsu M, Oya H, Shimizu W, Hosoda H, et al. Hemodynamic, renal, and hormonal effects of ghrelin infusion in patients with chronic heart failure. *J Clin Endocrinol Metab* 2001;**86**(12):5854–9.
84. Beiras-Fernandez A, Kreth S, Weis F, Ledderose C, Pottinger T, Dieguez C, et al. Altered myocardial expression of ghrelin and its receptor (GHSR-1a) in patients with severe heart failure. *Peptides* 2010;**31**(12):2222–8.
85. Ashby D, Choi P, Bloom S. Gut hormones and the treatment of disease cachexia. *Proc Nutr Soc* 2008;**67**(3):263–9.
86. Nagaya N, Uematsu M, Kojima M, Date Y, Nakazato M, Okumura H, et al. Elevated circulating level of ghrelin in cachexia associated with chronic heart failure: relationships between ghrelin and anabolic/catabolic factors. *Circulation* 2001;**104**(17):2034–8.
87. Xin X, Ren AJ, Zheng X, Qin YW, Zhao XX, Yuan WJ, et al. Disturbance of circulating ghrelin and obestatin in chronic heart failure patients especially in those with cachexia. *Peptides* 2009;**30**(12):2281–5.
88. Mitacchione G, Powers JC, Grifoni G, Woitek F, Lam A, Ly L, et al. The gut hormone ghrelin partially reverses energy substrate metabolic alterations in the failing heart. *Circ Heart Fail* 2014;**7**(4):643–51.
89. Soeki T, Niki T, Uematsu E, Bando S, Matsuura T, Kusunose K, et al. Ghrelin protects the heart against ischemia-induced arrhythmias by preserving connexin-43 protein. *Heart Vessels* 2013;**28**(6):795–801.
90. Schwenke DO, Tokudome T, Kishimoto I, Horio T, Shirai M, Cragg PA, et al. Early ghrelin treatment after myocardial infarction prevents an increase in cardiac sympathetic tone and reduces mortality. *Endocrinology* 2008;**149**(10):5172–6.

91. Schwenke DO, Tokudome T, Kishimoto I, Horio T, Cragg PA, Shirai M, et al. One dose of ghrelin prevents the acute and sustained increase in cardiac sympathetic tone after myocardial infarction. *Endocrinology* 2013;**153**(5):2436–43.
92. Mao Y, Tokudome T, Otani K, Kishimoto I, Miyazato M, Kangawa K. Excessive sympathoactivation and deteriorated heart function after myocardial infarction in male ghrelin knockout mice. *Endocrinology* 2013;**154**(5):1854–63.
93. Chang L, Zhao J, Li GZ, Geng B, Pan CS, Qi YF, et al. Ghrelin protects myocardium from isoproterenol-induced injury in rats. *Acta Pharmacol Sin* 2004;**25**(9):1131–7.
94. Chang L, Ren Y, Liu X, Li WG, Yang J, Geng B, et al. Protective effects of ghrelin on ischemia/reperfusion injury in the isolated rat heart. *J Cardiovasc Pharmacol* 2004;**43**(2):165–70.
95. Bell GI, Sanchez-Pescador R, Laybourn PJ, Najarian RC. Exon duplication and divergence in the human preproglucagon gene. *Nature* 1983;**304**(5924):368–71.
96. Deacon CF, Johnsen AH, Holst JJ. Degradation of glucagon-like peptide-1 by human plasma in vitro yields an N-terminally truncated peptide that is a major endogenous metabolite in vivo. *J Clin Endocrinol Metab* 1995;**80**(3):952–7.
97. Bose AK, Mocanu MM, Carr RD, Brand CL, Yellon DM. Glucagon-like peptide 1 can directly protect the heart against ischemia/reperfusion injury. *Diabetes* 2005;**54**(1):146–51.
98. Thorens B, Porret A, Buhler L, Deng SP, Morel P, Widmann C. Cloning and functional expression of the human islet GLP-1 receptor. Demonstration that exendin-4 is an agonist and exendin-(9-39) an antagonist of the receptor. *Diabetes* 1993;**42**(11):1678–82.
99. Bullock BP, Heller RS, Habener JF. Tissue distribution of messenger ribonucleic acid encoding the rat glucagon-like peptide-1 receptor. *Endocrinology* 1996;**137**(7):2968–78.
100. Richards P, Parker HE, Adriaenssens AE, Hodgson JM, Cork SC, Trapp S, et al. Identification and characterization of GLP-1 receptor-expressing cells using a new transgenic mouse model. *Diabetes* 2014;**63**(4):1224–33.
101. Kieffer TJ, Habener JF. The glucagon-like peptides. *Endocr Rev* 1999;**20**(6):876–913.
102. Holz GG, Leech CA, Heller RS, Castonguay M, Habener JF. cAMP-dependent mobilization of intracellular Ca2+ stores by activation of ryanodine receptors in pancreatic beta-cells. A Ca2+ signaling system stimulated by the insulinotropic hormone glucagon-like peptide-1-(7-37). *J Biol Chem* 1999;**274**(20):14147–56.
103. Hausenloy DJ, Yellon DM. New directions for protecting the heart against ischaemia-reperfusion injury: targeting the reperfusion injury salvage kinase (RISK)-pathway. *Cardiovasc Res* 2004;**61**(3):448–60.
104. Scrocchi LA, Marshall BA, Cook SM, Brubaker PL, Drucker DJ. Identification of glucagon-like peptide 1 (GLP-1) actions essential for glucose homeostasis in mice with disruption of GLP-1 receptor signaling. *Diabetes* 1998;**47**(4):632–9.
105. Gros R, You X, Baggio LL, Kabir MG, Sadi AM, Mungrue IN, et al. Cardiac function in mice lacking the glucagon-like peptide-1 receptor. *Endocrinology* 2003;**144**(6):2242–52.
106. Schirra J, Sturm K, Leicht P, Arnold R, Goke B, Katschinski M. Exendin(9-39)amide is an antagonist of glucagon-like peptide-1(7-36)amide in humans. *J Clin Invest* 1998;**101**(7):1421–30.
107. Green BD, Hand KV, Dougan JE, McDonnell BM, Cassidy RS, Grieve DJ. GLP-1 and related peptides cause concentration-dependent relaxation of rat aorta through a pathway involving KATP and cAMP. *Arch Biochem Biophys* 2008;**478**(2):136–42.
108. Ban K, Noyan-Ashraf MH, Hoefer J, Bolz SS, Drucker DJ, Husain M. Cardioprotective and vasodilatory actions of glucagon-like peptide 1 receptor are mediated through both glucagon-like peptide 1 receptor-dependent and -independent pathways. *Circulation* 2008;**117**(18):2340–50.
109. Nikolaidis LA, Elahi D, Shen YT, Shannon RP. Active metabolite of GLP-1 mediates myocardial glucose uptake and improves left ventricular performance in conscious dogs with dilated cardiomyopathy. *Am J Physiol Heart Circ Physiol* 2005;**289**(6):H2401–8.

110. Gutniak M, Orskov C, Holst JJ, Ahren B, Efendic S. Antidiabetogenic effect of glucagon-like peptide-1 (7-36)amide in normal subjects and patients with diabetes mellitus. *N Engl J Med* 1992;**326**(20):1316–22.
111. Xu G, Stoffers DA, Habener JF, Bonner-Weir S. Exendin-4 stimulates both beta-cell replication and neogenesis, resulting in increased beta-cell mass and improved glucose tolerance in diabetic rats. *Diabetes* 1999;**48**(12):2270–6.
112. Friedrichsen BN, Neubauer N, Lee YC, Gram VK, Blume N, Petersen JS, et al. Stimulation of pancreatic beta-cell replication by incretins involves transcriptional induction of cyclin D1 via multiple signalling pathways. *J Endocrinol* 2006;**188**(3):481–92.
113. Li Y, Cao X, Li LX, Brubaker PL, Edlund H, Drucker DJ. beta-Cell Pdx1 expression is essential for the glucoregulatory, proliferative, and cytoprotective actions of glucagon-like peptide-1. *Diabetes* 2005;**54**(2):482–91.
114. Jhala US, Canettieri G, Screaton RA, Kulkarni RN, Krajewski S, Reed J, et al. cAMP promotes pancreatic beta-cell survival via CREB-mediated induction of IRS2. *Genes Dev* 2003;**17**(13):1575–80.
115. Wang Q, Brubaker PL. Glucagon-like peptide-1 treatment delays the onset of diabetes in 8 week-old db/db mice. *Diabetologia* 2002;**45**(9):1263–73.
116. Imeryuz N, Yegen BC, Bozkurt A, Coskun T, Villanueva-Penacarrillo ML, Ulusoy NB. Glucagon-like peptide-1 inhibits gastric emptying via vagal afferent-mediated central mechanisms. *Am J Physiol* 1997;**273**(4 Pt 1):G920–7.
117. Turton MD, O'Shea D, Gunn I, Beak SA, Edwards CM, Meeran K, et al. A role for glucagon-like peptide-1 in the central regulation of feeding. *Nature* 1996;**379**(6560):69–72.
118. Gagnon J, Baggio LL, Drucker DJ, Brubaker PL. Ghrelin is a novel regulator of GLP-1 secretion. *Diabetes* 2015;**64**(5):1513–21.
119. Eng J, Kleinman WA, Singh L, Singh G, Raufman JP. Isolation and characterization of exendin-4, an exendin-3 analogue, from Heloderma suspectum venom. Further evidence for an exendin receptor on dispersed acini from guinea pig pancreas. *J Biol Chem* 1992;**267**(11):7402–5.
120. Knudsen LB, Nielsen PF, Huusfeldt PO, Johansen NL, Madsen K, Pedersen FZ, et al. Potent derivatives of glucagon-like peptide-1 with pharmacokinetic properties suitable for once daily administration. *J Med Chem* 2000;**43**(9):1664–9.
121. Gedulin BR, Smith P, Prickett KS, Tryon M, Barnhill S, Reynolds J, et al. Dose-response for glycaemic and metabolic changes 28 days after single injection of long-acting release exenatide in diabetic fatty Zucker rats. *Diabetologia* 2005;**48**(7):1380–5.
122. Christensen M, Knop FK, Holst JJ, Vilsboll T. Lixisenatide, a novel GLP-1 receptor agonist for the treatment of type 2 diabetes mellitus. *IDrugs* 2009;**12**(8):503–13.
123. Matthews JE, Stewart MW, De Boever EH, Dobbins RL, Hodge RJ, Walker SE, et al. Pharmacodynamics, pharmacokinetics, safety, and tolerability of albiglutide, a long-acting glucagon-like peptide-1 mimetic, in patients with type 2 diabetes. *J Clin Endocrinol Metab* 2008;**93**(12):4810–7.
124. Buse JB, Rosenstock J, Sesti G, Schmidt WE, Montanya E, Brett JH, et al. Liraglutide once a day versus exenatide twice a day for type 2 diabetes: a 26-week randomised, parallel-group, multinational, open-label trial (LEAD-6). *Lancet* 2009;**374**(9683):39–47.
125. Buse JB, Drucker DJ, Taylor KL, Kim T, Walsh B, Hu H, et al. DURATION-1: exenatide once weekly produces sustained glycemic control and weight loss over 52 weeks. *Diabetes Care* 2010;**33**(6):1255–61.
126. Klonoff DC, Buse JB, Nielsen LL, Guan X, Bowlus CL, Holcombe JH, et al. Exenatide effects on diabetes, obesity, cardiovascular risk factors and hepatic biomarkers in patients with type 2 diabetes treated for at least 3 years. *Curr Med Res Opin* 2008;**24**(1):275–86.
127. Garber A, Henry R, Ratner R, Garcia-Hernandez PA, Rodriguez-Pattzi H, Olvera-Alvarez I, et al. Liraglutide versus glimepiride monotherapy for type 2 diabetes (LEAD-3 Mono): a randomised, 52-week, phase III, double-blind, parallel-treatment trial. *Lancet* 2009;**373**(9662):473–81.
128. Ratner R, Han J, Nicewarner D, Yushmanova I, Hoogwerf BJ, Shen L. Cardiovascular safety of exenatide BID: an integrated analysis from controlled clinical trials in participants with type 2 diabetes. *Cardiovasc Diabetol* 2011;**10**:22.

129. Marso SP, Poulter NR, Nissen SE, Nauck MA, Zinman B, Daniels GH, et al. Design of the liraglutide effect and action in diabetes: evaluation of cardiovascular outcome results (LEADER) trial. *Am Heart J* 2013;**166**(5):823–30.
130. Marguet D, Baggio L, Kobayashi T, Bernard AM, Pierres M, Nielsen PF, et al. Enhanced insulin secretion and improved glucose tolerance in mice lacking CD26. *Proc Natl Acad Sci U S A* 2000;**97**(12):6874–9.
131. Nagakura T, Yasuda N, Yamazaki K, Ikuta H, Yoshikawa S, Asano O, et al. Improved glucose tolerance via enhanced glucose-dependent insulin secretion in dipeptidyl peptidase IV-deficient Fischer rats. *Biochem Biophys Res Commun* 2001;**284**(2):501–6.
132. Ahren B, Landin-Olsson M, Jansson PA, Svensson M, Holmes D, Schweizer A. Inhibition of dipeptidyl peptidase-4 reduces glycemia, sustains insulin levels, and reduces glucagon levels in type 2 diabetes. *J Clin Endocrinol Metab* 2004;**89**(5):2078–84.
133. Matsubara J, Sugiyama S, Sugamura K, Nakamura T, Fujiwara Y, Akiyama E, et al. A dipeptidyl peptidase-4 inhibitor, des-fluoro-sitagliptin, improves endothelial function and reduces atherosclerotic lesion formation in apolipoprotein E-deficient mice. *J Am Coll Cardiol* 2012;**59**(3):265–76.
134. Vittone F, Liberman A, Vasic D, Ostertag R, Esser M, Walcher D, et al. Sitagliptin reduces plaque macrophage content and stabilises arteriosclerotic lesions in Apoe (-/-) mice. *Diabetologia* 2012;**55**(8):2267–75.
135. Satoh-Asahara N, Sasaki Y, Wada H, Tochiya M, Iguchi A, Nakagawachi R, et al. A dipeptidyl peptidase-4 inhibitor, sitagliptin, exerts anti-inflammatory effects in type 2 diabetic patients. *Metabolism* 2013;**62**(3):347–51.
136. Makino Y, Fujita Y, Haneda M. Dipeptidyl peptidase-4 inhibitors in progressive kidney disease. *Curr Opin Nephrol Hypertens* 2015;**24**(1):67–73.
137. Barragan JM, Eng J, Rodriguez R, Blazquez E. Neural contribution to the effect of glucagon-like peptide-1-(7-36) amide on arterial blood pressure in rats. *Am J Physiol* 1999;**277**(5 Pt 1):E784–91.
138. Yamamoto H, Lee CE, Marcus JN, Williams TD, Overton JM, Lopez ME, et al. Glucagon-like peptide-1 receptor stimulation increases blood pressure and heart rate and activates autonomic regulatory neurons. *J Clin Invest* 2002;**110**(1):43–52.
139. Zhao T, Parikh P, Bhashyam S, Bolukoglu H, Poornima I, Shen YT, et al. Direct effects of glucagon-like peptide-1 on myocardial contractility and glucose uptake in normal and postischemic isolated rat hearts. *J Pharmacol Exp Ther* 2006;**317**(3):1106–13.
140. Ussher JR, Drucker DJ. Cardiovascular biology of the incretin system. *Endocr Rev* 2012;**33**(2):187–215.
141. Noyan-Ashraf MH, Momen MA, Ban K, Sadi AM, Zhou YQ, Riazi AM, et al. GLP-1R agonist liraglutide activates cytoprotective pathways and improves outcomes after experimental myocardial infarction in mice. *Diabetes* 2009;**58**(4):975–83.
142. Nystrom T, Gonon AT, Sjoholm A, Pernow J. Glucagon-like peptide-1 relaxes rat conduit arteries via an endothelium-independent mechanism. *Regul Pept* 2005;**125**(1–3):173–7.
143. Vila Petroff MG, Egan JM, Wang X, Sollott SJ. Glucagon-like peptide-1 increases cAMP but fails to augment contraction in adult rat cardiac myocytes. *Circ Res* 2001;**89**(5):445–52.
144. Nguyen TD, Shingu Y, Amorim PA, Schwarzer M, Doenst T. Glucagon-like peptide-1 reduces contractile function and fails to boost glucose utilization in normal hearts in the presence of fatty acids. *Int J Cardiol* 2013;**168**(4):4085–92.
145. Inoue T, Inoguchi T, Sonoda N, Hendarto H, Makimura H, Sasaki S, et al. GLP-1 analog liraglutide protects against cardiac steatosis, oxidative stress and apoptosis in streptozotocin-induced diabetic rats. *Atherosclerosis* 2015;**240**(1):250–9.
146. Balteau M, Van Steenbergen A, Timmermans AD, Dessy C, Behets-Wydemans G, Tajeddine N, et al. AMPK activation by glucagon-like peptide-1 prevents NADPH oxidase activation induced by hyperglycemia in adult cardiomyocytes. *Am J Physiol Heart Circ Physiol* 2014;**307**(8):H1120–33.
147. Liu J, Liu Y, Chen L, Wang Y, Li J. Glucagon-like peptide-1 analog liraglutide protects against diabetic cardiomyopathy by the inhibition of the endoplasmic reticulum stress pathway. *J Diabetes Res* 2013;**2013**: 630537.

148. Ozyazgan S, Kutluata N, Afsar S, Ozdas SB, Akkan AG. Effect of glucagon-like peptide-1(7-36) and exendin-4 on the vascular reactivity in streptozotocin/nicotinamide-induced diabetic rats. *Pharmacology* 2005;**74**(3):119–26.
149. Monji A, Mitsui T, Bando YK, Aoyama M, Shigeta T, Murohara T. Glucagon-like peptide-1 receptor activation reverses cardiac remodeling via normalizing cardiac steatosis and oxidative stress in type 2 diabetes. *Am J Physiol Heart Circ Physiol* 2013;**305**(3):H295–304.
150. Nystrom T, Gutniak MK, Zhang Q, Zhang F, Holst JJ, Ahren B, et al. Effects of glucagon-like peptide-1 on endothelial function in type 2 diabetes patients with stable coronary artery disease. *Am J Physiol Endocrinol Metab* 2004;**287**(6):E1209–15.
151. Best JH, Hoogwerf BJ, Herman WH, Pelletier EM, Smith DB, Wenten M, et al. Risk of cardiovascular disease events in patients with type 2 diabetes prescribed the glucagon-like peptide 1 (GLP-1) receptor agonist exenatide twice daily or other glucose-lowering therapies: a retrospective analysis of the LifeLink database. *Diabetes Care* 2011;**34**(1):90–5.
152. Paul SK, Klein K, Maggs D, Best JH. The association of the treatment with glucagon-like peptide-1 receptor agonist exenatide or insulin with cardiovascular outcomes in patients with type 2 diabetes: a retrospective observational study. *Cardiovasc Diabetol* 2015;**14**:10.
153. Sonne DP, Engstrom T, Treiman M. Protective effects of GLP-1 analogues exendin-4 and GLP-1(9-36) amide against ischemia-reperfusion injury in rat heart. *Regul Pept* 2008;**146**(1–3):243–9.
154. Matsubara M, Kanemoto S, Leshnower BG, Albone EF, Hinmon R, Plappert T, et al. Single dose GLP-1-Tf ameliorates myocardial ischemia/reperfusion injury. *J Surg Res* 2011;**165**(1):38–45.
155. Timmers L, Henriques JP, de Kleijn DP, Devries JH, Kemperman H, Steendijk P, et al. Exenatide reduces infarct size and improves cardiac function in a porcine model of ischemia and reperfusion injury. *J Am Coll Cardiol* 2009;**53**(6):501–10.
156. Kristensen J, Mortensen UM, Schmidt M, Nielsen PH, Nielsen TT, Maeng M. Lack of cardioprotection from subcutaneously and preischemic administered liraglutide in a closed chest porcine ischemia reperfusion model. *BMC Cardiovasc Disord* 2009;**9**:31.
157. Nikolaidis LA, Doverspike A, Hentosz T, Zourelias L, Shen YT, Elahi D, et al. Glucagon-like peptide-1 limits myocardial stunning following brief coronary occlusion and reperfusion in conscious canines. *J Pharmacol Exp Ther* 2005;**312**(1):303–8.
158. Nikolaidis LA, Mankad S, Sokos GG, Miske G, Shah A, Elahi D, et al. Effects of glucagon-like peptide-1 in patients with acute myocardial infarction and left ventricular dysfunction after successful reperfusion. *Circulation* 2004;**109**(8):962–5.
159. Sokos GG, Bolukoglu H, German J, Hentosz T, Magovern Jr. GJ, Maher TD, et al. Effect of glucagon-like peptide-1 (GLP-1) on glycemic control and left ventricular function in patients undergoing coronary artery bypass grafting. *Am J Cardiol* 2007;**100**(5):824–9.
160. Mussig K, Oncu A, Lindauer P, Heininger A, Aebert H, Unertl K, et al. Effects of intravenous glucagon-like peptide-1 on glucose control and hemodynamics after coronary artery bypass surgery in patients with type 2 diabetes. *Am J Cardiol* 2008;**102**(5):646–7.
161. Read PA, Hoole SP, White PA, Khan FZ, O'Sullivan M, West NE, et al. A pilot study to assess whether glucagon-like peptide-1 protects the heart from ischemic dysfunction and attenuates stunning after coronary balloon occlusion in humans. *Circ Cardiovasc Interv* 2011;**4**(3):266–72.
162. Read PA, Khan FZ, Dutka DP. Cardioprotection against ischaemia induced by dobutamine stress using glucagon-like peptide-1 in patients with coronary artery disease. *Heart* 2012;**98**(5):408–13.
163. Scholte M, Timmers L, Bernink FJ, Denham RN, Beek AM, Kamp O, et al. Effect of additional treatment with exenatide in patients with an acute myocardial infarction (EXAMI): study protocol for a randomized controlled trial. *Trials* 2011;**12**:240.
164. Bernink FJ, Timmers L, Diamant M, Scholte M, Beek AM, Kamp O, et al. Effect of additional treatment with exenatide in patients with an acute myocardial infarction: the EXAMI study. *Int J Cardiol* 2013;**167**(1):289–90.

165. Sauve M, Ban K, Momen MA, Zhou YQ, Henkelman RM, Husain M, et al. Genetic deletion or pharmacological inhibition of dipeptidyl peptidase-4 improves cardiovascular outcomes after myocardial infarction in mice. *Diabetes* 2010;**59**(4):1063–73.
166. Zaruba MM, Zhu W, Soonpaa MH, Reuter S, Franz WM, Field LJ. Granulocyte colony-stimulating factor treatment plus dipeptidylpeptidase-IV inhibition augments myocardial regeneration in mice expressing cyclin D2 in adult cardiomyocytes. *Eur Heart J* 2012;**33**(1):129–37.
167. Inthachai T, Lekawanvijit S, Kumfu S, Apaijai N, Pongkan W, Chattipakorn SC, et al. Dipeptidyl peptidase-4 inhibitor improves cardiac function by attenuating adverse cardiac remodelling in rats with chronic myocardial infarction. *Exp Physiol* 2015;**100**(6):667–79.
168. Chinda K, Palee S, Surinkaew S, Phornphutkul M, Chattipakorn S, Chattipakorn N. Cardioprotective effect of dipeptidyl peptidase-4 inhibitor during ischemia-reperfusion injury. *Int J Cardiol* 2013;**167**(2):451–7.
169. Read PA, Khan FZ, Heck PM, Hoole SP, Dutka DP. DPP-4 inhibition by sitagliptin improves the myocardial response to dobutamine stress and mitigates stunning in a pilot study of patients with coronary artery disease. *Circ Cardiovasc Imaging* 2010;**3**(2):195–201.
170. Theiss HD, Brenner C, Engelmann MG, Zaruba MM, Huber B, Henschel V, et al. Safety and efficacy of SITAgliptin plus GRanulocyte-colony-stimulating factor in patients suffering from Acute Myocardial Infarction (SITAGRAMI-Trial)--rationale, design and first interim analysis. *Int J Cardiol* 2010;**145**(2):282–4.
171. Scirica BM, Braunwald E, Raz I, Cavender MA, Morrow DA, Jarolim P, et al. Heart failure, saxagliptin, and diabetes mellitus: observations from the SAVOR-TIMI 53 randomized trial. *Circulation* 2014;**130**(18):1579–88.
172. White WB, Cannon CP, Heller SR, Nissen SE, Bergenstal RM, Bakris GL, et al. Alogliptin after acute coronary syndrome in patients with type 2 diabetes. *N Engl J Med* 2013;**369**(14):1327–35.
173. Erdogdu O, Eriksson L, Xu H, Sjoholm A, Zhang Q, Nystrom T. Exendin-4 protects endothelial cells from lipoapoptosis by PKA, PI3K, eNOS, p38 MAPK, and JNK pathways. *J Mol Endocrinol* 2013;**50**(2):229–41.
174. Sheikh A. Direct cardiovascular effects of glucagon like peptide-1. *Diabetol Metab Syndr* 2013;**5**(1):47.
175. Dokken BB, La Bonte LR, Davis-Gorman G, Teachey MK, Seaver N, McDonagh PF. Glucagon-like peptide-1 (GLP-1), immediately prior to reperfusion, decreases neutrophil activation and reduces myocardial infarct size in rodents. *Horm Metab Res* 2011;**43**(5):300–5.
176. Dokken BB, Hilwig WR, Teachey MK, Panchal RA, Hubner K, Allen D, et al. Glucagon-like peptide-1 (GLP-1) attenuates post-resuscitation myocardial microcirculatory dysfunction. *Resuscitation* 2010;**81**(6):755–60.
177. Ban K, Kim KH, Cho CK, Sauve M, Diamandis EP, Backx PH, et al. Glucagon-like peptide (GLP)-1(9-36) amide-mediated cytoprotection is blocked by exendin(9-39) yet does not require the known GLP-1 receptor. *Endocrinology* 2010;**151**(4):1520–31.
178. Poornima I, Brown SB, Bhashyam S, Parikh P, Bolukoglu H, Shannon RP. Chronic glucagon-like peptide-1 infusion sustains left ventricular systolic function and prolongs survival in the spontaneously hypertensive, heart failure-prone rat. *Circ Heart Fail* 2008;**1**(3):153–60.
179. Liu Q, Anderson C, Broyde A, Polizzi C, Fernandez R, Baron A, et al. Glucagon-like peptide-1 and the exenatide analogue AC3174 improve cardiac function, cardiac remodeling, and survival in rats with chronic heart failure. *Cardiovasc Diabetol* 2010;**9**:76.
180. Yu M, Moreno C, Hoagland KM, Dahly A, Ditter K, Mistry M, et al. Antihypertensive effect of glucagon-like peptide 1 in Dahl salt-sensitive rats. *J Hypertens* 2003;**21**(6):1125–35.
181. Liu Q, Adams L, Broyde A, Fernandez R, Baron AD, Parkes DG. The exenatide analogue AC3174 attenuates hypertension, insulin resistance, and renal dysfunction in Dahl salt-sensitive rats. *Cardiovasc Diabetol* 2010;**9**:32.
182. Nikolaidis LA, Elahi D, Hentosz T, Doverspike A, Huerbin R, Zourelias L, et al. Recombinant glucagon-like peptide-1 increases myocardial glucose uptake and improves left ventricular performance in conscious dogs with pacing-induced dilated cardiomyopathy. *Circulation* 2004;**110**(8):955–61.
183. Vyas AK, Yang KC, Woo D, Tzekov A, Kovacs A, Jay PY, et al. Exenatide improves glucose homeostasis and prolongs survival in a murine model of dilated cardiomyopathy. *PLoS One* 2011;**6**(2):e17178.

184. Thrainsdottir I, Malmberg K, Olsson A, Gutniak M, Ryden L. Initial experience with GLP-1 treatment on metabolic control and myocardial function in patients with type 2 diabetes mellitus and heart failure. *Diab Vasc Dis Res* 2004;**1**(1):40–3.
185. Sokos GG, Nikolaidis LA, Mankad S, Elahi D, Shannon RP. Glucagon-like peptide-1 infusion improves left ventricular ejection fraction and functional status in patients with chronic heart failure. *J Card Fail* 2006;**12**(9):694–9.

CHAPTER

FAT HORMONES, ADIPOKINES

7

I. Kyrou[1,2,3,4], H.S. Mattu[2,3], K. Chatha[4] and H.S. Randeva[1,2,3,4]

[1]Aston University, Birmingham, United Kingdom [2]University Hospitals Coventry and Warwickshire (UHCW) NHS Trust, Coventry, United Kingdom [3]University of Warwick, Coventry, United Kingdom [4]Walsall Manor Hospital Walsall Healthcare NHS Trust, Walsall, United Kingdom

INTRODUCTION

Adipose tissue was traditionally regarded as a passive energy storage depot. However, currently it is well-established that adipocytes secrete a plethora of hormones, factors, cytokines, and cytokine-like proteins that are collectively described as adipokines or adipocytokines.[1,2] Although leptin and adiponectin are the prototype adipokines, the number of identified adipokines is constantly growing with newer members such as resistin, visfatin, chemerin, vaspin, and omentin. Moreover, adipocytes express an array of receptors that enable the adipose tissue to directly respond to various external signals/factors (e.g., nutritional and hormonal signals from the periphery). As such, adipose tissue plays a broader and dynamic physiologic role, acting as an endocrine organ (Fig. 7.1).[3,4] The endocrine function of adipocytes reflects the metabolic status of various adipose tissue depots and relays this information to the central nervous system (CNS) and to other peripheral tissues including the heart.[1,3,5] Hence, adipose tissue constitutes a key station within an interconnected multileveled network regulating metabolic homeostasis. Dysregulation and impaired function of this network was implicated in the pathophysiology of obesity and obesity-related complications, including cardiovascular disease (CVD).[1,2]

Indeed, adipokine expression is altered in obesity leading to increased secretion of adipokines, which exert adverse cardio-metabolic effects and decreased and/or dysregulated secretion of adipokines with protective properties. This adverse adipokine secretion profile in obesity strongly correlates to the clinical manifestations of the metabolic syndrome (Fig. 7.2).[1–3] Of note, most of the adipokines that exhibit amplified secretion in obesity and exert detrimental cardio-metabolic effects are more potently expressed in central/visceral adipose tissue and have proinflammatory properties.[1,2,6] This chapter presents an overview of the endocrine function of adipose tissue in obesity and focuses on selected adipokines implicated in obesity-related CVD and directly and/or indirectly affect the cardiovascular function.

Endocrinology of the Heart in Health and Disease. DOI: http://dx.doi.org/10.1016/B978-0-12-803111-7.00007-5

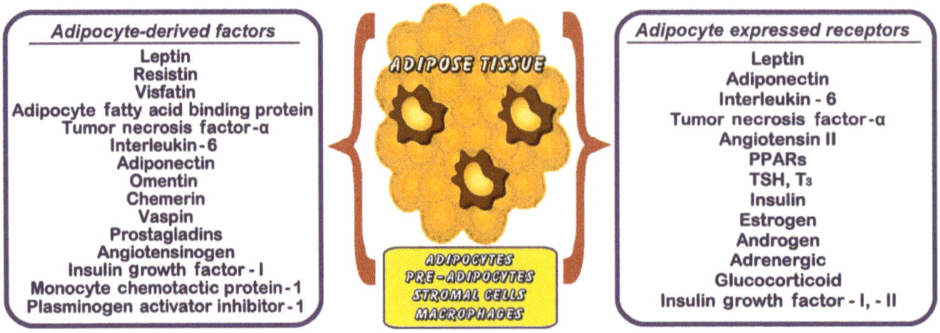

FIGURE 7.1

Adipose tissue as an endocrine organ. Adipocytes synthesize and secrete a plethora of proteins, factors, cytokines, and hormones (e.g., leptin, adiponectin, angiotensinogen, and plasminogen activator inhibitor-1) which exert autocrine, paracrine, and endocrine effects. Furthermore, adipocytes also express multiple receptors (e.g., leptin, adiponectin, insulin, and peroxisome proliferator-activated receptors), which receive signals from adjacent cells and the periphery. Although mature adipocytes constitute the primary cell population within adipose tissue depots, other cell types are also present, including preadipocytes, stromal cells, and resident macrophages. Obesity induces an expansion and remodeling of the adipose tissue and amplifies its endocrine function with marked changes in the local milieu and cellular composition. TSH: thyroid stimulating hormone; T3: triiodothyronine; PPARs: peroxisome proliferator-activated receptors.

OBESITY AS A CHRONIC PROINFLAMMATORY STATE

Adipose tissue exhibits a remarkable adaptive capacity to grow in size during periods of positive body energy balance. Accordingly, significant weight gain induces an expansion and remodeling of the adipose tissue depots with marked changes in the local milieu and cellular composition. Thus, obesity is characterized by both adipose tissue hyperplasia (increased number of adipocytes) and hypertrophy (increased mass/size of adipocytes) as preadipocytes proliferate and differentiate (stimulated adipogenesis), while small adipocytes accumulate lipid droplets and increase in size (stimulated lipogenesis). The hypertrophic and hyperplastic growth of adipose tissue is also supported by increased local vascularization and stromal cell proliferation.[7] It is noteworthy that enlarged mature adipocytes in obesity were found to be more lipolytic and insulin-resistant compared to small adipocytes, exhibiting an overall secretory function which promotes metabolic dysregulation and inflammation. Hence, the accumulation of excess adipose tissue in obesity induces the proliferation/differentiation of preadipocytes, as well as insulin resistance and proinflammatory responses in adipocytes.[8–11]

In parallel, circulating mononuclear cells were found to transmigrate from the circulation into the expanding adipose tissue, increasing the local population of macrophages.[12–14] As such, increased adiposity associated with a local (within adipose tissue depots) and systemic low-grade inflammatory state primarily mediated by the increased secretion of proinflammatory adipokines and cytokines, including tumor necrosis factor-α (TNF-α) and intrerleukin-6 (IL-6).[8–10] The chronic, low-grade inflammatory response driven by the adipose tissue increased proportionally to the accumulated adipose tissue

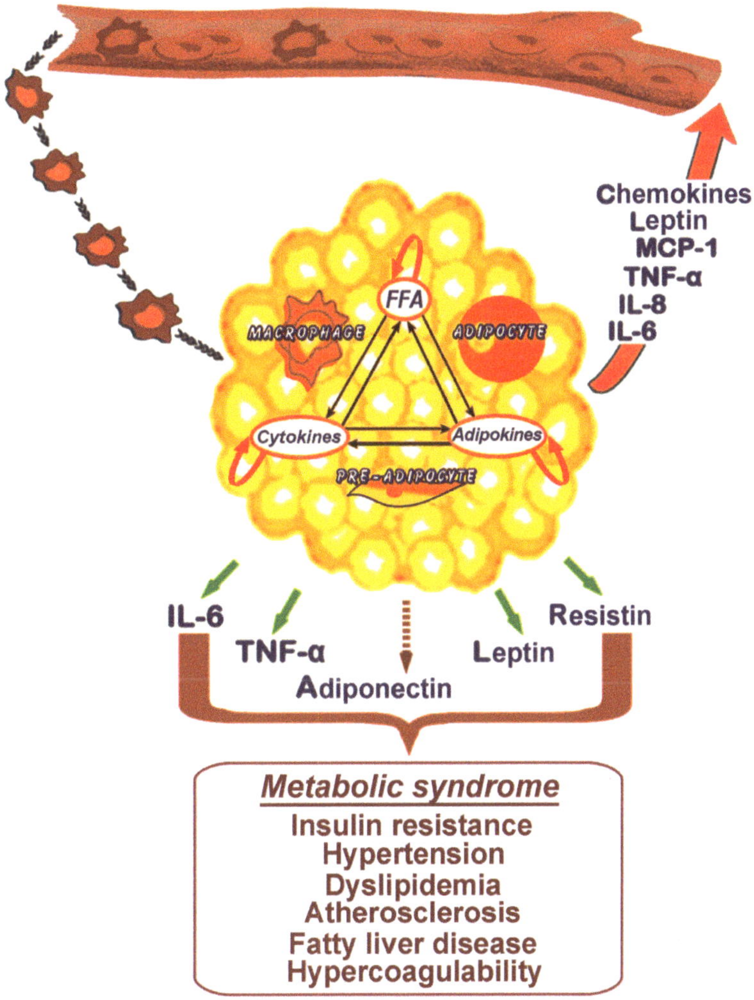

FIGURE 7.2

Development of a chronic, low-grade inflammatory state in obesity. Accumulation of excess adipose tissue, particularly in visceral adipose tissue depots, enhances the secretion of proinflammatory adipokines and chemokines into the systemic circulation. In parallel, obesity is characterized by either decreased or dysregulated secretion of anti-inflammatory adipokines (e.g., adiponectin and omentin). This creates a significantly altered circulating adipokine profile that favors the activation of proinflammatory pathways. Furthermore, in response to chemotactic stimuli, circulating mononuclear cells transmigrate into the growing adipose tissue, increasing the population of resident macrophages. In turn, these adipose tissue macrophages become the major source of local cytokine secretion (e.g., TNF-α, IL-1, and IL-6) and amplify the proinflammatory local milieu. Hence, a feed-forward vicious cycle is formed within adipose tissue depots with adipocyte-derived free fatty acids (FFA) and adipokines stimulating macrophages to secrete cytokines and vice versa. This interconnection fuels a chronic subclinical inflammation within adipose tissue depots, which persists for as long as the excess fat mass is maintained and progressively leads to a generalized, systemic inflammatory state due to the unremitting secretion of proinflammatory adipokines. The detrimental cardio-metabolic effects of this process contribute to the development of the metabolic syndrome and cardiovascular disease. MCP-1: monocyte chemotactic protein-1; TNF-α: tumor necrosis factor-α, IL-8: interleukin 8, IL-6: interleukin-6.

mass and exhibited positive correlations with both the body mass index (BMI) and central/visceral adiposity.[8,9,15] Overall, obesity triggers an inflammatory cascade that evolves within adipose tissue and progressively becomes generalized with systemic complications as the amplified secretion of proinflammatory adipokines persists for as long as the increased adiposity is maintained. Importantly, obesity-dependent activation of inflammatory signaling pathways is linked to the development of type 2 diabetes (T2DM), hypertension, dyslipidemia, atherosclerosis, thrombosis, and CVD.[16–19]

The underlying mechanisms promoting a chronic proinflammatory state in obesity rely on a feed-forward cycle between preadipocytes, mature adipocytes, and macrophages within adipose tissue depots (Fig. 7.2). Indeed, accumulation of excess fat induces adipogenesis and increases the secretion of proinflammatory adipokines and chemokines (e.g., IL-6 and monocyte chemotactic protein-1, MCP-1) from mature adipocytes into the systemic circulation. In response to persistent chemotactic stimuli, mononuclear cells are recruited from the bloodstream and transmigrate into the accumulated adipose tissue, where they are activated and function as resident macrophages.[11–13] Subsequently, resident macrophages in adipose tissue secrete cytokines (e.g., IL-6 and TNF-α) that further amplify the adverse proinflammatory and insulin resistant profile of mature adipocytes.[8–10,20] Hence, adipose tissue accumulation activates proinflammatory pathways and establishes an unremitting inflammatory state within the expanding adipose tissue that perpetuates locally via interactions between increasing populations of adipocytes and macrophages. This cascade progressively generates a chronic, low-grade, systemic inflammatory state in obesity, mediated by a persistent and amplified release of proinflammatory adipokines of adipocyte and/or macrophage origin.[8–10,21] Collectively, this inflammatory state results in a range of detrimental effects on peripheral tissues and organs (e.g., liver, skeletal muscles, vascular endothelium, and heart), promoting enhanced secretion of acute-phase reactants (e.g., fibrinogen and C-reactive protein, CRP), hepatic, skeletal muscle, and myocardial insulin resistance, hypertension, atherosclerosis, hypercoagulability, thrombosis, and cardiac dysfunction. The specific role of selected adipokines mediating the adverse adipokine profile in obesity are described in the following sections, focusing on identified links to CVD and potential direct actions on the heart.

PROINFLAMMATORY ADIPOKINES

LEPTIN

Leptin is a 16-kDa protein primarily secreted from adipocytes and represents the prototype for all subsequently identified adipokines.[22] Since its discovery in 1994, extensive research focused on identifying the physiologic role of leptin, revealing a wide range of functions (Fig. 7.3). Accordingly, leptin is now considered a pleiotropic hormone interacting with most of the major endocrine axes and plays a vital role not only in metabolic homeostasis but also in the regulation of reproduction, puberty, and fertility.[25]

Among its many actions, the primary effect of leptin is to suppress appetite and enhance energy expenditure in the hypothalamus.[26] Circulating leptin levels were shown to correlate with BMI in normal-weight and obese subjects and are strongly proportional to the percentage of body fat.[27] As such, leptin directly relays information regarding changes in peripheral fat/energy stores from the adipose tissue depots to the CNS. High circulating leptin concentrations in obesity constitute a pathophysiologic paradox which is explained, at least partly, by a degree of underlying leptin resistance.[28–30]

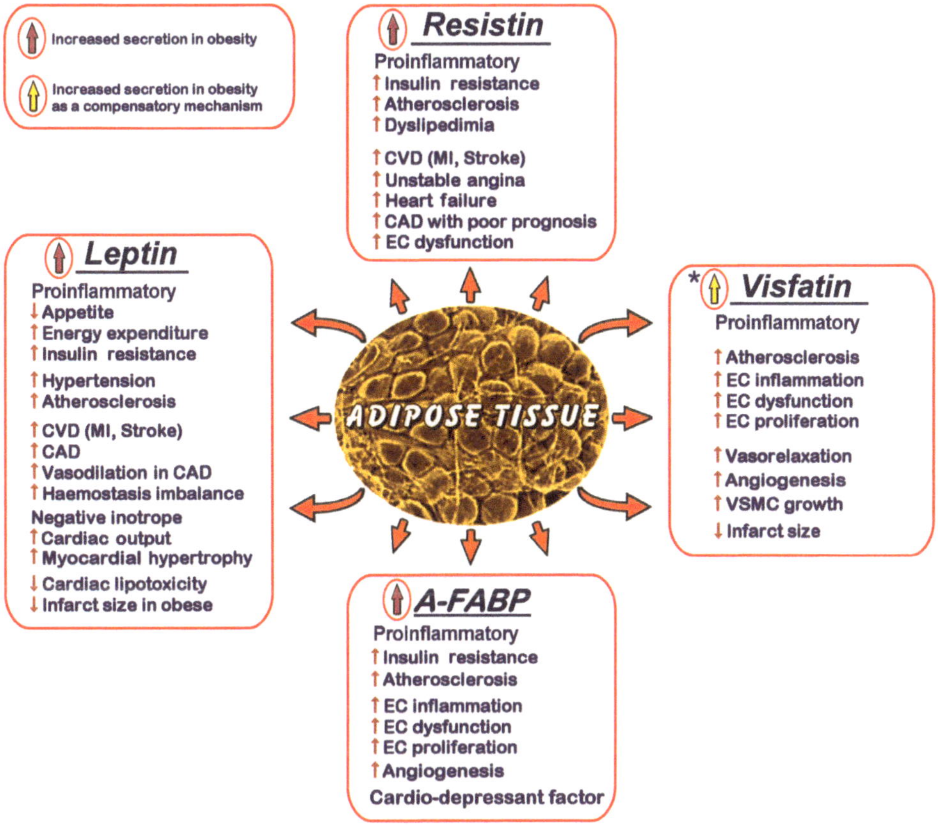

FIGURE 7.3

Effects of selected proinflammatory adipokines. *Although there are conflicting data in the literature, visfatin plasma levels appear to be increased in patients with obesity, metabolic syndrome, type 2 diabetes, and cardiovascular disease and exhibit a positive association with insulin resistance.[23] This association suggests that visfatin secretion may be stimulated by hyperglycemia in the context of a compensatory mechanism as there are data indicating that visfatin can increase insulin secretion and insulin receptor phosphorylation in mouse pancreatic β-cells.[24] EC: endothelial cells; VSMC: vascular smooth muscle cells; CVD: cardiovascular disease; CAD: coronary artery disease; MI: myocardial infraction.

This resistance is attributed to a number of extra- and intracellular factors, including increased levels of intracellular leptin signaling inhibitors such as the suppressor of cytokine signaling 3 (SOCS3) and other related molecules.[28–31] Indeed, leptin acts on target cells through binding to and activating specific cell membrane leptin receptors (LEPR) that exist in six isoforms (i.e., LEPRa, b, c, d, e, and f) due to alternative mRNA splicing.[28,29] Leptin signaling is mediated via modulation of the Janus Kinases/Signal Transducers and Activators of Transcription (JAK/STAT) and AMP-activated protein kinase (AMPK) pathways (Fig. 7.4). Negative feedback on the JAK/STAT and AMPK pathways is mediated by SOCS3, which is also induced by leptin, thereby completing the inhibitory feedback loop.[29,30,32–35]

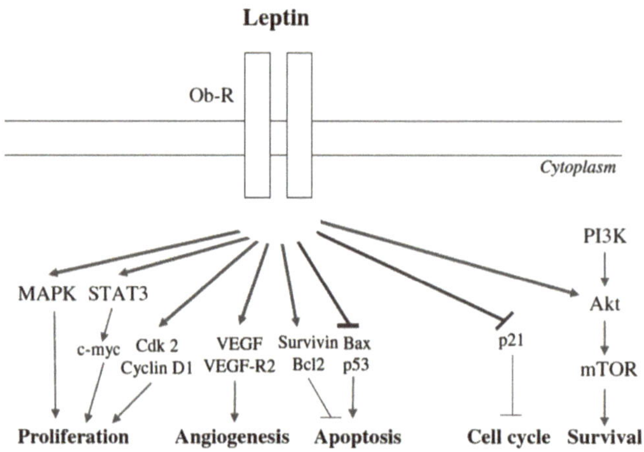

FIGURE 7.4

Schematic representation of leptin induced signaling pathways. Ob-R: leptin receptor; MAPK: mitogen-activated protein kinase; STAT3: signal transducer and activator of transcription 3; Cdk2: cyclin-dependent kinase 2; VEGF: vascular endothelial growth factor; VEGF-R: vascular endothelial growth factor receptor; Bcl2: B-cell lymphoma 2; PI3K: phosphoinositide 3-kinase; mTOR: mammalian target of rapamycin.

*Modified from Delort L, Rossary A, Farges M-C, et al. Leptin, adipocytes and breast cancer: focus on inflammation and anti-tumor immunity, Life Sci 2015;***140***(1):37–48.*

Of note, in addition to these pathways, leptin also acts via the phosphatidylinositol-3-kinase (PI3K)-Akt and the mitogen-activated protein kinase (MAPK) pathways involved in the Reperfusion Injury Salvation Kinase (RISK) pathway.[34–38] The latter protects the myocardium against ischemia/reperfusion (I/R) injury.

Leptin structurally belongs to the type I cytokine superfamily and exhibits proinflammatory and immune-modulating properties, potentially activating both adaptive and innate immunity.[39,40] Thus, leptin provides a functional bridge between energy homeostasis regulation and the immune system, offering important insight into the immune dysregulation noted in obesity and malnutrition.[40,41] Interestingly, mice lacking LEPR (*db/db* mice) exhibit thymus atrophy, while mice lacking leptin (*ob/ob* mice) are also immuno-deficient.[42] Such an interaction explains the immune-suppression of the murine immune system by acute starvation and reduced food intake, which result in low circulating leptin levels and also why administration of exogenous recombinant leptin appears to protect against these immune-suppressing effects.[43] Overall, the proinflammatory actions of leptin contribute to the development of CVD. Clinical data indicate that hyperleptinemia independently associated with CVD even after adjustment for CRP, while increased concentrations of both leptin and CRP conferred the highest CVD risk.[44,45]

Hyperleptinemia is also closely associated with atherosclerosis.[45,46] Notably, leptin appears to play a central role in early atherogenic stages by inducing mitochondrial superoxide production and MCP-1 expression in endothelial cells, and, thus, initiating macrophage and leukocyte recruitment into the endothelial wall.[47,48] Moreover, leptin is suggested to exert additional proatherogenic effects mainly by stimulating the hypertrophy and proliferation of vascular smooth muscle cells, inducing

CRP expression in coronary artery endothelial cells, and enhancing the secretion of proatherogenic lipoprotein lipase from macrophages.[46,48–50] Leptin also promotes the production of proliferative and profibrogenic cytokines and other mediators of vascular inflammation (e.g., TNF-α, IL-6, and IL-2) from endothelial cells.[46,48,49,51] Clinical studies demonstrated that circulating leptin levels were positively correlated to plasminogen activator inhibitor-1, Von Willebrand factor and fibrinogen plasma levels, whereas leptin was inversely related to circulating levels of protein C and coagulation inhibitors such as the tissue factor pathway inhibitor.[30] These findings suggest that leptin is also prothrombotic, contributing to the hypercoagulability and increased platelet aggregation/activity observed in obesity and the metabolic syndrome.[30,45,46]

Similarly, several studies reported a positive association between plasma leptin levels and blood pressure, suggesting leptin promotes arterial hypertension in obesity.[49] Interestingly, leptin induced the phosphorylation of endothelial nitric oxide (NO) synthase (eNOS) leading to NO release, while the intra-arterial administration of leptin in humans caused a vasoactive response independent of NO.[52–54] In addition, leptin exerted a direct endothelial-independent vasorelaxant effect on vascular smooth muscle cells in both animal and human studies.[55,56] As such, acute hyperleptinemia induced vasodilation which seemingly contradicts the evidence supporting the association between hypertension and hyperleptinemia in obesity. This may be attributed, at least partly, to different acute and chronic leptin effects on the vasculature. Studies in rats have shown that chronic intravenous infusion of leptin can increase both the mean arterial blood pressure and the heart rate due to sympathetic nervous system activation and release of catecholamines.[57–59] Importantly, hyperleptinemia also induced endothelial dysfunction, perhaps contributing to the differential vascular actions of leptin. Indeed, leptin induced oxidative stress by increasing the formation of reactive oxygen species (ROS) and decreasing the NO bioavailability in both endothelial and vascular smooth muscle cells, key mediators of endothelial dysfunction.[51,60]

Although leptin is primarily an adipocyte-derived protein, it is also produced by other tissues, including the heart. Hence, leptin can exert direct autocrine/paracrine effects on cardiac function.[61,62] Leptin has been shown to attenuate cardiac contraction in rat ventricular myocytes,[63] while hyperleptinemia appears to prevent lipotoxic cardiomyopathy in acyl CoA synthase transgenic mice.[64] Moreover, leptin was implicated in the regulation of the contractility, metabolism, cellular growth/size, and extracellular matrix production of cardiomyocytes.[65–67] Experiments in cultured myocytes from a one- to four-day-old neonatal rat heart ventricles showed that 24 hours of exposure to leptin produces cardiomyocyte hypertrophy via activation of the MAPK pathway, including p38 and p44/42 signaling.[68] Furthermore, inhibitors of PI3K-Akt and p44/42 MAPK signaling can prevent leptin-mediated cardiomyocyte proliferation.[69] Accordingly, studies in isolated mouse hearts demonstrated that leptin (at levels comparable to those circulating in obese patients) reduced the infarct size via prosurvival kinases, including the PI3K-Akt and p44/42 MAPK pathways.[70] Hence, leptin exerted a cardio-protective effect against I/R injury, through mechanisms involving JAK/STAT signaling and activation of the RISK pathway.[71] Moreover, leptin seems to protect cardiomyocytes from hypoxia-induced damage.[72] Such direct cardio-protective effects of leptin may be a contributing factor to the clinical manifestation of the "obesity paradox" phenomenon in which an unexpected reduction in CVD mortality and morbidity is documented in obese patients.[61] However, hyperleptinemia is associated with an overall adverse CVD profile in obesity due to the aforementioned proinflammatory, proatherogenic, and prothrombotic effects of leptin (Fig. 7.3). Thus, increased circulating leptin levels are associated with a higher risk of both myocardial infraction (MI) and stroke, independently of BMI and other CVD risk factors, due to the insulin resistance, hypercoagulability, atherosclerosis, and vascular inflammation and dysfunction in obesity.[73,74]

RESISTIN

Resistin, also referred to as ADSF (adipocyte-secreted factor) and FIZZ3 (found in inflammatory zone 3), is a 12.5-kDa peptide hormone and belongs to the family of cysteine-rich secretory proteins.[75,76] Resistin is primarily secreted from adipose tissue in rodents; however, inflammatory cells (e.g., macrophages) are considered the main source of resistin in humans.[76–79] Resistin exhibited proinflammatory properties such as increasing the expression of several cytokines (e.g., IL-1, IL-6, IL-12, and TNF-α) while inhibiting glucose uptake in various cell types, including cardiomyocytes (Fig. 7.3).[80–82] Recombinant resistin administration impairs glucose tolerance in wild-type mice, and neutralization of endogenous resistin with resistin antiserum improved insulin sensitivity in diet-induced obese mice, while adenovirus-mediated high expression of resistin caused dyslipidemia in C57BL/6 mice.[75–77,83] Moreover, plasma resistin levels were positively correlated to insulin resistance, circulating proinflammatory markers, and to other CVD risk factors indices (e.g., increased triglycerides and low-density lipoproteins (LDL) cholesterol levels) in obese patients.[84–88] As such, high circulating resistin levels were reported in obesity, T2DM, and metabolic syndrome.[82,89,90] Of note, patients with acute coronary syndrome (ACS) also exhibited increased concentrations of resistin in the circulation, potentially from ruptured atherosclerotic plaques, and correlated to both CRP plasma levels and to the number of significantly stenosed coronary vessels (>50% stenosis).[91–93] Circulating resistin levels appeared to associated with future cardiovascular death in patients with documented coronary artery disease (CAD) and with higher 5-year mortality/morbidity risk after athero-thrombotic ischemic stroke.[94,95]

The overall effects of resistin appear to be both proinflammatory and proatherogenic.[82,93] In animal models of atherosclerosis resistin levels were proportional to the severity of the atherosclerotic lesions, while in humans resistin secretion by macrophages in atheromas were linked to atherogenesis.[41,96] This local secretion of resistin can induce the release of endothelin-1, vascular cell adhesion molecule-1 (VCAM-1), intercellular adhesion molecule-1 (ICAM-1), and MCP-1 by vascular endothelial cells, affecting the endothelial function and vascular smooth muscle cell migration. Indeed, resistin promoted the proliferation of human aortic smooth muscle cells via PI3K-Akt and p44/42 signaling and increased the migration and proliferation of endothelial cells derived from human coronary arteries via stimulated p38 and p44/42 signaling.[97,98] Moreover, resistin induced endothelial dysfunction in isolated coronary artery rings.[99] Interestingly, it was suggested that there is a degree of crosstalk between the effects of resistin and other adipokines such as leptin and adiponectin.[77,100] For example, the induction of VCAM-1 and ICAM-1 (both key molecules implicated in leukocyte recruitment and early proatherosclerotic events) by resistin in vascular endothelial cells can be inhibited by adiponectin, suggesting that the relative balance between such adipokines determine their effects on the vasculature in obesity.[100]

In cardiomyocytes, further to inhibiting glucose uptake and promoting myocardial insulin resistance, resistin caused hypertrophy and contractile dysfunction with impaired calcium handling.[101,102] Additional studies in rat cardiomyocytes showed that resistin overexpression induces ROS production and promotes inflammation (e.g., increased TNF-α secretion), fibrosis, and apoptosis.[103] These effects indicate that resistin contributes to cardiomyocyte dysfunction and pathological cardiac remodeling. Moreover, in isolated perfused rat hearts resistin worsened cardiac I/R injury indicated by impaired cardiac recovery following ischemia.[104] However, other studies in a mouse heart perfusion model demonstrated that pretreatment with resistin exerts cardio-protective effects against I/R injury, mediated by PI3K-Akt-Protein kinase C (PKC) dependent pathways.[105] Further research is required to clarify the pathophysiologic role of resistin with respect to cardiac I/R injury and the downstream effects of resistin-mediated activation of the PI3K-Akt and p38 MAPK pathways in cardiomyocytes.

VISFATIN

Visfatin, also referred to as nicotinamide phosphoribosyltransferase (Nampt), was originally identified as a 52-kDa protein/cytokine expressed in lymphocytes (initially known as pre-B cell colony enhancing factor (PBEF)).[106,107] In 2005, visfatin was first reported as an adipokine predominantly produced in the visceral fat of both mice and humans, and was also reported to exert insulin-mimetic, glucose-lowering effects in mice.[108] However, subsequent studies were unable to reproduce these hypoglycemic effects in humans, it is now known that visfatin is also expressed in other adipose tissue depots, including subcutaneous, as well as perivascular and epicardial fat.[107] The latter suggests that visfatin also exerts direct effects on cardiovascular function in a paracrine manner. Adipocytes are not the only source of visfatin within the adipose tissue, as visfatin is released by activated resident macrophages isolated from human visceral white adipose tissue.[109] More recent human studies indicated that visfatin is also expressed in both hepatocytes and myoblasts, which constitute additional sources of secreted visfatin in the circulation.[110,111] Of note, secreted circulating/extracellular visfatin exhibited an enzymatic activity as a nicotinamide phosphoribosyltransferase (Nampt) and is identical to the intracellular Nampt, an enzyme necessary for nicotinamide adenine dinucleotide (NAD) synthesis and implicated in the regulation of cellular metabolism and survival.[106,107]

To date, several studies documented increased plasma visfatin levels in various cohorts of patients with obesity and/or other components of the metabolic syndrome. However, there are also conflicting data from studies that reported plasma concentrations of visfatin remain unchanged or are lower in obese patients compared to normal-weight healthy individuals. Results from a metaanalysis examining this controversy by systematically reviewing the available literature showed that circulating visfatin levels were higher in patients with obesity, metabolic syndrome, T2DM, and CVD and were also positively associated with insulin resistance.[23] This association suggests that visfatin secretion is stimulated by hyperglycemia in the context of a compensatory mechanism given that visfatin increased insulin secretion and insulin receptor phosphorylation in mouse pancreatic beta-cells.[24]

Besides being a surrogate biomarker in obesity, visfatin is now considered to exert proinflammatory and proatherogenic effects and is directly implicated in vascular dysfunction and inflammation (Fig. 7.3).[107] Indeed, visfatin expression in carotid atherosclerotic plaques was higher in patients with symptomatic carotid artery disease compared to asymptomatic individuals and appeared to be mainly localized in lesions that are unstable and rich in lipid-loaded macrophages.[112] These findings suggest that visfatin plays a role in plaque inflammation and destabilization, involving an increased population of foam cell macrophages within unstable atherosclerotic lesions. Notably, in vitro and in vivo experiments reveal that visfatin promoted macrophage survival through a nonenzymatic IL-6/STAT3 signaling mechanism.[113] Furthermore, visfatin directly induced vascular dysfunction and inflammation by: (1) increasing VCAM-1 and ICAM-1 expression through ROS-dependent NF-kB activation in endothelial cells; and (2) activating proinflammatory signaling through its Nampt activity and upregulating the inducible nitric oxide synthase (iNOS) expression in human vascular smooth muscle cells (iNOS: a proinflammatory enzyme contributing to vascular injury via dysregulated NO production) (Fig. 7.5).[112,114,115]

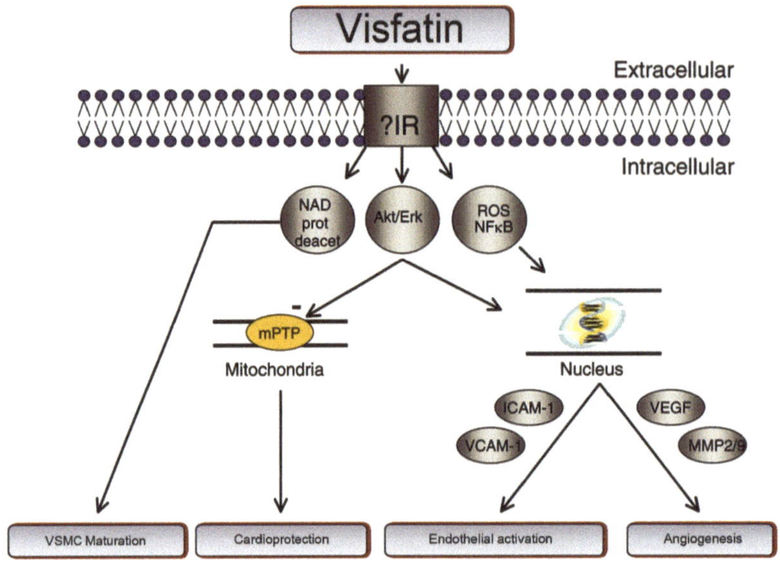

FIGURE 7.5

Schematic representation of visfatin-induced signaling pathways, potentially involving the insulin receptor (IR). NAD: nicotinamide adenine dinucleotide; ERK: extracellular signal-regulated kinase; Akt: a serine/threonine kinase also known as protein kinase B; ROS: reactive oxygen species; NF-κB: Nuclear Factor-kappaB; mPTP mitochondrial permeability transition pore; ICAM-1: intercellular adhesion molecule-1; VCAM-1: vascular cell adhesion molecule-1; VEGF: vascular endothelial growth factor; MMP: matrix metalloproteinases; VSMC, vascular smooth muscle cell.

*From Hausenloy DJ. Drug discovery possibilities from visfatin cardioprotection? Curr Opin Pharmacol 2009;***9***(2):202–7.*

In addition, visfatin stimulated endothelial proliferation and capillary tube formation in human umbilical vein endothelial cells (HUVECs) via increased production of vascular endothelial growth factor (VEGF) and matrix metalloproteinases (MMP-2 and MMP-9) mediated by MAPK/PI3K-Akt/VEGF signaling pathways.[116] Visfatin also stimulated vascular smooth muscle cell proliferation via nicotinamide mononucleotide-mediated activation of extracellular signal-regulated kinase (ERK 1/2) and p38 signaling pathways.[117] Interestingly, visfatin reduced apoptosis in HUVECs and induced maturation in human vascular smooth muscle cells.[116,118] In accord with the aforementioned effects in endothelial and vascular smooth muscle cells, clinical data documented that plasma visfatin levels were negative correlated with vascular endothelial function in T2DM patients.[119] Finally, visfatin exerted an endothelium-dependent vasodilating effect on isolated rat blood vessels that is not mediated via insulin receptors, but rather through endothelium-derived NO.[120]

Existing evidence also suggests that visfatin exerts direct cardio-protective effects. Visfatin reduced myocardial injury and cell death when administered at the time of myocardial reperfusion in experimental studies using an in situ murine heart model and in isolated ventricular murine cardiomyocytes subjected to hypoxia/reoxygenation.[121] This effect appears to involve the activation of the PI3K and MAPK kinase 1 and 2 (MEK1/2) pathways and the inhibition of the mitochondrial permeability transition pore (mPTP;

a nonspecific mitochondrial channel, whose opening in the first minutes of reperfusion is a key determining factor of cardiomyocyte death).[36–38,121] Notably, cardiac-specific overexpression of Nampt in mice increased cardiomyocytes resistance to oxidative stress and prevented myocardial injury in response to myocardial ischemia and reperfusion;[122] hence, Nampt is suggested to play a critical role in mediating cell survival by inhibiting apoptosis and stimulating autophagic flux in cardiomyocytes.[122] More recent data demonstrated that visfatin-induced cardio-protection involves suppression of myocardial apoptosis via AMPK activation.[123] Further research is needed to fully understand the complex signaling pathways that mediate the protective effects of visfatin on cardiomyocytes. Despite the potential cardio-protective effects of visfatin on the heart, in vivo studies using cardiac-specific overexpressing Nampt transgenic mice and various in vitro approaches have shown that visfatin secreted from cardiomyocytes promotes development of cardiac hypertrophy and adverse ventricular remodeling.[124] This further highlights that visfatin/Nampt functions as a rate-limiting enzyme in the NAD salvage pathway inside the cell (iNampt), while on the other hand, acts as a proinflammatory cytokine outside the cell (eNampt/visfatin).

ADIPOCYTE–FATTY ACID BINDING PROTEIN

Adipocyte–Fatty Acid Binding Protein (A-FABP), also known as adipocyte protein 2 (aP2), adipocyte lipid-binding protein and fatty acid binding protein 4 (FABP4), is a 14.6-kDa polypeptide of 132 amino acids that belongs to the family of intracellular lipid-binding proteins and acts as a chaperone for long-chain nonesterified fatty acids (NEFAs) (Fig. 7.6).[125,126] A-FABP has various endogenous ligands (e.g., retinoic, oleic, and arachidonic acid) and constitutes up to 5–6% of the total cytosolic protein in mature

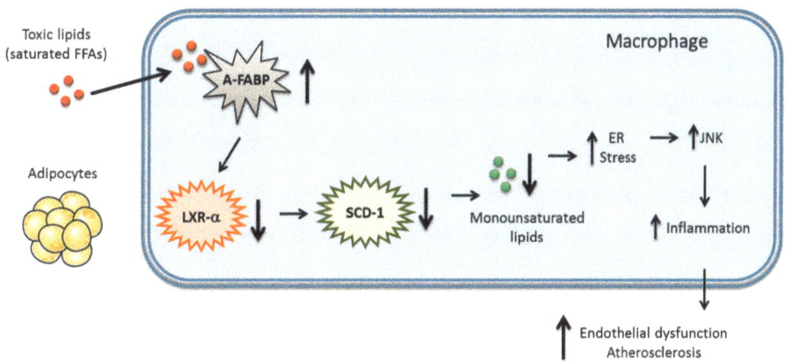

FIGURE 7.6

Adipocyte–fatty acid binding protein (A-FABP) acting as a lipid sensor which mediates toxic lipids-induced inflammation through endoplasmic reticulum (ER) stress in macrophages. In obesity, toxic lipids (e.g., palmitate) released from the adipose tissue bind to A-FABP and also induce A-FABP expression, which in turn suppresses Stearoyl-CoA desaturase-1 (SCD1) expression via inhibition of the nuclear receptor liver X receptor-α (LXR-α). This consequently leads to impaired production of monounsaturated lipids and ER stress. ER stress induces c-Jun N-terminal kinase (JNK) activation and inflammation in macrophages, resulting in vascular dysfunction and atherosclerosis.

*From Xu A, Wang Y, Lam KS, Vanhoutte PM. Vascular actions of adipokines molecular mechanisms and therapeutic implications. Adv Pharmacol 2010;**60**:229–55.*

adipocytes, although smaller amounts are also produced in dendritic cells, monocytes, macrophages, and endothelial cells.[126–130] In adipocytes A-FABP production is induced during differentiation and its expression is upregulated by fatty acids, insulin, and peroxisome proliferator-activated receptor gamma (PPARγ) agonists (e.g., thiazolidinediones that activate PPARγ-inducing, insulin-sensitizing, and proadipogenic effects).[131–134] Of note, it appears that there are regional differences in adipose tissue A-FABP expression that may be influenced by obesity.[135] As such, higher A-FABP expression and production has been detected in subcutaneous than visceral adipose tissue in obese patients.[135] In macrophages, A-FABP acts as a regulator of inflammatory responses and its expression is induced by proinflammatory stimuli, including oxidized low-density lipoproteins (Ox-LDL) and toll-like receptor agonists.[129,136–138]

A-FABP was first described as an adipokine in 2006 when it was identified as a circulating biomarker closely associated to obesity and components of the metabolic syndrome.[139] The exact mechanisms that mediate the secretion/release of A-FABP from cells have not been fully clarified. No secretory signal sequence has been identified in the structure of this protein, thus it is proposed that A-FABP is released from adipocytes into the systemic circulation through other mechanisms potentially involving adipocyte-derived microvesicles and/or lysis of large mature adipocytes.[125,139,140]

Multiple cross-sectional studies have linked circulating A-FABP to obesity-related cardio-metabolic disease in humans.[125,126] Indeed, compared to healthy controls, higher A-FABP plasma levels have been documented in several cohorts of patients with obesity and/or metabolic syndrome manifestations, exhibiting independent positive correlations to BMI, waist circumference, blood pressure, dyslipidemia, insulin resistance indices, fasting glucose and insulin levels, and oxidation and inflammation biomarkers.[134,139,141,142] In addition, elevated plasma A-FABP levels have been also found in patients with nonalcoholic fatty liver disease (NAFLD; an independent CVD risk factor regarded as the hepatic component of the metabolic syndrome), correlating with subcutaneous, but not visceral fat mass, and independently predicting hepatic inflammation and fibrosis.[143]

Notably, population genetic studies have identified that a single nucleotide polymorphism (SNP) in the 5′ promoter region of A-FABP in humans, i.e., a T-87C SNP that represents a loss of function mutation, results in a favorable cardio-metabolic phenotype characterized by lower triglyceridemia and decreased risk of T2DM and CAD.[144] Moreover, circulating A-FABP appears to be an independent determinant of carotid atherosclerosis in Chinese women,[145] which is associated to plaque instability and adverse outcome in patients with carotid atherosclerosis and acute ischemic stroke.[146] Furthermore, elevated plasma levels have been shown in CAD patients, exhibiting independent correlations to the burden of coronary atherosclerosis and the risk of heart failure.[147–151] Interestingly, a cross-sectional study utilizing [(18)F]-fluorodeoxyglucose positron emission tomography showed that circulating A-FABP levels are an independent risk factor for vascular inflammation in Korean men without previously diagnosed T2DM or CVD.[152]

Prospective data from clinical studies in the past decade further indicate that circulating A-FABP is independently associated with the risk of developing metabolic syndrome and CVD. A 5-year prospective study, following nondiabetic adults from the population-based Hong Kong Cardiovascular Risk Factor Prevalence Study, showed that circulating A-FABP predicts the development of metabolic syndrome independently of adiposity and insulin resistance.[153] This association was also noted in a cohort of Korean boys that was prospectively followed for 3 years, with baseline plasma A-FABP levels predicting the development of metabolic syndrome independently of pubertal status, adiposity, and insulin resistance.[154] In addition, the 10-year follow-up data in nondiabetic adults from the Hong Kong Cardiovascular Risk Factor Prevalence Study cohort documented that baseline circulating

A-FABP levels are associated with glucose dysregulation and predict T2DM development, independently of obesity, insulin resistance, and glycemic indices.[155] Furthermore, a 12-year prospective study following a community-based cohort of Chinese subjects without previous CVD recruited from the Hong Kong Cardiovascular Risk Factors Prevalence Study 2 (CRISPS 2) showed that plasma A-FABP levels are independently associated with CVD development.[156] Of note, a 10-year prospective in patients with prevalent coronary heart disease revealed that baseline circulating A-FABP exhibits a positive correlation to CVD-related death even after multivariable adjustment.[157] Similar data further support an independent association between circulating A-FABP and the occurrence and prognosis of ischemic stroke and other adverse cardiovascular events.[146,158,159] Finally, a number of studies have documented significantly decreased A-FABP levels after weight loss achieved through bariatric surgery or lifestyle interventions.[160–162] Moreover, atorvastatin treatment (40 mg/day for 12 weeks) was also followed by decreased circulating A-FABP levels in statin-naive patients with atherosclerosis.[163]

In accord with the aforementioned clinical data, mounting experimental evidence strongly suggests that A-FABP plays a key role in obesity-related CVD, primarily through effects promoting insulin resistance, atherogenesis, lipid-induced inflammation, and vascular endothelial dysfunction (Fig. 7.3).[125,126] Studies in mice have shown that a null mutation in *aP2*, the gene encoding A-FABP, is protective against the development of obesity-induced insulin resistance and T2DM, while increasing glucose-stimulated and decreasing lipolysis-induced insulin secretion from pancreatic β-cells.[164–167] These *aP2*-deficient mice are developmentally and metabolically normal and can develop diet-induced obesity, but they exhibit diminished obesity-induced TNF-α expression in adipose tissue and fail to develop insulin resistance or T2DM.[164] Similarly, *aP2* deletion in *ob/ob* mice (leptin-deficient mice: a genetic model of extreme obesity) results in increased peripheral insulin sensitivity, preserved pancreatic β-cell function and improved lipid metabolism, despite further increasing obesity.[166] It is suggested that *aP2* null mice exhibit both remodeling of the balance between lipolysis and lipogenesis and reprogramming of adipokine expression in adipocytes (e.g., increased adiponectin expression) which, despite the increased fat mass, results in decreased lipolysis, increased muscle glucose oxidation, and attenuated insulin resistance.[167] The in vivo investigation of fatty acid metabolism in aP2-deficient mice documented both reduced adipose tissue NEFA efflux and preferential utilization of glucose relative to fatty acids.[168]

In addition to the impact on insulin sensitivity and secretion, A-FABP is directly implicated in proinflammatory and proatherogenic processes. Genetic elimination of *aP2* in macrophages reduces both the intracellular cholesterol ester accumulation and the capacity to secrete proinflammatory cytokines (e.g., IL-6, MCP-1, and TNF-α) when exposed to modified lipoproteins.[169] A subsequent study further showed that A-FABP-deficient macrophages have altered lipid composition and enhanced PPARγ activity, and, in parallel, exhibit suppressed proinflammatory functions due to reduced IκB kinase and NF-κB activity.[170] Furthermore, A-FABP deficiency protects from atherosclerosis in apolipoprotein E (ApoE) deficient mice (a well-established experimental model of atherosclerosis).[169] Importantly, comparable reductions in atherosclerotic lesions were documented in ApoE null mice with total/whole-body A-FABP deficiency and in ApoE null mice, which, through bone-marrow transplantations, were generated to have A-FABP-deficient macrophages, but A-FABP-expressing adipocytes.[169] These data indicate that macrophage A-FABP expression plays an independent role in atherogenesis.[169]

Pharmacological inhibition of A-FABP was effective against severe atherosclerosis and T2DM in mouse models, involving suppression of c-Jun N-terminal kinase (JNK; a member of the MAPK family) activity.[138] Supporting the potential of this pharmacological inhibition of A-FABP against atherosclerosis, more recent findings have shown that a finely tuned positive-feedback loop is formed between A-FABP, JNK, and activator protein-1 (AP-1; a key transcription factor mediating inflammatory responses and proinflammatory cytokine production) that perpetuates inflammatory responses in macrophages.[171] Moreover, A-FABP has been identified as the predominant regulator of lipid-induced endoplasmic reticulum (ER) stress in macrophages, with A-FABP inhibition providing protection against macrophage ER stress, cell death, and atherosclerosis.[172] Of note, A-FABP was found to be highly expressed in vivo in macrophage/foam cells of human atherosclerotic plaques, and A-FABP overexpression in human THP-1 macrophages induced foam cell formation by enhancing intracellular cholesterol ester accumulation.[129,173] This macrophage-to-foam-cell transformation can be reduced by an A-FABP inhibitor, with A-FABP inhibitor-treated macrophages exhibiting significantly increased cholesterol efflux and reduced cholesterol ester accumulation.[138] Finally, atorvastatin also prevents the increase in A-FABP expression caused by Ox-LDL in human macrophages.[174]

Recent studies have also indicated that A-FABP is implicated in the regulation of endothelial cell proliferation and angiogenesis, thus playing a significant role in obesity-induced vascular endothelial dysfunction. Marked A-FABP expression has been identified in the endothelial cells of capillaries and small veins in several mouse and human tissues, including the heart.[130] In endothelial cells, A-FABP expression can be potently induced by vascular endothelial growth factor-A (VEGF-A) and basic fibroblast growth factor (bFGF) treatment, whereas it is inhibited by knockdown of the VEGF-receptor-2 (VEGFR2).[130] These findings indicate A-FABP constitutes a target of the VEGF/VEGFR2 pathway. Furthermore, A-FABP knockdown in endothelial cells can significantly reduce their proliferation in vitro under basal conditions and in response to VEGF and bFGF, suggesting that A-FABP is a positive regulator of endothelial cell proliferation.[130] In addition, A-FABP appears to have proangiogenic effects modulating important signaling pathways of angiogenesis, including the stem cell factor/c-kit pathway.[175] As such, A-FABP-deficient HUVECs have been shown to exhibit increased susceptibility to apoptosis and decreased migration and capillary network formation.[175] In the same study, aortic rings from A-FABP-deficient mice demonstrated decreased angiogenic sprouting, which was recovered by reconstitution of A-FABP. Notably, increased A-FABP expression in endothelial cells appears to contribute to their dysfunction both in vivo and in vitro.[176] Indeed, chronic administration of an A-FABP inhibitor resulted in improved endothelial function in ApoE-deficient mice and in cultured human endothelial cells by improving eNOS phosphorylation, NO production, and endothelium-dependent relaxation. These findings suggest a direct link between A-FABP and lipid-induced suppression of eNOS activation that results in vascular endothelial dysfunction.[176] Moreover, A-FABP inhibition appears to also prevent the selective dysfunction of G(i) protein-mediated relaxation to serotonin and the neointimal thickening resulting from endothelial regeneration.[177]

Finally, it must be highlighted that A-FABP released from adipocytes can have a direct effect on the heart acting as a cardio-depressant factor.[140] In isolated rat cardiomyocytes A-FABP has been shown to acutely depress the shortening amplitude and the intracellular systolic peak of calcium in a dose-dependent manner.[140] The N-terminal amino acids 1–20 of A-FABP appear to be the most effective cardio-depressive domain. Of note, in this study, A-FABP was shown to represent 1.8–8.1% of the total protein in the conditioned medium from adipocytes obtained from different individuals, whereas the microvesicle fraction prepared from this adipocyte-conditioned medium was also found to exert significant, although less potent, cardio-depressant effects on rat cardiomyocytes.[140] Taken together these findings suggest that A-FABP is implicated in cardiac contractile dysfunction in obese subjects, since the increased A-FABP levels released from the various adipose tissue depots, including epicardial fat, can directly exert acute calcium-dependent cardio-depressant effects.

ANTI-INFLAMMATORY ADIPOKINES

ADIPONECTIN

Equally significant to the discovery of leptin was the identification of adiponectin in 1995–6 by four independent research groups (initially reported as Acrp30, AdipoQ, apM1, and GBP28).[178–181] This adipokine is a secretory protein of 244–247 amino acids (dependent on species) encoded by the *ADIPOQ* gene and is synthesized almost exclusively by adipocytes; although it can be also produced by myocytes, endothelial cells, and cardiomyocytes.[1,182,183] Adiponectin is one of the most abundant circulating adipokines accounting for approximately 0.01% of the total plasma protein and plays a pleiotropic protective role highlighting the endocrine nature of adipose tissue (Fig. 7.7).[1,182,183,186,187]

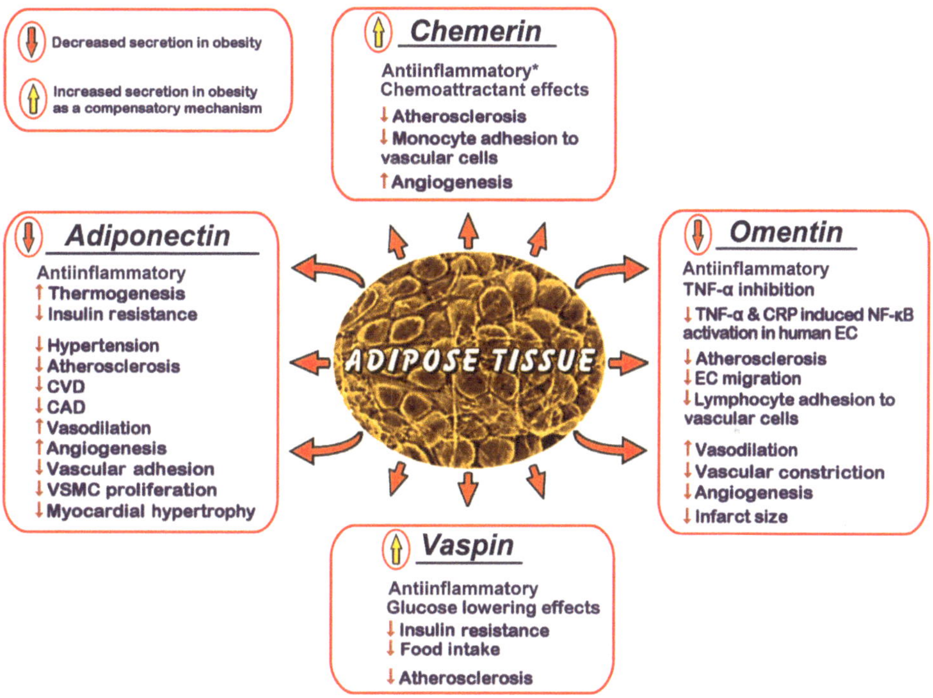

FIGURE 7.7

Effects of selected anti-inflammatory adipokines. *Chemerin is secreted as an inactive precursor, i.e., prochemerin, which is activated through proteolytic cleavage in the C-terminal region mediated by serine proteases of the coagulation, fibrinolytic and inflammatory cascades.[184,185] This enzymatic proteolysis of prochemerin can produce active chemerin forms with either chemotactic or anti-inflammatory properties, suggesting that chemerin may be implicated in both the initiation and resolution of inflammation.[185] Furthermore, the effects of chemerin appear to depend on the targeted cell type. *EC*: endothelial cells; *VSMC*: vascular smooth muscle cells; *TNF-α*: tumor necrosis factor-α; *CRP*: C-reactive protein; *NF-κB*: Nuclear factor kappa B; *CVD*: cardiovascular disease; *CAD*: coronary artery disease.

A sexual dimorphism has been noted regarding circulating adiponectin with lower plasma levels in men, potentially due to suppression by androgens.[188]

Adiponectin consists of four distinct domains, i.e., a short N-terminal signal sequence peptide that is cleaved upon entering the ER; a hypervariable region that exhibits the highest amino acid sequence divergence between species; followed by a collagenous domain with sequence and structural homology to collagen; and a C-terminal globular domain with striking homology to a number of proteins (e.g., complement factor C1q) that are involved in receptor binding.[178–181] Several SNPs of the *ADIPOQ* gene have been identified that modulate the function and circulating levels of adiponectin and are associated with insulin sensitivity, T2DM, and CVD complications of obesity.[189] Adiponectin undergoes extensive posttranslational modifications within the ER and the Golgi apparatus of adipocytes resulting in multimerization.[190,191] Thus, it is secreted as oligomers of trimmers, which are found in the circulation as low molecular weight (LMW: trimers), medium molecular weight (MMW: hexamers; alternatively LMW refers to both trimers and hexamers) and high molecular weight (HMW: 18- to 36-mers) multimers.[1,190,191] HMW adiponectin predominates in plasma and is considered to have more biological activity in insulin action.[191,192] Interestingly, a globular form of adiponectin (gAD), which may exert distinct biological effects compared to the full-length adiponectin peptide (fAD), can be also found in very low concentrations in the circulation, produced through cleavage of the globular domain from fAD by leukocyte elastase secreted from activated monocytes and/or neutrophils.[183,193,194]

In contrast to proinflammatory adipokines, adiponectin exhibits markedly reduced expression and secretion from adipocytes in obesity, particularly in central/visceral adipose tissue depots.[1,182,183,186,187] Notably, proinflammatory cytokines (e.g., IL-6 and TNF-α) inhibit adiponectin synthesis in adipocytes, highlighting the underlying interplay between different adipokines/cytokines in obesity-related inflammation (Fig. 7.2).[41] Thus, obesity, insulin resistance, T2DM, and metabolic syndrome are characterized by decreased circulating adiponectin concentrations (hypoadiponectinemia), while weight loss, various dietary interventions, and insulin sensitizing medications (e.g., thiazolidinediones) increase adiponectin expression and plasma levels.[1,182,183,186,187,195]

Adiponectin exerts its actions by binding to distinct specific receptors (Fig. 7.8), namely AdipoR1: a seven-transmembrane receptor that is ubiquitously expressed with the highest expression in skeletal muscle; AdipoR2: a seven-transmembrane receptor that is also expressed in several tissues, but predominantly in the liver; and to T-cadherin: a glycosylphosphatidylinositol-anchored extracellular protein without an intracellular domain that is highly expressed in the heart, skeletal muscle, and the vasculature, including pericytes and endothelial and vascular smooth muscle cells.[186,196–199] Of note, AdipoR1 and AdipoR2 are also expressed in several cardiovascular-relevant cells (e.g., monocytes, endothelial, and vascular smooth muscle cells) and in the heart where the former exhibits greater expression compared to the latter.[186,196,198,200] Importantly, T-cadherin is highly expressed in endothelial and smooth muscle cells at sites of vascular injury and exhibits affinity for the hexameric and HMW form of adiponectin, but not for the trimeric or globular form.[199] Hence, these adiponectin forms interact directly with T-cadherin and are abundantly present on vascular and muscle tissue surfaces, whereas adiponectin fails to associate with T-cadherin deficient tissues (e.g., with the cardiac tissue in T-cadherin deficient mice).[186,196,201] This interaction appears to be crucial for the cardio-protective and revascularization effects of adiponectin and for its role in atherosclerosis.[186,196,201] However, further research is required to elucidate the mechanism(s) mediating the effects of this adiponectin-binding protein on adiponectin cellular signaling and function.

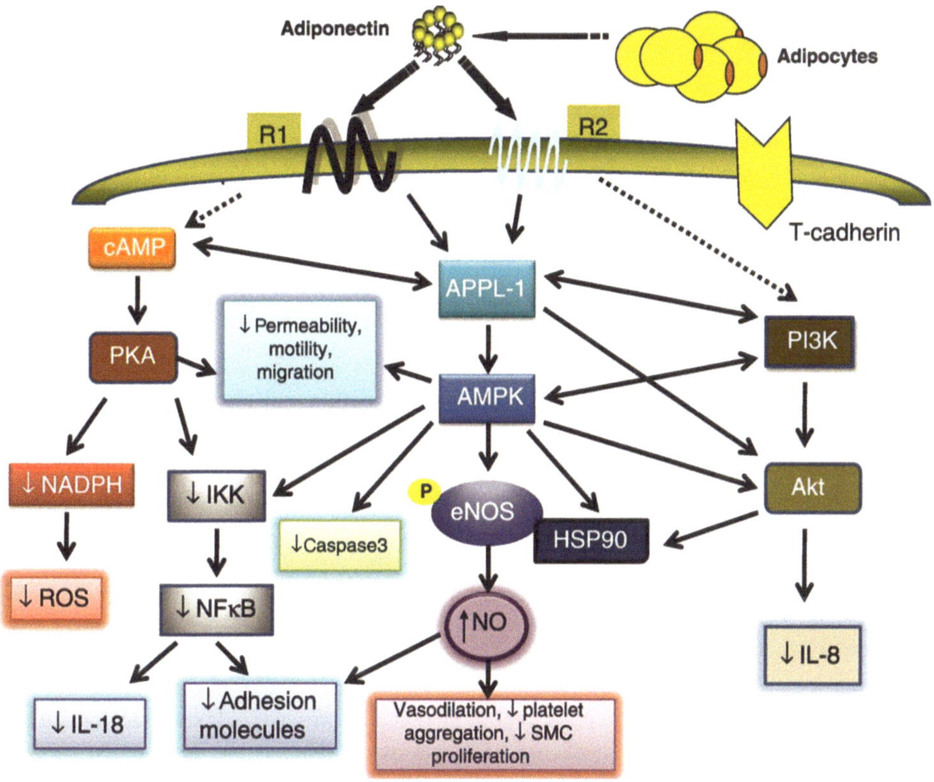

FIGURE 7.8

Schematic representation of adiponectin induced signaling pathways in the vascular endothelium. *AMPK*: including AMP-activated protein kinase; *APPL-1*: adaptor protein containing PH domain; *cAMP*: cyclic adenosine monophosphate; *eNOS*: endothelial nitric oxide synthase; *HSP-90*: heat shock protein 90; *IKK*: Iκ-kinase; *IL*: interleukin; *NADPH*: nicotinamide adenine dinucleotide phosphate; *NF-κB*: nuclear factor κB; *NO*: nitric oxide; *PI3K-Akt*: phosphatidylinositol-3-kinase-Akt; *PKA*: protein kinase A; *R1*: receptor 1; *R2*: receptor 2; *ROS*: reactive oxygen species.

*From Vaiopoulos AG, Marinou K, Christodoulides C, Koutsilieris M. The role of adiponectin in human vascular physiology. Int J Cardiol 2012;***155***(2):188–93.*

Improved insulin sensitivity is the most recognized beneficial metabolic effect of adiponectin, since, via AMPK phosphorylation, it stimulates glucose uptake in skeletal muscle, inhibits glucose production in the liver and induces fatty acid oxidation in both these tissues.[202–204] In addition, a strong body of clinical and experimental evidence has further revealed that adiponectin exhibits a wider spectrum of anti-inflammatory, antiatherogenic, and cardio-protective properties with significant impact on endothelial function, atherosclerosis, and CVD (Fig. 7.7).[1,182,183,186,205]

As aforementioned, reduced NO production in endothelial and vascular smooth muscle cells is considered a key mediator of endothelial dysfunction, which is a crucial step in the progression of atherosclerosis.[60] Circulating adiponectin constitutes a useful biomarker of endothelial dysfunction in hypertensive patients with hypoadiponectinemia being associated to impaired endothelium-dependent vasorelaxation.[206] In the same study, adiponectin knockout mice developed obesity, hyperglycemia, and hypertension after 4 weeks on an atherogenic diet and had significantly reduced endothelium-dependent vasodilation, while the endothelium-independent vasodilation was not affected.[206] In accord with these findings, adiponectin appears to have vasodilator actions by directly stimulating NO production in endothelial cells through PI3K-Akt dependent pathways, involving phosphorylation of eNOS by AMPK.[207] Furthermore, these adiponectin effects on eNOS phosphorylation and NO production were abolished when both AdipoR1 and AdipoR2 expression was simultaneously reduced in HUVECs.[208] APPL1, an intracellular adaptor protein, appears to act as a common downstream effector of AdipoR1 and AdipoR2 mediating adiponectin-induced endothelial NO production and endothelium-dependent vasodilation with *db/db* diabetic mice exhibiting decreased APPL1 expression and adiponectin-stimulated vasodilation.[208]

In patients with essential hypertension, hypoadiponectinemia and pronounced low-grade inflammation have an additive detrimental effect on aortic stiffness, accelerating vascular ageing.[209] It is now evident that, anti-inflammatory effects of adiponectin play a crucial protective role against endothelial dysfunction and atherosclerosis.[210] Indeed, adiponectin inhibits the proinflammatory cascade by suppressing TNF-α induced IκB phosphorylation and subsequent NF-κB activation through crosstalk between the NF-κB signaling pathway and both AMPK and protein kinase A [PKA; or cyclic AMP (cAMP)-dependent protein kinase] signaling in endothelial cells.[211–213] Of note, adiponectin can also suppress excess ROS production induced by high-glucose conditions or Ox-LDL in endothelial cells via a cAMP/PKA-dependent pathway, highlighting the significance of this adipokine for the protection of the vasculature in T2DM.[213]

Furthermore, adiponectin-deficient mice exhibit markedly increased leukocyte rolling and leukocyte adhesion in the microcirculation with decreased levels of endothelial NO and increased expression of E-selectin and VCAM-1 in the vascular endothelium.[214] Systemic administration of recombinant gAD in these mice attenuated the increased leukocyte-endothelium interactions and adhesion molecule expression while restoring physiologic levels of endothelial NO.[214] Interestingly, adiponectin-induced eNOS activation and increased NO production by endothelial cells is implicated in the anti-inflammatory action of adiponectin since pharmacological blockade of eNOS in mice abolishes the inhibitory effect of systemic gAD administration on TNF-α induced leukocyte adhesion.[214] In addition to protecting against endothelial dysfunction and activation of the endothelial adhesion molecular cascade that facilitates the macrophage entry into the vascular wall, adiponectin also suppresses macrophage-to-foam-cell transformation, acting as a crucial modulator of this process.[215] Moreover, adiponectin suppresses the proliferation and migration of human aortic smooth muscle cells by direct binding to platelet-derived growth factor (PDGF)-BB and inhibiting growth factor-stimulated ERK signaling, suggesting that adiponectin further acts as a modulator of vascular remodeling.[216] Importantly, in vivo experiments documented that adiponectin reduces development of atherosclerosis in ApoE-deficient mice.[217]

Adiponectin is also implicated in endothelial angiogenesis with in vitro data indicating it can stimulate new blood vessel growth by promoting crosstalk between AMPK and Akt signaling within endothelial cells, potentially forming an adiponectin-AMPK-PI3K-Akt-eNOS signaling axis.[218] Animal studies in adiponectin knockout mice reveal adiponectin can stimulate angiogenesis in response to ischemic stress by promoting AMPK signaling.[219] Notably, AMPK signaling plays an key role in upregulating VEGF and studies involving overexpression of adiponectin in the mouse brain have documented that this overexpression promotes focal angiogenesis following middle cerebral artery occlusion, thus attenuating ischemia-induced brain atrophy and improving neurological function.[220] In contrast, it must be noted that there are also data showing that adiponectin can suppress VEGF-stimulated migration of human coronary artery endothelial cells through cAMP/PKA-dependent signaling.[221] Furthermore, adiponectin-induced antiangiogenesis and antitumor activity appears to involve caspase-mediated endothelial cell apoptosis.[222] Interestingly, in vivo studies in an orthotopic liver cancer model in mice and in vitro functional experiments in endothelial and liver cancer cells showed that adiponectin treatment can inhibit liver tumor growth and metastasis by suppression of tumor angiogenesis and down-regulation of the Rho kinase/IFN-inducible protein 10/MMP9 pathway.[223]

Finally, mounting data strongly indicate that adiponectin exerts direct cardio-protective effects against ischemic myocardial damage, cardiac hypertrophy, and heart failure.[61,186,201,205,224] Indeed, adiponectin can protect against myocardial I/R injury through the regulation of independent signaling pathways involving both AMPK-mediated antiapoptotic actions and COX-2-mediated anti-inflammatory actions.[224,225] As such, cardiac ischemia/reperfusion produces a larger myocardial infarct associated with increased myocardial cell apoptosis and TNF-α expression in adiponectin knockout mice, compared with wild-type mice. Conversely, adiponectin administration diminishes the infarct size, apoptosis, and TNF-α production in both adiponectin-deficient and wild-type mice.[225]

Interestingly, another study in adiponectin knockdown/knockout and wild-type mice showed that treatment with the PPARγ agonist rosiglitazone increased adipocyte expression and plasma levels of adiponectin and reduced infarct size and apoptosis following coronary artery ligation in wild-type mice, whereas these effects are blunted in adiponectin knockdown/knockout mice and completely lost in adiponectin-null mice.[226] Therefore, potential cardio-protective effects of PPARγ agonists against ischemic heart injury appear to be critically dependent on their adiponectin stimulatory action, suggesting that when adiponectin expression is impaired (e.g., under pathological conditions such as advanced T2DM) the detrimental cardiovascular effects of these agonists may outweigh their cardio-protective benefits.[226] In accord with this, treatment with pioglitazone, another clinically available PPARγ agonist, was shown to attenuate angiotensin II-induced cardiac hypertrophy and interstitial fibrosis in wild-type mice through adiponectin-dependent effects involving ERK 1/2 and AMPK phosphorylation, while these effects were diminished in adiponectin-deficient mice.[227] Furthermore, adiponectin can also modulate hypertrophic signals in the heart as the adiponectin-AMPK signaling pathway negatively regulates changes in intracellular signaling and metabolism, which are linked to myocardial hypertrophy progression.[224,228] Finally, studies on cardiac remodeling after myocardial infarction in mice have documented that adiponectin protects against the development of systolic dysfunction postmyocardial infarction by suppressing cardiac hypertrophy and interstitial fibrosis and protecting against capillary and cardiomyocyte loss.[229]

Overall, adiponectin is one of the most extensively studied adipokines with well-established beneficial cardio-metabolic actions that are mediated through its direct insulin sensitizing, antidiabetic, anti-inflammatory, antiatherogenic, and cardio-protective effects (Fig. 7.7). Current research is focusing on developing effective approaches to modulate adiponectin and its downstream signaling pathways for the treatment of metabolic syndrome, T2DM, and CVD.[230]

OMENTIN

Omentin is a protein of 313 amino acids with two homologs (omentin-1 and omentin-2; 83% amino acid homology) that are respectively encoded by two genes that are located adjacent to each other in a region of chromosome 1 (1q22–q23) linked to T2DM.[231–233] In the context of this chapter, omentin refers to omentin-1 as this constitutes the main circulating omentin homolog.[232,233] This protein was first identified in the Paneth cells of the small intestine and it was later detected in endothelial cells in various tissues (e.g., in the small intestine, colon, thymus, and heart); thus, it was initially named intelectin and was also known as intestinal lactoferrin receptor, galactofuranose-binding lectin, and endothelial lectin.[232–235] The genomic structure details of the human omentin gene were described in 2005, revealing complete amino acid sequence homology between human omentin and intelectin.[236] Subsequently, in 2006, omentin was first described as a circulating adipokine that is predominantly expressed in omental (visceral) adipose tissue with barely detectable expression in subcutaneous fat.[237] Of note, omentin specifically expressed in stromal vascular cells, but not in adipocytes, isolated from omental adipose tissue.[237] Significant omentin expression has also been detected in human epicardial adipose tissue, which has a common embryological origin with the omental and mesenteric adipose tissue (intra-abdominal, visceral fat depots), derived from the splanchnopleuric mesoderm.[238] As such, omentin, like other locally produced adipokines, may exert direct paracrine effects on the underlying myocardium and vessels since the absence of a fibrous fascial layer between the epicardial adipose tissue and the heart allows a close anatomic relationship and diffusion of various factors between these tissues (e.g., free fatty acids and adipokines).[239,240] To date, omentin specific receptors have not been identified. However, this adipokine increases Akt phosphorylation and insulin-stimulated glucose uptake in adipocytes, regulating insulin action, but it also has anti-inflammatory effects (Fig. 7.7).[232,233]

Omentin expression in adipose tissue and circulating levels are decreased in obesity, exhibiting negative correlations with BMI, waist circumference, insulin resistance indices, and circulating leptin, and positive correlations with adiponectin and HDL plasma levels.[231] Decreased circulating omentin levels have also been documented in patients with T2DM or other components of the metabolic syndrome.[241–246] Notably, a study in healthy (asymptomatic) prepubertal children documented an association between increased circulating omentin levels and parameters indicating a less favorable metabolic profile, including family history of T2DM, higher levels of insulin resistance, fasting triacylglycerol, systolic and diastolic blood pressure, and lower levels of HMW adiponectin.[247] The study posited that this may be attributed, at least partly, to a compensatory mechanism whereby omentin is increased at an early stage in children to protect against metabolic dysfunction. Furthermore, interventional clinical studies have shown that omentin levels increase in the circulation after weight loss-induced improvement of insulin sensitivity achieved through restricted caloric intake or aerobic training.[248,249] Elevated plasma omentin levels have also been reported, although not consistently, following bariatric surgery.[250,251] Interestingly, an increase in circulating omentin was observed even before weight loss or insulin sensitivity improvement (as early as the first 24 hours) after biliopancreatic diversion with duodenal switch in most of the studied patients, while a decrease in plasma omentin levels at the first postoperative day was associated with higher CVD risk.[250] Moreover, omentin levels increased with metformin treatment and decreased in response to pharmacologic doses of metreleptin.[241,252]

In addition, strong clinical data further indicate a close association between circulating omentin and CVD. Indeed, circulating omentin appears to be a useful biomarker of endothelial dysfunction with an independent association to endothelium-dependent vasodilation.[244] Furthermore, compared to metabolic syndrome patients without atherosclerosis, patients with both metabolic syndrome and atherosclerosis exhibit even lower omentin plasma levels that negatively correlate to carotid intima-media thickness and arterial stiffness.[253] Similarly, T2DM patients with carotid plaques exhibit lower omentin levels compared to those without, and circulating omentin is an independent predictor of carotid atherosclerosis and arterial stiffness in T2DM.[254] Circulating omentin is also independently associated with CAD, with decreased levels in stable angina patients compared to healthy controls, and even lower levels in patients with ACS.[255,256] In accord with this, low plasma omentin levels were associated with both the presence and severity of CAD in metabolic syndrome patients and in postmenopausal women.[257,258] Of note, compared to healthy controls, patients with acute myocardial infarction had lower circulating omentin levels at admission, which significantly increased 6 months postinfarction.[259] Finally, decreased plasma omentin levels are also associated with a poor cardiac outcome in heart failure patients, independently predicting the risk of cardiac events.[260]

An increasing body of experimental evidence supports the association between decreased circulating omentin levels and both atherogenesis and endothelial dysfunction. As such, omentin has been shown to induce vasodilation in rat isolated blood vessels.[261] Omentin produced an endothelium-dependent relaxation in endothelium-intact rat isolated aorta that was mediated by endothelium-derived NO via increased eNOS phosphorylation and independent of PI3K/Akt and tyrosine phosphorylation.[261] This omentin-induced vasorelaxation was also observed in rat isolated mesenteric artery, suggesting that omentin is also effective on mesenteric resistance vessels.[261] Interestingly, in the same study, omentin inhibited noradrenaline-induced contraction even in endothelium-removed aorta, indicating that omentin induces vasorelaxation via additional endothelium-independent mechanisms (e.g., potentially through activating smooth muscle potassium channels).[261]

Furthermore, omentin exerts anti-inflammatory effects on vascular endothelial cells.[262–265] In vitro experiments in human microvascular endothelial cells showed that omentin attenuated CRP- and VEGF-induced migration and angiogenesis by suppressing NF-kB activation.[262] Omentin inhibited TNF-α-induced COX-2 expression in HUVECs via inhibiting JNK activation (decreased JNK phosphorylation), presumably through activation of AMPK/eNOS/NO pathways.[263] As an additional unpublished observation, the authors of this study further reported that omentin-induced AMPK activation could directly inhibit p38-mediated E-selectin induction and the subsequent lymphocyte adhesion to vascular endothelial cells.[264] Similarly, omentin appears to inhibit TNF-α-induced VCAM-1 expression in smooth muscle cells in a concentration-dependent manner via preventing p38 and JNK activation through inhibition of superoxide production.[265] In addition, omentin can inhibit PDGF-BB-induced vascular smooth muscle cell migration through an antioxidative mechanism and, thus, may protect against hypertension by inhibiting vascular structural remodeling.[266] Moreover, in HUVECs, omentin promotes endothelial cell function and revascularization in response to ischemia by stimulating an Akt/eNOS signaling pathway.[267]

More recently, a number of studies have also examined potential direct effects of omentin on cardiomyocytes and cardiac function.[268–270] The findings of a study combining clinical data with in vivo and in vitro experiments indicate that omentin can ameliorate acute ischemic injury in the heart by suppressing myocyte apoptosis via both AMPK- and Akt-dependent pathways.[268] In patients with acute myocardial infarction recruited in this study, high circulating omentin levels were associated with a decrease in heart damage and improved cardiac function after reperfusion therapy. In addition, systemic administration of human omentin in mice reduced the myocardial infarct size and apoptosis after I/R by enhancing AMPK and Akt phosphorylation in the ischemic heart.[268] Transgenic overexpression of human omentin in a fat-specific manner in mice also prevented myocardial ischemic damage and apoptosis in the heart.[268] In agreement, in vitro experiments in cultured cardiomyocytes documented that human omentin at physiological concentrations can suppress hypoxia/reoxygenation-induced apoptosis, an effect that can be blocked by inactivation of AMPK or Akt.[268] Furthermore, in vivo and in vitro data suggest that omentin can also attenuate myocardial hypertrophy via AMPK activation.[269] Interestingly, omentin was shown to prevent doxorubicin-induced apoptosis in rat cardiomyoblasts through inhibition of mitochondrial ROS production, thus protecting against the cardiac cytotoxicity of this anticancer drug.[270]

Taken together, the aforementioned insulin sensitizing, anti-inflammatory, and cardio-protective effects strongly indicate that omentin constitutes an additional link between diabesity, inflammation, and CVD, with an overall protective role against atherogenesis and endothelial and cardiac dysfunction.

CHEMERIN

Chemerin, also known as retinoic acid receptor responder protein 2 (RARRES2) and tazarotene induced gene 2, is a 16-kDa protein that was first identified as the product of a gene of unknown function that was upregulated in skin cells by the synthetic retinoid tazarotene.[271] Chemerin is secreted as an inactive precursor, i.e., prochemerin, which becomes active upon proteolytic cleavage in the C-terminal region mediated by serine proteases of the coagulation, fibrinolytic, and inflammatory cascades.[184,185] Importantly, the enzymatic proteolysis of this precursor can produce active chemerin forms with either chemotactic or anti-inflammatory properties, suggesting that chemerin may be implicated in both the initiation and resolution of inflammation (Fig. 7.7).[185] Indeed, chemerin was initially described as a chemokine exerting potent chemoattractant effects on various immune cells, such as dendritic cells and macrophages, which are both antigen-presenting cells with key roles in the innate and adaptive immunity.[272] In 2007 chemerin was further described as a novel adipokine that is expressed in mouse and human adipocytes and associated with obesity and factors contributing to the development of the metabolic syndrome (e.g., blood pressure and circulating triglycerides).[273,274] Subsequent studies have also reported that plasma chemerin levels are increased in morbidly obese patients and correlate to insulin resistance and biomarkers of fatty liver disease, while a marked decrease in circulating chemerin is observed after bariatric surgery.[275]

Chemerin acts on target cells through binding to and activating specific seven-transmembrane receptors, i.e., chemokine-like receptor 1 (CMKLR1; also known as ChemR23, ChemerinR; and DEZ)[184,185,272] These are G protein-coupled receptors expressed in various cell types, including dendritic cells, macrophages, adipocytes, cardiomyocytes, and endothelial and skeletal muscle cells.[184,185,272,274,276–279] Chemerin also binds to two other orphan G protein-coupled receptors, i.e., GPR1 and chemokine (C-C motif) receptor-like 2, although the downstream effects of this binding remain to be elucidated.[185] Accordingly, the exact range of chemerin actions is still not fully clarified, and the role of chemerin appears to depend on the targeted cell type. As such, chemerin has been shown to inhibit glucose uptake and induce insulin resistance in human skeletal muscle cells,[277] while it exerts the opposite effects in mature 3T3-L1 adipocytes increasing insulin-stimulated glucose uptake.[278] Moreover, targeted knockdown of chemerin or CMKLR1 expression can impair differentiation of 3T3-L1 cells into adipocytes, alter metabolic functions in mature adipocytes and decrease the expression of adipocyte genes regulating glucose and lipid homeostasis.[273] Of note, knockdown of chemerin or CMKLR1 expression arrests the adipogenic clonal expansion of bone marrow mesenchymal stem cells, while forced expression of PPARγ significantly induced chemerin expression and secretion in these cells, but failed to completely rescue this block in adipogenesis.[280] Upregulation of both chemerin and CMKLR1mRNA expression levels in adipose tissue were also noted in mice on a high-fat diet.[276]

In addition to promoting adipogenesis, existing data strongly indicate that chemerin also plays a role in the stimulation of endothelial angiogenesis.[279,281] Indeed, CMKLR1 is expressed in human vascular endothelial cells and its expression levels are upregulated by proinflammatory cytokines (e.g., TNF-α, IL-1β, and IL-6).[279] Moreover, chemerin exhibits potent angiogenic effects and can induce the production of MMP-2 and MMP-9 as well as key angiogenic and cell survival cascades (e.g., activation of PI3K-Akt and MAPK pathways) in endothelial cells.[279] Further studies have also shown that chemerin activates ERK1 and ERK2 (p42/44) of the MAPK pathway, while its angiogenic effects in endothelial cells are dependent on p42/44 MEK activation.[281,282] More recently, chemerin was reported to increase vascular contractile responses to phenylephrine and endothelin-1 via ERK 1/2 activation.[283] Arterial stiffness also appears associated to circulating chemerin levels even after adjusting for other CVD risk factors.[284] Notably, although chemerin positively correlates to circulating markers of inflammation, no association between chemerin levels and coronary atherosclerotic plaque burden and morphology has been reported.[285] Another study has documented higher chemerin levels in peri-aortic and epicardial adipose tissue of CAD patients and a positive correlation between coronary atherosclerosis and the peri-coronary fat expression of both chemerin and visfatin.[286] However, more extensive research is required to fully understand the direct role and relative contribution of such locally produced adipokines in the progression of aortic and coronary atherosclerosis. Finally, chemerin exerts anti-inflammatory effects in human vascular endothelial cells by preventing TNF-α-induced VCAM-1 expression and inhibiting monocyte adhesion to TNF-α-stimulated endothelial cells.[287] These effects are mediated via stimulated Akt/eNOS signaling and NO production, which suppress NF-κB and p38 activation.[287] Interestingly, iptakalim, an endothelial protective agent that induces the opening of K_{ATP} channels, has been shown to improve endothelial function in rat aortic endothelial cells by inducing the endothelial chemerin/CMKLR1 axis and NO production.[288]

Overall, chemerin appears to have protective properties on the endothelial function by promoting angiogenesis and reducing inflammation and monocyte adhesion to the endothelial wall (Fig. 7.7). However, to fully characterize the CVD risk profile of this relatively novel adipokine, the effects of chemerin (both direct effects and in relation to other adipokines) on cardiomyocytes and cardiac function need to be further studied.

VASPIN

Vaspin (visceral adipose tissue-derived serine protease inhibitor; also known as Serpin A12) is a 47-kDa protein of 415 amino acids that belongs to the serine protease inhibitor (serpin) family.[289,290] In 2005 vaspin was first found to be highly expressed in the visceral white adipose tissue of Otsuka Long-Evans Tokushima Fatty rats at the age of 30 weeks when obesity and insulin plasma levels reach a peak (OLETF rats: an animal model of abdominal/visceral obesity with T2DM).[291] Subsequently, it was shown that vaspin is expressed in both visceral and subcutaneous adipose tissue depots of obese humans and that its expression may be regulated in an adipose tissue depot-specific manner associated with parameters of obesity, glucose metabolism, and insulin resistance.[292] More recent data in women have further indicated that the expression of vaspin in abdominal adipose tissue is adipocyte-specific and that vaspin expression in subcutaneous adipose tissue decreases as the mass of visceral adipose tissue increases.[293] Of note, a sexual dimorphism characterizes circulating vaspin, since gender is an independent predictor of plasma vaspin levels, which are significantly higher in women.[294,295] A study in children further showed that vaspin levels increase with age and pubertal stage in girls, whereas there is a lack of change in circulating vaspin with development in boys.[296] Interestingly, vaspin expression has also been detected in other tissues, including the hypothalamus, stomach, skin, and pancreatic islets.[289]

Intraperitoneal administration of vaspin to obese mice fed a high-fat and high-sucrose diet resulted in improved glucose tolerance and insulin sensitivity and in reversal of the altered expression of genes implicated in insulin resistance (e.g., leptin, resistin, TNF-α, glucose transporter-4, and adiponectin gene expression).[291] As such, vaspin is considered to play an insulin-sensitizing role as part of a compensatory mechanism against insulin resistance and to also exert anti-inflammatory effects by inhibiting the expression of proinflammatory adipokines (e.g., leptin, resistin, and TNF-α) (Fig. 7.7).[289–291] Accordingly, elevated plasma vaspin levels and upregulated vaspin expression in adipose tissue have a positive association to obesity, insulin resistance, and metabolic syndrome parameters in humans.[289,290] Indeed, it has been shown that increased circulating vaspin levels are associated with obesity and impaired insulin sensitivity, while T2DM appears to negate the correlation between elevated vaspin levels and both high BMI and increased insulin resistance.[295] Furthermore, modest weight loss in obese patients, achieved through a 12-week lifestyle modification program and adjuvant treatment with the antiobesity agent orlistat, was accompanied by a decrease in circulating vaspin levels.[297] This decrease also correlated to changes in anthropometric and metabolic parameters based on the underlying insulin sensitivity status (more potent correlations were observed in the most insulin resistant group of obese patients).[297]

Importantly, peripheral (intraperitoneal) and central (intracerebroventricular) vaspin administration in different mouse models has been shown to cause both sustained glucose-lowering effects and reduced food intake (Fig. 7.7)[298] It has been proposed that these beneficial metabolic effects of vaspin are mediated by its ability to inhibit proteases that degrade factors with hypoglycemic and/or anorexigenic effects.[289,298] Kallikrein 7, a protease that can cleave human insulin in vitro, has been suggested as a vaspin target.[299] Vaspin can inhibit kallikrein 7 via its serpin activity, with both proteins being coexpressed in murine pancreatic β-cells and vaspin/kallikrein seven complexes being detected in human plasma.[299] Hence, vaspin-induced improvement of glucose homeostasis could be, at least in part, attributed to decreased insulin degradation in the circulation resulting in increased plasma insulin levels.

To date, there are limited clinical data on the association between vaspin and obesity-related CVD. Reduced coronary flow reserve appears associated to the combination of higher circulating vaspin levels and increased epicardial adipose tissue thickness in NAFLD patients.[300] Moreover, plasma vaspin levels have been reported to have a positive association with the presence and severity of coronary artery stenosis in women, but not in men, whereas in the same study higher circulating vaspin concentrations were associated with metabolic syndrome only in men.[301] Interestingly, data in patients with carotid stenosis undergoing carotid endarterectomy showed that vaspin levels were significantly lower in the patients with a recent ischemic event (within 3 months before surgery) compared to previously asymptomatic CAD patients, despite lack of association between circulating vaspin and parameters of atherosclerosis severity.[302] Moreover, lower vaspin and higher visfatin plasma levels were detected in patients with angiographically proven stable, asymptomatic CAD compared to matched healthy controls without CVD, with statin-free patients exhibiting an even greater decrease in circulating vaspin than statin-treated patients.[303] Data in children have also shown that, independently of gender, age and BMI, circulating vaspin exhibits a negative correlation to 24-hour systolic blood pressure, with lower plasma vaspin levels also being related to endothelial dysfunction as evaluated by the reactive hyperemia index.[296]

The potential direct effects of vaspin in atherogenesis and endothelial and cardiac function have not been adequately explored. A study on the relation of aortic and coronary atherosclerosis to the differential expression of adipokines in peri-aortic, peri-coronary, and epicardial adipose tissue has documented that vaspin is expressed in adipocytes and stromal vascular cells in fat samples from all these sites.[286] According to the results of this study vaspin expression was also detected in aortic and coronary vascular smooth muscle cells, as well as in macrophage foam cells of coronary and aortic atherosclerotic lesions. In the latter lesions vaspin expression in macrophage foam cells exhibited positive correlations to both leptin and chemerin expression levels.[286] These findings suggest that vaspin has the potential to act in an autocrine/paracrine manner on the cardiovascular system. A study focusing on the insulin-signaling pathway in endothelial cells has indicated that vaspin may have beneficial effects on atherogenesis by protecting human aortic endothelial cells against free fatty acid–induced apoptosis through upregulation of the PI3K-Akt signaling pathway.[304] Only a few studies have examined potential anti-inflammatory effects of vaspin in vascular cells. For example, in HUVECs vaspin appears to have no effect on both basal morphology and TNF-α–induced morphological damage, since it only inhibited TNF-α–induced Akt phosphorylation to a small degree (nonsignificant trend towards inhibition) without decreasing the TNF-α activation of JNK, p38 and NF-kB signaling and the expression of molecules related to inflammation and/or endothelial cell dysfunction (e.g., VCAM-1, ICAM-1, and MCP-1).[305] Conversely, in rat vascular smooth muscle cells vaspin inhibits the TNF-α–induced expression of ICAM-1 through preventing ROS generation and subsequent activation of NF-κB and PKCθ signaling.[306] Further research is clearly needed to expand the limited existing evidence regarding the exact mechanisms mediating the effects of vaspin in various organs/tissues and to better understand the potential of this adipokine as a biomarker and/or a therapeutic agent for obesity-related cardiometabolic disease.

CONCLUSION

The discovery of leptin and adiponectin revived the research interest in adipose tissue biology. To date, hundreds of adipokines have been identified highlighting the complexity of the adipose tissue as an endocrine organ. As such, it is now well-established that through secreted adipokines the adipose tissue signals its metabolic and inflammatory status in a dynamic way with profound impact on the CNS and organs/tissues of the periphery, including the heart and vasculature. Compelling data link the chronic, low-grade inflammation and the proinflammatory circulating adipokine profile in obesity to the development of CVD. However, the exact role of adipose tissue in the regulation of cardiac function in health and disease is still not completely understood. Emerging evidence indicates that several adipokines can exert direct effects on the heart regulating myocardial contractility, ischemic damage, remodeling, hypertrophy, and heart failure. Importantly, overlapping and opposing effects of different adipokines have been documented on the cardiovascular function, thus it is critical to clarify not only the exact effects of each single adipokine, but also how their combined action in the context of the obesity-related adverse adipokine profile results in the development of CVD. Current research is focusing on addressing these questions and clarifying the underlying mechanisms mediating the adipokine effects on the heart, which could potentially lead to novel approaches for the prevention and/or treatment of CVD.

REFERENCES

1. Fasshauer M, Blüher M. Adipokines in health and disease. *Trends Pharmacol Sci* 2015;**36**(7):461–70.
2. Deng Y, Scherer PE. Adipokines as novel biomarkers and regulators of the metabolic syndrome. *Ann N Y Acad Sci* 2010;**1212**:E1–E19.
3. Galic S, Oakhill JS, Steinberg GR. Adipose tissue as an endocrine organ. *Mol Cell Endocrinol* 2010;**316**(2):129–39.
4. Ahima RS. Adipose tissue as an endocrine organ. *Obesity (Silver Spring)* 2006;**14**(Suppl. 5):242S–9S.
5. Fortuño A, Rodríguez A, Gómez-Ambrosi J, et al. Adipose tissue as an endocrine organ: role of leptin and adiponectin in the pathogenesis of cardiovascular diseases. *J Physiol Biochem* 2003;**59**(1):51–60.
6. Matsuzawa Y, Funahashi T, Nakamura T. The concept of metabolic syndrome: contribution of visceral fat accumulation and its molecular mechanism. *J Atheroscler Thromb* 2011;**18**(8):629–39.
7. Hausman DB, DiGirolamo M, Bartness TJ, et al. The biology of white adipocyte proliferation. *Obes Rev* 2001;**2**(4):239–54.
8. Makki K, Froguel P, Wolowczuk I. Adipose tissue in obesity–related inflammation and insulin resistance: cells, cytokines, and chemokines. *ISRN Inflamm* 2013;**2013**:139239.
9. Gregor MF, Hotamisligil GS. Inflammatory mechanisms in obesity. *Annu Rev Immunol* 2011;**29**:415–45.
10. Maury E, Brichard SM. Adipokine dysregulation, adipose tissue inflammation and metabolic syndrome. *Mol Cell Endocrinol* 2010;**314**:1–16.
11. Le Lay S, Krief S, Farnier C, et al. Cholesterol, a cell size-dependent signal that regulates glucose metabolism and gene expression in adipocytes. *J Biol Chem* 2001;**276**(20):16904–10.
12. Lee J. Adipose tissue macrophages in the development of obesity-induced inflammation, insulin resistance and type 2 diabetes. *Arch Pharm Res* 2013;**36**:208–22.
13. Weisberg SP, McCann D, Desai M, et al. Obesity is associated with macrophage accumulation in adipose tissue. *J Clin Invest* 2003;**112**:1796–808.
14. Xu H, Barnes GT, Yang Q, et al. Chronic inflammation in fat plays a crucial role in the development of obesity-related insulin resistance. *J Clin Invest* 2003;**112**(12):1821–30.
15. Weiss R. Fat distribution and storage: how much, where, and how? *Eur J Endocrinol* 2007;**157**(Suppl. 1): S39–45.
16. Samad F, Ruf W. Inflammation, obesity, and thrombosis. *Blood* 2013;**122**:3415–22.
17. Després JP. Abdominal obesity and cardiovascular disease: is inflammation the missing link? *Can J Cardiol* 2012;**28**(6):642–52.
18. Rocha VZ, Libby P. Obesity, inflammation, and atherosclerosis. *Nat Rev Cardiol* 2009;**6**:399–409.
19. Shoelson SE, Lee J, Goldfine AB. Inflammation and insulin resistance. *J Clin Invest* 2006;**116**:1793–801.
20. Wellen KE, Hotamisligil GS. Obesity–induced inflammatory changes in adipose tissue. *J Clin Invest* 2003;**112**:1785–8.
21. Tilg H, Moschen AR. Adipocytokines: mediators linking adipose tissue, inflammation and immunity. *Nat Rev Immunol* 2006;**6**:772–83.
22. Zhang Y, Proenca R, Maffei M, et al. Positional cloning of the mouse obese gene and its human homologue. *Nature* 1994;**372**(6505):425–32.
23. Chang YH, Chang DM, Lin KC, et al. Visfatin in overweight/obesity, type 2 diabetes mellitus, insulin resistance, metabolic syndrome and cardiovascular diseases: a meta-analysis and systemic review. *Diabetes Metab Res Rev* 2011;**27**(6):515–27.
24. Brown JE, Onyango DJ, Ramanjaneya M, et al. Visfatin regulates insulin secretion, insulin receptor signalling and mRNA expression of diabetes-related genes in mouse pancreatic beta-cells. *J Mol Endocrinol* 2010;**44**(3):171–8.
25. Mantzoros CS, Magkos F, Brinkoetter M, et al. Leptin in human physiology and pathophysiology. *Am J Physiol Endocrinol Metab* 2011;**301**(4):E567–84.

26. Ahima RS. Central actions of adipocyte hormones. *Trends Endocrinol Metab* 2005;**16**(7):307–13.
27. Considine RV, Sinha MK, Heiman ML, et al. Serum immunoreactive-leptin concentrations in normal-weight and obese humans. *N Engl J Med* 1996;**334**(5):292–5.
28. Sáinz N, Barrenetxe J, Moreno-Aliaga MJ, et al. Leptin resistance and diet–induced obesity: central and peripheral actions of leptin. *Metabolism* 2015;**64**(1):35–46.
29. Zhou Y, Rui L. Leptin signaling and leptin resistance. *Front Med* 2013;**7**(2):207–22.
30. Martin SS, Qasim A, Reilly MP. Leptin resistance: a possible interface of inflammation and metabolism in obesity-related cardiovascular disease. *J Am Coll Cardiol* 2008;**52**(15):1201–10.
31. Enriori PJ, Evans AE, Sinnayah P, et al. Leptin resistance and obesity. *Obesity (Silver Spring)* 2006;**14** (Suppl. 5):254S–8S.
32. Zabeau L, Lavens D, Peelman F, et al. The ins and outs of leptin receptor activation. *FEBS Lett* 2003;**546**(1):45–50.
33. Minokoshi Y, Kim YB, Peroni OD, et al. Leptin stimulates fatty-acid oxidation by activating AMP-activated protein kinase. *Nature* 2002;**415**(6869):339–43.
34. Frühbeck G. Intracellular signalling pathways activated by leptin. *Biochem J* 2006;**393**(Pt 1):7–20.
35. Ren J. Leptin and hyperleptinemia - from friend to foe for cardiovascular function. *J Endocrinol* 2004;**181**(1):1–10.
36. Hausenloy DJ, Yellon DM. Survival kinases in ischemic preconditioning and postconditioning. *Cardiovasc Res* 2006;**70**(2):240–53.
37. Hausenloy DJ, Yellon DM. Cardioprotective growth factors. *Cardiovasc Res* 2009;**83**(2):179–94.
38. Yellon DM, Hausenloy DJ. Myocardial reperfusion injury. *N Engl J Med* 2007;**357**(11):1121–35.
39. Procaccini C, Jirillo E, Matarese G. Leptin as an immunomodulator. *Mol Aspects Med* 2012;**33**(1):35–45.
40. Naylor C, Petri Jr. WA. Leptin regulation of immune responses. *Trends Mol Med* 2016;**22**(2):88–98. pii: S1471–4914(15)00231–2.
41. Lago F, Dieguez C, Gómez-Reino J, et al. The emerging role of adipokines as mediators of inflammation and immune responses. *Cytokine Growth Factor Rev* 2007;**18**(3–4):313–25.
42. Kimura M, Tanaka S, Isoda F, et al. T lymphopenia in obese diabetic (db/db) mice is non-selective and thymus independent. *Life Sci* 1998;**62**(14):1243–50.
43. Howard JK, Lord GM, Matarese G, et al. Leptin protects mice from starvation-induced lymphoid atrophy and increases thymic cellularity in ob/ob mice. *J Clin Invest* 1999;**104**(8):1051–9.
44. Romero-Corral A, Sierra-Johnson J, Lopez-Jimenez F, et al. Relationships between leptin and C-reactive protein with cardiovascular disease in the adult general population. *Nat Clin Pract Cardiovasc Med* 2008;**5**(7):418–25.
45. Dong M, Ren J. What fans the fire: insights into mechanisms of leptin in metabolic syndrome–associated heart diseases. *Curr Pharm Des* 2014;**20**(4):652–8.
46. Wang H, Luo W, Eitzman DT. Leptin in thrombosis and atherosclerosis. *Curr Pharm Des* 2014;**20**(4):641–5.
47. Yamagishi SI, Edelstein D, Du XL, et al. Leptin induces mitochondrial superoxide production and monocyte chemoattractant protein-1 expression in aortic endothelial cells by increasing fatty acid oxidation via protein kinase A. *J Biol Chem* 2001;**276**(27):25096–100.
48. Beltowski J. Leptin and atherosclerosis. *Atherosclerosis* 2006;**189**(1):47–60.
49. Beltowski J. Role of leptin in blood pressure regulation and arterial hypertension. *J Hypertens* 2006;**24**(5):789–801.
50. Singh P, Hoffmann M, Wolk R, et al. Leptin induces C-reactive protein expression in vascular endothelial cells. *Arterioscler Thromb Vasc Biol* 2007;**27**(9):e302–7.
51. Bouloumie A, Marumo T, Lafontan M, et al. Leptin induces oxidative stress in human endothelial cells. *FASEB J* 1999;**13**(10):1231–8.
52. Vecchione C, Maffei A, Colella S, et al. Leptin effect on endothelial nitric oxide is mediated through Akt-endothelial nitric oxide synthase phosphorylation pathway. *Diabetes* 2002;**51**(1):168–73.

53. Matsuda K, Teragawa H, Fukuda Y, et al. Leptin causes nitric-oxide independent coronary artery vasodilation in humans. *Hypertens Res* 2003;**26**(2):147–52.
54. Rodríguez A, Fortuño A, Gómez-Ambrosi J, et al. The inhibitory effect of leptin on angiotensin II-induced vasoconstriction in vascular smooth muscle cells is mediated via a nitric oxide-dependent mechanism. *Endocrinology* 2007;**148**(1):324–31.
55. Fortuño A, Rodríguez A, Gómez-Ambrosi J, et al. Leptin inhibits angiotensin II-induced intracellular calcium increase and vasoconstriction in the rat aorta. *Endocrinology* 2002;**143**(9):3555–60.
56. Momin AU, Melikian N, Shah AM, et al. Leptin is an endothelial-independent vasodilator in humans with coronary artery disease: evidence for tissue specificity of leptin resistance. *Eur Heart J* 2006;**27**(19):2294–9.
57. Satoh N, Ogawa Y, Katsuura G, et al. Sympathetic activation of leptin via the ventromedial hypothalamus: leptin-induced increase in catecholamine secretion. *Diabetes* 1999;**48**(9):1787–93.
58. Shek EW, Brands MW, Hall JE. Chronic leptin infusion increases arterial pressure. *Hypertension* 1998;**31**(1 Pt 2):409–14.
59. Shirasaka T, Takasaki M, Kannan H. Cardiovascular effects of leptin and orexins. *Am J Physiol Regul Integr Comp Physiol* 2003;**284**(3):R639–51.
60. Hare JM, Stamler JS. NO/redox disequilibrium in the failing heart and cardiovascular system. *J Clin Invest* 2005;**115**(3):509–17.
61. Karmazyn M, Purdham DM, Rajapurohitam V, et al. Signalling mechanisms underlying the metabolic and other effects of adipokines on the heart. *Cardiovasc Res* 2008;**79**(2):279–86.
62. Purdham DM, Zou MX, Rajapurohitam V, et al. Rat heart is a site of leptin production and action. *Am J Physiol Heart Circ Physiol* 2004;**287**(6):H2877–84.
63. Nickola MW, Wold LE, Colligan PB, et al. Leptin attenuates cardiac contraction in rat ventricular myocytes. Role of NO. *Hypertension* 2000;**36**(4):501–5.
64. Lee Y, Naseem RH, Duplomb L, et al. Hyperleptinemia prevents lipotoxic cardiomyopathy in acyl CoA synthase transgenic mice. *Proc Natl Acad Sci U S A* 2004;**101**(37):13624–9.
65. Dong F, Zhang X, Ren J. Leptin regulates cardiomyocyte contractile function through endothelin-1 receptor-NADPH oxidase pathway. *Hypertension* 2006;**47**(2):222–9.
66. Palanivel R, Eguchi M, Shuralyova I, et al. Distinct effects of short- and long-term leptin treatment on glucose and fatty acid uptake and metabolism in HL-1 cardiomyocytes. *Metabolism* 2006;**55**(8):1067–75.
67. Madani S, De Girolamo S, Muñoz DM, et al. Direct effects of leptin on size and extracellular matrix components of human pediatric ventricular myocytes. *Cardiovasc Res* 2006;**69**(3):716–25.
68. Rajapurohitam V, Gan XT, Kirshenbaum LA, et al. The obesity-associated peptide leptin induces hypertrophy in neonatal rat ventricular myocytes. *Circ Res* 2003;**93**(4):277–9.
69. Tajmir P, Ceddia RB, Li RK, et al. Leptin increases cardiomyocyte hyperplasia via extracellular signal-regulated kinase- and phosphatidylinositol 3-kinase-dependent signaling pathways. *Endocrinology* 2004;**145**(4):1550–5.
70. Smith CC, Mocanu MM, Davidson SM, et al. Leptin, the obesity-associated hormone, exhibits direct cardioprotective effects. *Br J Pharmacol* 2006;**149**(1):5–13.
71. Smith CC, Dixon RA, Wynne AM, et al. Leptin-induced cardioprotection involves JAK/STAT signaling that may be linked to the mitochondrial permeability transition pore. *Am J Physiol Heart Circ Physiol* 2010;**299**(4):H1265–70.
72. Erkasap N, Ikizler M, Shneyvays V, et al. Leptin protects the cardiac myocyte cultures from hypoxic damage. *Life Sci* 2006;**78**(10):1098–102.
73. Sierra-Johnson J, Romero-Corral A, Lopez-Jimenez F, et al. Relation of increased leptin concentrations to history of myocardial infarction and stroke in the United States population. *Am J Cardiol* 2007;**100**(2):234–9.
74. Wannamethee SG, Tchernova J, Whincup P, et al. Plasma leptin: associations with metabolic, inflammatory and haemostatic risk factors for cardiovascular disease. *Atherosclerosis* 2007;**191**(2):418–26.
75. Steppan CM, Bailey ST, Bhat S, et al. The hormone resistin links obesity to diabetes. *Nature* 2001;**409**(6818):307–12.

76. Steppan CM, Brown EJ, Wright CM, et al. A family of tissue-specific resistin-like molecules. *Proc Natl Acad Sci U S A* 2001;**98**(2):502–6.
77. Rajala MW, Qi Y, Patel HR, et al. Regulation of resistin expression and circulating levels in obesity, diabetes, and fasting. *Diabetes* 2004;**53**(7):1671–9.
78. Patel L, Buckels AC, Kinghorn IJ, et al. Resistin is expressed in human macrophages and directly regulated by PPAR gamma activators. *Biochem Biophys Res Commun* 2003;**300**(2):472–6.
79. Fain JN, Cheema PS, Bahouth SW, et al. Resistin release by human adipose tissue explants in primary culture. *Biochem Biophys Res Commun* 2003;**300**(3):674–8.
80. Silswal N, Singh AK, Aruna B, et al. Human resistin stimulates the pro-inflammatory cytokines TNF-alpha and IL-12 in macrophages by NF-kappaB-dependent pathway. *Biochem Biophys Res Commun* 2005;**334**(4):1092–101.
81. Graveleau C, Zaha VG, Mohajer A, et al. Mouse and human resistins impair glucose transport in primary mouse cardiomyocytes, and oligomerization is required for this biological action. *J Biol Chem* 2005;**280**(36):31679–85.
82. Kusminski CM, McTernan PG, Kumar S. Role of resistin in obesity, insulin resistance and Type II diabetes. *Clin Sci (Lond)* 2005;**109**(3):243–56.
83. Sato N, Kobayashi K, Inoguchi T, et al. Adenovirus-mediated high expression of resistin causes dyslipidemia in mice. *Endocrinology* 2005;**146**(1):273–9.
84. Silha JV, Krsek M, Skrha JV, et al. Plasma resistin, adiponectin and leptin levels in lean and obese subjects: correlations with insulin resistance. *Eur J Endocrinol* 2003;**149**(4):331–5.
85. Reilly MP, Lehrke M, Wolfe ML, et al. Resistin is an inflammatory marker of atherosclerosis in humans. *Circulation* 2005;**111**(7):932–9.
86. Ohmori R, Momiyama Y, Kato R, et al. Associations between serum resistin levels and insulin resistance, inflammation, and coronary artery disease. *J Am Coll Cardiol* 2005;**46**(2):379–80.
87. Kunnari A, Ukkola O, Päivänsalo M, et al. High plasma resistin level is associated with enhanced highly sensitive C-reactive protein and leukocytes. *J Clin Endocrinol Metab* 2006;**91**(7):2755–60.
88. de Luis DA, González Sagrado M, Conde R, et al. Circulating adipocytokines in morbid obese patients, relation with cardiovascular risk factors and anthropometric parameters. *Nutr Hosp* 2011;**26**(1):91–6.
89. Gerber M, Boettner A, Seidel B, et al. Serum resistin levels of obese and lean children and adolescents: biochemical analysis and clinical relevance. *J Clin Endocrinol Metab* 2005;**90**(8):4503–9.
90. Malo E, Ukkola O, Jokela M, et al. Resistin is an indicator of the metabolic syndrome according to five different definitions in the Finnish Health 2000 survey. *Metab Syndr Relat Disord* 2011;**9**(3):203–10.
91. Wang H, Chen DY, Cao J, et al. High serum resistin level may be an indicator of the severity of coronary disease in acute coronary syndrome. *Chin Med Sci J* 2009;**24**(3):161–6.
92. Chu S, Ding W, Li K, et al. Plasma resistin associated with myocardium injury in patients with acute coronary syndrome. *Circ J* 2008;**72**(8):1249–53.
93. Burnett MS, Lee CW, Kinnaird TD, et al. The potential role of resistin in atherogenesis. *Atherosclerosis* 2005;**182**(2):241–8.
94. Lubos E, Messow CM, Schnabel R, et al. Resistin, acute coronary syndrome and prognosis results from the AtheroGene study. *Atherosclerosis* 2007;**193**(1):121–8.
95. Efstathiou SP, Tsiakou AG, Tsioulos DI, et al. Prognostic significance of plasma resistin levels in patients with atherothrombotic ischemic stroke. *Clin Chim Acta* 2007;**378**(1–2):78–85.
96. Jung HS, Park KH, Cho YM, et al. Resistin is secreted from macrophages in atheromas and promotes atherosclerosis. *Cardiovasc Res* 2006;**69**(1):76–85.
97. Calabro P, Samudio I, Willerson JT, et al. Resistin promotes smooth muscle cell proliferation through activation of extracellular signal-regulated kinase 1/2 and phosphatidylinositol 3-kinase pathways. *Circulation* 2004;**110**(21):3335–40.
98. Mu H, Ohashi R, Yan S, et al. Adipokine resistin promotes in vitro angiogenesis of human endothelial cells. *Cardiovasc Res* 2006;**70**(1):146–57.

99. Dick GM, Katz PS, Farias III M, et al. Resistin impairs endothelium-dependent dilation to bradykinin, but not acetylcholine, in the coronary circulation. *Am J Physiol Heart Circ Physiol* 2006;**291**(6):H2997–3002.
100. Kawanami D, Maemura K, Takeda N, et al. Direct reciprocal effects of resistin and adiponectin on vascular endothelial cells: a new insight into adipocytokines-endothelial cell interactions. *Biochem Biophys Res Commun* 2004;**314**(2):415–9.
101. Kim M, Oh JK, Sakata S, et al. Role of resistin in cardiac contractility and hypertrophy. *J Mol Cell Cardiol* 2008;**45**(2):270–80.
102. Kang S, Chemaly ER, Hajjar RJ, et al. Resistin promotes cardiac hypertrophy via the AMP-activated protein kinase/mammalian target of rapamycin (AMPK/mTOR) and c-Jun N-terminal kinase/insulin receptor substrate 1 (JNK/IRS1) pathways. *J Biol Chem* 2011;**286**(21):18465–73.
103. Chemaly ER, Hadri L, Zhang S, et al. Long-term in vivo resistin overexpression induces myocardial dysfunction and remodeling in rats. *J Mol Cell Cardiol* 2011;**51**(2):144–55.
104. Rothwell SE, Richards AM, Pemberton CJ. Resistin worsens cardiac ischaemia-reperfusion injury. *Biochem Biophys Res Commun* 2006;**349**(1):400–7.
105. Gao J, Chang Chua C, Chen Z, et al. Resistin, an adipocytokine, offers protection against acute myocardial infarction. *J Mol Cell Cardiol* 2007;**43**(5):601–9.
106. Sommer G, Garten A, Petzold S, et al. Visfatin/PBEF/Nampt: structure, regulation and potential function of a novel adipokine. *Clin Sci (Lond)* 2008;**115**(1):13–23.
107. Romacho T, Sánchez-Ferrer CF, Peiró C. Visfatin/Nampt: an adipokine with cardiovascular impact. *Mediators Inflamm* 2013;**2013**:946427.
108. Fukuhara A, Matsuda M, Nishizawa M, et al. Visfatin: a protein secreted by visceral fat that mimics the effects of insulin. *Science* 2005;**307**(5708):426–30.
109. Curat CA, Wegner V, Sengenès C, et al. Macrophages in human visceral adipose tissue: increased accumulation in obesity and a source of resistin and visfatin. *Diabetologia* 2006;**49**(4):744–7.
110. Garten A, Petzold S, Barnikol-Oettler A, et al. Nicotinamide phosphoribosyltransferase (NAMPT/PBEF/visfatin) is constitutively released from human hepatocytes. *Biochem Biophys Res Commun* 2010;**391**(1):376–81.
111. Costford SR, Bajpeyi S, Pasarica M, et al. Skeletal muscle NAMPT is induced by exercise in humans. *Am J Physiol Endocrinol Metab* 2010;**298**(1):E117–26.
112. Dahl TB, Yndestad A, Skjelland M, et al. Increased expression of visfatin in macrophages of human unstable carotid and coronary atherosclerosis: possible role in inflammation and plaque destabilization. *Circulation* 2007;**115**(8):972–80.
113. Li Y, Zhang Y, Dorweiler B, et al. Extracellular Nampt promotes macrophage survival via a nonenzymatic interleukin-6/STAT3 signaling mechanism. *J Biol Chem* 2008;**283**(50):34833–43.
114. Romacho T, Azcutia V, Vázquez-Bella M, et al. Extracellular PBEF/NAMPT/visfatin activates pro-inflammatory signalling in human vascular smooth muscle cells through nicotinamide phosphoribosyltransferase activity. *Diabetologia* 2009;**52**(11):2455–63.
115. Kim SR, Bae YH, Bae SK, et al. Visfatin enhances ICAM-1 and VCAM-1 expression through ROS-dependent NF-kappaB activation in endothelial cells. *Biochim Biophys Acta* 2008;**1783**(5):886–95.
116. Adya R, Tan BK, Punn A, et al. Visfatin induces human endothelial VEGF and MMP-2/9 production via MAPK and PI3K/Akt signalling pathways: novel insights into visfatin-induced angiogenesis. *Cardiovasc Res* 2008;**78**(2):356–65.
117. Wang P, Xu TY, Guan YF, et al. Perivascular adipose tissue–derived visfatin is a vascular smooth muscle cell growth factor: role of nicotinamide mononucleotide. *Cardiovasc Res* 2009;**81**(2):370–80.
118. van der Veer E, Nong Z, O'Neil C, et al. Pre-B-cell colony-enhancing factor regulates NAD+ -dependent protein deacetylase activity and promotes vascular smooth muscle cell maturation. *Circ Res* 2005;**97**(1):25–34.
119. Takebayashi K, Suetsugu M, Wakabayashi S, et al. Association between plasma visfatin and vascular endothelial function in patients with type 2 diabetes mellitus. *Metabolism* 2007;**56**(4):451–8.

120. Yamawaki H, Hara N, Okada M, et al. Visfatin causes endothelium-dependent relaxation in isolated blood vessels. *Biochem Biophys Res Commun* 2009;**383**(4):503–8.
121. Lim SY, Davidson SM, Paramanathan AJ, et al. The novel adipocytokine visfatin exerts direct cardioprotective effects. *J Cell Mol Med* 2008;**12**(4):1395–403.
122. Hsu CP, Oka S, Shao D, et al. Nicotinamide phosphoribosyltransferase regulates cell survival through NAD+ synthesis in cardiac myocytes. *Circ Res* 2009;**105**(5):481–91.
123. Xiao J, Sun B, Li M, et al. A novel adipocytokine visfatin protects against H(2)O(2)-induced myocardial apoptosis: a missing link between obesity and cardiovascular disease. *J Cell Physiol* 2013;**228**(3):495–501.
124. Pillai VB, Sundaresan NR, Kim G, et al. Nampt secreted from cardiomyocytes promotes development of cardiac hypertrophy and adverse ventricular remodeling. *Am J Physiol Heart Circ Physiol* 2013;**304**(3):H415–26.
125. Kralisch S, Fasshauer M. Adipocyte fatty acid binding protein: a novel adipokine involved in the pathogenesis of metabolic and vascular disease? *Diabetologia* 2013;**56**(1):10–21.
126. Wu G, Li H, Zhou M, et al. Mechanism and clinical evidence of lipocalin-2 and adipocyte fatty acid-binding protein linking obesity and atherosclerosis. *Diabetes Metab Res Rev* 2014;**30**(6):447–56.
127. Makowski L, Hotamisligil GS. Fatty acid binding proteins-the evolutionary crossroads of inflammatory and metabolic responses. *J Nutr* 2004;**134**(9):2464S–8S.
128. Pelton PD, Zhou L, Demarest KT, et al. PPARgamma activation induces the expression of the adipocyte fatty acid binding protein gene in human monocytes. *Biochem Biophys Res Commun* 1999;**261**(2):456–8.
129. Fu Y, Luo N, Lopes-Virella MF, Garvey WT. The adipocyte lipid binding protein (ALBP/aP2) gene facilitates foam cell formation in human THP-1 macrophages. *Atherosclerosis* 2002;**165**(2):259–69.
130. Elmasri H, Karaaslan C, Teper Y, et al. Fatty acid binding protein 4 is a target of VEGF and a regulator of cell proliferation in endothelial cells. *FASEB J* 2009;**23**(11):3865–73.
131. Bernlohr DA, Bolanowski MA, Kelly Jr TJ, et al. Evidence for an increase in transcription of specific mRNAs during differentiation of 3T3-L1 preadipocytes. *J Biol Chem* 1985;**260**(9):5563–7.
132. Amri EZ, Bertrand B, Ailhaud G, et al. Regulation of adipose cell differentiation. I. Fatty acids are inducers of the aP2 gene expression. *J Lipid Res* 1991;**32**(9):1449–56.
133. Kletzien RF, Foellmi LA, Harris PK, et al. Adipocyte fatty acid–binding protein: regulation of gene expression in vivo and in vitro by an insulin–sensitizing agent. *Mol Pharmacol* 1992;**42**(4):558–62.
134. Cabré A, Lázaro I, Girona J, et al. Fatty acid binding protein 4 is increased in metabolic syndrome and with thiazolidinedione treatment in diabetic patients. *Atherosclerosis* 2007;**195**(1):e150–8.
135. Fisher RM, Eriksson P, Hoffstedt J, et al. Fatty acid binding protein expression in different adipose tissue depots from lean and obese individuals. *Diabetologia* 2001;**44**(10):1268–73.
136. Kazemi MR, McDonald CM, Shigenaga JK, et al. Adipocyte fatty acid-binding protein expression and lipid accumulation are increased during activation of murine macrophages by toll-like receptor agonists. *Arterioscler Thromb Vasc Biol* 2005;**25**(6):1220–4.
137. Shi H, Kokoeva MV, Inouye K, et al. TLR4 links innate immunity and fatty acid-induced insulin resistance. *J Clin Invest* 2006;**116**(11):3015–25.
138. Furuhashi M, Tuncman G, Görgün CZ, et al. Treatment of diabetes and atherosclerosis by inhibiting fatty-acid-binding protein aP2. *Nature* 2007;**447**(7147):959–65.
139. Xu A, Wang Y, Xu JY, et al. Adipocyte fatty acid-binding protein is a plasma biomarker closely associated with obesity and metabolic syndrome. *Clin Chem* 2006;**52**(3):405–13.
140. Lamounier-Zepter V, Look C, Alvarez J, et al. Adipocyte fatty acid-binding protein suppresses cardiomyocyte contraction: a new link between obesity and heart disease. *Circ Res* 2009;**105**(4):326–34.
141. Stejskal D, Karpisek M. Adipocyte fatty acid binding protein in a Caucasian population: a new marker of metabolic syndrome? *Eur J Clin Invest* 2006;**36**(9):621–5.
142. Cabré A, Lázaro I, Girona J, et al. Plasma fatty acid binding protein 4 is associated with atherogenic dyslipidemia in diabetes. *J Lipid Res* 2008;**49**(8):1746–51.

143. Milner KL, van der Poorten D, Xu A, et al. Adipocyte fatty acid binding protein levels relate to inflammation and fibrosis in nonalcoholic fatty liver disease. *Hepatology* 2009;**49**(6):1926–34.
144. Tuncman G, Erbay E, Hom X, et al. A genetic variant at the fatty acid-binding protein aP2 locus reduces the risk for hypertriglyceridemia, type 2 diabetes, and cardiovascular disease. *Proc Natl Acad Sci USA* 2006;**103**(18):6970–5.
145. Yeung DC, Xu A, Cheung CW, et al. Serum adipocyte fatty acid-binding protein levels were independently associated with carotid atherosclerosis. *Arterioscler Thromb Vasc Biol* 2007;**27**(8):1796–802.
146. Holm S, Ueland T, Dahl TB, et al. Fatty acid binding protein 4 is associated with carotid atherosclerosis and outcome in patients with acute ischemic stroke. *PLoS One* 2011;**6**(12):e28785.
147. Rhee EJ, Lee WY, Park CY, et al. The association of serum adipocyte fatty acid-binding protein with coronary artery disease in Korean adults. *Eur J Endocrinol* 2009;**160**(2):165–72.
148. Miyoshi T, Onoue G, Hirohata A, et al. Serum adipocyte fatty acid-binding protein is independently associated with coronary atherosclerotic burden measured by intravascular ultrasound. *Atherosclerosis* 2010;**211**(1):164–9.
149. Doi M, Miyoshi T, Hirohata S, et al. Association of increased plasma adipocyte fatty acid-binding protein with coronary artery disease in non-elderly men. *Cardiovasc Diabetol* 2011;**10**:44.
150. Bao Y, Lu Z, Zhou M, et al. Serum levels of adipocyte fatty acid-binding protein are associated with the severity of coronary artery disease in Chinese women. *PLoS One* 2011;**6**(4):e19115.
151. Huang CL, Wu YW, Wu CC, et al. Association between serum adipocyte fatty-acid binding protein concentrations, left ventricular function and myocardial perfusion abnormalities in patients with coronary artery disease. *Cardiovasc Diabetol* 2013;**12**:105.
152. Yoo HJ, Kim S, Park MS, et al. Serum adipocyte fatty acid-binding protein is associated independently with vascular inflammation: analysis with (18)F-fluorodeoxyglucose positron emission tomography. *J Clin Endocrinol Metab* 2011;**96**(3):E488–92.
153. Xu A, Tso AW, Cheung BM, et al. Circulating adipocyte-fatty acid binding protein levels predict the development of the metabolic syndrome: a 5-year prospective study. *Circulation* 2007;**115**(12):1537–43.
154. Choi KM, Yannakoulia M, Park MS, et al. Serum adipocyte fatty acid-binding protein, retinol-binding protein 4, and adiponectin concentrations in relation to the development of the metabolic syndrome in Korean boys: a 3-y prospective cohort study. *Am J Clin Nutr* 2011;**93**(1):19–26.
155. Tso AW, Xu A, Sham PC, et al. Serum adipocyte fatty acid binding protein as a new biomarker predicting the development of type 2 diabetes: a 10-year prospective study in a Chinese cohort. *Diabetes Care* 2007;**30**(10): 2667–72.
156. Chow WS, Tso AW, Xu A, et al. Elevated circulating adipocyte-fatty acid binding protein levels predict incident cardiovascular events in a community-based cohort: a 12-year prospective study. *J Am Heart Assoc* 2013;**2**(1):e004176.
157. von Eynatten M, Breitling LP, Roos M, et al. Circulating adipocyte fatty acid-binding protein levels and cardiovascular morbidity and mortality in patients with coronary heart disease: a 10-year prospective study. *Arterioscler Thromb Vasc Biol* 2012;**32**(9):2327–35.
158. Peeters W, de Kleijn DP, Vink A, et al. Adipocyte fatty acid binding protein in atherosclerotic plaques is associated with local vulnerability and is predictive for the occurrence of adverse cardiovascular events. *Eur Heart J* 2011;**32**(14):1758–68.
159. Tso AW, Lam TK, Xu A, et al. Serum adipocyte fatty acid-binding protein associated with ischemic stroke and early death. *Neurology* 2011;**76**(23):1968–75.
160. Simón I, Escoté X, Vilarrasa N, et al. Adipocyte fatty acid-binding protein as a determinant of insulin sensitivity in morbid-obese women. *Obesity (Silver Spring)* 2009;**17**(6):1124–8.
161. Choi KM, Kim TN, Yoo HJ, et al. Effect of exercise training on A-FABP, lipocalin-2 and RBP4 levels in obese women. *Clin Endocrinol (Oxf)* 2009;**70**(4):569–74.

162. Corripio R, Gónzalez-Clemente JM, Pérez-Sánchez J, et al. Weight loss in prepubertal obese children is associated with a decrease in adipocyte fatty-acid-binding protein without changes in lipocalin-2: a 2-year longitudinal study. *Eur J Endocrinol* 2010;**163**(6):887–93.
163. Wu YW, Kao HL, Huang CL, et al. The effects of 3-month atorvastatin therapy on arterial inflammation, calcification, abdominal adipose tissue and circulating biomarkers. *Eur J Nucl Med Mol Imaging* 2012;**39**(3):399–407.
164. Hotamisligil GS, Johnson RS, Distel RJ, et al. Uncoupling of obesity from insulin resistance through a targeted mutation in aP2, the adipocyte fatty acid binding protein. *Science* 1996;**274**(5291):1377–9.
165. Scheja L, Makowski L, Uysal KT, et al. Altered insulin secretion associated with reduced lipolytic efficiency in aP2-/- mice. *Diabetes* 1999;**48**(10):1987–94.
166. Uysal KT, Scheja L, Wiesbrock SM, et al. Improved glucose and lipid metabolism in genetically obese mice lacking aP2. *Endocrinology* 2000;**141**(9):3388–96.
167. Hertzel AV, Smith LA, Berg AH, et al. Lipid metabolism and adipokine levels in fatty acid-binding protein null and transgenic mice. *Am J Physiol Endocrinol Metab* 2006;**290**(5):E814–23.
168. Baar RA, Dingfelder CS, Smith LA, et al. Investigation of in vivo fatty acid metabolism in AFABP/aP2(-/-) mice. *Am J Physiol Endocrinol Metab* 2005;**288**(1):E187–93.
169. Makowski L, Boord JB, Maeda K, et al. Lack of macrophage fatty-acid-binding protein aP2 protects mice deficient in apolipoprotein E against atherosclerosis. *Nat Med* 2001;**7**(6):699–705.
170. Makowski L, Brittingham KC, Reynolds JM, et al. The fatty acid-binding protein, aP2, coordinates macrophage cholesterol trafficking and inflammatory activity. Macrophage expression of aP2 impacts peroxisome proliferator-activated receptor gamma and IkappaB kinase activities. *J Biol Chem* 2005;**280**(13):12888–95.
171. Hui X, Li H, Zhou Z, et al. Adipocyte fatty acid-binding protein modulates inflammatory responses in macrophages through a positive feedback loop involving c-Jun NH2-terminal kinases and activator protein-1. *J Biol Chem* 2010;**285**(14):10273–80.
172. Erbay E, Babaev VR, Mayers JR, et al. Reducing endoplasmic reticulum stress through a macrophage lipid chaperone alleviates atherosclerosis. *Nat Med* 2009;**15**(12):1383–91.
173. Fu Y, Luo L, Luo N, et al. Lipid metabolism mediated by adipocyte lipid binding protein (ALBP/aP2) gene expression in human THP-1 macrophages. *Atherosclerosis* 2006;**188**(1):102–11.
174. Llaverias G, Noé V, Peñuelas S, et al. Atorvastatin reduces CD68, FABP4, and HBP expression in oxLDL-treated human macrophages. *Biochem Biophys Res Commun* 2004;**318**(1):265–74.
175. Elmasri H, Ghelfi E, Yu CW, et al. Endothelial cell-fatty acid binding protein 4 promotes angiogenesis: role of stem cell factor/c-kit pathway. *Angiogenesis* 2012;**15**(3):457–68.
176. Lee MY, Li H, Xiao Y, et al. Chronic administration of BMS309403 improves endothelial function in apolipoprotein E–deficient mice and in cultured human endothelial cells. *Br J Pharmacol* 2011;**162**(7):1564–76.
177. Chan CK, Zhao Y, Liao SY, et al. A-FABP and oxidative stress underlie the impairment of endothelium-dependent relaxations to serotonin and the intima–medial thickening in the porcine coronary artery with regenerated endothelium. *ACS Chem Neurosci* 2013;**4**(1):122–9.
178. Scherer PE, Williams S, Fogliano M, et al. A novel serum protein similar to C1q, produced exclusively in adipocytes. *J Biol Chem* 1995;**270**(45):26746–9.
179. Maeda K, Okubo K, Shimomura I, et al. cDNA cloning and expression of a novel adipose specific collagen-like factor, apM1 (AdiPose Most abundant Gene transcript 1). *Biochem Biophys Res Commun* 1996;**221**(2):286–9.
180. Hu E, Liang P, Spiegelman BM. AdipoQ is a novel adipose-specific gene dysregulated in obesity. *J Biol Chem* 1996;**271**(18):10697–703.
181. Nakano Y, Tobe T, Choi-Miura NH, et al. Isolation and characterization of GBP28, a novel gelatin-binding protein purified from human plasma. *J Biochem* 1996;**120**(4):803–12.

182. Ahima RS. Metabolic actions of adipocyte hormones: focus on adiponectin. *Obesity (Silver Spring)* 2006;**14**(Suppl. 1):9S–15S.
183. Adya R, Tan BK, Randeva HS. Differential effects of leptin and adiponectin in endothelial angiogenesis. *J Diabetes Res* 2015;**2015**:648239.
184. Meder W, Wendland M, Busmann A, et al. Characterization of human circulating TIG2 as a ligand for the orphan receptor ChemR23. *FEBS Lett* 2003;**555**(3):495–9.
185. Du XY, Leung LL. Proteolytic regulatory mechanism of chemerin bioactivity. *Acta Biochim Biophys Sin (Shanghai)* 2009;**41**(12):973–9.
186. Parker-Duffen JL, Walsh K. Cardiometabolic effects of adiponectin. *Best Pract Res Clin Endocrinol Metab* 2014;**28**(1):81–91.
187. Arita Y, Kihara S, Ouchi N, et al. Paradoxical decrease of an adipose-specific protein, adiponectin, in obesity. *Biochem Biophys Res Commun* 1999;**257**(1):79–83.
188. Nishizawa H, Shimomura I, Kishida K, et al. Androgens decrease plasma adiponectin, an insulin-sensitizing adipocyte-derived protein. *Diabetes* 2002;**51**(9):2734–41.
189. Breitfeld J, Stumvoll M, Kovacs P. Genetics of adiponectin. *Biochimie* 2012;**94**(10):2157–63.
190. Simpson F, Whitehead JP. Adiponectin-it's all about the modifications. *Int J Biochem Cell Biol* 2010;**42**(6): 785–8.
191. Wang Y, Lam KS, Yau MH, et al. Post-translational modifications of adiponectin: mechanisms and functional implications. *Biochem J* 2008;**409**(3):623–33.
192. Pajvani UB, Hawkins M, Combs TP, et al. Complex distribution, not absolute amount of adiponectin, correlates with thiazolidinedione–mediated improvement in insulin sensitivity. *J Biol Chem* 2004;**279**(13):12152–62.
193. Waki H, Yamauchi T, Kamon J, et al. Generation of globular fragment of adiponectin by leukocyte elastase secreted by monocytic cell line THP-1. *Endocrinology* 2005;**146**(2):790–6.
194. Hattori Y, Hattori S, Akimoto K, et al. Globular adiponectin activates nuclear factor-kappaB and activating protein-1 and enhances angiotensin II-induced proliferation in cardiac fibroblasts. *Diabetes* 2007;**56**(3):804–8.
195. Lopez-Jaramillo P. The role of adiponectin in cardiometabolic diseases: effects of nutritional interventions. *J Nutr* 2016;**146**(2):422S–426SS.
196. Yamauchi T, Iwabu M, Okada-Iwabu M, et al. Adiponectin receptors: a review of their structure, function and how they work. *Best Pract Res Clin Endocrinol Metab* 2014;**28**(1):15–23.
197. Kadowaki T, Yamauchi T. Adiponectin and adiponectin receptors. *Endocr Rev* 2005;**26**(3):439–51.
198. Yamauchi T, Kamon J, Ito Y, et al. Cloning of adiponectin receptors that mediate antidiabetic metabolic effects. *Nature* 2003;**423**(6941):762–9.
199. Hug C, Wang J, Ahmad NS, et al. T-cadherin is a receptor for hexameric and high-molecular-weight forms of Acrp30/adiponectin. *Proc Natl Acad Sci U S A* 2004;**101**(28):10308–13.
200. Fujioka D, Kawabata K, Saito Y, et al. Role of adiponectin receptors in endothelin-induced cellular hypertrophy in cultured cardiomyocytes and their expression in infarcted heart. *Am J Physiol Heart Circ Physiol* 2006;**290**(6):H2409–16.
201. Denzel MS, Scimia MC, Zumstein PM, et al. T-cadherin is critical for adiponectin-mediated cardioprotection in mice. *J Clin Invest* 2010;**120**(12):4342–52.
202. Kadowaki T, Yamauchi T, Kubota N, et al. Adiponectin and adiponectin receptors in insulin resistance, diabetes, and the metabolic syndrome. *J Clin Invest* 2006;**116**(7):1784–92.
203. Yamauchi T, Kamon J, Minokoshi Y, et al. Adiponectin stimulates glucose utilization and fatty-acid oxidation by activating AMP–activated protein kinase. *Nat Med* 2002;**8**(11):1288–95.
204. Tomas E, Tsao TS, Saha AK, et al. Enhanced muscle fat oxidation and glucose transport by ACRP30 globular domain: acetyl-CoA carboxylase inhibition and AMP-activated protein kinase activation. *Proc Natl Acad Sci USA* 2002;**99**(25):16309–13.
205. Caselli C, D'Amico A, Cabiati M, et al. Back to the heart: the protective role of adiponectin. *Pharmacol Res* 2014;**82**:9–20.

206. Ouchi N, Ohishi M, Kihara S, et al. Association of hypoadiponectinemia with impaired vasoreactivity. *Hypertension* 2003;**42**(3):231–4.
207. Chen H, Montagnani M, Funahashi T, et al. Adiponectin stimulates production of nitric oxide in vascular endothelial cells. *J Biol Chem* 2003;**278**(45):45021–6.
208. Cheng KK, Lam KS, Wang Y, et al. Adiponectin-induced endothelial nitric oxide synthase activation and nitric oxide production are mediated by APPL1 in endothelial cells. *Diabetes* 2007;**56**(5):1387–94.
209. Tsioufis C, Dimitriadis K, Selima M, et al. Low-grade inflammation and hypoadiponectinaemia have an additive detrimental effect on aortic stiffness in essential hypertensive patients. *Eur Heart J* 2007;**28**(9):1162–9.
210. Hopkins TA, Ouchi N, Shibata R, et al. Adiponectin actions in the cardiovascular system. *Cardiovasc Res* 2007;**74**(1):11–18.
211. Ouchi N, Kihara S, Arita Y, et al. Adiponectin, an adipocyte-derived plasma protein, inhibits endothelial NF-kappaB signaling through a cAMP-dependent pathway. *Circulation* 2000;**102**(11):1296–301.
212. Hattori Y, Nakano Y, Hattori S, et al. High molecular weight adiponectin activates AMPK and suppresses cytokine-induced NF-kappaB activation in vascular endothelial cells. *FEBS Lett* 2008;**582**(12):1719–24.
213. Ouedraogo R, Wu X, Xu SQ, et al. Adiponectin suppression of high-glucose-induced reactive oxygen species in vascular endothelial cells: evidence for involvement of a cAMP signaling pathway. *Diabetes* 2006;**55**(6):1840–6.
214. Ouedraogo R, Gong Y, Berzins B, et al. Adiponectin deficiency increases leukocyte-endothelium interactions via upregulation of endothelial cell adhesion molecules in vivo. *J Clin Invest* 2007;**117**(6):1718–26.
215. Ouchi N, Kihara S, Arita Y, et al. Adipocyte-derived plasma protein, adiponectin, suppresses lipid accumulation and class A scavenger receptor expression in human monocyte–derived macrophages. *Circulation* 2001;**103**(8):1057–63.
216. Arita Y, Kihara S, Ouchi N, et al. Adipocyte-derived plasma protein adiponectin acts as a platelet-derived growth factor-BB-binding protein and regulates growth factor-induced common postreceptor signal in vascular smooth muscle cell. *Circulation* 2002;**105**(24):2893–8.
217. Okamoto Y, Kihara S, Ouchi N, et al. Adiponectin reduces atherosclerosis in apolipoprotein E-deficient mice. *Circulation* 2002;**106**(22):2767–70.
218. Ouchi N, Kobayashi H, Kihara S, et al. Adiponectin stimulates angiogenesis by promoting cross-talk between AMP-activated protein kinase and Akt signaling in endothelial cells. *J Biol Chem* 2004;**279**(2):1304–9.
219. Shibata R, Ouchi N, Kihara S, et al. Adiponectin stimulates angiogenesis in response to tissue ischemia through stimulation of amp-activated protein kinase signaling. *J Biol Chem* 2004;**279**(27):28670–4.
220. Shen L, Miao J, Yuan F, et al. Overexpression of adiponectin promotes focal angiogenesis in the mouse brain following middle cerebral artery occlusion. *Gene Ther* 2013;**20**(1):93–101.
221. Mahadev K, Wu X, Donnelly S, et al. Adiponectin inhibits vascular endothelial growth factor-induced migration of human coronary artery endothelial cells. *Cardiovasc Res* 2008;**78**(2):376–84.
222. Bråkenhielm E, Veitonmäki N, Cao R, et al. Adiponectin-induced antiangiogenesis and antitumor activity involve caspase-mediated endothelial cell apoptosis. *Proc Natl Acad Sci USA* 2004;**101**(8):2476–81.
223. Man K, Ng KT, Xu A, et al. Suppression of liver tumor growth and metastasis by adiponectin in nude mice through inhibition of tumor angiogenesis and downregulation of Rho kinase/IFN-inducible protein 10/matrix metalloproteinase 9 signaling. *Clin Cancer Res* 2010;**16**(3):967–77.
224. Ouchi N, Shibata R, Walsh K. Cardioprotection by adiponectin. *Trends Cardiovasc Med* 2006;**16**(5):141–6.
225. Shibata R, Sato K, Pimentel DR, et al. Adiponectin protects against myocardial ischemia-reperfusion injury through AMPK- and COX-2-dependent mechanisms. *Nat Med* 2005;**11**(10):1096–103.
226. Tao L, Wang Y, Gao E, et al. Adiponectin: an indispensable molecule in rosiglitazone cardioprotection following myocardial infarction. *Circ Res* 2010;**106**(2):409–17.
227. Li P, Shibata R, Unno K, et al. Evidence for the importance of adiponectin in the cardioprotective effects of pioglitazone. *Hypertension* 2010;**55**(1):69–75.
228. Shibata R, Ouchi N, Ito M, et al. Adiponectin-mediated modulation of hypertrophic signals in the heart. *Nat Med* 2004;**10**(12):1384–9.

229. Shibata R, Izumiya Y, Sato K, et al. Adiponectin protects against the development of systolic dysfunction following myocardial infarction. *J Mol Cell Cardiol* 2007;**42**(6):1065–74.
230. Fisman EZ, Tenenbaum A. Adiponectin: a manifold therapeutic target for metabolic syndrome, diabetes, and coronary disease? *Cardiovasc Diabetol* 2014;**13**:103.
231. de Souza Batista CM, Yang RZ, Lee MJ, et al. Omentin plasma levels and gene expression are decreased in obesity. *Diabetes* 2007;**56**(6):1655–61.
232. Tan BK, Adya R, Randeva HS. Omentin: a novel link between inflammation, diabesity, and cardiovascular disease. *Trends Cardiovasc Med* 2010;**20**(5):143–8.
233. Tan YL, Zheng XL, Tang CK. The protective functions of omentin in cardiovascular diseases. *Clin Chim Acta* 2015;**448**:98–106.
234. Tsuji S, Uehori J, Matsumoto M, et al. Human intelectin is a novel soluble lectin that recognizes galactofuranose in carbohydrate chains of bacterial cell wall. *J Biol Chem* 2001;**276**(26):23456–63.
235. Lee JK, Schnee J, Pang M, et al. Human homologs of the Xenopus oocyte cortical granule lectin XL35. *Glycobiology* 2001;**11**(1):65–73.
236. Schäffler A, Neumeier M, Herfarth H, et al. Genomic structure of human omentin, a new adipocytokine expressed in omental adipose tissue. *Biochim Biophys Acta* 2005;**1732**(1–3):96–102.
237. Yang RZ, Lee MJ, Hu H, et al. Identification of omentin as a novel depot-specific adipokine in human adipose tissue: possible role in modulating insulin action. *Am J Physiol Endocrinol Metab* 2006;**290**(6):E1253–61.
238. Fain JN, Sacks HS, Buehrer B, et al. Identification of omentin mRNA in human epicardial adipose tissue: comparison to omentin in subcutaneous, internal mammary artery periadventitial and visceral abdominal depots. *Int J Obes (Lond)* 2008;**32**(5):810–5.
239. Sacks HS, Fain JN. Human epicardial adipose tissue: a review. *Am Heart J* 2007;**153**(6):907–17.
240. Fitzgibbons TP, Czech MP. Epicardial and perivascular adipose tissues and their influence on cardiovascular disease: basic mechanisms and clinical associations. *J Am Heart Assoc* 2014;**3**(2):e000582.
241. Tan BK, Adya R, Farhatullah S, et al. Omentin-1, a novel adipokine, is decreased in overweight insulin-resistant women with polycystic ovary syndrome: ex vivo and in vivo regulation of omentin-1 by insulin and glucose. *Diabetes* 2008;**57**(4):801–8.
242. Pan HY, Guo L, Li Q. Changes of serum omentin-1 levels in normal subjects and in patients with impaired glucose regulation and with newly diagnosed and untreated type 2 diabetes. *Diabetes Res Clin Pract* 2010;**88**(1):29–33.
243. Auguet T, Quintero Y, Riesco D, et al. New adipokines vaspin and omentin. Circulating levels and gene expression in adipose tissue from morbidly obese women. *BMC Med Genet* 2011;**12**:60.
244. Moreno-Navarrete JM, Ortega F, Castro A, et al. Circulating omentin as a novel biomarker of endothelial dysfunction. *Obesity (Silver Spring)* 2011;**19**(8):1552–9.
245. El-Mesallamy HO, El-Derany MO, Hamdy NM. Serum omentin-1 and chemerin levels are interrelated in patients with Type 2 diabetes mellitus with or without ischaemic heart disease. *Diabet Med* 2011;**28**(10):1194–200.
246. Jialal I, Devaraj S, Kaur H, et al. Increased chemerin and decreased omentin-1 in both adipose tissue and plasma in nascent metabolic syndrome. *J Clin Endocrinol Metab* 2013;**98**(3):E514–7.
247. Prats-Puig A, Bassols J, Bargalló E, et al. Toward an early marker of metabolic dysfunction: omentin-1 in prepubertal children. *Obesity (Silver Spring)* 2011;**19**(9):1905–7.
248. Moreno-Navarrete JM, Catalán V, Ortega F, et al. Circulating omentin concentration increases after weight loss. *Nutr Metab (Lond)* 2010;**7**:27.
249. Saremi A, Asghari M, Ghorbani A. Effects of aerobic training on serum omentin-1 and cardiometabolic risk factors in overweight and obese men. *J Sports Sci* 2010;**28**(9):993–8.
250. Lapointe M, Poirier P, Martin J, et al. Omentin changes following bariatric surgery and predictive links with biomarkers for risk of cardiovascular disease. *Cardiovasc Diabetol* 2014;**13**:124.

251. Urbanová M, Dostálová I, Trachta P, et al. Serum concentrations and subcutaneous adipose tissue mRNA expression of omentin in morbid obesity and type 2 diabetes mellitus: the effect of very-low-calorie diet, physical activity and laparoscopic sleeve gastrectomy. *Physiol Res* 2014;**63**(2):207–18.
252. Hamnvik OP, Thakkar B, Chamberland J, et al. Omentin-1 levels are reduced by pharmacologic doses of leptin, but remain unaffected by energy deprivation and display no day-night variation. *Int J Obes (Lond)* 2015;**39**(2):260–4.
253. Liu R, Wang X, Bu P. Omentin-1 is associated with carotid atherosclerosis in patients with metabolic syndrome. *Diabetes Res Clin Pract* 2011;**93**(1):21–5.
254. Yoo HJ, Hwang SY, Hong HC, et al. Association of circulating omentin-1 level with arterial stiffness and carotid plaque in type 2 diabetes. *Cardiovasc Diabetol* 2011;**10**:103.
255. Shibata R, Ouchi N, Kikuchi R, et al. Circulating omentin is associated with coronary artery disease in men. *Atherosclerosis* 2011;**219**(2):811–4.
256. Zhong X, Zhang HY, Tan H, et al. Association of serum omentin-1 levels with coronary artery disease. *Acta Pharmacol Sin* 2011;**32**(7):873–8.
257. Shang FJ, Wang JP, Liu XT, et al. Serum omentin-1 levels are inversely associated with the presence and severity of coronary artery disease in patients with metabolic syndrome. *Biomarkers* 2011;**16**(8):657–62.
258. Onur I, Oz F, Yildiz S, et al. Serum omentin 1 level is associated with coronary artery disease and its severity in postmenopausal women. *Angiology* 2014;**65**(10):896–900.
259. Kadoglou NP, Tahmatzidis DK, Giannakoulas C, et al. Serum levels of novel adipokines, omentin-1 and chemerin, in patients with acute myocardial infarction: KOZANI STUDY. *J Cardiovasc Med (Hagerstown)* 2015;**16**(5):341–6.
260. Narumi T, Watanabe T, Kadowaki S, et al. Impact of serum omentin-1 levels on cardiac prognosis in patients with heart failure. *Cardiovasc Diabetol* 2014;**13**:84.
261. Yamawaki H, Tsubaki N, Mukohda M, et al. Omentin, a novel adipokine, induces vasodilation in rat isolated blood vessels. *Biochem Biophys Res Commun* 2010;**393**(4):668–72.
262. Tan BK, Adya R, Farhatullah S, et al. Metformin treatment may increase omentin-1 levels in women with polycystic ovary syndrome. *Diabetes* 2010;**59**(12):3023–31.
263. Yamawaki H, Kuramoto J, Kameshima S, et al. Omentin, a novel adipocytokine inhibits TNF-induced vascular inflammation in human endothelial cells. *Biochem Biophys Res Commun* 2011;**408**(2):339–43.
264. Yamawaki H. Vascular effects of novel adipocytokines: focus on vascular contractility and inflammatory responses. *Biol Pharm Bull* 2011;**34**(3):307–10.
265. Kazama K, Usui T, Okada M, et al. Omentin plays an anti-inflammatory role through inhibition of TNF-α-induced superoxide production in vascular smooth muscle cells. *Eur J Pharmacol* 2012;**686**(1–3): 116–23.
266. Kazama K, Okada M, Yamawaki H. A novel adipocytokine, omentin, inhibits platelet-derived growth factor-BB-induced vascular smooth muscle cell migration through antioxidative mechanism. *Am J Physiol Heart Circ Physiol* 2014;**306**(12):H1714–9.
267. Maruyama S, Shibata R, Kikuchi R, et al. Fat-derived factor omentin stimulates endothelial cell function and ischemia-induced revascularization via endothelial nitric oxide synthase-dependent mechanism. *J Biol Chem* 2012;**287**(1):408–17.
268. Kataoka Y, Shibata R, Ohashi K, et al. Omentin prevents myocardial ischemic injury through AMP-activated protein kinase- and Akt-dependent mechanisms. *J Am Coll Cardiol* 2014;**63**(24):2722–33.
269. Matsuo K, Shibata R, Ohashi K, et al. Omentin functions to attenuate cardiac hypertrophic response. *J Mol Cell Cardiol* 2015;**79**:195–202.
270. Kazama K, Okada M, Yamawaki H. Adipocytokine, omentin inhibits doxorubicin-induced H9c2 cardiomyoblasts apoptosis through the inhibition of mitochondrial reactive oxygen species. *Biochem Biophys Res Commun* 2015;**457**(4):602–7.

271. Nagpal S, Patel S, Jacobe H, et al. Tazarotene-induced gene 2 (TIG2), a novel retinoid-responsive gene in skin. *J Invest Dermatol* 1997;**109**(1):91–5.
272. Wittamer V, Franssen JD, Vulcano M, et al. Specific recruitment of antigen-presenting cells by chemerin, a novel processed ligand from human inflammatory fluids. *J Exp Med* 2003;**198**(7):977–85.
273. Goralski KB, McCarthy TC, Hanniman EA, et al. Chemerin, a novel adipokine that regulates adipogenesis and adipocyte metabolism. *J Biol Chem* 2007;**282**(38):28175–88.
274. Bozaoglu K, Bolton K, McMillan J, et al. Chemerin is a novel adipokine associated with obesity and metabolic syndrome. *Endocrinology* 2007;**148**(10):4687–94.
275. Sell H, Divoux A, Poitou C, et al. Chemerin correlates with markers for fatty liver in morbidly obese patients and strongly decreases after weight loss induced by bariatric surgery. *J Clin Endocrinol Metab* 2010;**95**(6):2892–6.
276. Roh SG, Song SH, Choi KC, et al. Chemerin - a new adipokine that modulates adipogenesis via its own receptor. *Biochem Biophys Res Commun* 2007;**362**(4):1013–8.
277. Sell H, Laurencikiene J, Taube A, et al. Chemerin is a novel adipocyte-derived factor inducing insulin resistance in primary human skeletal muscle cells. *Diabetes* 2009;**58**(12):2731–40.
278. Takahashi M, Takahashi Y, Takahashi K, et al. Chemerin enhances insulin signaling and potentiates insulin-stimulated glucose uptake in 3T3-L1 adipocytes. *FEBS Lett* 2008;**582**(5):573–8.
279. Kaur J, Adya R, Tan BK, et al. Identification of chemerin receptor (ChemR23) in human endothelial cells: chemerin-induced endothelial angiogenesis. *Biochem Biophys Res Commun* 2010;**391**(4):1762–8.
280. Muruganandan S, Parlee SD, Rourke JL, et al. Chemerin, a novel peroxisome proliferator-activated receptor gamma (PPARgamma) target gene that promotes mesenchymal stem cell adipogenesis. *J Biol Chem* 2011;**286**(27):23982–95.
281. Bozaoglu K, Curran JE, Stocker CJ, et al. Chemerin, a novel adipokine in the regulation of angiogenesis. *J Clin Endocrinol Metab* 2010;**95**(5):2476–85.
282. Zabel BA, Zuniga L, Ohyama T, et al. Chemoattractants, extracellular proteases, and the integrated host defense response. *Exp Hematol* 2006;**34**(8):1021–32.
283. Lobato NS, Neves KB, Filgueira FP, et al. The adipokine chemerin augments vascular reactivity to contractile stimuli via activation of the MEK-ERK1/2 pathway. *Life Sci* 2012;**91**(13–14):600–6.
284. Yoo HJ, Choi HY, Yang SJ, et al. Circulating chemerin level is independently correlated with arterial stiffness. *J Atheroscler Thromb* 2012;**19**(1):59–66. discussion 67–8.
285. Lehrke M, Becker A, Greif M, et al. Chemerin is associated with markers of inflammation and components of the metabolic syndrome but does not predict coronary atherosclerosis. *Eur J Endocrinol* 2009;**161**(2):339–44.
286. Spiroglou SG, Kostopoulos CG, Varakis JN, et al. Adipokines in periaortic and epicardial adipose tissue: differential expression and relation to atherosclerosis. *J Atheroscler Thromb* 2010;**17**(2):115–30.
287. Yamawaki H, Kameshima S, Usui T, et al. A novel adipocytokine, chemerin exerts anti-inflammatory roles in human vascular endothelial cells. *Biochem Biophys Res Commun* 2012;**423**(1):152–7.
288. Zhao RJ, Wang H. Chemerin/ChemR23 signaling axis is involved in the endothelial protection by K(ATP) channel opener iptakalim. *Acta Pharmacol Sin* 2011;**32**(5):573–80.
289. Blüher M. Vaspin in obesity and diabetes: pathophysiological and clinical significance. *Endocrine* 2012;**41**(2):176–82.
290. Dimova R, Tankova T. The role of vaspin in the development of metabolic and glucose tolerance disorders and atherosclerosis. *Biomed Res Int* 2015;**2015**:823481.
291. Hida K, Wada J, Eguchi J, et al. Visceral adipose tissue-derived serine protease inhibitor: a unique insulin-sensitizing adipocytokine in obesity. *Proc Natl Acad Sci U S A* 2005;**102**(30):10610–5.
292. Klöting N, Berndt J, Kralisch S, et al. Vaspin gene expression in human adipose tissue: association with obesity and type 2 diabetes. *Biochem Biophys Res Commun* 2006;**339**(1):430–6.

293. Lee JA, Park HS, Song YS, et al. Relationship between vaspin gene expression and abdominal fat distribution of Korean women. *Endocr J* 2011;**58**(8):639–46.
294. Seeger J, Ziegelmeier M, Bachmann A, et al. Serum levels of the adipokine vaspin in relation to metabolic and renal parameters. *J Clin Endocrinol Metab* 2008;**93**(1):247–51.
295. Youn BS, Klöting N, Kratzsch J, et al. Serum vaspin concentrations in human obesity and type 2 diabetes. *Diabetes* 2008;**57**(2):372–7.
296. Körner A, Neef M, Friebe D, et al. Vaspin is related to gender, puberty and deteriorating insulin sensitivity in children. *Int J Obes (Lond)* 2011;**35**(4):578–86.
297. Chang HM, Lee HJ, Park HS, et al. Effects of weight reduction on serum vaspin concentrations in obese subjects: modification by insulin resistance. *Obesity (Silver Spring)* 2010;**18**(11):2105–10.
298. Klöting N, Kovacs P, Kern M, et al. Central vaspin administration acutely reduces food intake and has sustained blood glucose-lowering effects. *Diabetologia* 2011;**54**(7):1819–23.
299. Heiker JT, Klöting N, Kovacs P, et al. Vaspin inhibits kallikrein 7 by serpin mechanism. *Cell Mol Life Sci* 2013;**70**(14):2569–83.
300. Yilmaz Y, Kurt R, Gurdal A, et al. Circulating vaspin levels and epicardial adipose tissue thickness are associated with impaired coronary flow reserve in patients with nonalcoholic fatty liver disease. *Atherosclerosis* 2011;**217**(1):125–9.
301. Choi SH, Kwak SH, Lee Y, et al. Plasma vaspin concentrations are elevated in metabolic syndrome in men and are correlated with coronary atherosclerosis in women. *Clin Endocrinol (Oxf)* 2011;**75**(5):628–35.
302. Aust G, Richter O, Rohm S, et al. Vaspin serum concentrations in patients with carotid stenosis. *Atherosclerosis* 2009;**204**(1):262–6.
303. Kadoglou NP, Gkontopoulos A, Kapelouzou A, et al. Serum levels of vaspin and visfatin in patients with coronary artery disease - Kozani study. *Clin Chim Acta* 2011;**412**(1–2):48–52.
304. Jung CH, Lee WJ, Hwang JY, et al. Vaspin protects vascular endothelial cells against free fatty acid-induced apoptosis through a phosphatidylinositol 3-kinase/Akt pathway. *Biochem Biophys Res Commun* 2011;**413**(2):264–9.
305. Fu BD, Yamawaki H, Okada M, et al. Vaspin can not inhibit TNF-alpha-induced inflammation of human umbilical vein endothelial cells. *J Vet Med Sci* 2009;**71**(9):1201–7.
306. Phalitakul S, Okada M, Hara Y, et al. Vaspin prevents TNF-α-induced intracellular adhesion molecule-1 via inhibiting reactive oxygen species-dependent NF-κB and PKCθ activation in cultured rat vascular smooth muscle cells. *Pharmacol Res* 2011;**64**(5):493–500.

CHAPTER

NEURONAL HORMONES AND THE SYMPATHETIC/ PARASYMPATHETIC REGULATION OF THE HEART

8

M.J. Ranek[1], A. Vu[2], M.S. Willis[3] and A. Lymperopoulos[2]

[1]The Johns Hopkins Medical Institutes, Baltimore, MD, United States [2]Nova Southeastern University College of Pharmacy, Fort Lauderdale, FL, United States [3]University of North Carolina, Chapel Hill, NC, United States

INTRODUCTION

The heart serves as the pump that moves blood through blood vessels thereby providing the needed oxygen and nutrients to the body. To achieve this goal, the heart must beat regularly and continuously for an entire lifetime. To promptly respond to the changing requirements of the body and its environment, heart rate and contractility are modulated by the autonomic nervous system, several peripheral glands, and other hormones.

ELECTRICAL SYSTEM OF THE HEART

The heart is a functional syncytium that pumps blood most effectively with a synchronous contraction, coordinated by the electrical system of the heart (Fig. 8.1). Organized contraction begins with depolarization of the sinoatrial (SA) node that transmits an electrical signal impulse to the right atrium. The signal then spreads throughout the right atrium by the anterior and middle internodal tracts and spread to the left atrium via Bachmann's bundle.[1] Cardiomyocytes allow an electrical current flow through themselves to neighboring cardiomyocytes to facilitate all cardiomyocytes of the atrium contracting at once.[2,3] While the atria pump blood into the ventricles, the action potential reaches the termination point of the internodal tracts of the right atrium, the atrioventricular (AV) node, which is located at the base of the right atrium, will depolarize and continue the spread of the electrical signal to the ventricles. The electrical signal enters the ventricles via the bundle of HIS, which carries the signal to the ventricular septum where it then divides into the right and left bundle branches to transmit the action potential to the right and left ventricles, respectively. The electrical impulse is then transmitted throughout the ventricles via Purkinje fibers and cardiomyocyte-to-cardiomyocyte junctions, allowing the ventricle to contract at once.[1,4] Heart rate and transmission velocity of the electrical signal throughout the heart is modulated by innervation from the autonomic nervous system (sympathetic and parasympathetic nervous systems) and by hormonal regulation.[5]

Endocrinology of the Heart in Health and Disease. DOI: http://dx.doi.org/10.1016/B978-0-12-803111-7.00008-7

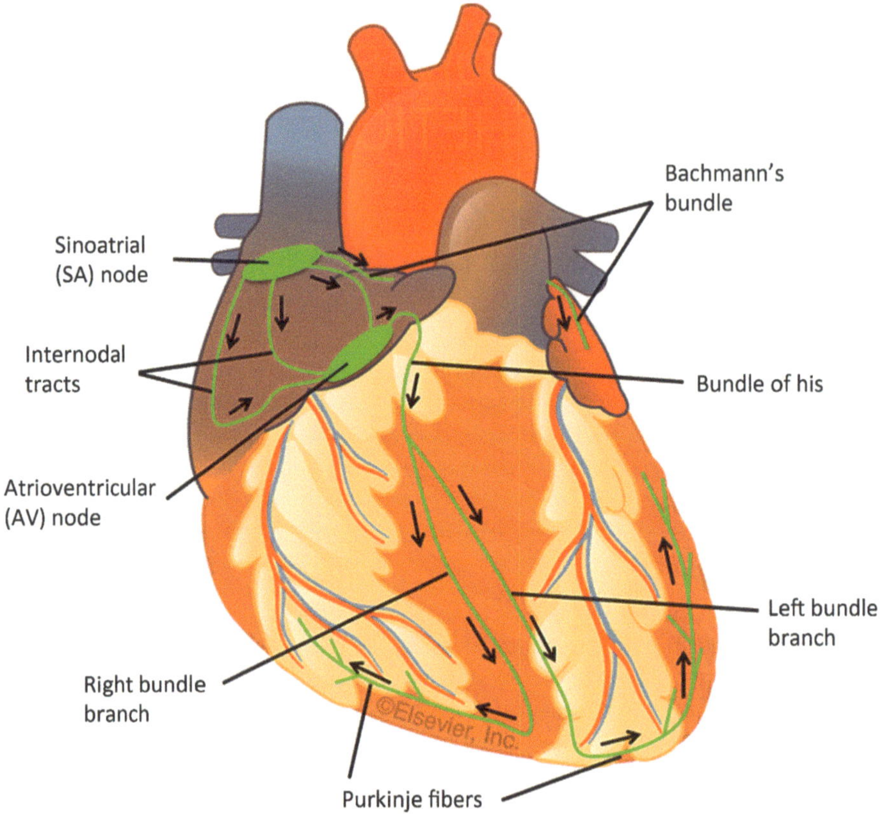

FIGURE 8.1

A schematic diagram of the electrical current flow (direction shown by arrows) from the sinoatrial node spreading throughout the heart.

SYMPATHETIC NERVOUS SYSTEM OF THE HEART

The sympathetic nervous system, responsible for orchestrating the body's response to situations of stress or emergency ("fight-or-flight"), forms cardiac sympathetic ganglia along the side of the viscera column (paravertebral ganglia).[5] These ganglia comprise the sympathetic trunks with their connecting fibers (Fig. 8.2). The postganglionic fibers extend to the heart. In general, sympathetic preganglionic neurons are shorter than sympathetic postganglionic neurons.[5] The (postganglionic) sympathetic neurotransmitter is norepinephrine (NE), although the neurotransmitter of the preganglionic neurons of both the sympathetic and parasympathetic systems is acetylcholine (ACh).[6] Thus, these sympathetic postganglionic fibers are called (nor)adrenergic neurons. NE and its close relative epinephrine (Epi) exert their actions through three α_1, three α_2, and three β adrenergic receptor (AR) subtypes (see chapter: Adrenergic Receptors for more detailed information on ARs), which are all G protein–coupled receptors (GPCRs).[7]

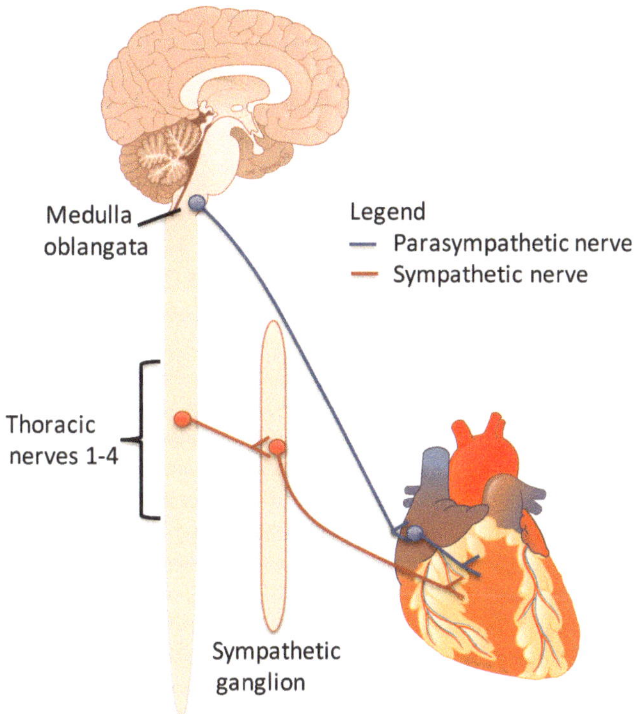

FIGURE 8.2

Illustration of parasympathetic and sympathetic innervation of the heart.

β_1ARs are expressed in the heart (in the sinoatrial and atrioventricular nodes, and in atrial and ventricular cardiomyocytes). Their activation increases heart rate (positive chronotropy), contractility (positive inotropy), and atrioventricular node conduction velocity (positive dromotropy).[8] β_1AR is also present in the juxtaglomerular apparatus cells of the kidney where it induces renin release to activate the renin-angiotensin-aldosterone system (RAAS) (see also below and chapter: Renin Angiotensin Aldosterone System and Heart Function). β_2ARs expression is found primarily in vascular smooth muscle, skeletal muscle, and in the coronary circulation.[8] Their activation elicits vasodilatation, which, in turn increases blood perfusion to target organs. These receptors are not innervated and thus are primarily stimulated by circulating epinephrine secreted by the adrenal medulla (see below).[8] There is also a low level of expression of β_2ARs in cardiomyocytes. α_1ARs are expressed in vascular smooth muscle proximal to sympathetic nerve terminals and they mediate vasoconstriction.[9] Cardiac myocytes also express small numbers of α_1ARs. Finally, α_2ARs are expressed in vascular smooth muscle distal to sympathetic nerve terminals where they also elicit vasoconstriction. Additionally, α2ARs are present in the central nervous system mediating autoinhibition of sympathetic outflow and in the adrenal medulla mediating autoinhibition of NE and Epi secretion.[10] Myocardial contractility is the ability of the heart to increase force of contraction, determined by the strength of the actomyosin filament interaction, which, in turn, depends on the cytoplasmic Ca^{2+} concentration of the myocyte. Catecholamine binding to the β_1AR is among the most powerful stimuli for elevation of intracellular Ca^{2+} concentration in the cardiomyocyte, and, consequently, for contraction of both the atria and ventricles (see below).[11]

As mentioned above, all ARs are GPCRs. Agonist-induced activation of βARs catalyzes the exchange of guanosine triphosphate for guanosine diphosphate on the G_α subunit of heterotrimeric G proteins, resulting in the dissociation of the heterotrimer into active G_α and free $G_{\beta\gamma}$ subunits (always associated together, i.e., a heterodimer that functions as a monomer), which can transduce intracellular signals independently of each other.[12] The most powerful physiologic mechanism to increase cardiac performance is activation of cardiomyocyte β_1ARs and β_2ARs, which, in turn, activate G_s proteins (stimulatory G proteins), as shown in Fig. 8.3. G_s protein signaling stimulates the effector adenylate cyclase (AC), which converts adenosine triphosphate (ATP) to the second messenger adenosine 3′,5′-monophosphate or cyclic AMP (cAMP), which in turn binds to and activates the cAMP-dependent protein kinase (protein kinase A, PKA). PKA is the major effector of cAMP by phosphorylating a variety of substrates, it ultimately results in significant raise in free intracellular Ca^{2+} concentration, which is the master regulator of cardiac muscle contraction.[13] Among the main targets of PKA phosphorylation in the cardiomyocyte are: (1) the cell membrane-located L-type calcium channels and the sarcoplasmic reticulum (SR)-located ryanodine receptors, both leading to an increase in Ca^{2+} entry into the cell[13];

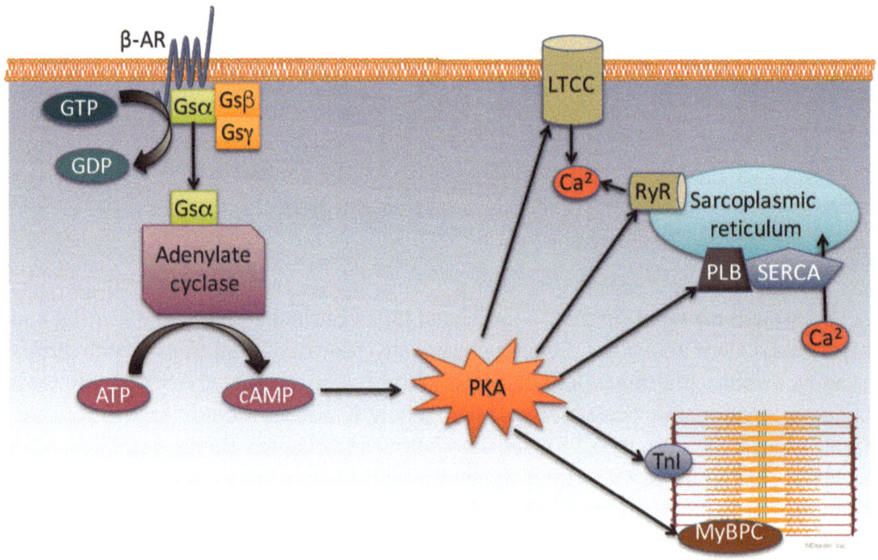

FIGURE 8.3

An illustration of protein kinase A (PKA) activation and protein it phosphorylates. Abbreviations: beta-adrenergic receptor (β-AR), guanosine triphosphate (GTP), guanosine diphosphate (GDP), G stimulatory protein subunit alpha (Gsα), G stimulatory protein subunit beta (Gsβ), G stimulatory protein subunit gamma (Gsγ), adenosine triphosphate (ATP), cyclic adenosine monophosphate (cAMP), L-type calcium channel (LTCC), calcium (Ca^2), ryanodine receptor (RyR), phospholamban (PLB), sarcoplasmic/endoplasmic reticulum calcium ATPase (SERCA), troponin I (TnI), and myosin binding protein-C (MyBPC).

(2) phospholamban (PLB), a negative modulator of SERCA (Sarcoplasmic/endoplasmic reticulum Ca^{2+}-ATPase), whose phosphorylation by PKA uninhibits SERCA activity, thus accelerating Ca^{2+} reuptake by the SR after contraction and increasing SR Ca^{2+} stores available for the next contraction[13]; (3) hyperpolarization-activated cyclic nucleotide-gated channels that generate the hyperpolarization-activated cation inward current (If) affecting the initiation and modulation of rhythmic activity in cardiac pacemaker cells[14]; (4) troponin I and myosin binding protein-C that reduce myofilament sensitivity to Ca^{2+}, thereby accelerating the relaxation of myofilaments[15]; and (5) phosphomman (PLM), an inhibitor of the Na^{+}/K^{+}-ATPase, and phosphorylation of PLM relieves Na^{+}/K^{+}-ATPase inhibition and stimulates the sodium pump, thereby accelerating cardiac muscle repolarization and relaxation.[16] Moreover, PKA can phosphorylate the βARs themselves (and other GPCRs) in the heart, causing G protein uncoupling and functional desensitization of the receptor (heterologous or agonist-independent desensitization).[17]

Of note, the β_2AR also mediates catecholamine effects in the heart, but in a qualitatively different manner from β_1AR, as it can also couple to the AC inhibitory G protein (G_i). This switching of β_2AR signaling from G_s to G_i proteins is postulated to be induced by the phosphorylation of the β_2AR by PKA.[17] It is generally accepted that in the heart, β_2AR signals and functions in a substantially different way compared to β_1AR.[18–20] For example, whereas β_1AR activation enhances cardiomyocyte apoptosis, β_2AR exerts antiapoptotic effects in the heart.[18–22] This essential difference between the two receptor subtypes is ascribed to the signal of β_2AR through G_i proteins.[20] Studies using transgenic mice, β_2AR-selective stimulation, and adenoviral-mediated β_2AR overexpression, have demonstrated the protective effects of β_2AR signaling in the myocardium, including improved cardiac function and decreased apoptosis. Conversely, hyperstimulation or overexpression of β_1AR has detrimental effects in the heart.[21,22]

Both α_2- and βARs, like the majority of GPCRs, are subject to agonist-promoted (homologous) desensitization and downregulation, a regulatory process that diminishes receptor response to continuous or repeated agonist stimulation.[23,24] At the molecular level, this process is initiated by receptor phosphorylation by a family of kinases, termed GPCR kinases (GRKs), followed by binding of βarrestins (βarrs) to the GRK-phosphorylated receptor (see below). The βarrs then uncouple the receptor from its cognate G proteins, sterically hinder its further binding to them (functional desensitization) and subsequently target the receptor for internalization.[23,24] Across all mammalian species, GRK2 and GRK5 are the most physiologically important members of the GRK family because they are expressed ubiquitously and regulate the vast majority of GPCRs. They are particularly abundant in the heart and neuronal tissues.[25,26]

Of note, the differences between the two predominant cardiac βARs, i.e., β_1AR & β_2AR, in terms of their signaling properties, might take a quite different shape and have a much bigger bearing on pathophysiologic implications in the setting of human heart failure: for instance, and as discussed in more detail in subsequent sections, β_1AR is selectively downregulated (i.e., functional receptor number reduced) in human heart failure, thus shifting the above mentioned stoichiometry of β_1AR:β_2AR towards 50:50 in the failing heart from ~75%:~20% in the normal, healthy heart.[27,28] However, β_2AR is also nonfunctional and does not signal properly in the failing heart. In addition, emerging evidence suggests that β_2AR signaling in the failing heart is quite different from that in the normal heart, i.e., is more diffuse and noncompartmentalized and resembles more the proapoptotic "diffuse" cAMP signaling pattern of the β_1AR.[29] Therefore, this stoichiometric shift in favor of the supposedly "good" β_2AR in heart failure appears unable to complete compensate and return heart structure and function back to baseline.

The human heart also expresses α_{1A}- and α_{1B}ARs, albeit at much lower levels than βARs (~20% of total βARs).[30] How important a role cardiac α_1ARs play in cardiac physiology is still a matter of debate. In contrast, their role in regulating blood flow by inducing constriction in the smooth muscle wall of major arteries (e.g., aorta, pulmonary arteries, mesenteric vessels, coronary arteries, etc.) is well known and unequivocal. The α_1ARs couple to the $G_{q/11}$ family of heterotrimeric G proteins, thereby activating phospholipase C (PLC)-β. PLCβ generates the second messenger intermediates inositol[31] trisphosphate (IP_3) and 2-diacylglycerol (DAG) from the cell membrane component phospholipid phosphatidylinositol (4,5)-bisphosphate (PIP_2).[32] IP_3 binds specific receptors in the SR membrane which cause release of Ca^{2+} from intracellular stores, whereas DAG activates protein kinase C (PKC) and transient receptor potential channels, raising intracellular [Ca^{2+}] and producing vasoconstriction.[32]

Finally, regarding α_2AR subtypes, α_{2B}ARs are present in vascular smooth muscle causing constriction of certain vascular beds, while centrally located α_{2A}ARs can inhibit sympathetic outflow (presynaptic inhibitory autoreceptors) and thus lower systemic blood pressure.[33,34] The release of NE from cardiac sympathetic nerve terminals is controlled by both presynaptic α_{2A}- and α_{2C}ARs,[35] and genetic deletion of both of these α_2AR subtypes leads to cardiac hypertrophy and heart failure due to chronically enhanced cardiac NE release, as well as enhanced NE and Epi secretion from the adrenal medulla.[36,37]

An important exception to the usual arrangement in sympathetic fibers is the set of preganglionic fibers that pass through the sympathetic ganglia and extend to the medulla of the adrenal glands (Fig. 8.4). These fibers terminate on the chromaffin cells, specialized hormone-synthesizing and secreting cells that release NE (~20%) and mainly Epi (80%).[38–40] Epi is produced from the amino acid tyrosine and released from chromaffin cells in the adrenal medulla of the adrenal glands. It can stimulate all nine ARs.[38–40] Epi at low concentrations is relatively β_2-selective, producing mainly vasodilatation (reduces blood pressure), but at high concentrations it stimulates all ARs equipotently, producing vasoconstriction (through α_1- and α_2ARs) and increases heart rate and contractility (through β_1ARs).[38–40] Epi serves to initiate the fight-or-flight response system by boosting the oxygen and glucose supplies to the brain and skeletal muscle through increased cardiac output and vasodilatation. All of the Epi in the body and a significant amount of circulating NE derive from the adrenal medulla, and the total amount of catecholamines presented to cardiac ARs at any given time is composed of circulating NE and Epi as well as NE released locally from sympathetic nerve terminals within the heart.[38–40] The secretion of catecholamines from the bilateral adrenal glands is regulated in a complex manner by a variety of cell membrane receptors present in chromaffin cells. Many of these receptors are GPCRs, including α_2ARs that inhibit secretion (inhibitory presynaptic autoreceptors), and βARs that enhance it (facilitatory presynaptic autoreceptors).[41] Of note, although various presynaptic auto- and hetero-receptors increase adrenal catecholamine secretion, e.g., βARs, muscarinic cholinergic receptors (mAChRs), angiotensin II-ergic, histaminergic, and adrenomedullin receptors, the α_2AR is the only receptor type reported to date to inhibit adrenal catecholamine secretion.[41]

Adrenal α_2AR-dependent catecholamine inhibition is tightly regulated by GRK2 (described above). Specifically, studies over the past few years have established that GRK2 upregulation is responsible for severe adrenal α_2AR dysfunction in chronic heart failure that causes a loss of the sympathoinhibitory function of these receptors in the adrenal gland, and catecholamine secretion is thus chronically elevated.[42–45] This emerging role for adrenal GRK2 in heart failure is underlined by the observation that specific inhibition of GRK2 via adenoviral-mediated βARKct adrenal gene delivery (see below), leads to a reduction in circulating catecholamine levels, restoring not only adrenal but also cardiac function

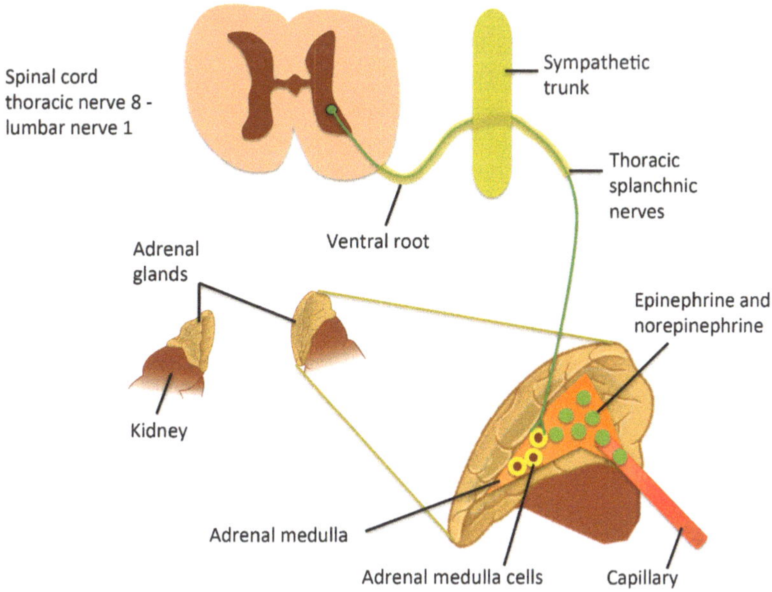

FIGURE 8.4

An illustration of sympathetic innervation of the adrenal gland.

in heart failure. Additional evidence for the role of adrenal GRK2 regulating α_2ARs in controlling adrenal sympathetic tone in heart failure comes from the phenylethanolamine-*N*-methyl transferase-driven GRK2 KO (knockout) mice that do not express GRK2 in their adrenal medulla from birth.[43] These mice display decreased ANS outflow and circulating catecholamines in response to myocardial infarction translating to preserved cardiac function and morphology over the course of the ensuing heart failure.[43]

PARASYMPATHETIC NERVOUS SYSTEM OF THE HEART

The parasympathetic nervous system, in most (but not all) cases, is antagonistic to the sympathetic system in regulating heart function.[12] Parasympathetic preganglionic fibers innervate organs of the thorax and upper abdomen as parts of the vagus nerve, which carries ~75% of all parasympathetic nerve fibers passing to the heart and many other visceral organs.[12] The short postganglionic neurons reside essentially inside or very close to the effector organs. Unlike the sympathetic ones, most parasympathetic preganglionic fibers reach the target organs and form the peripheral ganglia in the wall of the organ.[12] The preganglionic fibers synapse within the ganglion and short postganglionic fibers leave the ganglia to the target organ. Thus, in the parasympathetic system, preganglionic neurons are generally longer than postganglionic neurons.[46] ACh is the neurotransmitter of both preganglionic and postganglionic parasympathetic neurons, and are referred to as cholinergic neurons. ACh exerts its effects via two types of cholinergic receptors: nicotinic receptors (nAChRs) and muscarinic receptors (mAChRs).[12] mAChRs are GPCRs located in the membranes of effector cells at the end of postganglionic parasympathetic nerves and at the ends of cholinergic sympathetic fibers. Responses from these receptors are excitatory and relatively slow.[12] The nAChRs are ligand-gated ion channels located at synapses between pre- and postganglionic neurons of the sympathetic and parasympathetic pathways. Because they are ion channels, nAChRs produce rapid, excitatory responses, in contrast to mAChRs.[12] Out of the five different known subtypes of mAChRs, the M_2 receptors are expressed in the heart, being particularly abundant in nodal and atrial tissue, with little or no expression in the ventricles.[46] Thus, binding of ACh to M_2 receptors slows heart rate and atrioventricular conduction (negative chronotropy and dromotropy, respectively) and also reduces the contractility of atrial cardiomyocytes (negative inotropy). However, given the small contribution of the atrial muscle into the overall myocardial contractility, the inhibitory effect of ACh on cardiac inotropy is negligible.[12] The M_3 receptor subtype is expressed primarily in vascular endothelium and mediates nitric oxide-dependent vasodilatation.[12] In conclusion, the parasympathetic system opposes the effects of the sympathetic nervous system on heart rate and nodal conduction but the effect of the parasympathetic system on myocardial contractility is minimal.

MEASURING AUTONOMIC NERVOUS SYSTEM REGULATION OF THE HEART

An imbalance of the autonomic nervous system is linked to cardiac mortality, such as sudden cardiac death. An increase and decrease in sympathetic and parasympathetic nervous system modulation, respectively, increases the propensity for arrhythmias.[47–50] This observation increased the demand for a quantitative measurement of the autonomic nervous system regulation of the heart. Heart rate variability (HRV) was proven to be an effective and reliable measurement of autonomic activity.[51,52] HRV is the variation of beat-to-beat intervals, also known as the R-to-R intervals. In the mid-1960s HRV was first documented from recording fetal distress that preceded beat-to-beat variation without any noticeable change in heart rate overall.[53] Then, in 1977, Wolf et al. reported an association of reduced HRV with postmyocardial infarction mortality.[54] These results were later confirmed that HRV was a strong predictor of mortality following acute myocardial infarction.[55]

HRV can be calculated by a variety of methods, which in the simplest sense is determined from heart rate and rhythm tracked via an electrocardiogram (ECG). Heart rate and rhythm are controlled by the vagal nerve releasing acetylcholine (parasympathetic nervous system) and epinephrine release (sympathetic nervous system) onto the sinoatrial node. The HRV is then calculated by the R-to-R interval dictated by the balance in activities of the parasympathetic and sympathetic regulation of the sinoatrial node.[56,57] Monitoring HRV over a 24-hour ambulatory period is sufficient to assess HRV in normal subjects,[58] postinfarction patients,[59] and in ventricular arrhythmia patients.[59]

Heart rate and rhythm are a function of autonomic nervous activity, making HRV a reliable index of autonomic nervous regulation of the heart. Notably, a reduction in HRV has been reported in patients with several cardiac etiologies.[56,60] A decreased HRV following a myocardial infarction may indicate a reduction in vagal activity and a corresponding increase in sympathetic predominance over the heart, contributing to cardiac electrical instability.[61] Human heart failure patients also had decreased HRV and were characterized by increased sympathetic activity as evidenced by a faster heart rate and increased circulating catecholamines.[51,60,62,63]

Fortunately, there are methods that are thought to increase HRV while also decreasing cardiovascular mortality and sudden cardiac death. One such method is exercise, thought to be capable of balancing the autonomic regulation of the heart. Regular exercise can increase regulation of the heart by the parasympathetic nervous system.[64–67] Furthermore, a study performed on dogs subjected to myocardial infarction subsequently separated into either exercise or nonexercise groups demonstrated that the exercise group increased HRV by 74%. The animals in the exercise arm of this study also had reduced incidence of sudden death.[68]

CIRCADIAN RHYTHM REGULATION OF THE AUTONOMIC SYSTEM

The mechanism of alterations in autonomic control of the heart are related to sleep may be mediated by changes in the circadian rhythm. The circadian rhythm is the approximately 24-hour cycle governing several physiological processes in animals, including humans. Circadian rhythms are endogenously generated but are modulated by external cues such as food, sunlight, and temperature. Diurnal variations in autonomic nervous system activity, plasma cortisol, and renin-angiotensin activity are well known in the pathogenesis of cardiovascular disease.[69] Transcriptional-translational feedback loops of the circadian genes within cells constitute a molecular clock system.[69] At a molecular level, this clock is composed of two transcription factors named CLOCK and BMAL that form a heterodimer and bind to the E-box upstream of the *Per* and *Cry* genes encoding the PERIOD and CRYPTOCHROME 1 proteins, respectively.[69] The mammalian central clock is located in the pituitary suprachiasmatic nucleus (SCN) region of the brain and responds to light/dark systems by modulating body temperature and releasing cortisol and melatonin. The central clock regulates peripheral clocks via the autonomic nervous system, circulating hormones, or metabolic cues (Fig. 8.5(A)).

How the autonomic nervous system centrally regulates peripheral tissue circadian rhythms such as the heart requires an understanding of the cardiomyocyte's own circadian rhythm machinery. Microarray analysis of cardiomyocytes has identified that 8–10% of transcripts have circadian expression patterns in the heart.[70] Like the SCN cells, the cardiomyocyte has clock genes that respond to serum shock or norepinephrine (Fig. 8.5(B)).[71] In response to these stimuli, cardiomyocyte CLOCK and BMAL proteins form a heterodimer, which transcribes *Per* and *Cry* genes (Fig. 8.5(B), left). The resulting PER protein acts to negatively inhibit CLOCK/BMAL1 activity (negative feedback look) which CRY is eventually phosphorylated by casein kinase-1 epsilon and degraded by the proteasomal pathway. This negative feedback loop, primarily the proteasomal-dependent degradation of the PER and CRY proteins are thought to account for the 24-hour internal rhythm that exists intrinsically in cardiomyocytes.[69] In addition to the PER/CRY negative feedback loop, the CLOCK/BMAL1 complex regulate several circadian-related genes (Fig. 8.5(B), right) involved in intracellular metabolism or electrophysiological activity, including pyruvate dehydrogenase kinase isoenzyme-4 (*Pdk-4*), glucose transporters 1 and 4 (*Slc2a1, Slc2a4*), and the potassium channels *Kcna5* and *Kcnd2*.[72–74] Hence, the CLOCK/BMAL1-self regulation through PER/CRY is complemented by regulation of critical genes integral to cardiac performance.

While the autonomic nervous system, plasma cortisol, and RAAS show intraday diurnal variation, resulting in 24-hour variances in blood pressure, cardiomyocytes have a circadian expression of cardioprotective genes, such as atrial natriuretic peptide (*Anp*) that may offset these diurnal changes, anticipating and adapting to the external environment. The rise in blood pressure that occurs in the morning may be met by morning increases in *Anp*. A key question that remains unanswered is whether the peripheral cardiomyocyte clock is at fault, making the heart more susceptible by not adapting to the autonomic changes that regularly occur.

In rat hearts subjected to pressure overload-induced hypertrophy, the circadian expression of PAR transcription factors (*Dbp, Hlf*), and *Anp* are significantly attenuated.[74] Expression of the

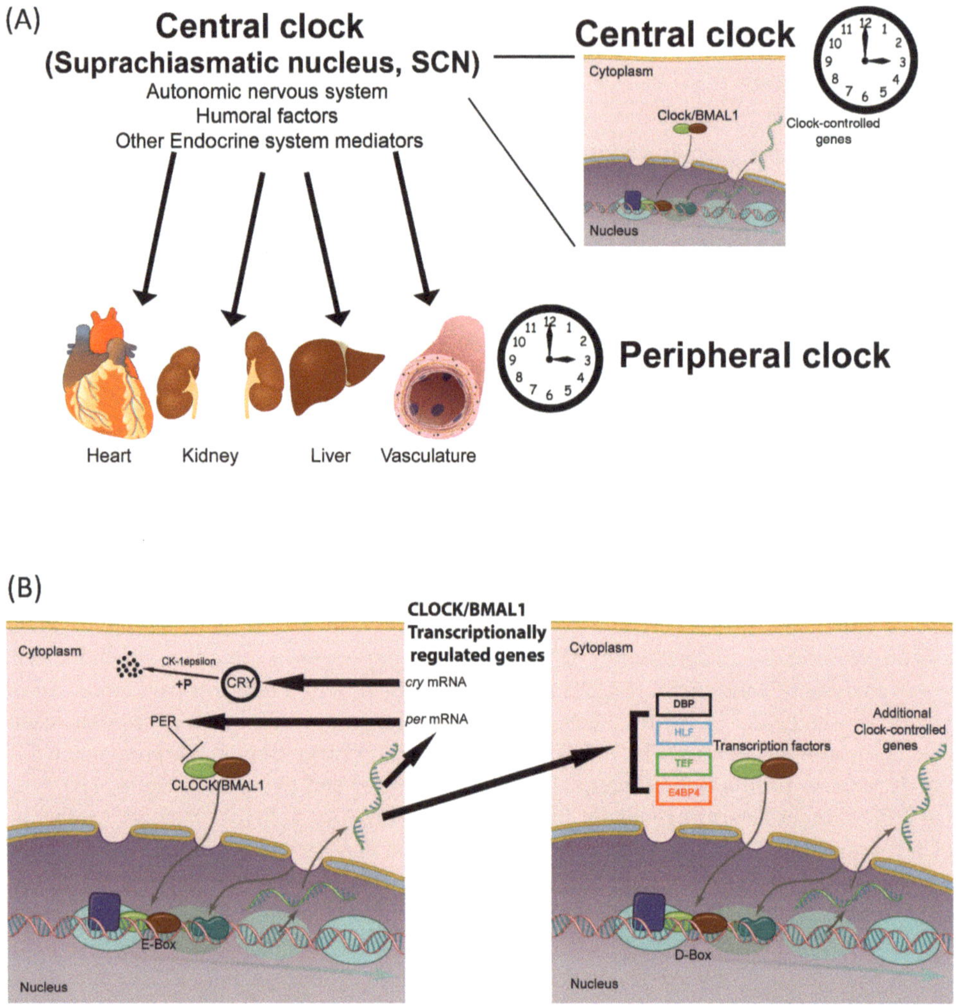

FIGURE 8.5

The central clock is found in the hypothalamic suprachiasmatic nucleus (SCN), where molecular clock machinery regulates the peripheral clock. (A) The autonomic nervous system and humoral factors both regulate the peripheral clock found in various tissues, including the heart. (B) The proteins CLOCK and BMAL1 form a heterodimer, binding to the Per and Cry E-box to initiate transcription of the PER and CRY proteins. PER and CRY are posttranslationally phosphorylated by casein kinase-1 epsilon and degraded by the proteasome. They also accumulate and inhibit the transcription of per and cry genes, which occurs in a 24-hour loop responsible for the internal rhythm of the tissue. Other PER/BMAL1-regulated genes including the D-element binding proteins (dbp), hepatic leukemia factor (hlf), and thyrotrophic embryonic factor (tef).

*Adapted from Takeda N, Maemura K. The role of clock genes and circadian rhythm in the development of cardiovascular diseases Cell Mol Life Sci 2015;**72**:3225–34.*

cardiomyocyte core clock genes is affected in myocardial ischemia; expression of *Nfil3* (also known as E4BP4) increases in I/R and antagonizes the circadian PAR family transcription factors.[75] In the diabetic heart, the diurnal variation was reported to be altered.[76] Interpreted together, the misreading of the physiological (or pathophysiological) cues by the cardiomyocyte clock system may contribute to disease susceptibility by preventing central circadian cues from the autonomic system to elicit the proper response in the heart.

Our understanding of the molecular basis of altered circadian rhythm in cardiomyocytes is in its infancy. However, recent studies uncovered aspects of altered rhythms seen in diabetes/metabolic syndrome and the effect of sleep deprivation on cardiovascular disease, as discussed above. As an example, we present the process of posttranslational modification of proteins by monosaccharides of O-linked beta-*N*-acetylglucosamine (O-GlcNAc) (Fig. 8.6). The addition of monosaccharides by O-GlcNAc occurs in a process of O-GlcNAcylation, which completes with phosphorylation reactions on serine and threonine residues.[69] The two enzymes that regulate this process, O-GlcNAc transferase and O-GlcNAcase are transcriptionally regulated and both genes have a circadian oscillation, whereby diurnal variation of protein O-GlcNAcylation modifications are seen in the heart,[77] representing differential signaling environments depending on the time of day. Furthermore, in diabetes, hyperglycemia contributes to an increase in O-GlcNAc modification.[78] Conceptually, alterations in critical signaling pathways involved in cardiovascular disease could be caused by diurnal variations in the central SCN signal (e.g., in response to sleep deprivation), which is seen routinely with increases in myocardial infarction incidence when shifts to and from daylight savings time occurs, increasing 24% the Monday following spring time changes and a 21% reduction in the Tuesday following fall changes.[79,80]

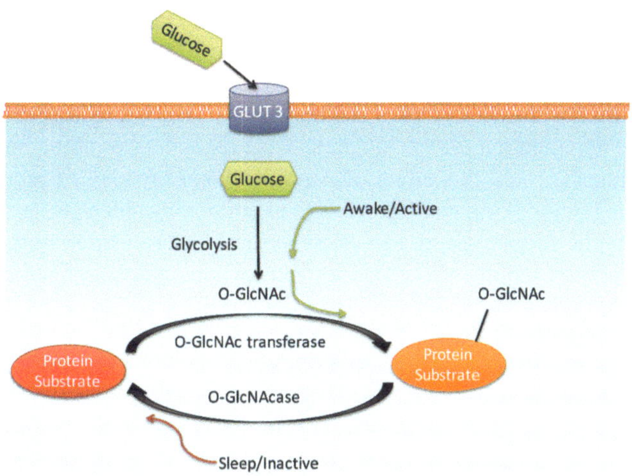

FIGURE 8.6

A schematic diagram of addition (O-GlcNAcylation) and subtraction of O-GlcNAc to and from a protein substrate during the circadian rhythm.

OTHER ENDOCRINE ORGANS AND THE HEART: POSTERIOR PITUITARY

Vasopressin (antidiuretic hormone) is another hormone that modulates cardiac function and is released by the parvocellular neurosecretory neurons of the posterior pituitary gland, albeit synthesized in the hypothalamus.[5] Within the kidney, vasopressin causes water retention via V_2 receptors and results in increasing water permeability of the distal tubule and collecting duct cells.[9,10] Within the cardiovascular system, via V_1 receptors vasopressin is a vasoconstrictor that results in increased blood pressure.[9,10] An increase in blood volume results in increased cardiac output and improved cardiovascular function, provided the cardiovascular system is healthy and intact.

MISCELLANEOUS HORMONES AND THE HEART

Another important hormonal system regulating cardiac function is the RAAS. The RAAS (shown in Fig. 8.7 in the context of the other systems discussed in this chapter) mainly regulates blood pressure and fluid balance during instances of hypovolemia or blood loss. The RAAS (see chapter: Renin Angiotensin Aldosterone System and Heart Function for more detailed content) is activated either by baroreceptors within the carotid sinus that detect decreases in blood pressure, decreases in sodium chloride concentration, and/or a decreased in the rate of blood flow through the macula densa of the kidney (juxtaglomerular apparatus).[5] Once a decrease in blood volume is detected, renin is released and angiotensinogen (produced in the liver) is cleaved to angiotensin I. Angiotensin I is biologically inert and is converted to angiotensin II (Ang II) by ACE (angiotensin converting enzyme). Angiotensin II acts upon the proximal tubules to increase sodium reabsorption, thus helping the body to retain water while maintaining the glomerular filtration rate and blood pressure.[5] Angiotensin II reduces renal medullary blood flow and also constricts the renal arteries, as well as afferent and efferent arterioles and mesangial cells, thereby decreasing the filtration rate of the kidneys. Angiotensin II also causes the adrenal cortex (zona glomerulosa) to release aldosterone, a hormone that causes sodium retention and potassium excretion; this Ang II signaling event requires not only G protein activation by the Ang II AT_1 receptor but also the aforementioned adapter protein βarr1 (see above).[38] Specifically, βarr1 signaling results in the upregulation of steroidogenic acute regulatory protein, the most critical enzyme in aldosterone biosynthesis,[81] and this effect of βarr1 is independent of G proteins.[81] In vivo, βarr1 appears to be a major regulator of physiological levels of circulating aldosterone, since the upregulation of βarr1, specifically in the adrenal gland, can cause hyperaldosteronism in normal healthy animals.[81] Importantly, in chronic heart failure, also characterized by hyperaldosteronism, adrenal βarr1 overexpression/overactivity promotes increased circulating aldosterone levels, accelerated adverse cardiac remodeling, and deterioration of heart function.[82] Moreover, the cardiotoxic effects of aldosterone in heart failure are prevented by inhibiting adrenal βarr1 activity in vivo[82] and βarr1-knockout mice progressing to heart failure did not have elevated circulating aldosterone levels.[83]

Angiotensin II has three major cardiac effects: (1) as a potent vasoconstrictor (second only to endothelin), resulting in increased systemic blood pressure,[5] (2) as prothrombotic, stimulating platelet aggregation and inducing production of plasminogen activator inhibitor (PAI)-1 and -2,[84] and (3) as a powerful prohypertrophic signal in cardiac myocytes, causing cell growth, ventricular dilatation, and cardiac fibrosis through fibroblast activation and proliferation, the so-called "adverse remodeling" of the heart.[6]

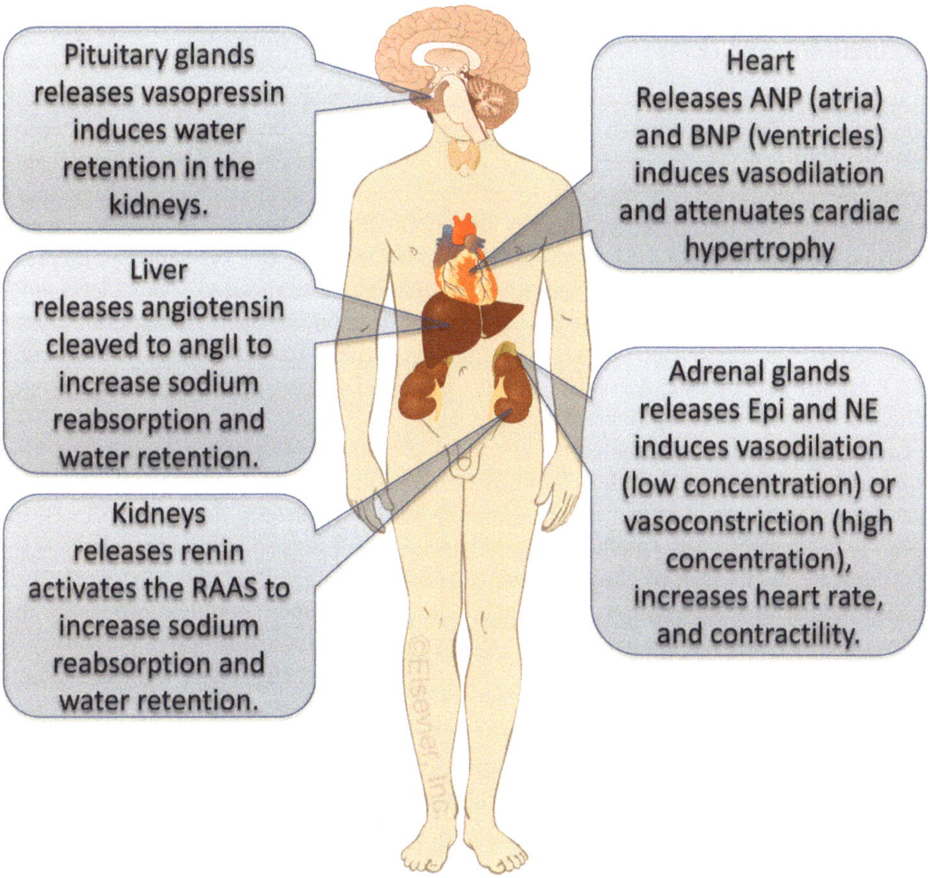

FIGURE 8.7

An illustration of the endocrine organs and their regulation on the cardiovascular system.

Two other hormones regulating cardiac function are produced and secreted by the myocardium itself: ANP, produced by atrial cardiomyocytes, and brain (or B-type) natriuretic peptide (BNP), produced by ventricular cardiomyocytes (see chapter: Cardiac Natriuretic Peptides for a complete discussion). ANP is released in response to atrial distention (hypervolemia), β-adrenergic stimulation, hypernatremia, and Ang II or endothelin elevations.[85] Atrial natriuretic peptide causes vasodilatation, reducing blood pressure, and inhibiting cardiac hypertrophy; ANP also exerts cardioprotective effects demonstrated by preventing ischemia-reperfusion injury-related fibrosis.[86] Brain natriuretic peptide is secreted by the ventricles in response to excessive stretching of ventricular myocytes, and BNP levels are typically increased in patients with left ventricular dysfunction.[87] Clinically, BNP levels are used as biomarker of human heart failure, as elevated BNP levels are indicative of poor left ventricular function and heart failure.[88]

PHYSIOLOGY AND PATHOPHYSIOLOGY OF CARDIOVASCULAR FUNCTION INVOLVING THE AUTONOMIC SYSTEM: PREGNANCY AND THE BAROREFLEX

The baroreceptor reflex is the mechanism by which arterial pressure is maintained through autonomic regulation within a set range, although this set range can shift during physiological and pathophysiological conditions (Fig. 8.8). During pregnancy, the cardiovascular system undergoes significant changes to appropriately serve the developing fetus. In early gestation, the mother's blood volume and cardiac output increases by 30–50%; however, there is also a reduction in arterial pressure. Reduced arterial pressure is due to suppression of the baroreflex response, which decreases systemic vascular resistance. The baroreflex dysfunction that occurs during pregnancy is due to reduced sympathetic modulation of the vasculature, thus limiting the response to vasoconstriction and increased arterial pressure.[89,90] The mechanism for the diminished baroreflex response is attributed to (1) reduced insulin acting in the brain that normally supports the baroreflex and (2) increased levels of the neurosteroid progesterone metabolite, 3α-hydroxy-dihydroprogesterone (3α-OH-DHP).[91]

The baroreflex response is mediated by afferent and efferent innervations to and from the brainstem. Afferent nerves for the baroreflex response terminate in the nucleus tractus solitarius, project to the caudal ventrolateral medulla that projects to the rostral ventrolateral medulla (RVLM). Efferents then project to the baroreflex receptors. During pregnancy, there is a reduction of insulin action, which facilitates the placental transfer of glucose to the fetus by increasing circulating glucose levels. Insulin enhances the baroreflex response, thus when insulin is decreased the baroreflex response is impaired. The concentration of the neurosteroid, 3α-OH-DHP in the blood, increases during pregnancy. 3α-OH-DHP acts on the RVLM to inhibit efferent signaling originating in the RVLM.[91] In turn, the diminished

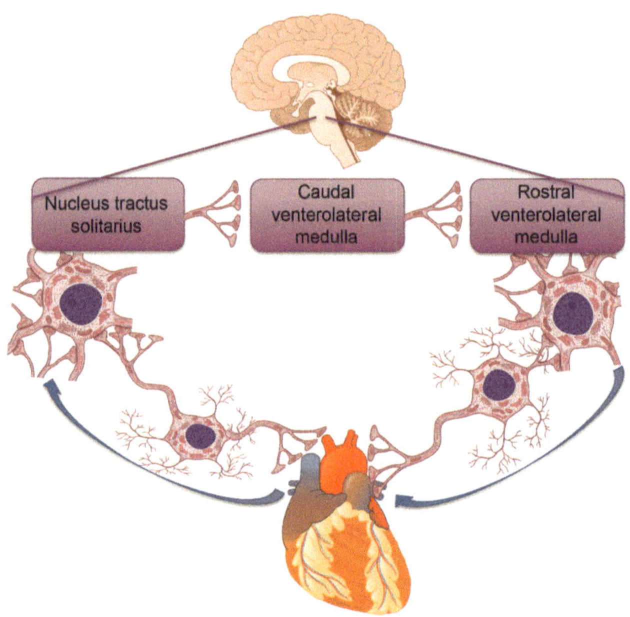

FIGURE 8.8

A schematic overview of the baroreflex response.

baroreflex response signals back to the vasculature to increase arterial pressure. Collectively, these mechanisms suppress the baroreflex response during pregnancy.

DIABETIC AUTONOMIC DYSFUNCTION/METABOLIC SYNDROME (A SYMPATHETIC DISEASE?) AND ITS EFFECTS ON THE HEART

An imbalance in the autonomic regulation of the heart (decreased HRV) is magnified in the presence of diabetes or metabolic syndrome. There is increased morbidity and mortality in people with metabolic syndrome and with autonomic dysregulation, specifically increased sympathetic drive and decreased parasympathetic tone.[92] Notably there is evidence that increased sympathetic drive is a complication for individuals with a history of diabetes, but also increased sympathetic drive is involved in the pathogenesis leading to the development of the diabetes.[93–96] Autonomic imbalance in people with metabolic syndrome had increased resting heart rates and exercise intolerances.[92,97]

Lifestyle changes and therapeutic interventions are recommended for individuals with metabolic syndrome to combat autonomic dysregulation of the heart. As mentioned above, exercise can restore autonomic balance and increase HRV. Diet and exercise reduced the risk of autonomic dysfunction by 25% in participants of the diabetes Prevention Program designated as high risk of developing diabetes (i.e., BMI> 24 kg/m^2, fasting glucose 5.3–6.9 mmol/L, and 2-hour glucose 7.8–11.0 mmol/L).[98,99] Various therapeutic approaches can be used to help restore autonomic balance including antioxidant therapy, ACE inhibitors, angiotensin receptor blockers, and beta-blockers. The restoration of autonomic balance via increased parasympathetic tone and decreased sympathetic drive, increased HRV, decreased cardiac events, and improved patient outcomes.[100–102]

POSTURAL TACHYCARDIA

Postural tachycardia syndrome (POTS) is a heterogeneous group of disorders that are characterized primarily by an increased heart rate on standing; however, exercise intolerance and fatigue are also symptoms. These symptoms are typically relieved by recumbence. Individuals with POTS see a heart rate increase of at least 30 beats per minute or a heart rate that exceeds 120 beats per minute from standing.[103,104] POTS is caused by the inability of the peripheral vasculature, particularly the peripheral nervous system, to maintain adequate vascular resistance during the increased gravitational stress experienced during standing. In an attempt to compensate, heart rate is increased. An underlying mechanism for this loss of function is a continuous increase in adrenergic stimulation, termed the hyperadrenergic state. These patients typically have elevated serum NE levels.[104–106]

Treatment options for POTS are centered on correcting this autonomic imbalance. An acetylcholinesterase inhibitor blocks the degradation of acetylcholine, allowing this parasympathetic neurotransmitter to stimulate its receptors longer, thus increasing parasympathetic tone. Another treatment option is to block the effects of NE. A combined alpha- and beta-receptor blocker was also shown to be a useful treatment.[103–105]

EFFECT OF SLEEP DEPRIVATION ON CARDIOVASCULAR REGULATION

Sleep deprivation can have profound effects on the cardiovascular system and its regulation. Increased cardiovascular morbidity is often reported in people whose sleep is disrupted or insufficient, such as shift workers.[107] Resting blood pressure, specifically diastolic blood pressure, is elevated by sleep deprivation.[108]

Increase in blood pressure is thought to be due to a resetting of the arterial baroreflex response to a higher setpoint along with decreased baroreflex sensitivity (reduced beat-to-beat adaptation ability). The mechanism for these pathophysiological changes is caused by increased sympathetic stimulation and decreased parasympathetic modulation of the cardiovascular system.[108,109] Better sleep quality and longer sleep duration corrected the autonomic imbalance experienced by sleep deprivation.[107,110]

CONCLUDING REMARKS

The heart is built to promptly respond to acute and chronic disturbances in blood pressure and body homeostasis and environment. A plethora of biological players, from the central nervous system (brain) to the peripheral neuroendocrine system with the adrenal glands and the renal juxtaglomerular apparatus, and even the heart's own endocrine system consisting of several heart-secreted peptide factors participate in the fine-tuning of cardiac function at any given time. The amazing coordination of the effects of all of these factors results in the remarkable ability of the cardiovascular system to properly respond to any external or internal stimulus towards the goal of sustaining body homeostasis at all costs.

REFERENCES

1. Bonke FI, Kirchhof CJ, Allessie MA, Wit AL. Impulse propagation from the SA-node to the ventricles. *Experientia* 1987;**43**:1044–9.
2. Rohr S. Role of gap junctions in the propagation of the cardiac action potential. *Cardiovasc Res* 2004;**62**:309–22.
3. Spach MS, Kootsey JM. The nature of electrical propagation in cardiac muscle. *Am J Physiol* 1983;**244**:H3–22.
4. Kleber AG, Rudy Y. Basic mechanisms of cardiac impulse propagation and associated arrhythmias. *Physiol Rev* 2004;**84**:431–88.
5. Gordan R, Gwathmey JK, Xie LH. Autonomic and endocrine control of cardiovascular function. *World J Cardiol* 2015;**7**:204–14.
6. Somers VK.. In: Mann DL, Zipes DP, Libby P, Bonow RO, Philadelphia PA, editors. *Braunwald's heart disease: a textbook of cardiovascular medicine*. Saunders, an imprint of Elsevier, Inc.; 2015. p. 1931–43.
7. Brodde OE, Michel MC. Adrenergic and muscarinic receptors in the human heart. *Pharmacol Rev* 1999;**51**:651–90.
8. Lymperopoulos A, Rengo G, Koch WJ. Adrenergic nervous system in heart failure: pathophysiology and therapy. *Circ Res* 2013;**113**:739–53.
9. Capote LA, Mendez Perez R, Lymperopoulos A. GPCR signaling and cardiac function. *Eur J Pharmacol* 2015;**763**:143–8.
10. Lymperopoulos A, Garcia D, Walklett K. Pharmacogenetics of cardiac inotropy. *Pharmacogenomics* 2014;**15**:1807–21.
11. Lymperopoulos A, Bathgate A. Pharmacogenomics of the heptahelical receptor regulators G-protein-coupled receptor kinases and arrestins: the known and the unknown. *Pharmacogenomics* 2012;**13**:323–41.
12. Lohse MJ, Engelhardt S, Eschenhagen T. What is the role of beta-adrenergic signaling in heart failure? *Circ Res* 2003;**93**:896–906.
13. Bers DM. Calcium cycling and signaling in cardiac myocytes. *Annu Rev Physiol* 2008;**70**:23–49.
14. Ludwig A, Zong X, Jeglitsch M, Hofmann F, Biel M. A family of hyperpolarization-activated mammalian cation channels. *Nature* 1998;**393**:587–91.

15. Sulakhe PV, Vo XT. Regulation of phospholamban and troponin-I phosphorylation in the intact rat cardiomyocytes by adrenergic and cholinergic stimuli: roles of cyclic nucleotides, calcium, protein kinases and phosphatases and depolarization. *Mol Cell Biochem* 1995;**149–150**:103–26.
16. Despa S, Bossuyt J, Han F, Ginsburg KS, Jia LG, Kutchai H, et al. Phospholemman-phosphorylation mediates the beta-adrenergic effects on Na/K pump function in cardiac myocytes. *Circ Res* 2005;**97**:252–9.
17. Daaka Y, Luttrell LM, Lefkowitz RJ. Switching of the coupling of the beta2-adrenergic receptor to different G proteins by protein kinase A. *Nature* 1997;**390**:88–91.
18. Communal C, Singh K, Sawyer DB, Colucci WS. Opposing effects of beta(1)- and beta(2)-adrenergic receptors on cardiac myocyte apoptosis : role of a pertussis toxin-sensitive G protein. *Circulation* 1999;**100**: 2210–2.
19. Chesley A, Lundberg MS, Asai T, Xiao RP, Ohtani S, Lakatta EG, et al. The beta(2)-adrenergic receptor delivers an antiapoptotic signal to cardiac myocytes through G(i)-dependent coupling to phosphatidylinositol 3′-kinase. *Circ Res* 2000;**87**:1172–9.
20. Zhu WZ, Zheng M, Koch WJ, Lefkowitz RJ, Kobilka BK, Xiao RP. Dual modulation of cell survival and cell death by beta(2)-adrenergic signaling in adult mouse cardiac myocytes. *Proc Natl Acad Sci USA* 2001;**98**:1607–12.
21. Liggett SB, Tepe NM, Lorenz JN, Canning AM, Jantz TD, Mitarai S, et al. 2nd: Early and delayed consequences of beta(2)-adrenergic receptor overexpression in mouse hearts: critical role for expression level. *Circulation* 2000;**101**:1707–14.
22. Dorn II GW, Tepe NM, Lorenz JN, Koch WJ, Liggett SB. Low- and high-level transgenic expression of beta2-adrenergic receptors differentially affect cardiac hypertrophy and function in Galphaq-overexpressing mice. *Proc Natl Acad Sci U S A* 1999;**96**:6400–5.
23. Reiter E, Lefkowitz RJ. GRKs and beta-arrestins: roles in receptor silencing, trafficking and signaling. *Trends Endocrinol Metab* 2006;**17**:159–65.
24. Ferguson SS. Evolving concepts in G protein-coupled receptor endocytosis: the role in receptor desensitization and signaling. *Pharmacol Rev* 2001;**53**:1–24.
25. Rockman HA, Koch WJ, Lefkowitz RJ. Seven-transmembrane-spanning receptors and heart function. *Nature* 2002;**415**:206–12.
26. Arriza JL, Dawson TM, Simerly RB, Martin LJ, Caron MG, Snyder SH, et al. The G-protein-coupled receptor kinases beta ARK1 and beta ARK2 are widely distributed at synapses in rat brain. *J Neurosci* 1992;**12**:4045–55.
27. Bristow MR, Ginsburg R, Umans V, Fowler M, Minobe W, Rasmussen R, et al. Beta 1- and beta 2-adrenergic-receptor subpopulations in nonfailing and failing human ventricular myocardium: coupling of both receptor subtypes to muscle contraction and selective beta 1-receptor down-regulation in heart failure. *Circ Res* 1986;**59**:297–309.
28. Bristow MR, Ginsburg R, Minobe W, Cubicciotti RS, Sageman WS, Lurie K, et al. Decreased catecholamine sensitivity and beta-adrenergic-receptor density in failing human hearts. *N Engl J Med* 1982;**307**:205–11.
29. Nikolaev VO, Moshkov A, Lyon AR, Miragoli M, Novak P, Paur H, et al. Beta2-adrenergic receptor redistribution in heart failure changes cAMP compartmentation. *Science* 2010;**327**:1653–7.
30. Woodcock EA, Du XJ, Reichelt ME, Graham RM. Cardiac alpha 1-adrenergic drive in pathological remodelling. *Cardiovasc Res* 2008;**77**:452–62.
31. Iellamo F, Legramante JM, Massaro M, Raimondi G, Galante A. Effects of a residential exercise training on baroreflex sensitivity and heart rate variability in patients with coronary artery disease: a randomized, controlled study. *Circulation* 2000;**102**:2588–92.
32. Shannon R, Chaudhry M. Effect of alpha1-adrenergic receptors in cardiac pathophysiology. *Am Heart J* 2006;**152**:842–50.
33. Philipp M, Hein L. Adrenergic receptor knockout mice: distinct functions of 9 receptor subtypes. *Pharmacol Ther* 2004;**101**:65–74.

34. Philipp M, Brede M, Hein L. Physiological significance of alpha(2)-adrenergic receptor subtype diversity: one receptor is not enough. *Am J Physiol Regul Integr Comp Physiol* 2002;**283**:R287–95.
35. Johnson RM, Kirkwood DH. Loss of resealing ability in erythrocyte membranes. Effect of divalent cations and spectrin release. *Biochim Biophys Acta* 1978;**509**:58–66.
36. Brede M, Nagy G, Philipp M, Sorensen JB, Lohse MJ, Hein L. Differential control of adrenal and sympathetic catecholamine release by alpha 2-adrenoceptor subtypes. *Mol Endocrinol* 2003;**17**:1640–6.
37. Brede M, Wiesmann F, Jahns R, Hadamek K, Arnolt C, Neubauer S, et al. Feedback inhibition of catecholamine release by two different alpha2-adrenoceptor subtypes prevents progression of heart failure. *Circulation* 2002;**106**:2491–6.
38. McCrink KA, Brill A, Lymperopoulos A. Adrenal G protein-coupled receptor kinase-2 in regulation of sympathetic nervous system activity in heart failure. *World J Cardiol* 2015;**7**:539–43.
39. Lymperopoulos A, Rengo G, Koch WJ. GRK2 inhibition in heart failure: something old, something new. *Curr Pharm Des* 2012;**18**:186–91.
40. Rengo G, Lymperopoulos A, Leosco D, Koch WJ. GRK2 as a novel gene therapy target in heart failure. *J Mol Cell Cardiol* 2011;**50**:785–92.
41. Lymperopoulos A, Rengo G, Koch WJ. Adrenal adrenoceptors in heart failure: fine-tuning cardiac stimulation. *Trends Mol Med* 2007;**13**:503–11.
42. Lymperopoulos A, Rengo G, Funakoshi H, Eckhart AD, Koch WJ. Adrenal GRK2 upregulation mediates sympathetic overdrive in heart failure. *Nat Med* 2007;**13**:315–23.
43. Lymperopoulos A, Rengo G, Gao E, Ebert SN, Dorn II GW, Koch WJ. Reduction of sympathetic activity via adrenal-targeted GRK2 gene deletion attenuates heart failure progression and improves cardiac function after myocardial infarction. *J Biol Chem* 2010;**285**:16378–86.
44. Rengo G, Leosco D, Zincarelli C, Marchese M, Corbi G, Liccardo D, et al. Adrenal GRK2 lowering is an underlying mechanism for the beneficial sympathetic effects of exercise training in heart failure. *Am J Physiol Heart Circ Physiol* 2010;**298**:H2032–8.
45. Lymperopoulos A, Rengo G, Zincarelli C, Soltys S, Koch WJ. Modulation of adrenal catecholamine secretion by in vivo gene transfer and manipulation of G protein-coupled receptor kinase-2 activity. *Mol Ther* 2008;**16**:302–7.
46. Lymperopoulos A, Koch WJ. Autonomic pharmacology. In: Waldman SA, Terzic A, editors. *Pharmacology and therapeutics: principles to practice* 1st ed.. Philadelphia, PA: Saunders/Elsevier; 2009.
47. Pogwizd SM, Corr PB. Mechanisms of arrhythmogenesis during myocardial ischemia and reperfusion: a perspective of our current understanding. *J Mol Cell Cardiol* 1986;**18**(Suppl. 4):43–7.
48. Du XJ, Dart AM. Role of sympathoadrenergic mechanisms in arrhythmogenesis. *Cardiovasc Res* 1999;**43**:832–4.
49. Ripplinger CM, Noujaim SF, Linz D. The nervous heart. *Prog Biophys Mol Biol* 2016;**120**(1–3):199–209.
50. Schwartz PJ, La Rovere MT, Vanoli E. Autonomic nervous system and sudden cardiac death. Experimental basis and clinical observations for post-myocardial infarction risk stratification. *Circulation* 1992;**85**:I77–91.
51. Heart rate variability for risk stratification of life-threatening arrhythmias. American College of Cardiology Cardiovascular Technology Assessment Committee. J Am Coll Cardiol 1993;**22**:948–50.
52. Goldberger JJ, Cain ME, Hohnloser SH, Kadish AH, Knight BP, Lauer MS, et al. American Heart Association/American College of Cardiology Foundation/Heart Rhythm Society scientific statement on noninvasive risk stratification techniques for identifying patients at risk for sudden cardiac death: a scientific statement from the American Heart Association Council on Clinical Cardiology Committee on Electrocardiography and Arrhythmias and Council on Epidemiology and Prevention. *Circulation* 2008;**118**:1497–518.
53. Welford NT, Sontag LW, Phillips W, Phillips D. Individual differences in heart rate variability in the human fetus. *Am J Obstet Gynecol* 1967;**98**:56–61.

54. Wolf MM, Varigos GA, Hunt D, Sloman JG. Sinus arrhythmia in acute myocardial infarction. *Med J Aust* 1978;**2**:52–3.
55. Akselrod S, Gordon D, Ubel FA, Shannon DC, Berger AC, Cohen RJ. Power spectrum analysis of heart rate fluctuation: a quantitative probe of beat-to-beat cardiovascular control. *Science* 1981;**213**:220–2.
56. Kamath MV, Fallen EL. Power spectral analysis of heart rate variability: a noninvasive signature of cardiac autonomic function. *Crit Rev Biomed Eng* 1993;**21**:245–311.
57. Montano N, Ruscone TG, Porta A, Lombardi F, Pagani M, Malliani A. Power spectrum analysis of heart rate variability to assess the changes in sympathovagal balance during graded orthostatic tilt. *Circulation* 1994;**90**:1826–31.
58. Kleiger RE, Bigger JT, Bosner MS, Chung MK, Cook JR, Rolnitzky LM, et al. Stability over time of variables measuring heart rate variability in normal subjects. *Am J Cardiol* 1991;**68**:626–30.
59. Bigger Jr. JT, Fleiss JL, Rolnitzky LM, Steinman RC. Stability over time of heart period variability in patients with previous myocardial infarction and ventricular arrhythmias. The CAPS and ESVEM investigators. *Am J Cardiol* 1992;**69**:718–23.
60. Malik M, Camm AJ. Heart rate variability and clinical cardiology. *Br Heart J* 1994;**71**:3–6.
61. Casolo GC, Stroder P, Signorini C, Calzolari F, Zucchini M, Balli E, et al. Heart rate variability during the acute phase of myocardial infarction. *Circulation* 1992;**85**:2073–9.
62. Tsuji H, Larson MG, Venditti FJ, Manders ES, Evans JC, Feldman CL, et al. Impact of reduced heart rate variability on risk for cardiac events. The Framingham Heart Study. *Circulation* 1996;**94**:2850–5.
63. Musialik-Łydka A, Sredniawa B, Pasyk S. Heart rate variability in heart failure. *Kardiol Pol* 2003;**58**:10–16.
64. Routledge FS, Campbell TS, McFetridge-Durdle JA, Bacon SL. Improvements in heart rate variability with exercise therapy. *Can J Cardiol* 2010;**26**:303–12.
65. Figueiredo T, Rhea MR, Peterson M, Miranda H, Bentes CM, dos Reis VM, et al. Influence of number of sets on blood pressure and heart rate variability after a strength training session. *J Strength Cond Res* 2015;**29**:1556–63.
66. Masson GS, Nair AR, Silva Soares PP, Michelini LC, Francis J. Aerobic training normalizes autonomic dysfunction, HMGB1 content, microglia activation and inflammation in hypothalamic paraventricular nucleus of SHR. *Am J Physiol Heart Circ Physiol* 2015;**309**:H1115–22.
67. Sloan RP, Shapiro PA, DeMeersman RE, Bagiella E, Brondolo EN, McKinley PS, et al. The effect of aerobic training and cardiac autonomic regulation in young adults. *Am J Public Health* 2009;**99**:921–8.
68. Hull SS, Evans AR, Vanoli E, Adamson PB, Stramba-Badiale M, Albert DE, et al. Heart rate variability before and after myocardial infarction in conscious dogs at high and low risk of sudden death. *J Am Coll Cardiol* 1990;**16**:978–85.
69. Takeda N, Maemura K. The role of clock genes and circadian rhythm in the development of cardiovascular diseases. *Cell Mol Life Sci* 2015;**72**:3225–34.
70. Storch KF, Lipan O, Leykin I, Viswanathan N, Davis FC, Wong WH, et al. Extensive and divergent circadian gene expression in liver and heart. *Nature* 2002;**417**:78–83.
71. Durgan DJ, Hotze MA, Tomlin TM, Egbejimi O, Graveleau C, Abel ED, et al. The intrinsic circadian clock within the cardiomyocyte. *Am J Physiol Heart Circ Physiol* 2005;**289**:H1530–41.
72. Yamashita T, Sekiguchi A, Iwasaki YK, Sagara K, Iinuma H, Hatano S, et al. Circadian variation of cardiac K+ channel gene expression. *Circulation* 2003;**107**:1917–22.
73. Young ME, Razeghi P, Cedars AM, Guthrie PH, Taegtmeyer H. Intrinsic diurnal variations in cardiac metabolism and contractile function. *Circ Res* 2001;**89**:1199–208.
74. Young ME, Razeghi P, Taegtmeyer H. Clock genes in the heart: characterization and attenuation with hypertrophy. *Circ Res* 2001;**88**:1142–50.
75. Kung TA, Egbejimi O, Cui J, Ha NP, Durgan DJ, Essop MF, et al. Rapid attenuation of circadian clock gene oscillations in the rat heart following ischemia-reperfusion. *J Mol Cell Cardiol* 2007;**43**:744–53.

76. Young ME, Wilson CR, Razeghi P, Guthrie PH, Taegtmeyer H. Alterations of the circadian clock in the heart by streptozotocin-induced diabetes. *J Mol Cell Cardiol* 2002;**34**:223–31.
77. Durgan DJ, Pat BM, Laczy B, Bradley JA, Tsai JY, Grenett MH, et al. O-GlcNAcylation, novel post-translational modification linking myocardial metabolism and cardiomyocyte circadian clock. *J Biol Chem* 2011;**286**:44606–19.
78. Durning SP, Flanagan-Steet H, Prasad N, Wells L. O-Linked beta-*N*-acetylglucosamine (O-GlcNAc) Acts as a Glucose Sensor to Epigenetically Regulate the Insulin Gene in Pancreatic Beta Cells. *J Biol Chem* 2016;**291**:2107–18.
79. Sandhu A, Seth M, Gurm HS. Daylight savings time and myocardial infarction. *Open Heart* 2014;**1**:e000019.
80. Jiddou MR, Pica M, Boura J, Qu L, Franklin BA. Incidence of myocardial infarction with shifts to and from daylight savings time. *Am J Cardiol* 2013;**111**:631–5.
81. Lymperopoulos A, Rengo G, Zincarelli C, Kim J, Soltys S, Koch WJ. An adrenal beta-arrestin 1-mediated signaling pathway underlies angiotensin II-induced aldosterone production in vitro and in vivo. *Proc Natl Acad Sci U S A* 2009;**106**:5825–30.
82. Lymperopoulos A, Rengo G, Zincarelli C, Kim J, Koch WJ. Adrenal beta-arrestin 1 inhibition in vivo attenuates post-myocardial infarction progression to heart failure and adverse remodeling via reduction of circulating aldosterone levels. *J Am Coll Cardiol* 2011;**57**:356–65.
83. Bathgate-Siryk A, Dabul S, Pandya K, Walklett K, Rengo G, Cannavo A, et al. Negative impact of beta-arrestin-1 on post-myocardial infarction heart failure via cardiac and adrenal-dependent neurohormonal mechanisms. *Hypertension* 2014;**63**:404–12.
84. Skurk T, Lee YM, Hauner H. Angiotensin II and its metabolites stimulate PAI-1 protein release from human adipocytes in primary culture. *Hypertension* 2001;**37**:1336–40.
85. De Bold AJ. Atrial natriuretic factor: a hormone produced by the heart. *Science* 1985;**230**:767–70.
86. Kasama S, Furuya M, Toyama T, Ichikawa S, Kurabayashi M. Effect of atrial natriuretic peptide on left ventricular remodelling in patients with acute myocardial infarction. *Eur Heart J* 2008;**29**:1485–94.
87. Don-Wauchope AC, McKelvie RS. Evidence based application of BNP/NT-proBNP testing in heart failure. *Clin Biochem* 2015;**48**:236–46.
88. Sun RR, Lu L, Liu M, Cao Y, Li XC, Liu H, et al. Biomarkers and heart disease. *Eur Rev Med Pharmacol Sci* 2014;**18**:2927–35.
89. Brooks VL, Cassaglia PA, Zhao D, Goldman RK. Baroreflex function in females: changes with the reproductive cycle and pregnancy. *Gend Med* 2012;**9**:61–7.
90. Blake MJ, Martin A, Manktelow BN, Armstrong C, Halligan AW, Panerai RB, et al. Changes in baroreceptor sensitivity for heart rate during normotensive pregnancy and the puerperium. *Clin Sci (Lond)* 2000;**98**:259–68.
91. Brooks VL, Dampney RA, Heesch CM. Pregnancy and the endocrine regulation of the baroreceptor reflex. *Am J Physiol Regul Integr Comp Physiol* 2010;**299**:R439–51.
92. Schlaich M, Straznicky N, Lambert E, Lambert G. Metabolic syndrome: a sympathetic disease? *Lancet Diabetes Endocrinol* 2015;**3**:148–57.
93. Grassi G. Sympathetic overdrive and cardiovascular risk in the metabolic syndrome. *Hypertens Res* 2006;**29**:839–47.
94. Grassi G, Quarti-Trevano F, Seravalle G, Dell'Oro R. Cardiovascular risk and adrenergic overdrive in the metabolic syndrome. *Nutr Metab Cardiovasc Dis* 2007;**17**:473–81.
95. Mancia G, Bousquet P, Elghozi JL, Esler M, Grassi G, Julius S, et al. The sympathetic nervous system and the metabolic syndrome. *J Hypertens* 2007;**25**:909–20.
96. Palatini P. Heart rate and the cardiometabolic risk. *Curr Hypertens Rep* 2013;**15**:253–9.
97. Garruti G, Giampetruzzi F, Vita MG, Pellegrini F, Lagioia P, Stefanelli G, et al. Links between metabolic syndrome and cardiovascular autonomic dysfunction. *Exp Diabetes Res* 2012;**2012**:615835.

98. Carnethon MR, Prineas RJ, Temprosa M, Zhang ZM, Uwaifo G, Molitch ME, Diabetes prevention program research G The association among autonomic nervous system function, incident diabetes, and intervention arm in the Diabetes Prevention Program. *Diabetes Care* 2006;**29**:914–9.
99. Vinik AI, Maser RE, Ziegler D. Autonomic imbalance: prophet of doom or scope for hope? *Diabet Med* 2011;**28**:643–51.
100. Stuckey MI, Tulppo MP, Kiviniemi AM, Petrella RJ. Heart rate variability and the metabolic syndrome: a systematic review of the literature. *Diabetes Metab Res Rev* 2014;**30**:784–93.
101. Grundy SM, Cleeman JI, Daniels SR, Donato KA, Eckel RH, Franklin BA, et al. National Heart Ln, and Blood Institute: diagnosis and management of the metabolic syndrome: an American Heart Association/National Heart, Lung, and Blood Institute Scientific Statement. *Circulation* 2005;**112**:2735–52.
102. Grundy SM. Metabolic syndrome: therapeutic considerations. *Handb Exp Pharmacol* 2005:107–33.
103. Grubb BP. Postural tachycardia syndrome. *Circulation* 2008;**117**:2814–7.
104. Raj SR. Postural tachycardia syndrome (POTS). *Circulation* 2013;**127**:2336–42.
105. Agarwal AK, Garg R, Ritch A, Sarkar P. Postural orthostatic tachycardia syndrome. *Postgrad Med J* 2007;**83**:478–80.
106. Raj SR. Highlights in clinical autonomic neurosciences: treatment insights for postural tachycardia syndrome and inappropriate sinus tachycardia. *Auton Neurosci* 2013;**177**:72–3.
107. Vgontzas AN, Liao D, Pejovic S, Calhoun S, Karataraki M, Basta M, et al. Insomnia with short sleep duration and mortality: the Penn State cohort. *Sleep* 2010;**33**:1159–64.
108. Ogawa Y, Kanbayashi T, Saito Y, Takahashi Y, Kitajima T, Takahashi K, et al. Total sleep deprivation elevates blood pressure through arterial baroreflex resetting: a study with microneurographic technique. *Sleep* 2003;**26**:986–9.
109. Elsenbruch S, Harnish MJ, Orr WC. Heart rate variability during waking and sleep in healthy males and females. *Sleep* 1999;**22**:1067–71.
110. Calhoun DA, Harding SM. Sleep and hypertension. *Chest* 2010;**138**:434–43.

CHAPTER

RENIN ANGIOTENSIN ALDOSTERONE SYSTEM AND HEART FUNCTION

9

W.C. De Mello

University of Puerto Rico, San Juan, PR, United States

THE CONVENTIONAL RENIN ANGIOTENSIN ALDOSTERONE SYSTEM

The activation of the conventional renin angiotensin aldosterone system (RAAS) plays a seminal role on the regulation of blood volume and blood pressure and is involved in the regulation of cardiac function and remodeling during hypertension, heart failure, and myocardial ischemia including LVH, fibrosis as well as vascular damage. Renin, released from the kidney, converts angiotensinogen from liver to the decapeptide angiotensin (Ang)-I, which undergoes proteolytic cleavage generating the octapeptide Ang-II—a process catalyzed by angiotensin converting enzyme (ACE), which is found not only on the endothelial lining of blood vessels in the lungs but also by epithelial cells in the kidney (Fig. 9.1). Ang II is a potent vasoconstrictor peptide that stimulates the synthesis and secretion of the mineralocorticoid aldosterone from the outer region (zona glomerulosa) of the adrenal gland. Although other ACE cleavage products have been identified their physiological and clinical relevance is unclear. The most important changes induced by RAAS activation are related to Ang II, including variation in heart contractility and excitability, interstitial, and perivascular fibrosis as well as ventricular hypertrophy—all related to the activation of Ang II type I receptor (AT1) (Fig. 9.1). The AT1 is a seven-transmembrane spanning G protein–coupled receptor (GPCR) located at the plasma cell membrane that activates multiple intracellular signaling pathways mediating the major cardiovascular actions of Ang II.[1] Activation of the receptor stimulates phospholipase C (PLC) via Gq/11 increasing the cytoplasmic calcium concentrations that ultimately increases protein kinase C (PKC) activity. In humans only one form of AT1 receptor is expressed but two forms are seen in rodents (AT1A and AT1B). Experiments performed on AT1A receptor knockout mouse revealed that ventricular hypertrophy still occurs during pressure overload. As to the observation that hypertrophy still occurs in the absence of AT1A receptors, two possible explanations have been considered: (1) a contribution by AT1B or (2) a compensatory mechanism activated on AT1A gene deletion generated during embryonic development. On the other hand, experiments have demonstrate that splice variants harboring exon 2 accounts for at least 30% of all the hAT1R mRNA transcripts expressed in the human tissues investigated.

The location of AT1 receptors is not limited to the plasma cell membrane. Indeed, nuclear Ang II binding sites have been identified[2,3] suggesting an intracrine role for this peptide.[4] Down-regulation of AT1 receptors at both the level of protein and gene expression has been reported in the failing

Endocrinology of the Heart in Health and Disease. DOI: http://dx.doi.org/10.1016/B978-0-12-803111-7.00009-9

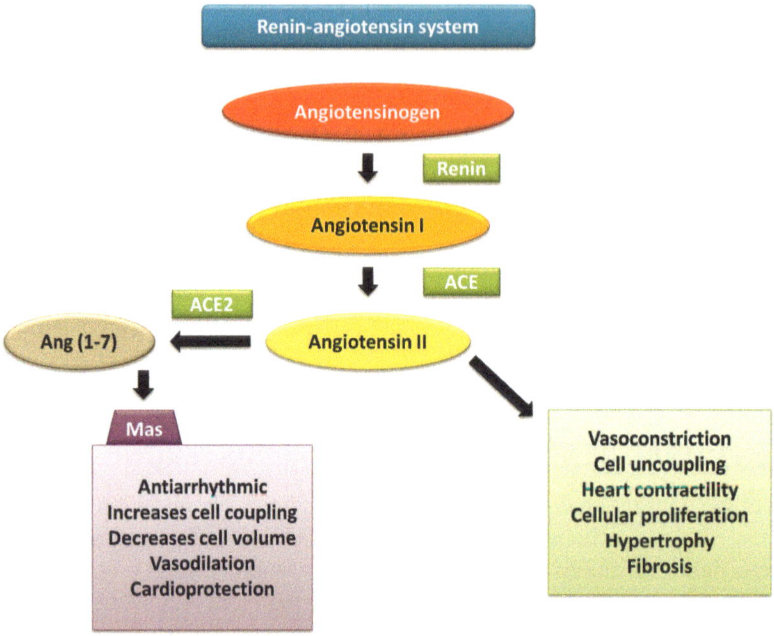

FIGURE 9.1

Renin angiotensin aldosterone system and the major effects of angiotensin II (Ang II) on the cardiovascular system.

heart[5]—the result of chronic stimulation by Ang II elicited by RAAS activation and upregulation of ACE.[6] In the human heart, the serine protease referred to as chymase seems to play an important role on the generation of Ang II during heart failure.[7]

Activation of AT1 receptors in cardiac myocytes phosphorylates several proteins including ion channels, contractile proteins as well as proteins involved in the regulation of gene expression and protein synthesis.[8] Second messengers like diacylglycerol (DAG), calcium as well as inositol phosphates are involved in this process. AT1 receptor activation also stimulates Ras that participates in the proliferative effect of Ang II on cardiac fibroblasts[9] and the Rho family that is related to ventricular hypertrophy induced by the peptide.[10] Activation of AT1 and AT2 receptors, which were cloned in 1993,[11] has different effects. While the AT2 receptor is also a GPCR, its activation enhances the action of some phosphatases and nitric oxide (NO) production, while AT1 receptors activate tyrosine kinases.[12] AT2 receptors are mainly expressed in fetal tissues, including the heart, but their density decreases in adult heart tissue.[13] The AT1 and AT2 receptors share a sequence identity of about 30% but have a similar affinity for Ang II.

There are several lines of evidence that AT1 receptors are involved in cardiac growth. Ang II, e.g., elicits ventricular hypertrophy—an effect suppressed by the AT1 receptor antagonist losartan,[14] which supports the role of AT1 receptors. AT2 receptors blockers, in contrast, enhance the stimulating effect of Ang II on protein synthesis.[15] AT1 receptor activates the major MAPK cascades in cardiac

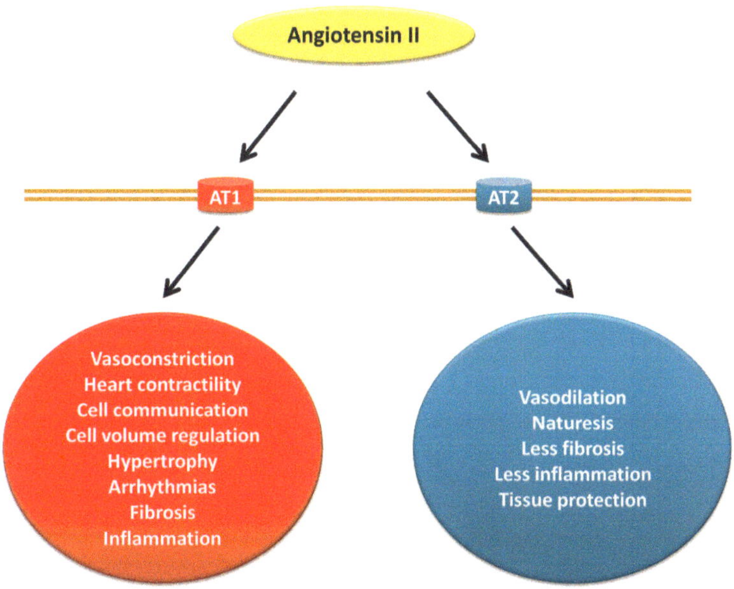

FIGURE 9.2

Activation of Ang II-AT1 and AT2 receptors in their respective effects in the heart and vessels.

myocytes and ERK via PKC, JNK via calcium, and PKC and p38 via NAD(P)H oxidase and ROS generation are also important signaling pathways related to AT1 activation.

Clinical trials have demonstrated that AT1 receptor blockade enhances cardiac function and reduces cardiac remodeling in patients with heart failure.[16,17] More recent studies have revealed that AT2 receptors seem to play an important role on the regulation of cardiac function. In AT2 knockout mice, for instance, the cardiac function was reduced[18] as well as the ventricular hypertrophy induced by pressure overload.[19] Conversely, AT2 receptor overexpression improves left ventricle systolic function, reduces the mass index at baseline, and preserves heart function postmyocardial infarction.[18] AT2 receptor activation seems to inhibit inflammation and apoptosis[20] (Fig. 9.2). The activation of the pathways related to AT1 receptors including MAP/endoplasmic reticulum (ER) kinase pathway, contributes to the generation of fibrosis, and recently evidence has been provided that AT2 receptors prevent cardiac remodeling after myocardial infarction.[21]

RAAS AND HEART CELL COMMUNICATION

Heart cells communicate through intercellular junctions (gap junctions) making possible the spread of electrical current and chemical signals from cell-to-cell. Hormones, cytokines, and growth factors that are released into the blood or generated locally influence intercellular coupling. Ang II plays a seminal role on the regulation of cell-to-cell communication and impulse conduction in the heart, impairing the spread of intercellular messages particularly under pathological conditions like hypertension and heart

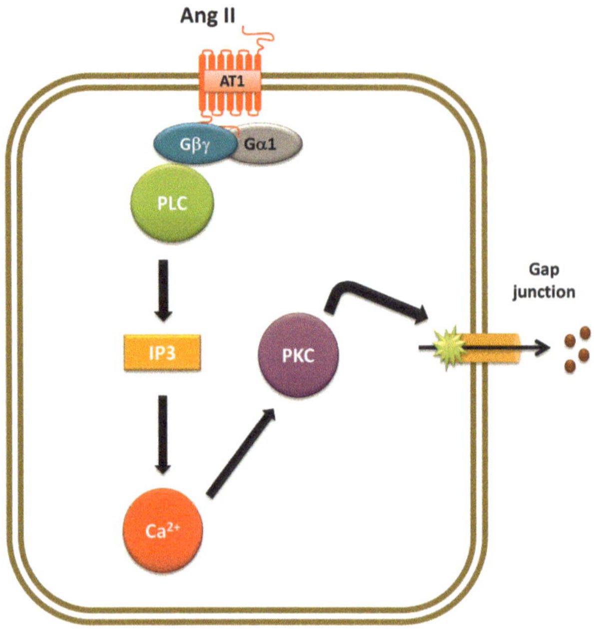

FIGURE 9.3

Signaling pathway involved in the effect of Ang II on the regulation of gap junction conductance. Gj is gap junction.

failure[20] with a consequent decrease of conduction velocity and the generation of reentrant rhythms[22] (Fig. 9.3). For example, in the heart of cardiomyopathic hamsters treated chronically with losartan an enhancement of the impulse propagation and reduction in the incidence of cardiac arrhythmias was found—an effect in part related to the decrease of interstitial fibrosis elicited by the AT1 blocker but also due to an increase in gap junction conductance.[23] The decline of gap junction communication caused by Ang II also impairs cell proliferation and metabolic cooperation between cardiac myocytes eliciting a derangement of cardiac function.[24,25] Cellular uncoupling elicited by Ang II involves binding to the AT1 receptor and PKC activation with consequent phosphorylation of Cx43 and a decrease of gap junction conductance.

AT1 RECEPTOR AS A MECHANOSENSOR

Acute mechanical stretch activates membrane channels with consequent changes in the electrical properties of the heart including shortening of the action potential, decrease of resting potential, and the generation of early after depolarizations.[26] On the other hand, stretch applied chronically activates intracellular pathways such as MAPK and second messengers responsible for cardiac remodeling.

A mechanical stimulus applied to the chest of a patient with cardiac arrest can reestablish the heart beat—the mechanoelectrical feedback. The intricate mechanisms involved in this process have been under investigation for several years, and it appears that the extracellular matrix, adherent junctions at intercalated discs, and costameric proteins at focal adhesions, are involved in the process of mechanosensing and transduction.[27] Moreover, membrane proteins including integrins and titin play an important role as mechanosensors.[28] Membrane proteins sense stretch and the information is transmitted to the nucleus with consequent change in cellular biochemistry including alteration of fetal gene expression.[29,30] Mechanical stress induces the activation of phospholipases with consequent increase in inositol tri-phosphate (IP3) and DAG leading to PKC activation and calcium influx in cardiomyocytes.[31]

Evidence has been presented that mechanical stress can activate AT1 receptors via a change in receptor conformation independently of Ang II[32,33]—an effect inhibited by an inverse agonist AT1 receptor blocker (ARB) like valsartan but not by neutral agonists like losartan.[34] Receptors exist in two states: (1) uncoupled or inactive and (2) coupled or active. The binding of the agonist activates the receptor. However, even when Ang II is unavailable, AT1 receptor can still be in the active state and hence the receptor exhibits constitutive activity. Evidence is available that an AT1 receptor can be activated by mechanical stretch of cardiac cells even in the absence of Ang II.[26,32,33] An inverse agonist is a compound that when binding to the receptor increases the number of the receptors that exist in an inactive state and reduces constitutive activity of the signaling pathway.

Experiments performed in vivo indicated that mechanical stress can activate AT1 receptors and induce ventricular hypertrophy—an effect prevented by AT1 blockers even in the absence of changes in plasma renin or Ang II. Mechanical stretch increases the potassium currents in adult rat cardiomyocytes that can be inhibited by valsartan.[26] This finding is noteworthy because the cardiac action potential involves Na and Ca inward currents and an outward potassium current, which is involved in the repolarization of the action potential. AT1 receptor activation changes the potassium conductance through PKC activation. It is then conceivable that experimental or clinical conditions characterized by an increased expression of AT1 receptors like hyperaldosteronism, lead to structural and electrical remodeling of the heart and facilitates the generation of cardiac arrhythmias.[35] Several signaling pathways including JAK-STAT, MAP kinases, and PI3K-Akt cascades can be activated by mechanical stress but the precise mechanosensors involved are not known.[27–29,35] These new concepts change our view of how ACE inhibitors benefit the heart. It is conceivable that the therapeutic advantage of valsartan as an inverse agonist AT1 receptor, is not limited to decreasing morphological remodeling, but can prevent changes in action potential duration and reduce the incidence of arrhythmias such as atrial fibrillation—an arrhythmia influenced by mechanical stress.

ROLE OF ACE INHIBITORS AND AT1 RECEPTOR BLOCKERS

The important role of Ang II on cardiac growth has been demonstrated by the ability of ACE inhibitors or ARBs to reduced ventricular hypertrophy in humans and animals.[17,27–29,36] AT1 antagonists such as losartan reduce remodeling postmyocardial infarct in the failing heart thereby decreasing mortality.[37] Patten and colleagues[36] reported that both ACE inhibitors and ARBs reduce the incidence of interstitial fibrosis by decreasing collagen I gene expression, which is an important factor in the etiology of left ventricular hypertrophy and diastolic dysfunction.[38] Indeed, treatment with ACE inhibitors in mice deficient for the AT1 prevented remodeling postmyocardial infarction and development of hypertension.[38] First attempted in animals[39] and later in clinical trials involving patients enrolled in the Survival and Ventricular Enlargement Trial, the use of ACE inhibitors proved to be of benefit [40] in patients with

LVH-associated and hypertension.[41,42] Studies have revealed that long-term intensive exercise practice induces myocardial fibrosis in rat and LV hypertrophy, an effect related to collagen deposition in the right ventricle.[43] Both effects were prevented by losartan, supporting the view that the activation of AT1 is involved in the development of fibrosis.[44]

The activation of the renin angiotensin system has a profound effect on cardiac excitability and impulse propagation. ACE inhibitors are of benefit in the failing heart by improving impulse conduction in depolarized fibers in part by activating the Na pump by a poorly defined mechanism, with a consequent increase of membrane potential but also by increasing the gap junction conductance.[24] The antiarrhythmic action of enalapril and other ACE inhibitors is now recognized particularly during atrial fibrillation.[22,24] The decrease of Ang II plasma levels induced by ACE inhibitors reduces vasoconstriction, ventricular hypertrophy, sympathetic stimulation, the plasminogen inhibitor levels as well as platelet aggregation. As a consequence of the decline of Ang II plasma levels, aldosterone secretion is decreased resulting in a reduction of the blood volume and fall in blood pressure as a result of the reduction in sodium reabsorption by the distal nephron.

ACE2/ANG (1-7) /MAS RECEPTOR AXIS ACTIVATION

Angiotensin-converting enzyme (ACE2) is an enzyme having a high homology to ACE and able to hydrolyze Ang II to the peptide angiotensin (1-7) Ang (1-7).[45,46] This heptapeptide has the Mas receptor as the endogenous binding protein[47] and counteracts many effects of Ang II including its pressor, proliferative, and profibrotic effects.[48–51] The most relevant signaling pathway of Mas receptors involves phospholipase A (PLA) with consequent generation of arachidonic acid and phosphoinositide 3 kinase (PI3K) as well as AKT to activate endothelial nitric oxide synthase (eNOS) (Fig. 9.4). Expression of Mas receptors has been described in cardiomyocytes in which acute stimulation elicited by Ang (1-7) promotes NO release by activation of eNOS. Cardiomyocytes from Mas knockout mice have a decrease in both peak calcium transient and cardiac function,[52] while intracellular injection of Ang (1-7) enhances the inward calcium current through PKA activation.[53] Ang (1-7) also reduces the incidence of heart failure after myocardial infarct in rats[49] and probably in humans,[48] enhances cardiac function, coronary perfusion, and aortic endothelial function[51,54] and increases the velocity of the electrical impulse in the failing heart[20] resulting in a decrease of slow conduction and reentry, which is an important cause of cardiac arrhythmias (Fig. 9.4).

Substantial experimental data derived from preclinical models confirm the beneficial effect of the heptapeptide, but the biological significance of ACE2-Ang (1-7)-Mas receptor axis activation in humans remains unclear.[55–58] Overexpression of ACE2, which e.g., occurs in the failing heart, does not prevent the progression of the disease.[59,60] Additionally, in the human coronary circulation, the levels of Ang (1-7) were found to be more closely associated to those of Ang I not Ang II, thereby implying no role of ACE2 on angiotensin II metabolism.[61] Furthermore, under some experimental conditions, Ang (1-7) may be harmful by exacerbating renal injury[62] and at higher doses causes abnormalities of cardiac rhythm.[58] A relationship between Ang (1–7) and diastolic pressure as well as vascular function may be sex-dependent,[62] but the precise cause of this difference is still uncertain. Contradictory results have been reported concerning the role of ACE2 in patients with coronary artery disease and heart failure due to variations in ethnicity, age, and possible polymorphism of ACE2 indicating that large-scale clinical studies are needed to confirm the role of ACE2 in human cardiovascular disease.

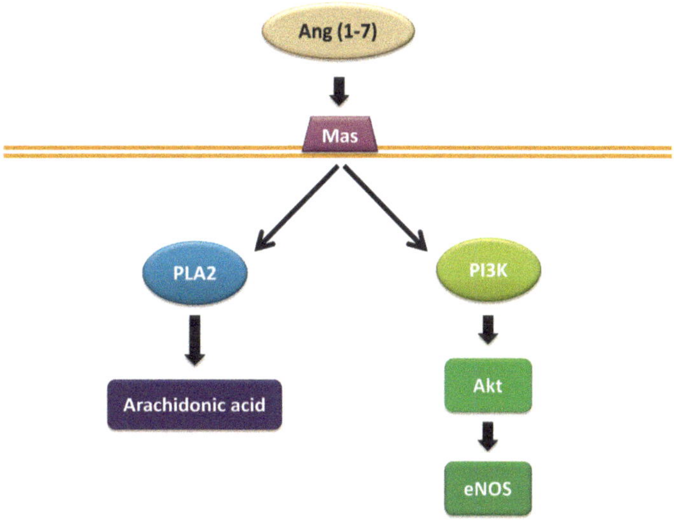

FIGURE 9.4

ACE2 converts Ang II to angiotensin (1-7) (Ang (1-7)), which has major beneficial effects in the heart mediated by Mas receptor activation.

The activation of the ACE2-Ang (1-7)-Mas receptor axis also reduces cardiac cell volume,[63] while Ang II had an opposite effect.[63,64] Cell swelling during myocardial ischemia activates the swelling-dependent chloride current ($I_{(Clswell)}$) with consequent changes of cardiac excitability. It is then reasonable to posit that the activation of the ACE2-Ang (1-7)-Mas receptor axis might potentially reduce cell volume and the activation of ionic channels[63] with a corresponding reduction of cardiac arrhythmias.

LOCAL CARDIAC RAAS, THE INTRACRINE COMPONENT

The concept that a local RAAS is present in different organs including the heart and kidney[4,35,65–72] has been substantiated by experimental and clinical evidence and opens a new window into understanding how the local RAAS contributes to local regulation of heart function. Several components of the RASS are present in the heart[73–75] including renin, angiotensinogen, ACE, and Ang II.[76] Uptake from plasma[74,75] or local synthesis of these compounds has been described especially during pathological conditions. Studies performed in the normal porcine heart demonstrated as much as 75% of cardiac Ang II is synthesized locally.[77] Moreover, cardiac Ang II levels were increased in patients with congestive heart failure[78] supporting an important role of the peptide on cardiac pathology. Experimental studies revealed that the internalization of the Ang II-AT1 receptor complex contributes significantly to the intracellular levels of the peptide and that the internalized AT1 receptor is displaced to different organelles including the nucleus and mitochondria.[79] The cytoplasmic tail of AT1 is involved in internalization of the receptor and may also target internalized receptor to the nucleus. The activation of AT1 receptor binding sites in the cell nuclei elicits an increase in calcium[80] and the expression of TGF-β1 and NHE-3.[81] Stimulation of cardiac nuclear Ang-II receptors by their ligands modulates NO and IP3, which participate in fine-tuning the regulation of local calcium release.[80]

Although several transgenic mouse models where cardiac-specific overexpression of Ang II have been developed to investigate the physiological significance of the local RAAS, the results from these studies of the pathophysiology related to Ang II expression in the heart per se are contradictory. For example, some models showed ventricular hypertrophy or fibrosis while others report no hypertrophy (see Ref. [20]). The conclusion was that cardiac remodeling is more dependent on hemodynamic changes than on local Ang II levels. In some models, the production of Ang II in cardiac muscle driven by a αMHC promoter increased the release of Ang II by 20-fold, but no hypertrophy was observed. In transgenic mouse lines overexpressing cardiac-specific angiotensinogen, Ang II was increased in cardiac muscle but not in plasma, and ventricular hypertrophy was found despite no change in blood pressure.[82] In this particular model the hypertrophy was abolished by ACE inhibitors or AT1 blockers[83] and supports a conceptual framework whereby the local RAAS contributes to cardiac remodeling. A possible explanation for these discrepant results[84] may be the different animal species or experimental conditions used. Furthermore, the primary endpoint used to define cardiac remodeling in many of these models was ventricular hypertrophy leaving aside other relevant aspects of cellular remodeling like changes in cell communication and fibrosis as well as expression and function of ionic channels that are involved in the generation of cardiac arrhythmias.

The presence of components of the RAAS in cardiac cells raised the question if they are synthesized intracellularly or reached the cell interior through internalization. Renin synthesized by cardiomyocytes appears to be of physiological importance as renin expression is increased after myocardial infarction[85] or after cardiomyocyte stretch.[84] Indeed, a renin transcript that does not encode a secretory signal and remains inside the heart cell is overexpressed during myocardial infarction[85] suggesting functional properties (Fig. 9.5). Further, cytosolic renin protein exerts functions different and even opposite to those of secretory renin that enhances necrotic death of cardiac cells while the cytosolic renin isoform protects cells from necrotic death.[85] The regulation of the secretory adrenal RAAS clearly is different from the regulation of the circulatory RAAS because under potassium load the activity of the renal and circulatory RAAS is suppressed, whereas activity of the adrenal RAAS is stimulated.[85]

The influence of intracellular renin and Ang II on cardiac cell function was demonstrated when both compounds were dialyzed into cardiac myocytes from the failing heart. Renin and particularly Ang II decreases cell communication by increasing the gap junction resistance through PKC activation and phosphorylation of connexins. Moreover, the inward calcium current in cardiac cells was reduced by intracellular Ang II.[4,22,24,66,67] The decrease of gap junction conductance elicited by intracellular Ang II impairs electrical coupling and mechanical synchronization generating slow conduction and cardiac arrhythmias.[22] Studies performed on the intact ventricle of normal rats reveal that intracellular renin depolarizes ventricular fibers and decreased the action potential duration at 50% and at 90% repolarization, respectively, while the cardiac refractoriness was decreased with consequent generation of triggered activity.[86] The intimate mechanism by which intracellular renin alters cardiac excitability is in part related to a change of potassium current, which is responsible for repolarization of the action potential.[86] Furthermore, the possible role of an intracellular renin receptor[87] that is activated by renin cannot be discarded.[86,87]

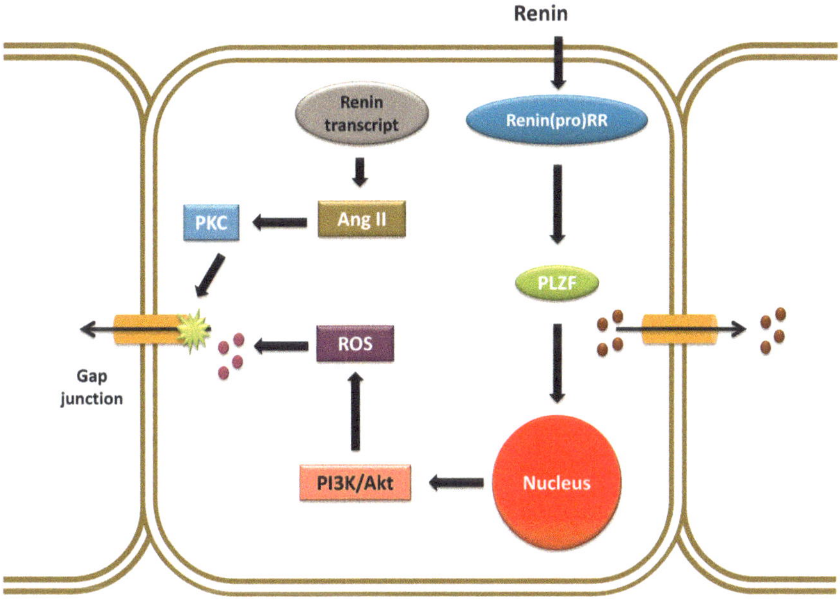

FIGURE 9.5

Role of intracellular renin due internalization or intracellular synthesis on gap junctional communication between heart cells. (pro)RR is the prorenin receptor.

INTRACELLULAR RENIN ALTERS CHEMICAL COMMUNICATION AND METABOLIC COOPERATION

The role of gap junctions is not limited to the spread of electrical current between cardiac cells but are also involved the process of chemical communication between the cardiomyocytes making possible the intercellular diffusion of nucleotides, amino acids, and other molecules small than approximately 1 kD.[88]

Intracellular renin and Ang II disrupt the chemical communication between cardiac cells impairing metabolic cooperation and generating a metabolic imbalance in cardiac muscle.[89,90] Of particular interest was the finding that glucose flows from cell-to-cell through gap junctions and that intracellular renin and Ang II impair the intercellular diffusion of glucose.[91] Furthermore, high glucose disrupts the intercellular flux of glucose[91] by eliciting a hyperphosphorylation of connexin43 that is the main connexin present in cardiac gap junctions.[91] The intercellular flow of glucose may regulate the homogenous distribution of glucose through the cardiac muscle preventing unequal generation of ATP and might be expected to have important implications for the diabetic heart.

MITOCHONDRIA, THE NUCLEUS AND THE INTRACRINE RENIN-ANGIOTENSIN SYSTEM

Evidence has been presented that different components of the RAAS including enzymes, angiotensins, and their receptors can be transported intracellularly via secretory vesicles to the cell surface, to mitochondria, or to the nucleus and that the activation of the mitochondrial Ang system is coupled to mitochondrial NO production.[92] The binding of Ang II to mitochondria AT2 receptors, for instance, stimulates NO formation suppressing mitochondrial oxygen consumption.[92] Nuclear Ang II can also stimulate NO formation through AT2 receptor activation. The pathophysiological significance of renin or Ang II in mitochondria is not known, but considering the role of Ang II in oxidative stress, it is conceivable that the activation of AT1 or AT2 receptors in mitochondria may be involved in the etiology of heart or kidney failure. In this regard, ROS can act as signaling molecules inducing gene expression and developing adaptation of the cell to low oxygen levels.[93–95] Conversely, enhanced oxidative stress is associated with heart disease and cardiomyopathy induced by Ang II infusion in rodents is related to increased mitochondrial ROS generation.[95] AT2 receptors localization in the mitochondrial inner membrane suggests their importance to NO production. Although these findings strongly support mitochondria as a component of the intracrine RAS their physiological role is not well defined.

ALDOSTERONE AND MINERALOCORTICOID RECEPTOR

Aldosterone is a central regulator of blood volume and blood pressure; however, available data also suggests that aldosterone has many effects independent of its regulatory role on blood volume. For example, aldosterone binds to the mineralocorticoid receptor (MR), which resides predominantly in the cytoplasm and upon ligand binding the MR acts as a transcription factor inducing cardiac remodeling including hypertrophy and fibrosis. Genomic and nongenomic effects of aldosterone have been described (Fig. 9.6). The transcription effects of aldosterone take more than 3 hours while rapid nongenomic effects can occur within minutes. Signaling pathways related to the rapid MR/aldosterone responses include the MAPK family as well as PKC as well as intracellular levels of calcium, cAMP and NO.

Aldosterone antagonists, like eplerenone, are beneficial to patients with heart failure by reducing cardiac remodeling. The randomized aldactone evaluation study trial indicated a beneficial effect of the aldosterone receptor antagonist spironolactone on morbidity and mortality of patients with heart failure mainly related to the decrease of fibrosis[96] (Fig. 9.7). Aldosterone, like Ang II, stimulates fibroblast growth and synthesis,[97] induces both oxidative stress and inflammation;[97] however, spironolactone inhibits both effects of the hormone and was beneficial to patients with heart failure in part by reducing myocardial fibrosis and improving diastolic dysfunction. As aldosterone synthesis in cardiac muscle is enhanced in the failing heart,[98,99] this supports the concept that aldosterone contributes to the effect of local RAAS.[20] Moreover, the MR antagonist eplerenone reduces cardiac remodeling, the incidence of cardiac arrhythmias and improves impulse propagation, an effect in part related to the antifibrotic effect of the drug but also to the activation of the electrogenic sodium pump.[100] These effects of eplerenone are not necessarily related to the blood pressure. Furthermore, the intracrine renin angiotensin component involves aldosterone and its receptor because eplerenone administered chronically to the failing heart abolished the intracellular action of Ang II on the inward calcium current,[56] an effect reversed by aldosterone and related to a decrease of intracellular AT1 receptor levels.[101]

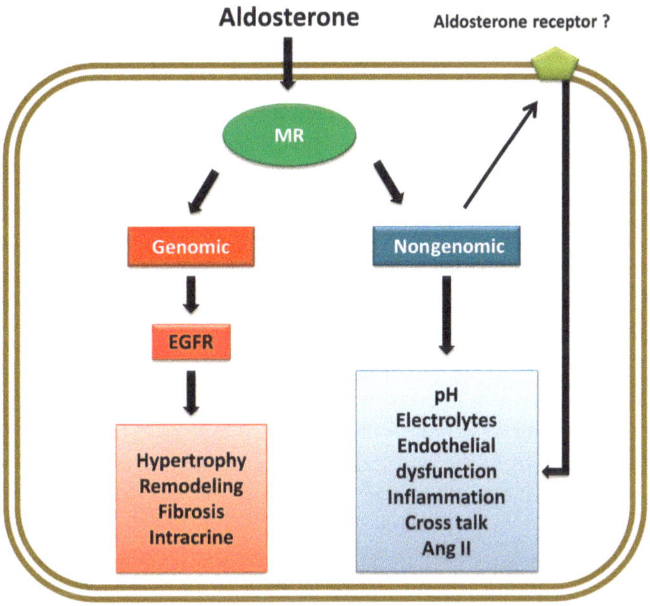

FIGURE 9.6

Genomic and nongenomic effects of aldosterone on cardiac muscle.

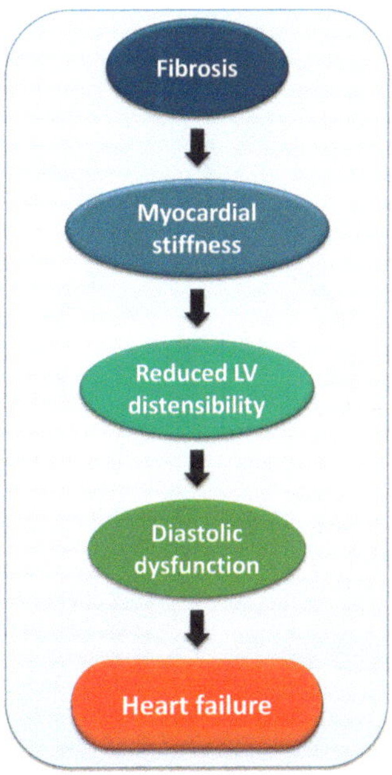

FIGURE 9.7

Interstitial fibrosis leads to ventricular stiffness with consequent generation of diastolic dysfunction and heart failure.

Activation of MR by aldosterone modulates the expression of membrane subunits of the epithelial Na+ channel in coordination with glucocorticoid-regulated kinase-1. The hormone also elicits a rapid "nongenomic" effect activating several protein kinases in cardiovascular and renal tissues. The nongenomic effect of the hormone, which can be mediated through MR activation or to a possible aldosterone receptor located at cell membrane, regulates pH, cell volume, electrolytes, and causes endothelial dysfunction, inflammation, and cardiac remodeling. In these complex set of events, there is a crosstalk with Ang II and epidermal growth factor.

NEW DEVELOPMENTS

ANGIOTENSIN (1-12)

Ang (1-12), a peptide containing a two-amino acid (Leu11-Tyr12) C-terminal extension of Ang I and initially isolated and identified from the rat small intestine, is present in high concentrations in several tissues, including the heart, kidney, and aorta.[102,103] The relevance of this finding is that Ang (1-12) might be a significant source of Ang II independently of renin[104] (Fig. 9.8). The enzyme responsible for angiotensinogen cleavage to Ang (1-12), however, is not known and further studies are needed to clarify this point. Possible candidates are chymase, cathepsins or the kallikrein-kinin system. Because

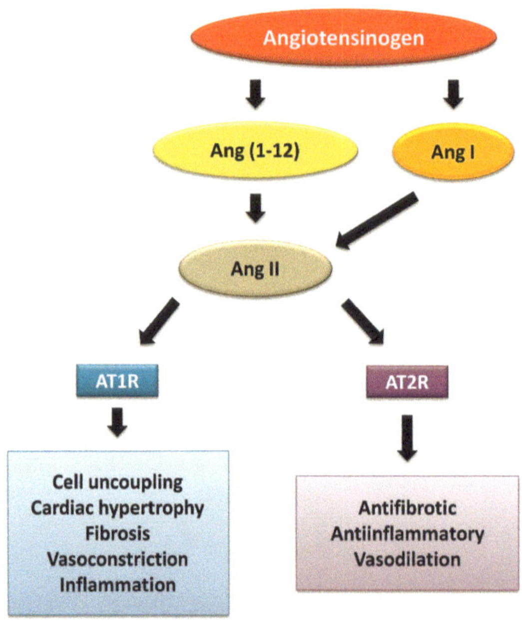

FIGURE 9.8

Formation of angiotensin (1-12) (Ang (1-12)) from angiotensinogen and the possible effect on the cardiovascular system mediated by Ang II.

the tissue levels of Ang (1-12) are not changed by bilateral nephrectomy or renin inhibition,[105] the possibility that the peptide plays an important role on the local generation of Ang II has been considered.[106] Recent observations revealed that higher Ang (1-12) expression and upregulation of chymase gene transcripts are found in the atrial appendages of subjects with left heart disease suggesting a role of Ang (1-12) in the process of atrial remodeling.[107] Because mechanical stress enhances the expression of angiotensinogen in cardiac cells, it has been posited that stretch of the atrial wall may promote the synthesis of Ang (1-12) with consequent alteration of atrial cell function.

NEPRILYSIN INHIBITORS

A new protocol for treatment of patients with heart failure was approved involving neprilysin inhibitors. The natriuretic peptides adrenomedullin and bradykinin can reduce vasoconstriction, sodium retention, and cardiac remodeling[108–110] and neprilysin—an enzyme responsible for the breakdown of these peptides—might benefit patients with cardiac diseases. The activity of neprilysin is found to be enhanced in the failing heart justifying the use of neprilysin inhibitors in patients with this condition.[111] Indeed, the PARADIGM-HF trial[112] revealed that a new drug involving the angiotensin receptor-neprilysin inhibitor is of benefit particularly in patients with heart failure with preserved ejection fraction and after myocardial infarction.

(PRO)RENIN RECEPTOR

Renin and prorenin bind to the (pro) renin receptor (P)RR, also named ATP6ap2.[113] This is an accessory protein of the vacuolar type H+ -ATPase (V-ATPase) present in membranes of intracellular components and is involved in protein degradation and vesicle trafficking. In addition, (P)RR can also induce ERK1/2 activation independent of the angiotensin signaling pathway. (P)RR knockout mice are lethal, and cardiac cell ablation of this receptor in mice causes death within weeks due to heart failure. Although the binding of prorenin to the (P)RR may be involved in the development of diabetic nephropathy, studies on the possible relation between (P)RR expression and the development of hypertension and other cardiac diseases yielded disappointing results showing no role of (P)RR on organ damage.[113] Further studies will be required to exclude the possible role of this receptor on cardiovascular pathophysiology.

RENIN INHIBITION

Although ACE inhibitors and ARBs proved to be of great benefit for patients with myocardial infarction and ischemic heart disease, mortality remains high. This might be related to the fact that complete blockade of the RAAS is not achieved with these drugs. Aliskiren, a direct renin inhibitor, has been introduced into the list of drugs useful in the treatment of hypertension and cardiac diseases. Experimental studies indicate that aliskiren reduces the left ventricular remodeling after myocardial infarction,[113] increases NO bioavailability, and inhibits atherosclerosis. Low-dose aliskiren also reduces the cardiac electrical remodeling in a hypertensive animal model.[114] Despite these beneficial effects of aliskiren in preclinical models, clinical trials have provided disappointing results. For example, the ASTRONAUT trial[52] reported there was no significant change of LV ejection fraction, cardiovascular death or re-hospitalization in the patients with acute heart failure after 6 months of treatment with aliskiren. Moreover, patients had a higher rate of hyperkalemia, worsening renal function and frequent episodes of hypotension. In contrast, other studies have report aliskiren to be a safe antihypertensive drug. Further studies are needed to support the use of this drug in the treatment of cardiac and vascular disease.

In summary, the activation of the conventional RAAS and the presence of RAAS components in the heart (the intracrine component) are responsible for regulation of cardiac contractility and excitability and contribute to cardiac pathology inducing structural and electrical remodeling. ACE inhibitors as well as ARBs are of benefit for patients with heart failure, hypertension, and myocardial ischemia. The activation of the ACE2/Ang (1-7)/Mas receptor axis counteracts many effects of the ACE/Ang II/AT1 receptor axis activation reducing cardiac remodeling, improving cell communication and impulse propagation with consequent decrease of cardiac arrhythmias. Furthermore, aldosterone antagonists reduce cardiac fibrosis with consequent increase of end diastolic volume and amelioration of diastolic heart failure. The presence of a local RAAS in the heart, by the expression or internalization of RAAS components, might be exploited for the development of therapeutic agents.

REFERENCES

1. Berry C, Touyz R, Dominiczak AE, Dominiczak AF, Webb RC, Johns DG. Angiotensin II receptors: signaling, vascular pathophysiology and interaction with ceramide. *Am J Physiol Heart Circ Physiol* 2001;**281**:H2337–65.
2. Tang SS, Schumaker R, Dzau VJ. Characterization of nuclear angiotensin II-binding sites in rat liver and comparison with plasma membrane receptors. *Endocrinology* 1992;**131**:374–80.
3. Zhuo JL, Ferrao FM, Zheng Y, Li XC. New frontiers in the intrarenal Renin-Angiotensin system: a critical review of classical and new paradigms. *Front Endocrinol (Lausanne)* 2013;**4**:166. http://dx.doi.org/10.3389/fendo.2013.00166. eCollection 2013.
4. De Mello WC. Is an intracellular renin angiotensin system involved in the control of cell communication in heart? *J Cardiovasc Pharmacol* 1994;**23**:640–6.
5. Asano K, Dutcher D, Port J, et al. Selective down regulation of the angiotensin II AT1 receptor subtype in failing human ventricular myocardium. *Circulation* 1997;**95**:1193–200.
6. Studer R, Reinecke H, Muller B, et al. Increase angiotensin I converting enzyme gene expression in the failing human heart. *J Clin Invest* 1994;**94**:301–10.
7. Zisman IS, Abraham WT, Meixell GE, et al. Angiotensin II formation in the intact human heart: predominance of the angiotensin converting enzyme pathway. *J Clin Invest* 1995;**95**:1490–8.
8. Guo DF, Sun YL, Hamet P, Inagami T. The angiotensin II type 1 receptor and receptor-associated proteins. *Cell Res* 2001;**11**(3):165–80.
9. Murazawa S, Mori Y, Nozawa Y, et al. Angiotensin II type I receptor-induced extracellular signal-regulated protein kinase activation is mediated by Ca2+ /calmodulin-dependent transactivation of epidermal growth factor receptor. *Circ Res* 1998;**82**:1338–48.
10. Aikawa R, Komuro I, Naggai R, Yazaki Y. Rho plays an important role in angiotensin II-induced hypertrophic responses in cardiac myocytes. *Mol Cell Biochem* 2000;**212**:177–82.
11. Kambayashi Y, Bardhan S, Takahashi K, et al. Molecular cloning of a novel angiotensin II receptor isoform involved in phosphotyrosine phosphatase inhibition. *J Biol Chem* 1993;**268**:24543–6.
12. Inagami T, Eguchi S, Numagushi K, et al. Cross talk between angiotensin receptor and the tyrosine kinases and phosphatases. *J Am Soc Nephrol* 1999;**10**(Suppl. 11):S57–61.
13. Unger T, Culman J, Gohlke P. Angiotensin II receptor blockade and end-organ protection: pharmacological rationale and evidence. *J Hypertens* 1998;**16**:S3–S9.

14. Liu Y, Leri A, Li B, et al. Angiotensin II stimulation in vitro induces hypertrophy of normal and postinfarcted ventricular myocytes. *Circ Res* 1998;**82**:1145–59.
15. Booz GW, Baker KM. Role of type 1 and type 2 angiotensin receptors in angioyensin II- induced cardiomyocyte hypertrophy. *Hypertension* 1996;**28**:635–40.
16. Pitt B, Poole-Wilson PA, Segal R, et al. Effect of losartan compared with captopril on mortality in patients with symptomatic heart failure: randomized trial-the Losartan Heart Failure Survavil Study ELITE II. *Lancet* 2000;**355**:1582–7.
17. Cohn JN, Tognoni G. A randomized trial of the angiotensin-receptor blocker valsartan in chronic heart failure. *New Engl J Med* 2001;**345**:1667–75.
18. Yang Z, Be CM, French BA, et al. Angiotensin II type 2 receptor overexpression preserves left ventricular function after myocardial infarction. *Circulation* 2002;**106**:106–11.
19. Susuki S, Kanazawa T, Iwai M, Horiuchi M. Angiotensin II AT2 receptors and cardiac function. In: De Mello WC, editor. *Renin angiotensin II and the heart.* West Sussex, UK: John Wiley and Sons; 2004. p. 85–99.
20. De Mello WC, Frohlich ED. Clinical perspectives and fundamental aspects of local cardiovascular and renal Renin-Angiotensin systems. *Front Endocrinol (Lausanne)* 2014;**5**:16. http://dx.doi.org/10.3389/fendo.2014.00016 eCollection 2014.
21. De Mello WC, Frohlich ED. On the local cardiac renin angiotensin system. Basic and clinical implications. *Peptides* 2011;**32**(8):1774–9. http://dx.doi.org/10.1016/j.peptides.2011.06.018. Epub 2011 Jun 25.
22. De Mello WC. Cardiac arrhythmias: the possible role of the renin-angiotensin system. *Mol Med (Berl)* 2001;**79**(2–3):103–8.
23. De Mello WC, Specht P. Chronic blockade of angiotensin II AT1-receptors increased cell-to-cell communication, reduced fibrosis and improved impulse propagation in the failing heart. *J Renin Angiotensin Aldosterone Syst* 2006;**7**(4):201–5.
24. De Mello WC. Cell coupling and impulse propagation in the failing heart. *J Cardiovasc Electrophysiol* 1999;**10**(10):1409–20.
25. De Mello WC. Intracellular angiotensin II disrupts chemical communication and impairs metabolic cooperation between cardiac myocytes. *Peptides* 2015;**72**:57–60. http://dx.doi.org/10.1016/j.peptides.2015.04.001. [Epub ahead of print].
26. De Mello WC. Mechanical stretch reduces the effect of angiotensin II on potassium current in cardiac ventricular cells of adult Sprague Dawley rats. On the role of AT1 receptors as mechanosensors. *J Am Soc Hypertens* 2012;**6**(6):369–74. http://dx.doi.org/10.1016/j.jash.2012.08.006. Epub 2012 Oct 11.
27. Linke WA. Sense and stretch ability: the role of titin and titin-associated proteins in myocardial stress-sensing and mechanical dysfunction. *Cardiovasc Res* 2008;**77**:637–48.
28. Linke WA, Knoll RH. Cardiac mechanosensation and clinical implications. *Eur J Cardiovasc Med* 2010;**1**:33–7.
29. Han B, Bai XH, Lodyga M, Xu J, Burton B, et al. Conversion of mechanical forces into biochemical signaling. *J Biol Chem* 2004;**279**:54793–5480.
30. Lang F, Busch GL, Ritter M, Volkl H, et al. Functional significance of cell volume regulatory mechanisms. *Physiol Rev* 1998;**78**:247–306.
31. Sadoshima J, Xu Y, Slayter HS, Izumo S. Autocrine release of angiotensin II mediates stretch-induced hypertrophy of cardiac myocytes in vitro. *Cell* 1993;**75**(5):977–84.
32. Yasuda N, Miura S, Akazawa H, Tanaka T, Qin Y, et al. Conformational switch of angiotensin II type 1 receptor underlying mechanical stress-induced activation. *EMBO Rep* 2008;**9**:179–86.
33. Zou Y, Akazawa H, Qin Y, Sano M, Takano H, et al. Mechanical stress activates angiotensin II type 1 receptor without the involvement of angiotensin II. *Nat Cell Biol* 2004;**6**:499–506.
34. Miura S. Angiotensin II receptor blocker as an inverse agonist: a current perspective. *Curr Hypertens Rev* 2005;**1**:115–21.

35. Re RN. The implication of intracrine hormone action for physiology and medicine. *Am J Physiol Heart Circ Physiol* 2003;**284**:H751–7.
36. Patten RD, Aronovitz MJ, Einstein M, Lambert M, Pandian NG, Mendelsohn ME, et al. Effects of angiotensin II receptor blockade versus angiotensin-converting-enzyme inhibition on ventricular remodeling following myocardial infarction in the mouse. *Clin Sci (Lond)* 2003;**104**:109–18. [PubMed].
37. Azevedo CF, Cheng S, Lima JA. Cardiac imaging to identify patients at risk for developing heart failure after myocardial infarction. *Curr Heart Fail Rep* 2005;**2**:183–8. [PubMed].
38. Jin Y, Han HC, Lindsey ML. ACE inhibitors to block MMP-9 activity: new functions for old inhibitors. *J Mol Cell Cardiol* 2007;**43**(6):664–6. Published online 2007 Sep 12. 10.1016/j.yjmcc.2007.09.002.
39. Pfeffer MA, Pfeffer JM, Braunwald E. Influence of chronic captopril therapy on the infarcted left ventricle of the rat. *Circ Res* 1985;**57**:84–95.http://dx.doi.org/10.1161/01.RES.57.1.84.
40. Pfeffer JM, Pfeffer MA, Mirsky I, Braunwald E. Regression of left ventricular hypertrophy and prevention of left ventricular dysfunction by captopril in the spontaneously hypertensive rat. *Proc Natl Acad Sci USA* 1982;**79**:3310–4.http://dx.doi.org/10.1073/pnas.79.10.3310.
41. Frohlich ED. Risk mechanisms in hypertensive heart disease. *Hypertension* 1999;**34**:782–910. 1161/01.HYP.34.4.782 [PubMed] [Cross Ref].
42. Diez J, Querejata R, Lopez B, Gonzalez A, Larman M, Martinez-Ubago JL. Losartan-dependent regression of myocardial fibrosis is associated with reduction of left ventricular chamber stiffness in hypertensive patients. *Circulation* 2002;**105**:2512–710. 1161/01.CIR.0000017264.66561.3D [PubMed] [Cross Ref].
43. Gay-Jordi G, Guash E, Benito B, Brugada J, Nattel S, Mont L, et al. Losartan prevents heart fibrosis induced by long-term intensive exercise in an animal model. *PLoS One* 2013;**8**(2):e55427.http://dx.doi.org/10.1371/journal.pone.0055427.
44. Dahlof B, Herlitz H, Aurell M, Hansson L. Reversal of cardiovascular structural changes when treating essential hypertension. The importance of the renin-angiotensin-aldosterone system. *Am J Hypertens* 1992;**5**:900–11. [PubMed].
45. Donoghue M, Hsieh F, Baronas E, Godbout K, Gosselin M, et al. A novel angiotensin converting enzyme related carboxypeptidase (ACE2) converts angiotensin I to angiotensin (1-9). *Circ Res* 2000;**87**:E1–E9.
46. Tipnis SR, Hooper NM, Hyde R, Karran E, Christie G, Turner AJ. A human homolog of angiotensin converting enzyme. Cloning and functional expression as as a captopril insensitive carboxypeptidase. *J Biol Chem* 2000;**275**:33238–43.
47. Santos RA, Simoes e Silva AC, Maric C, Silva DM, Machado RP, et al. Angiotensin-(1–7) is an endogenous ligand for the G protein-coupled receptor Mas. *Proc Natl Acad Sci U S A* 2003;**100**:8258–63.
48. Tallant EA, Diz DI, Ferrario CM. State-of-the-Art lecture. Antiproliferative actions of angiotensin-(1-7) in vascular smooth muscle. *Hypertension* 1999;**34**(4 Pt 2):950–7.
49. Wysocki J, Wilsbacher L, Batlle D. Angiotensins and the heart: is angiotensin-(1-7) cardioprotective? *Hypertension* 2015;**66**(2):260–2. http://dx.doi.org/10.1161/HYPERTENSIONAHA.115.05093. Epub 2015 Jun 15.
50. Patel VB, Takawale A, Ramprasath T, Das SK, Basu R, Grant MB, et al. Antagonism of angiotensin 1-7 prevents the therapeutic effects of recombinant human ACE2. *J Mol Med (Berl)* 2015;**93**(9):1003–13. http://dx.doi.org/10.1007/s00109-015-1285-z. Epub 2015 Apr 15.
51. Niu X, Xue Y, Li X, He Y, Zhao X, Xu M, et al. Effects of angiotensin-(1-7) on the proliferation and collagen synthesis of arginine vasopressin-stimulated rat cardiac fibroblasts: role of mas receptor-calcineurin-NF-κB signaling pathway. *J Cardiovasc Pharmacol* 2014;**64**(6):536–42.http://dx.doi.org/10.1097/FJC.0000000000000151.
52. Gomes ER, Santos RA, Guatimosim S. Angiotensin-(1-7)-mediated signaling in cardiomyocytes. *Int J Hypertens* 2012:493129.

53. De Mello WC. Intracellular angiotensin (1-7) increases the inward calcium current in cardiomyocytes. On the role of PKA activation. *Mol Cell Biochem* 2015;**407**(1–2):9–16. http://dx.doi.org/10.1007/s11010-015-2449-4. Epub 2015 May 16.
54. Zisman LS, Keller RS, Weaver B, Lin Q, Speth R, Bristow MR, et al. Increased angiotensin (1-7) forming activity in failing human heart ventricles: evidence for upregulation of the angiotensin converting enzyme homolog, ACE2. *Circulation* 2003;**108**:1707–12.
55. Ferrario CM, Chappell MC, Tallant EA, Brosnihan KB, Diz DI. Counterregulatory actions of angiotensin (1-7). *Hypertension* 1997;**30**:535–41.
56. Crackower MA, Sarao R, Oudit GY, Yagil C, Kozieradzki I, Scanga SE, et al. Angiotensin-converting enzyme 2 is an essential regulator of heart function. *Nature* 2002;**417**(6891):822–8.
57. Ferrario CM, Trask AJ, Jessup JA. Advances in biochemical and functional roles of angiotensin-converting enzyme 2 and angiotensin-(1-7) in regulation of cardiovascular function. *Am J Physiol Heart Circ Physiol* 2005;**289**:H2281–90.
58. De Mello WC, Ferrario CM, Jessup JA. Beneficial versus harmful effects of Angiotensin (1-7) on impulse propagation and cardiac arrhythmias in the failing heart. *J Renin Angiotensin Aldosterone Syst* 2007;**8**:74–80.
59. Burrell LM, Harrap SB, Velkoska E, Patel SK. The ACE2 gene: its potential as a functional candidate for cardiovascular disease. *Clin Sci (Lond)* 2013;**124**(2):65–76.
60. Zimmerman D, Burns KD. Angiotensin- (1–7) in kidney disease: a review of the controversies. *Clin Sci* 2012;**123**:333–46.
61. Campbell DJ, Zeitz CJ, Esler MD, Horowitz JD. Evidence against a major role for angiotensin converting enzyme-related carboxypeptidase (ACE2) in angiotensin peptide metabolism in the human coronary circulation. *J Hypertension* 2004;**22**:1971–6.
62. Sullivan JC, Rodriguez-Miguelez P, Zimmerman MA, Harris RA. Differences in angiotensin (1-7) between men and women. *Am J Physiol Heart Circ Physiol* 2015;**308**(9):H1171–6. http://dx.doi.org/10.1152/ajpheart.00897.2014. Epub 2015 Feb 6.
63. De Mello WC. Cell swelling, impulse conduction, and cardiac arrhythmias in the failing heart. Opposite effects of angiotensin II and angiotensin (1-7) on cell volume regulation. *Mol Cell Biochem* 2009;**330**(1–2):211–7. http://dx.doi.org/10.1007/s11010-009-0135-0. Epub 2009 May 30.
64. De Mello WC. Angiotensin (1-7) re-establishes heart cell communication previously impaired by cell swelling: implications for myocardial ischemia. *Exp Cell Res* 2014;**23**(2):359–65. http://dx.doi.org/10.1016/j.yexcr.2014.03.006. Epub 2014 Mar 18.
65. De Mello WC, Danser AHJ. Angiotensin II and the heart. On the intracrine renin angiotensin system. *Hypertension* 2000;**35**:1183–8.
66. De Mello WC. Influence of intracelular renin on heart cell communication. *Hypertension* 1995;**25**:1172–7.
67. De Mello WC. Intracellular angiotensin II regulates the inward calcium current in cardiac myocytes. *Hypertension* 1998;**32**:076–82.
68. De Mello WC. Novel aspects of angiotensin II action in the heart. Implications to myocardial ischemia and heart failure. *Regul Pept* 2011;**166**(1–3):9–14. http://dx.doi.org/10.1016/j.regpep.2010.10.003. Epub 2010 Oct 8.
69. Re RN, Cook JL. The basis of an intracrine physiology. *J Clin Pharmacol* 2008;**48**:344–50.
70. Kumar R, Singh VP, Baker KM. The intracellular renin angiotensin system: implications in cardiovascular remodeling. *Curr Opin Nephrol Hypertens* 2008;**17**:168–73.
71. De Mello WC. Intracellular angiotensin II increases the total potassium current and the resting potential of arterial myocytes from vascular resistance vessels of the rat. Physiological and pathological implications. *J Am Soc Hypertens* 2013;**7**(3):192–7. http://dx.doi.org/10.1016/j.jash.2013.02.003. Epub 2013 Mar 26.
72. De Mello WC, Gerena Y. Eplerenone inhibits the intracrine and extracellular actions of angiotensin II on the inward calcium current in the failing heart. On the presence of an intracrine renin angiotensin aldosterone system. *Regul Pept* 2008;**151**(1–3):54–60.

73. Bader M. Role of the local renin–angiotensin system in cardiac damage: a minireview focusing on transgenic animal models. *J Mol Cell Cardiol* 2002;**34**:1455–62.
74. Kurdi M, De Mello WC, Booz GW. Working outside the system: an uptodate on unconventional behavior of the renin angiotensin system components. *Int J Biochem Cell Biol* 2005;**37**:1357–67. 488.
75. Danser AH, van Kats JP, Admiraal PJ, Derkx FH, Lamers JM, Verdouw PD, et al. Cardiac renin and angiotensins. Uptake from plasma versus in situ synthesis. *Hypertension* 1994;**24**(1):37–48.
76. Zhou J, Allen AM, Yamada H, Sun Y, Mendelsohn FAO. Localization and properties of angiotensin converting enzyme and angiotensin receptors in the heart. In: Lindpaintner K, Ganten D. eds. *The Cardiac-Renin Angiotensin System*. Armonk, NY: Futura Publishing Co Inc. 1994:63–88.
77. Serneri GG, Boddi M, Cecioni I, Vanni S, Coppo M, Papa ML, et al. Cardiac angiotensin II formation in the clinical course of heart failure and its relationship with left ventricular function. *Circ Res* 2001;**88**:961–8. 531.
78. Gwathmey TM, Alzayadneh EM, Pendergrass KD, Chappell MC. Novel roles of nuclear angiotensin receptors and signaling mechanisms. *Am J Physiol Regul Integr Comp Physiol* 2012;**302**(5):R518–30.
79. Li XC, Zhuo JL. Intracellular Ang II directly induces in vitro transcription of TGF-B1, MCP-1 and NHE-3 mRNAs in isolated rat cortical nuclei via activation of nuclear AT1 receptor. *Am J Physiol Renal Physiol* 2008;**294**:C1034–45.
80. Tadevosyan A, Vaniotis G, Allen BG, Hébert TE, Nattel S. G protein-coupled receptor signaling in the cardiac nuclear membrane: evidence and possible roles in physiological and pathophysiological function. *J Physiol* 2012;**590**(Pt 6):1313–30.
81. Zhuo JL, Li XC, Garvin JL, Navar LG, Carretero OA. Intracellular Ang II induces cytosolic Ca2+ mobilization by stimulating intracellular AT1 receptors in proximal tubule cells. *Am J Physiol Renal Physiol* 2006;**290**:F1382–90.
82. Reudelhuber TL, Bernstein KE, Delafontaine P. Is angiotensin II a direct mediator of left ventricular hypertrophy? *Hypertension* 2007;**49**:1196–201.
83. Mazzolai L, Nussberger J, Aubert JF, Brunner DB, Gabbiani G, Brunner HR, et al. Blood pressure-independent cardiac hypertrophy induced by locally activated renin angiotensin system. *Hypertension* 1998;**31**:1324–30. 494.
84. Peters J. Cytosolic (pro) renin and the matter of intracellular renin actions. *Front Biosci (Schol Ed)* 2013;**1**(5):198–205.
85. De Mello WC. Intracellular renin alters the electrical properties of the intact heart ventricle of adult Sprague Dawley rats. *Regul Pept* 2013;**181**:45–9. http://dx.doi.org/10.1016/j.regpep.2012.12.015. Epub 2013 Jan 11.
86. Schefe JH, Menk M, Reinemund J, Effertz K, Hobbs RM, Pandolfi PP, et al. A novel signal transduction cascade involving direct physical interaction of the renin/prorenin receptor with the transcription factor promyelocytic zinc finger protein. *Circ Res* 2006;**99**:1355–66.
87. De Mello WC. On the pathophysiological implications of an intracellular renin receptor. *Circ Res* 2006;**99**:1285–6.
88. De Mello WC. Cell-to-cell diffusion of glucose in the mammalian heart is disrupted by high glucose. Implications for the diabetic heart. *Exp Cell Res* 2015;**334**(2):239–45. http://dx.doi.org/10.1016/j.yexcr.2015.01.021. Epub 2015 Feb 9.
89. De Mello WC. Intracellular renin disrupts chemical communication between heart cells. Pathophysiological implications. *Front Endocrinol (Lausanne)* 2015;**5**:238. http://dx.doi.org/10.3389/fendo.2014.00238. eCollection 2014.
90. Goodenough DA, Paul DL. Gap junctions. *Cold Spring Harb Perspect Biol* 2009;**1**(1):a002576.http://dx.doi.org/10.1101/cshperspect.a002576.
91. Abadir PM, Walston JD, Carey RM. Subcellular characteristics of functional intracellular renin-angiotensin systems. *Peptides* 2012;**38**(2):437–45. http://dx.doi.org/10.1016/j.peptides.2012.09.016 [PMC free article] [PubMed] [Cross Ref].

92. Chandel NS. Mitochondria as signaling organelles. *BMC Biol* 2014;**12** 34–12. 10.1186/1741-7007-12-34 [PMC free article] [PubMed] [Cross Ref].
93. Dai DF, Santana LF, Vermulst M, Tomazela DM, Emond MJ, MacCoss MJ, et al. Overexpression of catalase targeted to mitochondria attenuates murine cardiac aging. *Circulation* 2009;**119**:2789–97. 10.1161/CIRCULATIONAHA.108.822403 [PMC free article].
94. Vajapey R, Rini D, Walston J, Peter Abadir P. The impact of age-related dysregulation of the angiotensin system on mitochondrial redox balance. *Front Physiol* 2014;**5**:439.
95. Pitt B, Zannad F, Remme WJ, Randomized Aldactone Evaluation Study Investigators The effect of spironolactone on morbidity and mortality in patients with severe heart failure. *N Engl J Med* 1999;**341**:709–17.
96. Sun Y, Zhang J, Lu L, Chen SS, Quinn MT, Weber KT. Aldosterone-induced inflammation in the rat heart: role of oxidative stress. *Am J Pathol* 2002;**16**:1773–81.
97. Mizuno Y, Yoshimura M, Yasue H, Sakamoto T, Ogawa H, Kugiyama K, et al. Aldosterone production is activated in the failing ventricle in humans. *Circulation* 2001;**103**:72–710. 1161/01.CIR.103.1.72 [PubMed] [Cross Ref].
98. Messaoudi S, Azibani F, Delcayre C, Jaisser F. Aldosterone, mineralocorticoid receptor and heart failure. *Mol Cell Endocrinol* 2012;**350**(2):266–72. http://dx.doi.org/10.1016/j.mce.2011.06.038 [PubMed] [Cross Ref].
99. De Mello WC. Eplerenone reduces cardiac remodeling, the incidence of cardiac arrhythmias and improves impulse propagation, an effect in part related to the antifibrotic effect of the drug but also to the activation of the electrogenic sodium pump. *J Renin Angiotensin Aldosterone Syst* 2006;**7**(1):40–6.
100. De Mello WC, Gerena Y. Eplerenone inhibits the intracrine and extracellular actions of angiotensin II on the inward calcium current in the failing heart. On the presence of an intracrine renin angiotensin aldosterone system. *Regul Pept* 2008;**151**(1–3):54–60. http://dx.doi.org/10.1016/j.regpep.2008.06.003. Epub 2008 Jun 8.
101. Nagata S, Kato J, Sasaki K, Minamino N, Eto T, Kitamura K. Isolation and identification of proangiotensin-12, a possible component of the renin-angiotensin system. *Biochem Biophys Res Commun* 2006;**350**:1026–31.
102. Ahmad S, Wei CC, Tallaj J, Dell'Italia LJ, Moniwa N, Varagic J, et al. Chymase mediates angiotensin-(1-12) metabolism in normal human hearts. *J Am Soc Hypertens* 2013;**7**:128–36.
103. Moniwa N, Varagic J, Simington SW, Ahmad S, Nagata S, Von Cannon JL, et al. Primacy of angiotensin converting enzyme in angiotensin (1–12) metabolism. *Am J Physiol Heart Circ Physiol* 2013;**305**(5):H644–50.http://dx.doi.org/10.1152/ajpheart.00210.2013.
104. Ferrario CM, Varagic J, Habibi J, Nagata S, Kato J, Chappell MC, et al. Differential regulation of angiotensin-(1-12) in plasma and cardiac tissue in response to bilateral nephrectomy. *Am J Physiol Heart Circ Physiol* 2009;**296**:H1184–92.
105. McMurray JJV, Packer M, Desai AS, et al. Angiotensin-neprilisyn inhibition versus enalapril in heart failure. *N Engl J Med* 2014;**371**:993–1004.
106. Cataliotti A, Tonne JM, Bellavia D, Martin FL, Oehler EA, Harders GE, et al. Long-term cardiac pro-B-type natriuretic peptide gene delivery prevents the development of hypertensive heart disease in spontaneously hypertensive rats. *Circulation* 2011;**123**:1297–305.
107. Ye Y, Qian J, Castillo AC, Perez-Polo JR, Birnbaum Y. Aliskiren and valsartan reduce myocardial AT1 receptor expression and limit myocardial infarct size in diabetic mice. *Cardiovasc Drugs Ther* 2011;**25**:505–15.
108. Tonduangu D, Hittinger L, Ghaleh B, Le Corvoisier P, Sambin L, Champagne S, et al. Chronic infusion of bradykinin delays the progression of heart failure and preserves vascular endothelium-mediated vasodilation in conscious dogs. *Circulation* 2004;**109**:114–9.
109. Nakamura R, Kato J, Kitamura K, Onitsuka H, Imamura T, Cao Y, et al. Adrenomedullin administration immediately after myocardial infarction ameliorates progression of heart failure in rats. *Circulation* 2004;**110**:426–31.
110. McMurray JJ, Packer M, Desai AS, Gong J, Lefkowitz MP, Rizkala AR, et al. PARADIGM-HF investigators and committees. Angiotensin-neprilysin inhibition versus enalapril in heart failure. *N Engl J Med* 2014;**371**:993–1004.

111. Nagata S, Varagic J, Kon ND, Wang H, Groban L, Simington SW, et al. Differential expression of the angiotensin-(1-12)/chymase axis in human atrial tissue. *Ther Adv Cardiovasc Dis* 2015;**9**(4):168–80. http://dx.doi.org/10.1177/1753944715589717. Epub 2015 Jun 16.
112. Nguyen G, Delarue F, Burckle C, Bouzhir L, Giller T, Sraer JD. Pivotal role of the renin/prorenin receptor in angiotensin II production and cellular responses to renin. *J Clin Invest* 2002;**109**:1417–27.
113. De Mello W, Rivera M, Rabell A, Gerena Y. Aliskiren, at low doses, reduces the electrical remodeling in the heart of the TGR(mRen2)27 rat independently of blood pressure. *J Renin Angiotensin Aldosterone Syst* 2013;**14**(1):23–33. http://dx.doi.org/10.1177/1470320312463832. Epub 2012 Nov 1.
114. Gheorghiade M, Bohm M, Greene SJ, et al. Effect of aliskiren on postdischarge mortality and heart failure readmissions among patients hospitalized for heart failure: the ASTRONAUT randomized trial. *JAMA* 2013;**309**:1125–35.
115. Camargo de Andrade MC, Di Marco GS, de Paulo CI, Mortara RA, Sabatini RA, Pesquero JB, et al. Expression and localization of N-domain of Ang I converting enzymes in mesangial cells in culture from spontaneous hypertensive rats. *Am J Physiol Renal Physiol* 2006;**290**:F364–75.

CHAPTER

NUCLEAR RECEPTORS AND THE ADAPTIVE RESPONSE OF THE HEART

10

T. Parry[1], D. Ledee[2], M.S. Willis[1,3] and M.A. Portman[2]

[1]University of North Carolina, Chapel Hill, NC, United States [2]University of Washington and Seattle Children's Research Institute, Seattle, WA, United States [3]University of North Carolina, Chapel Hill, NC, United States

NUCLEAR RECEPTORS: INTRODUCTION

Nuclear receptors (NRs) are members of a large superfamily of evolutionarily related DNA-binding proteins with a primary function as transcription factors. These proteins regulate programs involved in a broad spectrum of physiological phenomena.[1,2] After sequencing of the human genome, at least 48 NRs were identified. These receptors classically have been characterized by their ability to bind DNA and regulate the expression of adjacent genes, and therefore are classified as transcription factors. Structurally, they have five domains: (1) an N-terminal A/B domain, (2) a C domain (also known as the DNA-binding domain), (3) a D domain (also known as the hinge region), (4) an # domain (also known as the ligand binding domain), and (5) the F C-terminal domain (Fig. 10.1(A)). Although their structural organization is highly evolutionarily conserved, the functions and mechanisms of action of the NRs are very diverse. Many of these receptors bind small lipophilic ligands and are therefore considered potential drug targets. Ligands trigger changes in the conformational and dynamic behavior of the receptors that in turn regulate the recruitment of coregulators, and chromatin-modifying machinery. The coregulator complex incorporates either corepressor molecules with histone deacetylase activity associated with "turned-off" conformation, or coactivator proteins with histone transacetylase activity associated with the "turned-on" conformation. Following DNA binding at site-specific response elements, the liganded NRs enhance the recruitment and/or function of the general transcription machinery[3] (Fig. 10.1(B)). However, many of the NRs are translated as splice variants that lack either the ligand binding or DNA-binding domains (DBDs). For example, splice variants of the NR thyroid hormone receptor (THR) without a ligand binding domain function as dominant negative proteins by preferentially binding to receptor DNA sites and bypassing ligand-dependent transactivation. DNA binding of variants lacking ligand binding domains can result in either transcriptional activation or repression depending on the particular receptor.

Many of the NRs bind to a wide variety of structurally diverse DNA response elements as either monomers or homodimers.[4] However, some NRs such as the peroxisome proliferator-activated receptors (PPARs) require a heterodimer partner to bind to DNA. PPARs have the ability to form heterodimers

Endocrinology of the Heart in Health and Disease. DOI: http://dx.doi.org/10.1016/B978-0-12-803111-7.00010-5

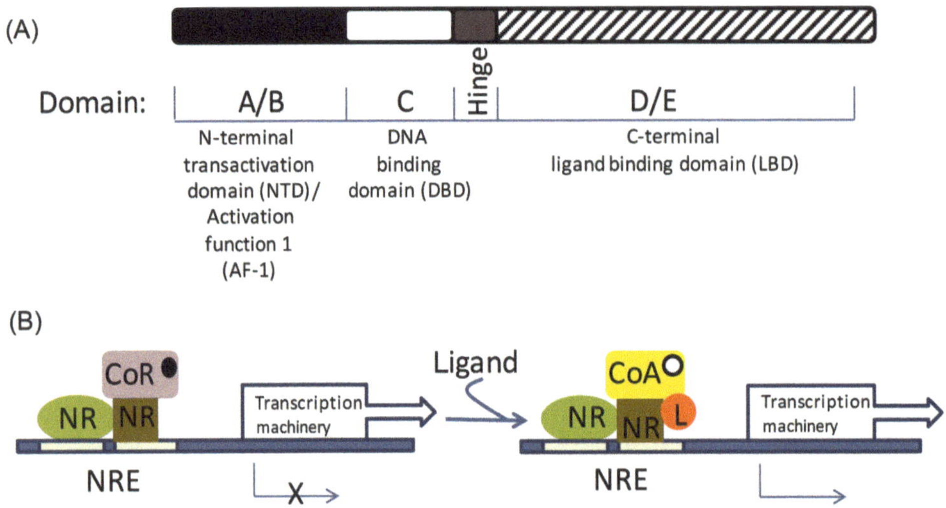

FIGURE 10.1

(A) Functional domains of NR receptors depicted schematically. (B) NRs mechanism of action. Ligand binds to NR complex and alters affinity and conformation of the complex making it compatible or incompatible to corepressors or coactivators thereby effecting changes in gene transcription. *NR*, Nuclear Receptor, *CoR*, Corepressor, *CoA*, Coactivator, *NRE*, nuclear receptor response element, ● histone deacetylase, ○ histone transdecetylase.

with the retinoid X receptor (RXR) and bind to response elements in the promoter regions of target genes. The DNA binding sequences for numerous NRs is highly variable leading to cross-reactivity and competition for these sites. Furthermore, non-DNA binding receptors can form heterodimers with other receptors either ligand or nonligand binding, thereby sequestering these away from DNA binding.[5] While these findings are fairly specific for the SHP orphan nuclear hormone receptor, it may suggest that both members of a heterodimer need to have DNA binding regions to act as a transcription factor.

NR binding to DNA in hormone response elements (HRE) depends on the spacer length between the direct repeats (DR). For instance, NRs as monomers[6,7] or heterodimers with RXRα activate (or repress) transcription of genes containing DR of AGGTCA with spacing of four base pairs (DR4), while other NRs bind at DR with different spacing. Recent studies revealed degeneracy of this spacer rule identifying substantial variability.[8] Thus, the competition between these receptors at various binding sites is highly dependent on their ability to recognize, discriminate, and bind to different (A/G) GGT(C/G/A)A core sequences.

Although the primary function of these receptors is regulation of nuclear DNA transcription, NRs also modify cellular functions independent of nuclear DNA binding. NRs are found within mitochondria and bind to response elements on mitochondrial DNA. Additionally, data suggest NRs interact with cytosolic proteins and directly regulate enzymatic function in either a ligand-dependent or—independent manner.

PGC COACTIVATORS IN THE DEVELOPING AND DISEASED HEART

Peroxisome proliferator-activated receptor γ coactivator-1α (PGC-1α) and PGC-1β are inducible, developmentally regulated transcriptional coregulators of cellular energy processes and fatty acid metabolism.[9] The coactivators bind to NRs and amplify their transcriptional activity. Three members of the PGC-1 family of transcriptional coactivators have been described: PGC-1α was first identified in a yeast two-hybrid screen as a PPARγ interaction protein after cold exposure in brown adipose tissue.[10] Two PGC-1α structural homologs were then identified including PGC-1β (also called PERC; PGC-1–related estrogen receptor coactivator) and PRC (PGC-1–related coactivator 1).[11,12] PGC-1α and PGC-1β are expressed predominantly in tissues with high mitochondrial content and high oxidative capacity, such as the heart, brown adipose tissue, skeletal muscle, and kidney. PGC-1α expression is induced during conditions that increase energy demand and mitochondrial ATP production, such as fasting, exercise, and cold exposure.[10,13,14] Additionally, PGC-1α mRNA expression is highly sensitive to thyroid stimulation. The postnatal thyroid hormone surge prompts a large increase in PGC-1 expression.[15]

PGC-1α and PGC-1β both regulate the expression of genes involved in oxidative phosphorylation via coactivation of the transcription factors NRF (nuclear respiratory factor) 1 and 2, mitochondrial transcription factor A (TFAm), and estrogen-related receptor (ERR) -α. NRF-1 and 2 regulate nuclear-encoded genes that encode proteins necessary for mitochondrial oxidative phosphorylation. PGC-1α and PGC-1β also bind to the TFAm promoter thereby coordinating the transcription of nuclear and mitochondrial target genes.[13] PGC-1α also regulates the expression of genes involved in fatty acid metabolism by coactivating the PPAR, ERR, and THR NRs[16] (discussed later). These NRs also regulate fatty acid uptake and oxidation in the heart and can form complexes with PGC-1 coactivators at specific DNA binding sites to promote transcriptional activation.

Cardiac Development. It is postulated that PGC-1 coactivators play an important role in mitochondrial biogenesis and metabolic regulation during fetal and postnatal cardiac development.[13] Initially, this role for PGC-1 coactivators was based primarily on changes in PCG-1 expression during the perinatal period in mice. Data from mice lacking PGC-1α and PGC-1β expression is limited due to lethal early postnatal cardiomyopathy induced by the loss of PGC-1 function. More recently, Martin et al. used a conditional PGC-1α/β knockout by crossing mice with skeletal muscle- and heart-specific disruption of the PGC-1β gene via Cre recombinase driven by an MCK promoter (PGC-1βf/f/MCK-Cre mice) to whole-body PGC-1α–deficient mice. MCK promoter expression is activated during the late fetal stages and, to a greater extent, the early postnatal period, resulting in mice with PGC-1β mRNA levels that were approximately one-third of control in the early postnatal period. Hearts from conditional PGC-1α/β–deficient mice exhibited mitochondrial structural derangements during postnatal growth, including fragmentation and elongation; these derangements were associated with the development of a lethal cardiomyopathy. The expression of genes involved in mitochondrial fusion (*Mfn1*, *Opa1*) and fission (*Drp1*, *Fis1*) was reduced in the hearts of PGC-1α/β–deficient mice. In unrelated studies, C2C12 myotubes and undifferentiated 10T1/2 cells (which express very low levels of endogenous ERRα and PGC-1α) as well as chromatin immunoprecipitation demonstrated that PGC-1α directly regulates *Mfn1* gene transcription by coactivating the ERRα on a conserved DNA element.[17] However, these studies may be species-specific or related to extremes due to the targeted gene strategy.

Cardiac Pathology and Heart Failure. Studies in conditional PGC-1α/β deficiency in the adult murine heart did not result in evidence of abnormal mitochondrial dynamics or heart failure.[17] However, transcriptional profiling demonstrated that PGC-1 coactivators are required for high-level expression of nuclear- and mitochondrial-encoded genes involved in mitochondrial dynamics and energy transduction. Conditional PGC-1α/β–deficient adult mice did exhibit an increase in cardiomyocyte lipid droplets, although the relevance of this finding on cardiac physiology is not known. These studies indicate that although adequate expression of PGC-1 is critical for postnatal mitochondrial biogenesis and function, the same is not true for the healthy adult murine myocardium. However, Riehle et al. found an accelerated development of heart failure in PCG-1β mice associated with increased oxidative stress and a more rapid decline in myocardial glucose utilization after transaortic constriction.[18] Furthermore, hearts from PGC-1β–deficient mice showed enhanced repression of a subset of oxidative phosphorylation genes. In summary, although PGC-1α/β deficiency does not appear to alter function or mitochondrial dynamics in normal myocardium, PGC-1β appears to be required for cardiac adaptation during pathological conditions such as pressure overload.

PGC-1 transitions during heart failure in humans have not been studied in detail due to difficulties in obtaining cardiac tissue at different time points in disease. However, Karamanlidis et al. observed mitochondrial DNA (mtDNA) depletion during the transition from right ventricular hypertrophy in infants undergoing surgery for congenital heart disease.[19] The mtDNA depletion was not due to downregulation of PGC-1 mRNA expression. Higher PGC-1 protein expression noted in failing right ventricle probably represented an attempt at compensation after mtDNA depletion through an alternative mechanism.

ESTROGEN RECEPTORS

Throughout much of their life, men are at greater risk for cardiovascular disease compared to age-matched women. However, once women reach menopause (and estrogen production rapidly declines) cardiovascular disease becomes more prevalent and risk increases, paralleling that of men.[20] This has led to the inference that estrogen is in fact cardioprotective, yet specific mechanisms for the cardioprotective effect of estrogens are lacking. Estrogen-dependent mechanisms are becoming better defined as new information emerges on how estrogen exerts activity through different receptors and how different cell types in the cardiovascular system regulate downstream signaling pathways after activation of these receptors.

STRUCTURE AND FUNCTION

Circulating hormones, including estrogen, directly influence cardiac function. Estrogen acts through four different estrogen receptors (ERs): (1) ERα, (2) ERβ, (3) a more recently identified G protein-coupled receptor 30 (GPER), and (4) a less defined ER-X in the brain.[21] ERs are widely expressed throughout the body in many tissues beyond reproductive organs, including the myocardium and vasculature, specifically endothelial cells and vascular smooth muscle cells (VSMCs).[21,22] ERα and ERβ are expressed in the extracellular plasma and nuclear membranes, while ERα is localized to the T-tubule membrane of the sarcolemma.[20] Binding of these receptors elicits both transcriptional (genomic) effects and rapid (nongenomic) cell signaling,[20,21,23,24] highlighting the multitude of possible estrogenic effects on the heart.

ESTROGEN CELL SIGNALING

In classic signaling, estrogen binding stimulates homo/heterodimerization of two ERs which then translocate to the nucleus and directly bind estrogen response elements (ERE), eliciting a transcriptional response (Fig. 10.2).[24] Nonclassical estrogen signaling occurs through direct protein–protein interactions instead of acting through the direct binding to ERE. In this environment, ERα and ERβ interact with transcription factors activating protein-1 (AP-1) and stimulating protein-1 (SP1) to indirectly

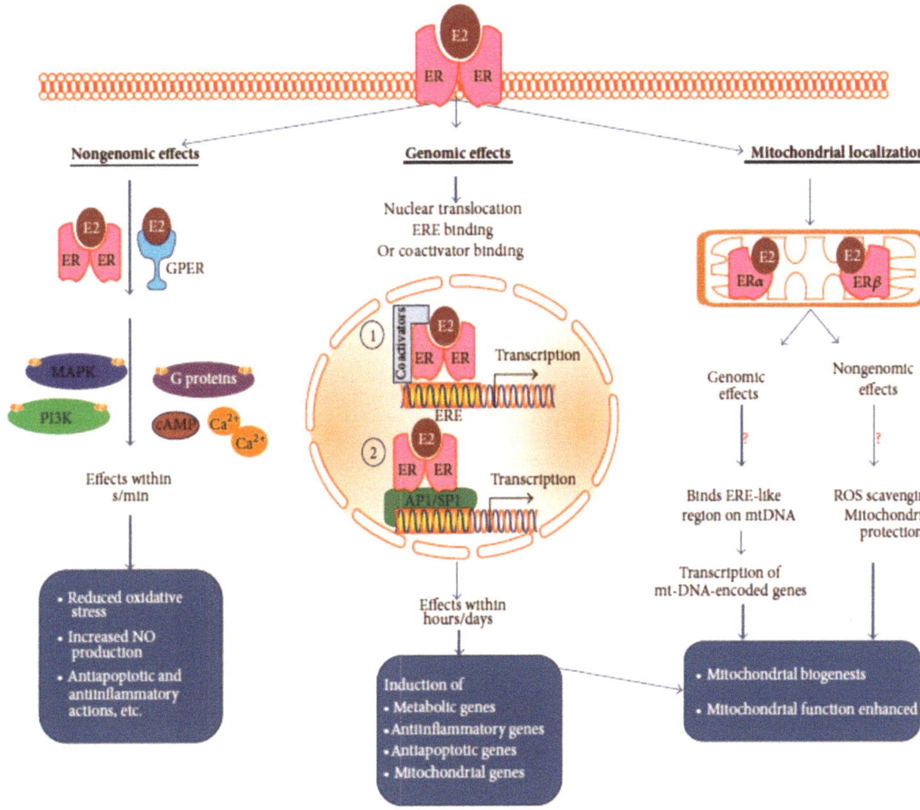

FIGURE 10.2

Estrogen receptor genomic and nongenomic signaling. Nongenomic effects may be mediated by estrogen (E2)–estrogen receptor (ER) or by E2 bound to G protein-coupled estrogen receptor (GPER) by activating signaling molecules like MAPK, PI3K, G-proteins, etc. to elicit immediate actions. Genomic effects are mediated by nuclear translocation of E2-ER complex and either (1) direct binding with estrogen response elements (ERE) along with coactivators to form a transcription complex or (2) binding to transcriptional coactivators to induced gene transcription indirectly. ERs may also localize to mitochondria to induce potentially genomic and nongenomic actions; however, the mechanisms are not well understood.

*From Gupte AA, Pownall HJ, Hamilton DJ, Estrogen: an emerging regulator of insulin action and mitochondrial function. J Diabetes Res 2015;***2015***:916585. Copyright © 2015 Anisha A. Gupte et al. Creative Commons Attribution License.*

(i.e., not directly interacting with DNA) modulate genomic signaling (Fig. 10.2).[21,24] Estrogen exerts nongenomic signaling through plasma membrane-associated ERs that interact with adaptor proteins, like c-Src, initiating intracellular signaling via PI3-K/Akt, mitogen-activated protein kinase (MAPK), and protein kinase C (PKC) pathways, stimulating downstream processes including cell death, protein synthesis, and metabolism (Fig. 10.1). Additionally, estrogen may act through GPER to initiate PI3-K/Akt and MAPK signaling, cAMP production, or calcium release and activation of calcium calmodulin-dependent kinases (Fig. 10.2).[20,23,24]

CALCIUM HANDLING

Since ERs are expressed in cardiomyocytes, it is not surprising that ERs affect cardiomyocyte contractility differentially in females based on circulating estrogen levels. Circulating estrogen modulates myocardial contractility through a negative inotropic effect, attributed to estrogen's ability to sensitize the myocardium to calcium (Ca^{2+}).[20] Evidence for this is derived from studies of cardiomyocytes isolated from female rats that function at lower levels of intracellular Ca^{2+} compared to cardiomyocytes isolated from male rats. Specifically, isolated female cardiomyocytes have a lower transient peak amplitude of cytosolic (activating) Ca^{2+} compared to isolated male cardiomyocytes.[25] Similarly, Ca^{2+} peaks measured in cardiomyocytes isolated from ovariectomized female rats (inhibited estrogen production) were significantly greater that of cardiomyocytes isolated from ovariectomized female rats supplemented with 17-beta estradiol.[26] These data suggest that estrogen possesses a unique ability to regulate Ca^{2+} handling within cardiomyocytes. Since calcium handling is central to cardiac intropy and thus function, and impaired calcium handling is associated with cardiac dysfunction, these findings may help explain why males and postmenopausal women experience cardiac complications.

Modulating cardiac intropy may be related to estrogen's action on the L-type Ca^{2+} channel (LTCC). The LTCC plays an important role in excitation–contraction coupling in muscle fibers. In cardiomyocytes, membrane depolarization causes the LTCC to release Ca^{2+}, which triggers the ryanodine receptor to release Ca^{2+} from the sarcoplasmic reticulum. This process is known as calcium-induced calcium release and is unique to cardiac myocytes. Estrogen has been shown to decrease expression of the Cav1.2 subunit of the LTCC while increasing sodium–calcium exchanger (NCX) protein expression. This would serve to decrease Ca^{2+} load and rate of contraction (effect of LTCC) and increase rate of relaxation (effect of NCX). Ovariectomization of rats increased Cav1.2 protein expression and reduced NCX-protein expression, which led to calcium overload; however, estrogen supplementation restored protein expression, assisting with cytosolic calcium clearance.[27] Additionally, female mouse hearts have a four-fold increase in NCX-protein expression compared to males, which was subsequently reduced upon ovariectomization of female mice.[28] Reduced Ca^{2+} clearing ability increases cytosolic calcium levels, leading to poor calcium handling, a characteristic of many types of cardiac dysfunction.[29] Alternatively, estrogen may suppress myocardial contractility by reducing the amount of Ca^{2+} released from the sarcoplasmic reticulum versus influencing actual LTCC Cav1.2 subunit expression.[30] This would result in a lower "gain" for Ca^{2+} release from the sarcoplasmic reticulum.[31]

REGULATION OF MITOCHONDRIAL MASS, Ca^{2+}, AND APOPTOSIS

In addition to the role of ERs in regulating cardiomyocyte contractility by sensitizing Ca^{2+} signaling in the sarcoplasmic reticulum, estrogen also plays an important regulatory role in mitochondrial function at multiple levels. Cardiomyocytes have a particularly high mitochondrial density (relative to most other cell types), which allows them to synthesize large amounts of ATP quickly, which is necessary for the ongoing high metabolic demands of the heart. In mitochondria, estrogen has a role in regulating mitochondrial biogenesis, lowering cytosolic Ca^{2+} concentrations, and increasing ATP production. Experimental evidence suggests the effects of estrogen on mitochondrial function occur through genomic and nongenomic mechanisms.[21,24] Transcriptional (genomic) regulation is evidenced by the ability of estrogen to increase protein levels of several components of the mitochondrial respiratory chain, including complex IV subunits and cytochrome c.[32] Additionally, estrogen binding to ERs stimulates critical transcription factors that regulate mitochondrial antioxidant systems (nuclear respiratory factor 1 (Nrf1), nuclear factor like 2 (Nrf2), TFAm and mitochondrial biogenesis (PGC1α).[33] This may occur sequentially, with estrogen-binding ERs, which enhance the Nrf1 transcription factor, which then activates TFAm.[34] The ERα and ERβ receptors were identified in the mitochondria and may elicit the action of estrogen directly, as both ERs bind mouse and human mtDNA encoding subunits for NADH-CoQ reductase, cytochrome oxidase, cytochrome b, and ATP synthase.[35] The nongenomic effects of estrogen may be attributed to cytosolic Ca^{2+} influx, which promotes mitochondrial sequestration of excess Ca^{2+}, allowing the adverse consequences of cytosolic Ca^{2+} overload and ultimately cell apoptosis to be avoided.[21] However, this mechanism may have negative consequences in other situations, as mitochondria are highly susceptible to reactive oxygen species (ROS)-mediated damage. Under pathological conditions, particularly oxidative stress, mitochondrial Ca^{2+} uptake may cause the mitochondrial transition pore to open, triggering the release of cytochrome c and initiate apoptotic pathways leading to cell death.[21,36] Together, these studies suggest that although estrogen may assist physiologically in mitochondrial-mediated cytosolic Ca^{2+} buffering to help delay cell death, in pathological conditions the effect of estrogen could negatively affect cardiomyocyte survival.

ISCHEMIC HEART DISEASE

In developed countries, ischemic heart disease remains the most common form of cardiovascular disease. In the United States, more women than men die of ischemic heart disease, most typically caused by coronary artery disease.[37] The growing rates of obesity, diabetes, and metabolic syndrome reflect the disproportionate effect these diseases influence ischemic heart disease in women.[37] While disease onset in women usually occurs 10 years after it does in men, the prevalence postmenopause increases rapidly such that it is comparable to men by their 80s.[38]

These sex-based observations reflect the differences in biology related to estrogen signaling in cardiomyocytes related to ER-regulated apoptosis, Akt signaling, and regulation of ROS production. The female myocardium is less susceptible to postischemic tissue necrosis, apoptosis, and overall contractile dysfunction compared to men.[20] Studies investigating heart hypertrophic rats (HHR) compared to normal heart rats (NHR) found that upon ischemia/reperfusion (I/R), female NHR had improved outcomes compared to male NHR, and associated with increased Akt expression in females. However, the Akt-mediated protection was lost when comparing I/R outcomes in female and male HHR.[39] This protective effect of phosphoinositide 3-kinase (PI3K)/Akt signaling may be related to augmented nitric oxide synthase (NOS), which has been shown to limit mitochondrial ROS production[40] while improving Ca^{2+} handling to reduce I/R injury.[41]

Estrogen may directly inhibit cardiac hypertrophy and protect against arrhythmias and ischemic heart disease. Over time, the extent of pathological cardiac hypertrophy is the most predictive risk factor for cardiovascular disease, which can lead to chronic heart failure and death. One underlying mechanism may be linked to the ability of estrogen to reduce cardiac hypertrophy, which may be ER-dependent. For example, activation of ERβ limits calcineurin activity, potentially by upregulating p38-MAPK and ERK1/2 signaling,[42] resulting in GPER suppressed hypertrophy markers atrial and brain natriuretic peptides (ANP, BNP).[43] Estrogen was also shown to protect against arrhythmias. NOS has been implicated to contribute to the antiarrhythmic effect of estrogen,[44] which may be secondary to PI3K/Akt signaling that is cardioprotective. Additionally, estrogen-induced improvements in Ca^{2+} handling may also be an underlying mechanism for cardioprotection[30] since Ca^{2+} drives cardiomyocyte contraction and relaxation.

ESTROGEN-RELATED RECEPTORS

STRUCTURE AND FUNCTION

In contrast to the gender-associated relationship between cardioprotection in females with the ER receptors and the presence of estrogen (the ER ligand), the ERRs have no known ligand to make this association. Therefore, the ERRs are classified as orphan NRs, a family of NRs that do not have identified endogenous ligands (orphan); the name "estrogen related" came about due to sequence homology with ERs—they do not bind estrogen.[45,46] While ERRs do not apparently bind to estrogen, or other nuclear steroid hormones that have been tested to date, the three ERR isoforms (ERRα, ERRβ, and ERRγ) are part of the NR 3 subfamily sharing 30–40% homology with the ligand binding domain of ERα.[45,46] In general, ERR structure is similar to that of typical NRs, however, the N-terminal/activation function (AF)-1 domain of all three isoforms contains conserved motifs subject to posttranslational by SUMOylation and phosphorylation, which serves to regulate transcriptional activity.[45,47]

While ERRs have a similar DBD as ERα, ERRs do not bind strongly to perfect palindromic to ER response elements. However, this does allow ERRs to either cooperate with ERα for full activation, or antagonize ERα to hinder activity.[45] ERRs have a DBD with two highly conserved zinc finger motifs that bind the ERR response element (ERRE) in the promoter of target genes. It has been shown that ERRs can bind to ERREs by forming homo- mono- or heterodimers. Since this DBD is nearly identical between ERRα, ERRβ, and ERRγ, ERR-regulated genes can be targeted by more than one ERR isoform.[45] Furthermore, ERRs activate or repress gene transcription without the addition of exogenous ligands, typical of NRs. This may be due to a conformation adopted by the LBD in the absence of a ligand that fosters recruitment of NR coactivators which appear to be important for ERR initiated gene transcription.[45,48] All three isoforms are upregulated in adult tissues in response to stimuli that increase oxidative capacity. In particular, ERRα and ERRγ expression and activity are highest in tissues that rely heavily on mitochondrial oxidative metabolism for ATP production, such as the heart, kidney, skeletal muscle, and brown adipose tissue.[45]

FATTY ACID OXIDATION

The first evidence that ERRs participate in regulating cardiac energy metabolism came from the observation that ERRα binds the promoter of *Acadm*, which encodes medium chain acyl-coenzyme A dehydrogenase (MCAD) enzyme and regulates the initiation of mitochondrial fatty acid oxidation

(FAO).[49,50] Since tissue MCAD expression dictates a tissue's FAO rate, MCAD levels are closely regulated and aerobic tissues like the myocardium naturally express high levels of MCAD. ERRα's recruitment of the *Acadm* promoter was later confirmed in vivo in mouse hearts by chromatin immunoprecipitation (ChIP) assays.[51] In these studies, PGC-1α increased MCAD expression in the presence of ERRα; this effect was abolished if ERRα was knocked down with siRNA illustrating the relationship between ERRα and MCAD expression.[52] Additionally, in both neonatal rat cardiomyocytes and mouse embryonic fibroblasts, ERRα led to increases in palmitate oxidation, indicating a direct effect of ERRα on mitochondrial FAO.[53]

TRANSCRIPTIONAL CONTROL OF METABOLISM

Additional studies of mouse hearts utilizing chromatin immunoprecipitation (ChIP) demonstrated that cardiac ERRα and ERRγ occupy promoter regions of genes involved in mitochondrial oxidative pathways (e.g. *Acadm*, creatine kinase mitochondrial 2, *Ckmt2*), fuel sensing (e.g. pyruvate dehydrogenase kinase isozyme 4, *Pdk4*), substrate uptake (e.g. fatty acid binding protein 4; *Fabp4*), and contractile proteins (e.g. α-myosin heavy chain, *Myh6*; β-myosin heavy chain, *Myh7*).[51] Both RRα and ERRγ target transcription factors involved in metabolism and metabolic signaling pathways, including CREB, NRF-1, and STAT3 in the adult heart.[51] ERRα was similarly shown to directly bind the PPARα promoter, activating PPARα gene expression, and contributing to ERRα regulated cardiac energy metabolism.[53] The importance of ERRs in the heart is exemplified in mice that lack ERRγ gene expression, resulting in the inhibition of myocardial transcription of glucose and fatty acid oxidative metabolic genes.[54] Together, these data provide convincing evidence for the regulation of myocardial metabolic gene transcription by ERRα and ERRγ.

ERRs regulate the transcription of other NRs previously discussed in this chapter, including thyroid hormone receptor (TRα) (see "Thyroid Hormone Receptors" section), the PGC-1 co-activator of PPAR (see "PGC Coactivators in the Developing and Diseased Heart" section), and receptor-interacting protein 140 (RIP140; also known as NR interacting protein (NRIP1)).[49] Therefore, we will discuss them only briefly in the context of ERRs. TRα plays an important role in regulating energy balance and thermogenesis in the heart.[49] In fact, the TRα1 isoform and ERRα are coexpressed in several tissues, including the heart.[49] While TRα1 does contain a perfect ERRE that is necessary and sufficient for ERRα-mediated promoter activation,[55] the deletion of the ERRE in the TRα1 promoter did not influence the ERR-mediated response to the TRα1 promoter, indicating that other sites or mechanisms may also be involved in ERRα promoter activaton.[56] The PGC-1 family of transcriptional coactivators partner with numerous nuclear and nonnuclear receptor transcription factors to stimulate the expression of genes involved in FAO, mitochondrial biogenesis, glycolysis, and gluconeogenesis in various tissues, namely those with high aerobic capacity like the heart.[57] As PGC-1α was only able to maximally activate *Acadm* transcription (encoding MCAD) and other ERRE containing genes in the presence of ERRα and ERRγ,[45,52,53] these studies indicate the codependence of multiple transcription factors on ERRs for the physiological regulation of metabolic gene expression. In a broader context, ERRs and their cooperative effects with other NRs such as THRs and the PGC-1 family of coactivators discussed in the previous sections are indicative of the widespread regulatory effect of ERRs on cardiac metabolism.

The NR cofactor RIP140 exhibits both coactivator and corepressor actions.[45] While loss of RIP140 function enhances myocyte expression of genes involved in FAO, oxidative phosphorylation, and mitochondrial biogenesis,[58] overexpression downregulates these same gene programs by repressing EERα or ERRγ binding.[59] Reduced metabolic flexibility (ability to switch from one fuel source to another) through inhibition of oxidative metabolic pathways impairs myocardial function by inducing hypertrophy and fibrosis, which reduces fractional shortening.[45] ERR's interaction with RIP140, to either enhance or reduce cardiac metabolism, further highlights the far reach of ERR's influence over cardiac metabolism and thus cardiac function.

PATHOLOGY

The progression of heart failure is clearly complex and multifactorial with many underlying mechanisms, but alterations in bioenergetics are an apparent and important part of the pathophysiology. During cardiac pressure overload, as seen clinically in hypertension, the heart undergoes pathological hypertrophy, altering the metabolic and contractile function to sustain systolic function in a compensated state. With continued stress, the heart progresses to a decompensated state, resulting in both systolic and diastolic dysfunction with inevitable metabolic deficiency.[45,49,60] In animal models of pathological hypertrophy, ERRα expression decreases in parallel with the decline in cardiac function, while mice lacking ERRα progress to heart failure more rapidly.[61] Therefore, it appears that ERRα slows metabolic decline during cardiac dysfunction, and that decreased EERα expression promotes metabolic dysregulation and cardiovascular decline. In support of this notion, ERRα and/or its PGC-1 coactivators are downregulated in various models of heart failure.[62,63] For example, pressure overload-induced cardiac hypertrophy in PGC-1α−/− and PGC-1β−/− mice resulted in an accelerated heart failure with decreased metabolic gene targets of ERR.[18,64] In humans, altered or downregulation of ERRα and/or its metabolic target genes is correlated with congestive, ischemic, and idiopathic heart failure.[65,66] Metabolic failure is also suspected to play a role in diabetic cardiomyopathy because these hearts exhibited impaired glycolysis and increased FAO with elevated triglyceride stores.[67] However, the mechanisms underlying these diseases are less defined. The downregulation of ERRα and PGC-1α cofactors may be linked to the upregulation of cofactors like RIP140 or sirtuin 1 (SIRT1), or by microRNAs, like microRNA-22, which serve to decrease EERα and its metabolic target genes.[59,62] Alternatively, SIRT1 and PPARα have been shown to form a complex that impedes binding of ERRα to ERRE and thus suppresses the expression of metabolic genes.[68]

GLUCOCORTICOID RECEPTORS

STRUCTURE AND FUNCTION

The word "glucocorticoid" is a portmanteau derived from a combination of glucose metabolism, their synthesis in the adrenal cortex, and their steroidal structure, that is: glucose+ cortex+ steroid. The glucocorticoid receptor (GR) is the receptor that binds cortisol and other glucocorticoids and, in turn, regulates gene expression. The GR is found throughout the body in every cell type, including cardiomyocytes. The DBD of the GR contains two zinc fingers that target the receptor to GR response elements, (GRE) found in the promoter region of GR target genes and can result in either activation of repression of the target genes. The NTD contains posttranslational modifications (PTMs) sites that can undergo phosphorylation, ubiquitination, SUMOylation, and acetylation that can alter the function of GR.[69] The NTD also contains the region of (AF1; transcriptional function and interacts with coactivators). The

C-terminus LBD comprises a hydrophobic glucocorticoid binding pocket and a second transcriptional activation function (AF2) for ligand-dependent interaction with coregulators. And finally, two nuclear localization signals, NL1 and NL2, are located within the DBD and the LBD.[69,70] By binding cortisol and other glucocorticoid to the LBD, the GR binds the promoter of specific genes by its DBD to regulate their expression and affect their antiinflammatory and other activities in vivo.

GENOMIC AND NONGENOMIC SIGNALING

In the absence of ligand, the GR resides in the cell cytoplasm as part of a large multiprotein complex that includes heat shock protein 90 (HSP90) (Fig. 10.3).[69,71] In this conformation, the GR is transcriptionally inactive, but readily binds glucocorticoid ligands when present. When cortisol (or other GR ligands) binds the LBD, a conformational change is induced resulting in GR dissociation from the

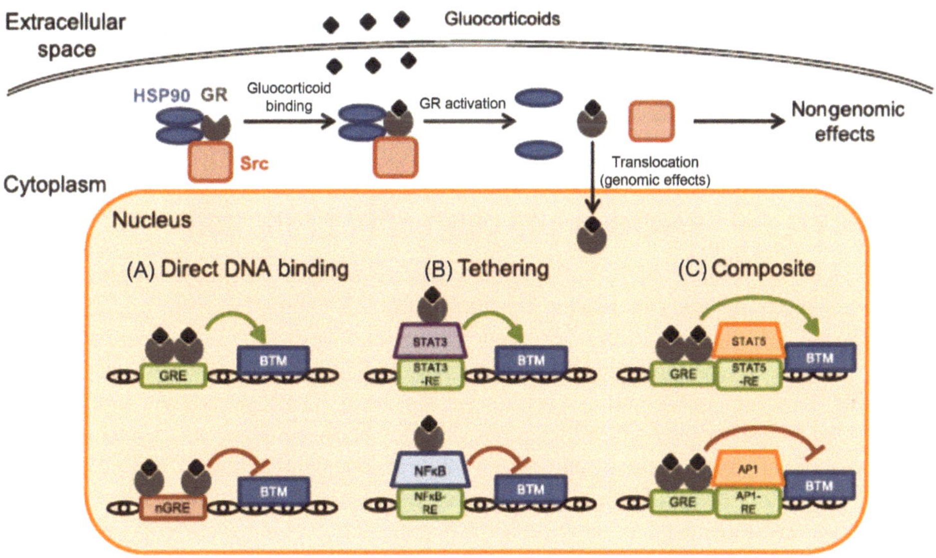

FIGURE 10.3

Glucocorticoid receptor genomic and nongenomic signaling. GR ligands induce biological changes by binding the glucocorticoid receptor (GR) and inducing genomic and nongenomic effects. Genomic effects of activated GR occur following nuclear translocation and manifest through three primary mechanisms: (A) direct binding of GR to DNA via glucocorticoid response elements (GRE) and nuclear GREs (nGREs) to activate or repress transcription, (B) tethering to DNA-bound transcription factors to modulate transcription indirectly, or (C) composite activity of DNA binding and interaction with adjacent DNA-bound transcription factors to affect transcription. Rapid nongenomic effects of GR ligation occur following ligand–induced dissociation of the GR multiprotein complex in the cytoplasm. BTM, basal transcription machinery.

*Used with permission © Elsevier 2015 (Cain DW, Cidlowski JA. Specificity and sensitivity of glucocorticoid signaling in health and disease. Best Pract Res Clin Endocrinol Metab 2015;***29***(4):545–56.*

multiprotein complex. The dissociation of GR from the multiprotein complex liberates other complex components for rapid nongenomic signaling while allowing the nuclear translocation of GR to exert genomic effects (Fig. 10.3).[69–71] Binding of GR to DNA results in conformational changes, leading to recruitment of coregulators and chromatin remodeling complexes to regulate the rate of transcription of target genes through RNA polymerase II regulation.[70,72] Many genetic and nongenetic factors influence the GR transcriptional response, including regulatory elements outside the GRE including chromatin context, and the amount of glucocorticoid bound to the LBD, respectively.[70,73] Additionally, GR interacts with other transcription factors such as AP-1, NF-κB, or the STAT family.[69,74] These interactions are either through GR-mediated "tethering" of a transcription factor and its bound response element or through composite activity where the bound GRE interacts with adjacent DNA-bound transcription factors to either activate or repress gene transcription.[69]

While the GR is encoded by a single gene, several functionally distinct isoforms exist due to alternative splicing and alternative translation initiation.[75] Exon 9 alternative splicing generates two receptor isoforms: GRα and GRβ. The GRα isoform exhibits classic hormone signaling by binding glucocorticoids and translocating to the nucleus to regulate the transcription of target genes.[74,76] Alternatively, the GRβ isoform resides in the nucleus constitutively and generally acts in opposition of GRα. The GRβ isoform can also directly regulate genes that are not controlled by the GRα isoform. In this way, GRβ negatively regulates the actions of GRα while exerting its own independent actions.[74] The differing activity of these modified GRs and GR isoforms explain the varying subcellular and tissue-specific responses of GR-mediated signaling.

CARDIOMYOCYTE Ca^{2+} HANDLING AND CONTRACTILE FUNCTION

The first clues to the role of GR in the cardiomyocyte came from a mouse model with increased human GR expression.[77] Experimentally increasing cardiomyocyte GR expression three fold the endogenous level results in only a minor reduction in ejection fraction and no change in myocardial contractility. Additionally, these hearts did not undergo adverse remodeling (as determined by hematoxylin and eosin and Sirius Red stains investigating morphological criteria: disarray, myocyte and nuclear hypertrophy, lesions, and mononuclear infiltration), nor did they show evidence of apoptosis, necrosis, or fibrosis. However, they did show electrophysiology abnormalities in the form of bradycardia and atrioventricular block. Further investigation of cardiomyocytes revealed decreases in sodium and potassium currents with increased transient Ca^{2+} amplitudes, L-Type calcium channel currents, and sarcoplasmic reticulum Ca^{2+} levels measured by whole cell patch clamp or fluorescent Ca^{2+} probes.[77] These data indicate that elevated levels of GR (and GR signaling) generate abnormal sinus node and conduction properties, but in the absence of cardiac dysfunction or adverse remodeling.

Alternatively, global GR deletion (GR−/−) in mice impaired cardiac function, with diastolic function being the most affected phenotype. Fetal cardiomyocytes from GR−/− mice were irregularly shaped, failed to align properly, and contained shortened disorganized myofibrils. Furthermore, these fetal cardiomyocytes failed to show normal developmental increases in contractile and calcium handling proteins: α myosin heavy chain (αMHC, Myh6), NCX, ryanodine receptor (Ryr2), and sarco-endoplasmic reticulum calcium ATPase (SERCA2a).[78] To control for the lack of glucocorticoid signaling the global GR−/− model, further studies were performed in conditional Cre-loxP mice with GR lacking in the myocardium and VSMC. Here, many phenotypes were similar to global GR−/− mice, but diastolic dysfunction was not present. Conditional GR−/− fetal cardiomyocytes also showed impaired alignment with short, disorganized myofibrils, and SERCA2a and Ryr2 expression were also dysregulated.[78] Together, these data indicate that GR signaling plays a role in Ca^{2+} handling and the contractile processes in the heart.

Mice lacking cardiomyocyte-specific GR (csGR−/−) were created to determine a specific role for GR in the heart. These mice developed normally, but died prematurely of heart failure at seven months of age.[79] Compared to wildtype controls, transthoracic echocardiography indicated that csGR−/− hearts were normal at one month of age in terms of cardiac function. However, by 3–6 months of age, conscious echocardiography revealed csGR−/− mice started to show signs of systolic dysfunction (reduced ejection fraction and fractional shortening percentages).[79] At six months of age, csGR−/− mice had enlarged hearts with left ventricular dilation, reduced ejection fraction and fractional shortening, without fibrosis.[79] With increases in βMHC (Myh7), skeletal muscle α-actin, smooth muscle α-actin, and BNP mRNA in the hearts of csGR−/− mice, cardiomyocyte GR is needed to maintain cardiomyocyte homeostasis and prevent pathological cardiac hypertrophy.[79] Mechanistically, hearts from csGR−/− mice demonstrated that GR supports genes responsible for maintaining myocardial contractility, repressing pathological cardiac hypertrophy, inhibiting inflammation, and promoting cardiomyocyte survival.[79] Taken together, these data convincingly demonstrate the importance of cardiomyocyte glucocorticoid signaling in the maintenance of normal cardiovascular function.

PATHOLOGY

Deficiency in glucocorticoid signaling has been linked to poor cardiac outcomes. Studies have shown that cortisol levels correlate with heart failure severity and the NYHA score and treadmill exercise capacity, but not with testosterone or cortisol/testosterone ratios.[80] This was first observed by Dr. Thomas Addison 150 years ago when patients with adrenal insufficiency (including suppressed glucocorticoid secretion) presented with "remarkable weakness" of the heart.[81] Today, Addison's disease is characterized by impaired adrenal function, including glucocorticoid production resulting in hyperglycemia, hyperkalemia, hyponatremia, hypercalcemia, and metabolic acidosis that can result in cardiac dysfunction.[70,82] Congenital adrenal hyperplasia (CAH) is an autosomal recessive disorder caused by a mutation in the gene encoding for 21-hydoxylase, an enzyme involved in the synthesis of cortisol and aldosterone, resulting in decreased glucocorticoid secretion and increased androgen secretion. Patients with CAH have an increased prevalence of insulin resistance, obesity, and hypertension,[83,84] increasing the risk of cardiac complications.[85] As these patients are treated with supraphysiological doses of glucocorticoids, these patients may also develop Cushing's syndrome, characterized by excessive glucocorticoids for prolonged periods of time, which can also result in an increased risk of cardiac complications due to treatment-induced metabolic abnormalities and hypertension.[70]

While glucocorticoids have the potential to augment cardiac hypertrophy via cardiac GRs to induce heart failure, alterations in glucocorticoid signaling may mediate these effects.[86] Polymorphisms in the GR gene have been associated with heart failure; a frequent haplotype of the GR is haplotype 3, associated with prevalent heart failure, systolic dysfunction, and subsequent hospitalization for heart failure and coronary heart disease.[87] Also associated with low-grade inflammation, the GR haplotype 3 may be a risk factor for cardiovascular disease for multiple reasons, yet to be delineated.[88]

MINERALOCORTICOID RECEPTORS

STRUCTURE AND FUNCTION

Mineralocorticoids are a class of steroid hormones that influence salt and water balance. The primary mineralocorticoid is aldosterone, but other endogenous hormones such as progesterone and deoxycorticosterone have mineralocorticoid function. Aldosterone, produced in the adrenal gland cortex, is induced primarily by angiotensin II (see Chapter 9, Renin Angiotensin Aldosterone System and Heart Function) and is regulated by adrenocorticotrophin hormone (ACTH) and potassium levels. The mineralocorticoid receptor (MR) is a NR found in the cytosol that crosses the lipid bilayer of the cell with equal affinity for mineralocorticoids and glucocorticoids (e.g., cortisol discussed in the previous section) equally. The MR consists of three domains: NTD, LBD, and DBD (Fig. 10.1(A)), of which the latter two are highly conserved among steroid receptors.[89] When ligand binds the MR LBD, the receptor–ligand complex translocates to the nucleus, where the MR DBD binds HRE in the promoter regions of target genes. In the absence of ligand, the MR interacts with heat shock proteins to prevent the transcription of these target genes.

MRs are expressed in many different tissues and cell types, including cardiomyocytes, vascular smooth muscle and coronary endothelial cells, fibroblasts, and inflammatory cells.[90] Interestingly, both aldosterone and cortisol (glucocorticoid) bind to the MR, and with similar affinity. This is surprising since plasma concentrations of cortisol are 100- to 1000-fold higher than aldosterone.[90] However, overstimulation of the MR is prevented by the enzymatic activity of 11β-hydroxysteroid dehydrogenase (11β-HSD2), which converts cortisol into cortisone, which has a lower affinity for the MR.[91] Notably, 11β-HSD2 is not coexpressed in all tissues with MR, but it is expressed in the kidney as well as VSMC and endothelial cells within the heart, but not the cardiomyocytes themselves.[92] In general, aldosterone and the MR regulate potassium secretion and sodium reabsorption at the kidney and thus influence blood pressure as well as water and electrolyte homeostasis.[89,90] However, aldosterone and the effect of the MR in the myocardium are less defined and appear to be unrelated to blood pressure regulation.

GENOMIC AND NONGENOMIC SIGNALING

Unbound MR resides in the cytoplasm, forming a multiprotein complex that involves chaperone proteins including Hsp90 and FK506-binding protein 4 (FKBP52). In the cytosol, Hsp90 stabilizes the MR and allows for ligand binding (similar to that of GRs, Fig. 10.3).[93] Upon ligand binding to the MR, it is not clear if Hsp90 dissociates from the complex or if Hsp90 assists with MR nuclear translocation.[93] However, after nuclear translocation, the MR forms a homodimer that allows binding to promoter regions of target genes [90] including response elements shared with the GR.[94] A number of coregulators interact with the MR to either enhance or suppress MR's transcriptional activity. Binding predominantly occurs through the NTD, but can also occur through the LBD.[89] Coactivators include PGC-1α, p300/CBP, and steroid receptor coactivator 1 (Src1),[95,96] while NF-YC has been shown to be a corepressor.[97] Alternatively, phosphorylation can increase or decrease MR transcriptional activity,[98] while acetylation decreases MR transcriptional activity,[99] thus altering genomic signaling.

Nongenomic signaling appears to be achieved through aldosterone's interaction with the G protein-coupled estrogen receptor 1 (GPER, discussed in "Estrogen Receptors" section) in VSMC and endothelial cells (Fig. 10.2). Through the GPER, aldosterone activates PI3K-dependent pathways leading to stimulation of the ERK signaling pathway, apoptosis, and cell proliferation.[100,101] However, the influence of aldosterone and the MR on these signaling pathways are poorly defined and more research is needed to elucidate the molecular interactions that regulate and shape them.

Cardiac and endothelial genetic targets of the MR and aldosterone include *Fkbp5* (FK506-binding protein 4; interacts with calcineurin), *Sgk1* (serum-glucocorticoid regulated kinase 1; regulates hormones, inflammation, fibrosis, cell proliferation, and apoptosis),[102] *Adamts1* (ADAM metallopeptidase with thrombospondin type 1; role in inflammation and tissue morphology), and *Pai-1* (plasminogen activator inhibitor 1; development of fibrosis).[103,104] Aldosterone and the MR may act in concert or independently to regulate inflammation, fibrosis, cell proliferation, and apoptosis in the vasculature and heart.

PATHOPHYSIOLOGY: INFLAMMATION AND FIBROSIS

The significance of cardiomyocyte MR in cardiac disease was first suggested as its expression is increased in patients with congestive heart failure and associated with poor cardiac outcomes.[105,106] The functional role of MRs in the myocardium has originated primarily from studies of mice with increased cardiac MR expression (MR Tg+) and mice lacking MR expression (MR−/−). MR Tg+ mice develop an abnormal ventricular remodeling, progression of heart failure, and arrhythmias in response to pressure overload or myocardial infarction.[107–109] Differently, MR−/− mice that are subject to pressure overload or myocardial infarction, show a reduction in cardiac hypertrophy, left ventricular dilation, and progression of heart failure.[107,108] When mice lacking cardiac-specific MR (csMR−/−) underwent permanent coronary artery ligation (to simulate myocardial infarction), csMR−/− mice exhibited reduced infarct size, less fibrosis and ventricular remodeling, and reduced functional decline as well as improved scar structure and matrix collagen organization after eight weeks postinfarction. Additionally, csMR−/− mouse hearts exhibited less apoptosis, attributed to reduced oxidative stress, matrix metalloproteinase (MMP) activity, and nuclear factor κB (NF-κB) signaling.[108] Since MMPs and NF-κB are associated with adverse tissue remodeling and inflammation, these studies illustrate the role of MR in myocardial infarction. Inhibiting MR activity postinfarction appears to be beneficial to cardiac function and may represent a therapeutic target to help with cardiac remodeling that occurs early after an ischemic event.

In contrast, the MR ligand aldosterone itself mediates a number of harmful outcomes. Mice lacking aldosterone exhibit increases in arrhythmia, cardiac hypertrophy, myocardial ischemia, impaired coronary blood flow, and cardiac injury including fibrosis.[90,110] Healthy rats treated with aldosterone and sodium showed an increased inflammatory response, including elevated tumor necrosis factor α (TNFα), transforming growth factor β (TGF-β), and interleukin-1β.[111] These mechanisms may be carried out through the transcriptional upregulation of SGK-1, NF-κB, and AP-1.[90,112] Similarly, administration of aldosterone has been shown to induce cardiac collagen synthesis and fibrosis through TGF-β, AP-1, MMP2, TNFα, and connective tissue growth factor in healthy mice.[90,112] Therefore, inflammation and fibrosis appear to play an important role in adrenal-mediated and MR-mediated cardiac pathophysiology.

Aldosterone and angiotensin II have been shown to increase oxidative stress, and oxidative stress, fibrosis, and inflammation have been shown in several models of various types of heart failure[90,105] (Chapter 9, Renin Angiotensin Aldosterone System and Heart Function). Furthermore, aldosterone-induced oxidative stress is dependent on MR activation of calmodulin kinase II, which can lead to cardiac aggravation and MMP2 and MMP9 activation.[113] MMP9 is associated with adverse cardiac remodeling[114] and is regulated by lipocalin 2, which forms a complex with MMP9 to inhibit its degradation.[115] Interestingly, cardiac MR activation regulates lipocalin 2, linking MR signaling to MMP activity.[103] Furthermore, lipocalin 2 is also regulated by aldosterone and enhanced by NF-κB.[89,115] These data further tie MR and aldosterone-mediated oxidative stress to mechanisms involving inflammation, fibrosis, and impaired calcium handling that ultimately negatively affect cardiovascular function, leading to myocardial dysfunction and poor clinical outcomes.

MINERALOCORTICOID ANTAGONISTS IN TREATING HEART FAILURE

MR antagonists are effective in reducing the total mortality in patients with heart failure and reduced ejection fraction.[116] As aldosterone levels decrease with age, the effectiveness of antagonists in patients ≥80 years of age where the greatest risk of heart failure with a preserved ejection fraction may not be intuitive.[116] Decreases in the enzyme 11β-HSD2 also decrease with age, allowing cortisol to stimulate the MR receptor, which in younger patients with higher 11β-HSD2 levels would not occur.[116] Increases in vascular MR occur with age, amplifying MR signals even in the context of lower aldosterone. Together, these findings suggest that inhibiting MR may therapeutically be beneficial in heart failure and has led to current clinical trials investigating their safety and efficacy[117–122] (more details in Chapter 9, Renin Angiotensin Aldosterone System and Heart Function).

THYROID HORMONE RECEPTORS

MECHANISMS OF THYROID HORMONE ACTION

THR Genomics. The actions of thyroid hormones (THs) are diverse, including regulation of basal metabolism in adults, cholesterol homeostasis and various myocardial events. One mode of TH activity is mediated through thyroid hormone receptors (THRs). THRs are members of the NR superfamily that function as T_3-induced transcription factors. THRs play a role in regulating expression of genes involved in metabolic homeostasis, tissue remodeling, cell proliferation, differentiation, and survival. Similar to other members of the NR family the THRs contain four domains: the amino-terminal A/B transactivation domain, the central DBD C, a small hinge region, and the hormone/ligand-binding domain (LBD) D/E (Fig. 10.1(A)). The THRs bind to DNA, thyroid hormone response elements (TREs) at the recognition sequence (A/G)GGT(G/C/A)A that occur alone or in pairs as DR, palindromes or inverted palindromes. Paired TREs allow dimerization between the THRs and other members of the receptor superfamily, such as retinoid X receptors (RXRs) (Fig. 10.5).[123] Additionally, THRs do not solely interact with NRs, they host a multitude of cellular proteins that bind and coregulate THRs based on TH induction. This combination of binding partner potential plus the multiple TREs sequence structure allows for diversity in modulating gene expression.[124]

THRs are encoded by two genes, THRα and THRβ, located on chromosomes 17 and 3, respectively. The THRα locus encodes THRα1 and THRΔ-αE6, which binds T_3 and THRα2, THRα3, THRΔ-α1 and THRΔ-α2 which do not.[125–127] THRα2 and THRα3 are splice variants that differ from THRα1 at 3′ end. THRΔ-α1 and THRΔ-α2 lack the amino-terminal A/B and DBDs being transcribed from an internal promoter in intron 7; and THRΔ-αE6 is the product of alternative splicing with exon 6b instead of exon

6. THRβ locus encodes THRβ1, THRβ2, THRβ3, THRΔβ3 and THRβ4. THRβ1, THRβ2, THRβ3 isoforms share high sequence homology in the DNA and LBD, but differ in length in the amino-terminal A/B domain. THRΔβ3 lacks the amino-terminal and DBD due to the internal usage of an ATG start site. THRβ4 is a truncated variant of THRβ1, lacking the LBD (Fig. 10.4).[128]

THRα and THRβ are widely expressed in all tissues but exhibit differential expression in developmental and tissue-specific patterns and in distinct ratios in adult tissue.[129–131] THRα1 is predominantly expressed in the heart, bone, intestine, and brain, whereas THRβ1 is highly expressed in skeletal muscle, kidney, thyroid, and liver.[132,133] THRβ2 has a more restrictive expression pattern in the hypothalamus, pituitary, and

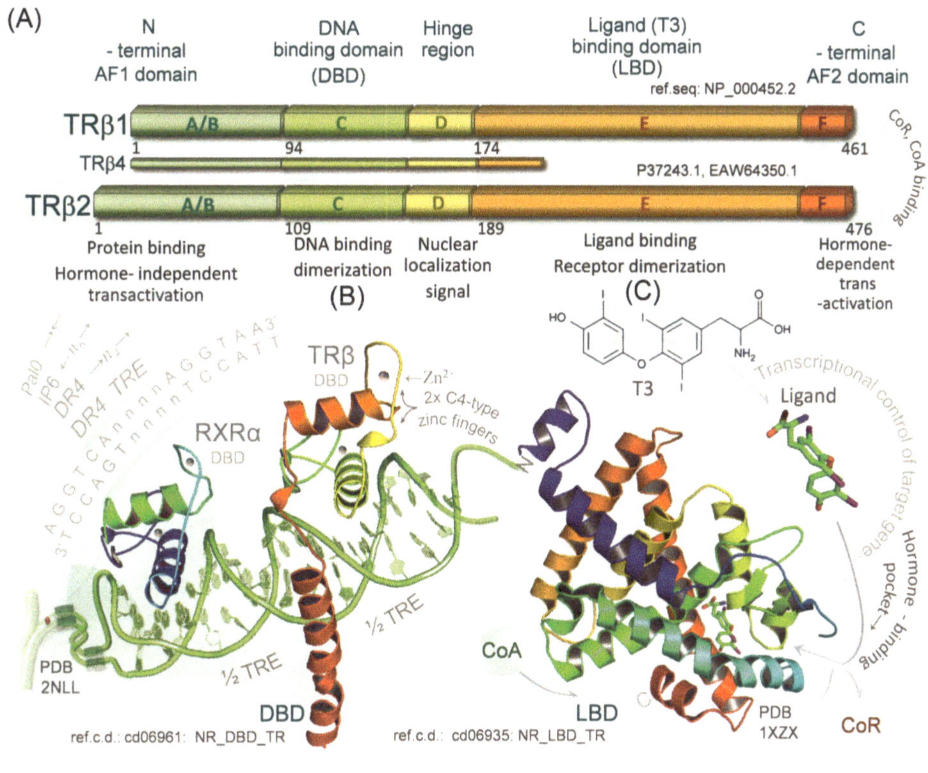

FIGURE 10.4

Structure and functional domains of TRβ isoforms. Three protein isoforms: TRβ1, TRβ2, and truncated variant TRβ4. (A) Functional domains: N-terminal AF1 domain (A/B), DNA-binding domain (C), hinge region (D), ligand (T3) binding domain (E), and C-terminal AF2 domain (F). (B) Crystallographic structure of heterodimer formed by the human thyroid hormone receptor DNA-binding domain and RXR DNA-binding domain (rainbow colored) complexed with double strained DNA (green). (C) Crystallographic structure of the ligand binding domain of the human thyroid hormone (T3) receptor beta (rainbow colored, N-terminus in blue, C-terminus in red) complexed with triiodothyronine (T3).

*From Master A, Nauman A. THRB (Thyroid Hormone Receptor, Beta). Atlas Genet Cytogenet Oncol Haematol 2014;***18***(6):400–33.*

retina.[134,135] Due to the high sequence homology, the isoforms of THRα and THRβ do share overlapping as well as distinct biological roles[136] and the distinct roles probably arise from the variants ability to bind ligands other than T_3 or recruit transcription factors into complexes with different transcriptional results.

PATHOPHYSIOLOGY

THs play an important role in the maintenance of cardiovascular health[137,138] and recovery from myocardial injury.[139] Altered heart rate and cardiac contractility are a few of the changes observed in patients with hypo- or hyperthyroidism.[140,141] T_3-induced cardiac hypertrophy is initially associated with compensated cardiac functional response;[142] however, chronic hyperthyroidism can stress the heart into a decompensated state and reduced cardiac function.[143] Hypothyroidism increases the risk of hypercholesterolemia, hypertension, atherosclerosis, and can result in congestive heart failure.[144–147] TH regulates much of these changes via binding to THRs affecting the transcriptional machinery. Therefore, cardiac-specific mice expressing cardiac THRβ$^{\Delta337}$ were created containing a mutation of the human THRB gene with impaired ligand binding. The resulting THRβ$^{\Delta337}$ hearts exhibit contractile deficits, altered carbohydrate oxidation in response to stress, and changes in developmental genes independent of changes in peripheral systems confirming THs role in cardiac function.[15,148,149] Macchia et al.[150] showed that changes in cardiac sensitivity to THs was dependent on the presence/interactions of the THRs. Using mice with deficiency in all THR isoforms (THR 1 and THR 2), THRα$^{o/o}$ mice compared to THRα$^{-/-}$ mice (lacking only THRα1 and THRα2) both exhibited lower heart rates than wildtype litter mates, but these mouse strains had different sensitivities to TH. The variable phenotypes observed for the different THR mutant models reinforce the importance of the type of mutation/deletion and the complexity of communication network of the THRs.

In concert with this tenet, several studies have shown that the THR isoform profile is altered in failing hearts;[151] however, the response is different in human hearts compared to other mammalian models. In human heart failure, THRα1 expression is decreased but THRα2 is upregulated. As THRα2 is a dominant negative, this model is consistent with a hypothyroid-like gene program frequently observed in several heart failure models. The antiarrhythmic drug amiodarone, via its main metabolite desethylamiodarone, exerts competitive inhibition of T_3 binding to THRα1 and noncompetitive inhibition of T_3 binding to THRβ1. The antiarrhythmic effect of amiodarone potentially induces a cardiac hypothyroid state by competitive inhibition at these receptors.

THR MUTATIONS

Resistance to thyroid hormone (RTH) is a clinical condition associated with impaired TH activity and involves cardiac changes. Patients with TH resistance present with mild cardiomyopathy,[152] and both bradycardia[153–155] and tachycardia.[156] Resistance to TH results predominately from mutations in the THRα or THRβ genes.[157,158] In >85% of the cases of RTH the THRβ is mutated. More than 120 mutations have been identified in THRβ1[128,158] in comparison to only nine mutations in the THRα1 gene.[152–154, 159–162] Interestingly, all the THR mutations cluster in the 3′ region of the ligand binding domain (Fig. 10.1(A)), and tend to show reduced T_3 affinity or abnormal cofactors interaction and loss of transcriptional activity.[153,154,163,164] It is proposed that THRα mutations may be more prevalent, but due to the lack of clear-cut overt clinical presentation be under diagnosed.

Mutations in THRs can also affect expression and function of other NRs, such as PPARs. A study by Buroker et al.[165] showed reduced levels of the THRα1, and RXRα proteins, and increased levels of PPARβ in the hearts of $THR\beta^{\Delta 337}$ mice, a cardiac-specific (cs) hypothyroid murine model.[166] The hearts of the $csTHR\beta^{\Delta 337}$ mice also had reduced mRNA levels for PPARα and its target gene (uncoupled protein 3) in response to the PPARα agonist WY-14643, supporting cross-talk between receptors. A study using the THRβ mutation knock-in mouse model, $THR\beta^{PV/PV}$ showed reduced PPARγ ligand–induced transcriptional activity due to the $THR\beta^{PV/PV}$ binding PPAR response element sites and coopting corepressors.[8] Therefore, THRs and PPARs competition for the RXR receptor and DNA binding sites demonstrates additional mechanisms for signal transduction.[167–169]

TH AND THR NONNUCLEAR REGULATION

The influence of TH in the heart is not restricted to actions within the nucleus. Several studies demonstrated the immediate beneficial action of systemic TH supplementation in subclinical sick euthyroid states (low serum levels of thyroid hormone), which cannot be attributed to genomic or nuclear action. Some nongenetic mechanisms include cellular protein interactions, localized in cytoplasm or at the plasma membrane, in a ligand-dependent or -independent manner. For example, Cyclin D_1, a regulator of cell cycle progression, interacts with THRβ1 at the LBD in a T_3-independent manner altering THRβ1 transcriptional activity;[170] whereas the plasma membrane receptor, integrin ανβ3, can bind TH and mediate cellular events such as activation of the MAPK/ERK pathways.[171] Both triiodothyronine and thyroxine (T_4) directly or indirectly activate PI3K, which phosphorylates phosphatidylinositols (PtdINS) (Fig. 10.5).[172] The PtdINS regulate downstream kinases such as Akt/PKB, a serine threonine protein kinase with a high sequence homology to protein kinase A. Akt/PKB regulates several downstream kinases, which directly control metabolic pathways. Upstream from Akt/PKB, activation of PI3K by TH involves novel protein to protein interaction with TRβ,[173] which can be modified by receptor mutation. The TRβPV mutation demonstrates greater binding affinity for PI3K p85 regulatory subunit, and increases PI3K activity more than does the wildtype TRβ1. Kenessey et al. also showed direct interaction of cytosol-localized thyroid hormone receptor TRα1 and the p85alpha subunit of PI3K in cardiomyocytes. T3 exposure rapidly elevated PI3K activity, resulting in increased phosphorylation of downstream kinases Akt and the mammalian target of rapamycin (mTOR).[174] Thus, these studies indicate that T_3 or T_4 bind to THRs, which interact with PI3K, and alter the enzyme's conformation and modify activity with substantial changes in several regulatory pathways for cardiac hypertrophy and metabolism.

PPAR FAMILY RECEPTORS

PPARs are ligand-activated transcription factors belonging to the NR superfamily. The PPAR family consists of three isoforms (PPAR α, β/δ, and γ), each encoded by different genes that show significant amino acid similarity, with shared and unique biological effects. PPARs heterodimerize with 9-cis-retinoic acid RXRs,[175,176] and in response to binding a specific ligand undergoes a conformational change, allowing the recruitment or release of accessory proteins that determine the functional state of the PPAR–RXR complex.[177,178]

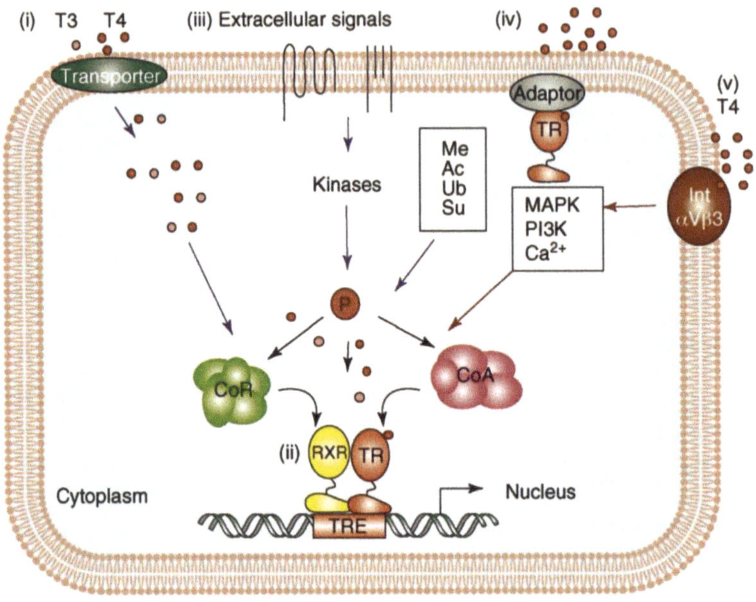

FIGURE 10.5

Mechanism of thyroid hormone receptor action. (i) Thyroid hormones, thyroxine (T4), and triiodothyronine (T3) enter the cell through transporter proteins. Although the major form of thyroid hormone in the blood is T4, it is converted to the more active hormone T3 within cells by 50 deiodinases. (ii) T3 binds to nuclear thyroid hormone receptors that regulate transcription by binding, generally as heterodimers with the RXR, to thyroid hormone response elements (*TREs*) located in regulatory regions of target genes. Activity is regulated by an exchange of corepressor (CoR) and coactivator (CoA) complexes. (iii) Receptor activity is also modulated by hormones and growth factors that stimulate diverse signal transduction pathways. Both receptors and coregulators are targets for phosphorylation (P) as well as for modifications, such as acetylation (Ac), methylation (Me), ubiquitination (Ub), or sumoylation (Su), that regulate their activity, levels, or localization. (iv) Binding of T3 to a subpopulation of receptors located outside the nuclei can also elicit a response; through interaction with adaptor proteins, rapid "nongenomic" effects lead to stimulation of kinase pathways. (v) T4 can also bind to putative membrane receptors, such as integrin aVb3, inducing MAPK activity.

*Copyright Elsevier 2009 (From Aranda A, et al. Thyroid receptor: roles in cancer. Trends Endocrinol Metab 2009;**20**(7):318–24. (Fig. 10.1). Used with Permission.*

DOMAIN STRUCTURE

PPARs, like other NRs, have a generally conserved domain structure (Fig. 10.1(A))[4,179]:

1. The N-terminal A/B domain is a poorly conserved region that contains the AF-1 transactivation domain, which allows interactions with coactivators and corepressors in a ligand independent manner.
2. The DBD, which is highly conserved and composed of two zinc finger motifs, is responsible for binding the repeated PPAR response element hexamer sequence (AGGTC) separated by one or two nucleotides.

3. A small hinge region allows for three-dimensional conformational changes allowing for recruitment or release of accessory molecules.
4. The LBD shows the greatest sequence variability and determines ligand affinity and receptor activity. In the C-terminus of the LBD domain is the ligand-dependent activating function (AF-2) domain.

PHYSIOLOGICAL FUNCTIONS

PPARα: The adult heart primarily relies on FAO as its primary source of energy and PPARα plays an important role in the regulation of genes involved in β-oxidation of fatty acids.[180,181] In addition to the heart, tissues high in PPARα include the liver, kidney, skeletal muscle and brown fat as well as several vascular cell types.[182–184] Activation of PPARα has been shown to lower triglyceride levels in vivo, and repress inflammation caused by cardiovascular disease.[185–189] Induction of PPARα activity substantially reduced the infarct size due to regional myocardial ischemia and reperfusion in rats[190] and suppressed hypertension-induced increase in adhesion molecules.[191] Interestingly, mice with cardiac-specific PPARα (csPPARα) overexpression developed a cardiomyopathy mimicking the diabetes mellitus condition. These mice showed ventricular dysfunction, increased myocyte fatty acid uptake and beta-oxidation, reduced glucose import and glycolysis, lipid accumulation, and cardiac hypertrophy.[192] The cardiomyopathy worsened when fed long-chain fatty acids (LCFAs) and reversed by lowering the LCFAs content of the diet.[193] Mitochondrial dysfunction correlated with the lipid accumulation supporting PPARα involvement in cardiac mitochondrial biogenesis. Duncan et al.[194] speculated that PPARα up-regulation in response to insulin resistance might be an adaptive response that becomes maladaptive with the development of diabetes/lipotoxic effects.

PPARβ/δ: PPAR β/δ has been the least studied of the three PPARs. It is almost ubiquitously expressed and has a potential role in FAO.[195] Activation of PPARβ/δ improves metabolic abnormalities in animal models of obesity, such as insulin resistance, dyslipidemia, and increasing FAO,[196–198] as well as having a positive inotropic effect.[199] PPARβ/δ activation induced rapid cardiac angiogenesis and cardiac muscle mass in adult mice hearts by direct transcriptional activation of calcineurin A.[200] Studies in humans and primates demonstrated that PPARβ/δ activation improved plasma lipid profiles.[201–203] Studies examining cardio-specific (cs) PPARβ/δ null mice reported severe cardiomyopathy and prematurely mortality due to heart failure.[204] The fatty acid phenotypes observed support PPARβ/δ as necessary for the hearts FAO potential similar to PPARα. However, in contrast to PPARα, hearts from csPPARβ/δ transgenic mice had an increased expression of myocardial glucose transport, oxidation and glycolytic genes; the increased myocardial glucose utilization had a cardioprotective effect to I/R injury.[205]

PPARγ: The PPARγ gene encodes three isoforms due to differential promoter usage: PPARγ-1, PPARγ-2 and PPARγ-3, all of which are found in mammals.[206] The translated products of PPARγ-1 and PPARγ-3 yield the same protein, whereas PPARγ-2 contains an additional 30 amino acid at it N-terminus. Additionally, the tissue distribution of the two distinct isoforms also differs. PPARγ-1/3 is more ubiquitously expressed, while PPARγ-2 is restricted to adipose tissue. PPARγ is critical for the differentiation of pre-adipocytes to adipocytes and is important in glucose homeostasis.[207] Inactivation of PPARγ in mature adipocytes led to insulin resistance through dysregulation of genes essential to insulin signaling and free fatty acid uptake.[208,209] PPARγ is expressed in myocardial cells albeit at relatively low levels, and evidence suggests PPARγ normalized glucose uptake and protected the heart from ischemic injury in obese rats.[210,211] The therapeutic effects of PPARγ agonist ligands is attributed primarily to their antiinflammatory properties.[212] Myocardial mRNA expression of inflammatory cytokines was suppressed in an autoimmune myocarditis model after admission of PPARγ ligands.[213] Additionally, treatments with PPARγ ligands resulted in a decrease in proinflammatory risk markers concurrent with improved platelet function and coagulation.[214] In the diabetic myocardium, the PPARγ synthetic ligand rosiglitazone decreased cardiac fibrosis and improved left ventricular diastolic dysfunction by inhibiting receptors for glycated end products and connective tissue growth factors;[215] whereas another PPARγ synthetic ligand, pioglitazone, improved the deterioration of ischemic preconditioning.[216] Increased expression of PPARγ lowered blood pressure in a hypertensive rodent model.[217,218] Dissimilar phenotypes have been reported for two independently created csPPARγ null mice lines. Duan et al.[219] reported a mild myocardial hypertrophy with preserved systolic function, whereas Ding et al.[220] reported progressive dilated cardiomyopathy and premature mortality. Transgenic mice that over-express csPPARγ developed cardiomyopathy[221]; and interestingly, the profiles for the csPPARγ transgenic mice resembled both the csPPARα and csPPARβ/δ transgenic, displaying both increased expression of genes involved in FAO and glucose transport.

PPAR LIGANDS

PPARs bind a host of endogenous and pharmacological ligands[222] and it is these variable interactions that alter the recruitment of cofactors to the PPAR–RXR complex allowing for the differences in transactivation of target genes within and between cell types.[223] Endogenous ligands of PPARs include: fatty acids and their derivatives, eicosanoids, phosphoinositides, sphingolipids, some cannabinoid-like molecules, certain prostanoids and oxidized alkyl phospholipids.[190,224] The synthetic ligands of the PPARs include two classes of drugs, the fibrates and thiazolidinedione (TZD), which predominately bind and activate PPARα and PPARγ, respectively.

Fibrates are used clinically as a cholesterol-lowering drug, decreasing triglyceride levels and increasing high-density lipoproteins. Fibrates effects are attributed to PPARα-mediated induction of the gene encoding ABCA1, a cholesterol efflux regulatory protein.[225] Given the prescribed use of fibrates and the strong association between elevated triglyceride levels and cardiovascular heart disease (CHD), the efficacy of fibrates in the treatment of cardiovascular disease was studied. In the Helsinki Heart Study (HHS), a randomized, placebo-controlled five-year trial in middle-aged men with dyslipidemia, showed that gemfibrozil was associated with a 34% reduction in CHD events at five years but not for CHD-related deaths.[226] The Veteran Affairs High-Density Lipoprotein Intervention Trial (VA-HIT) showed a 22% reduction in the primary endpoint of CHD death and nonfatal myocardial infarction and a 24% reduction in the combined outcome of death from CHD, nonfatal MI or confirmed stroke.[227] Analysis of combined data from a meta-analysis of 53 fibrate trials, including the HHS and VA-HIT, showed the risk of major coronary events was reduced by 25%, but there was no reduction in cardiovascular mortality or heart failure events.[228]

TZD drugs, also called glitazones, were initially used as a noninsulin treatment in type 2 diabetes mellitus (T2DM) patients for lowering glucose levels before being identified as PPARγ ligands.[229] Although these drugs showed positive cardiac effects, such as increased cardiac output in T2DM patients,[230] or protection from ischemic injury,[210] they were not without side effects, such as increased risk of myocardial infarction and congestive heart failure.[231,232] In several studies, diabetic patients on the TZD rosiglitazone showed an increased risk of ischemic stroke and heart failure.[233–235] In 2007, the U.S. Food and Drug Administration (USDA) significantly restricted the use of rosiglitazone to diabetics who could not adequately control their blood sugar levels with other medications. In comparison, the TZD drug pioglitazone demonstrated a significantly lower risk of death, myocardial infarction, or stroke in diabetic patients. Serious heart failure increased, but was not associated with an increase in mortality.[233,236,237] In 2013, based on the re-evaluation of the *R*osiglitazone *E*valuated for *C*ardiovascular *O*utcomes and *R*egulation of *G*lycemia in *D*iabetes (RECORD), the USDA removed the restriction stating there was no increased risk of heart attacks due to rosiglitazone compared to other standard type 2 diabetes medications.

Agonists targeting both PPARα/PPARγ isoforms, combining the glycemic and lipid control, were investigated for their potential clinical value. Dual-agonist, theoretically, would yield a more balanced phenotype with improved efficacy. However, late phase clinical trials for several of these dual-agonists—muraglitazar (Bristol-Myers Squibb/Merck), tesaglitazar (AstraZeneca), tesaglitazar (F. Hoffmann-La Roche)—were terminated due to adverse affects such as congestive heart failure, and renal and hepatotoxicity.[230,238,239]

POSTTRANSLATIONAL MECHANISMS OF PPAR REGULATION

Ligand binding is not the only mechanism by which PPAR can be regulated; post-translational modifications (PTMs) also control PPAR action.

Phosphorylation. Activation of kinases, such as MAPK, extracellular signal-regulated kinase 1/2 (ERK 1/2), or cyclin-dependent kinases (CDKs) result in PPAR phosphorylation at Ser112 of PPARγ-2 (Ser-82 of PPARγ1).[240–242] Phosphorylation at Ser112 is responsible for both inhibiting and activating PPARγ transcriptional activity based on the kinase involved. CDK5 phosphorylation of PPARγ at Ser-273 plays a role in regulating genes involved in glucose homeostasis, such as adiponectin and adipsin. The phosphorylation was blocked by antidiabetic PPARγ ligands, such as rosiglitazone and MRL24. The docking of Thrap3 (thyroid hormone receptor-associated protein 3) at the PPARγ phospho-Ser273 site controls the regulation of several diabetic genes.[243,244]

SUMOylation. SUMOylation (Small Ubiquitin-like Modifier (or SUMO) proteins) are a family of small proteins that attach covalently to other proteins and alter their function. SUMOylation of PPARγ occur at K107 (K77 in PPARγ-1) and K395 (K365 in PPARγ-1). SUMOylation strongly represses PPARγ transcriptional activity of direct and indirect target genes. Several examples establish a role in regulating whole body insulin sensitivity, FAO, and antiinflammatory responses.[245–247] PPARγ ligands negatively affect SUMOylation by interdomain communication offering a potential mechanism of action target for therapeutic ligands that bind PPARγ.[248]

Ubiquitination. Ubiquitination is the addition of ubiquitin, a small regulatory protein, that targets the protein to which it attaches to for degradation, relocation, or altered protein interaction. The ubiquitin ligase (muscle ring finger-1/MuRF1) has been shown to inhibit FAO by inhibiting PPARα, but not PPARβ/δ or PPARγ in cardiomyocytes in vitro. Rodriguez et al. [249] showed that transgenic MuRF1 hearts had decreased nuclear PPARα activity and acyl-carnitine intermediates, while MuRF1knockout hearts exhibited increased PPARα activity and acyl-carnitine intermediates. The MuRF1 protein directly interacts with and mono-ubiquitinates PPARα, resulting in nuclear export and thereby inhibiting FAO in a proteasome-independent manner.[249] MuRF2 was also identified as the first ubiquitin ligase to regulate cardiac PPARα and PPARγ1 activities in vivo via posttranslational modification without degradation.[250]

O-GlcNAcylation. O-GlcNAcylation is the posttranslational modification in which a single β-*O*-linked *N*-acetylGLucosamine (O-GLcNac) is added to the hydroxyl groups of serine and threonine residues of target proteins. Residue T54 in the AF-1 domain (T84 in PPARγ-2) is the only currently identified O-GLcNac site and inhibition of this modification decreased PPARγ transcriptional activity and adipocyte differentiation.[251]

Acetylation. Acetylation is the introduction of an acetyl group onto a protein molecule. Confirmed acetylation sites were identified in PPARγ at K268 and K293 (K238 and K263 in PPARγ-1). PPARγ deacetylation by SirT1, an NAD^+-dependent deacetylase, allowed the recruitment of PRDM16, a transcriptional coactivator of browning of white adipose tissue. Two additional sites, K154/155 of PPARγ-1, were found to be acetylated and required for the binding of SirT1and PPARγ-1 affected adipogenesis.[252] Since SirT1 is activated by energy deficiency,[253] influencing pathways such as FAO and gluconeogenesis, the deacetylation of PPARγ may promote energy expenditure and insulin sensitivity.[254]

The complex cycling of PPAR and its cointeractors is not based on a single PTM, but rather requires the coordinated actions of a myriad of PTM combinations. An example of this coordination is the recruitment of NCoR, a corepressor. NCoR recruitment requires acetylation of PPARγ, and subsequently the PPAR-NCoR interaction leads to CDK-5-mediated PPAR phosphorylation at Ser273 and the downstream expression of a host of metabolic genes. Exploiting PPARs PTMs offer an alternative target for drug development without the undesirable side effects. Choi et al.[255] developed a nonagonist PPARγ ligand that blocked CDK5 phosphorylation and demonstrated potent antidiabetic activity without many of the undesirable side effects of the TZD drugs.

EMERGING AND ASSOCIATED PLAYERS

VITAMIN D RECEPTORS

Vitamin D3 (cholecalciferol) is mainly produced nonenzymatically from precursors when skin is exposed to ultraviolet light. Vitamin D receptor (VDR) is a member of the NR superfamily with the active metabolite of vitamin D, 1α,25-dihydroxyvitamin D (1,25(OH)2D) as the principal ligand. VDR and its relationship to the cardiovascular system was recently and extensively reviewed.[256] VDR regulates numerous genes with promoters that contain vitamin D response elements. These genes regulate various processes of potential relevance to CVD, including cell proliferation and differentiation, apoptosis, oxidative stress, membrane transport, matrix homeostasis, tissue mineralization, and cell adhesion. VDRs have been found in all the major cardiovascular cell types, including VSMCs, endothelial cells, cardiomyocytes, most immune cells, and platelets.

VDR binds 1,25(OH)2D with high affinity and specificity, and like other members of this superfamily heterodimerizes, predominantly with RXR. VDR contains a short N-terminal domain before the DBD comprising two zinc fingers, the first conferring vitamin D response element specificity and the second providing a site for heterodimerization (Fig. 10.1(A)). The remainder of the receptor contains the lipophilic 1,25(OH)2D-binding domain and at the C-terminal, the coactivator-binding domain. Transcriptional activity induced or repressed by this receptor depends on complex formation with tissue-specific coactivators, including steroid receptor coactivators, and the silencing of corepressors that modify chromatin structure. These protein complexes influence target gene specificity that show relevance to the heart and the cardiovascular system. The VDR influences transcription of genes involved in multiple processes including inflammation and the renin-angiotensin system, which affect cardiovascular function.

Some evidence exists that VDR expressed in cardiomyocytes plays a role in ventricular remodeling after stress. The VDR KO mice exhibit ventricular hypertrophy and increased matrix turnover. However, this model also produces systemic hypertension and elevated parathyroid hormones, so that the mechanism for the development of hypertrophy remains unclear. Chen et al. demonstrated that selective cardiomyocyte deletion of VDR in mice does produce an anti-hypertrophic effect in vivo. VDR overexpression decreased myocardial infarct size and improved cardiac function through attenuating oxidative stress, and inhibiting apoptosis and autophagy dysfunction. Several studies in animal models show that VDR agonists such as paricalcitol or maxacalcitol prevent or reverse myocardial damage in disease processes such as diabetes, end-stage renal disease, and diabetes. However, results in clinical trials using Vitamin D or VDR activators are still lacking.

SUMMARY

Over the past decade, an evolving appreciation of the dynamic and critical roles of NRs in cardiomyocytes in the pathogenesis of heart failure has emerged. In this chapter, we introduced the structural conception of NRs, then reviewed the role of the cardiomyocyte ER, ERRs, the glucocorticoid receptor (GR), and MR in the static and diseased heart. Emerging roles of thyroid and PPAR family receptors were discussed along with relatively "new" studies implicating the vitamin D receptor in ventricular remodeling post-insult. With their complex interactions and dual agonist and repressor roles dependent upon context, they represent interesting pharmacological targets for disease therapy once their basic biology is better understood, particularly their PTMs that have been largely unexplored.

REFERENCES

1. Gronemeyer H, Gustafsson JA, Laudet V. Principles for modulation of the nuclear receptor superfamily. *Nat Rev Drug Discov* 2004;**3**(11):950–64.
2. Evans RM. The nuclear receptor superfamily: a rosetta stone for physiology. *Mol Endocrinol* 2005;**19**(6):1429–38.
3. Fondell JD, Ge H, Roeder RG. Ligand induction of a transcriptionally active thyroid hormone receptor coactivator complex. *Proc Natl Acad Sci USA* 1996;**93**(16):8329–33.
4. Desvergne B, Wahli W. Peroxisome proliferator-activated receptors: nuclear control of metabolism. *Endocr Rev* 1999;**20**(5):649–88.
5. Seol W, Choi HS, Moore DD. An orphan nuclear hormone receptor that lacks a DNA binding domain and heterodimerizes with other receptors. *Science* 1996;**272**(5266):1336–9.
6. Umesono K, et al. Direct repeats as selective response elements for the thyroid hormone, retinoic acid, and vitamin D3 receptors. *Cell* 1991;**65**(7):1255–66.
7. Hunter J, et al. Crosstalk between the thyroid hormone and peroxisome proliferator-activated receptors in regulating peroxisome proliferator-responsive genes. *Mol Cell Endocrinol* 1996;**116**(2):213–21.
8. Araki O, et al. Thyroid hormone receptor beta mutants: dominant negative regulators of peroxisome proliferator-activated receptor gamma action. *Proc Natl Acad Sci USA* 2005;**102**(45):16251–6.
9. Riehle C, Abel ED. PGC-1 proteins and heart failure. *Trends Cardiovasc Med* 2012;**22**(4):98–105.
10. Puigserver P, Spiegelman BM. Peroxisome proliferator-activated receptor-g co-activator 1a (PGC-1a): transcriptional co-activator and metabolic regulator. *Endocr Rev* 2003;**24**:78–90.

11. Andersson U, Scarpulla RC. Pgc-1-related coactivator, a novel, serum-inducible coactivator of nuclear respiratory factor 1-dependent transcription in mammalian cells. *Mol Cell Biol* 2001;**21**(11):3738–49.
12. Kressler D, et al. The PGC-1-related protein PERC is a selective coactivator of estrogen receptor alpha. *J Biol Chem* 2002;**277**(16):13918–25.
13. Kelly DP, Scarpulla RC. Transcriptional regulatory circuits controlling mitochondrial biogenesis and function. *Genes Dev* 2004;**18**:357–68.
14. Lehman JJ, et al. The transcriptional coactivator PGC-1alpha is essential for maximal and efficient cardiac mitochondrial fatty acid oxidation and lipid homeostasis. *Am J Physiol Heart Circ Physiol* 2008;**295**(1):H185–96.
15. Hyyti OM, et al. Cardioselective dominant-negative thyroid hormone receptor (Delta337T) modulates myocardial metabolism and contractile efficiency. *Am J Physiol Endocrinol Metab* 2008;**295**(2):E420–7.
16. Zhang Y, et al. Peroxisomal proliferator-activated receptor-gamma coactivator-1 alpha (PGC-1 alpha) enhances the thyroid hormone induction of carnitine palmitoyltransferase I (CPT-I alpha). *J Biol Chem* 2004;**279**(52):53963–71.
17. Martin OJ, et al. A role for peroxisome proliferator-activated receptor gamma coactivator-1 in the control of mitochondrial dynamics during postnatal cardiac growth. *Circ Res* 2014;**114**(4):626–36.
18. Riehle C, et al. PGC-1β deficiency accelerates the transition to heart failure in pressure overload hypertrophy. *Circ Res* 2011;**109**(7):783–93.
19. Karamanlidis G, et al. Defective DNA replication impairs mitochondrial biogenesis in human failing hearts. *Circ Res* 2010;**106**(9):1541–8.
20. Bell JR, et al. Sex and sex hormones in cardiac stress—mechanistic insights. *J Steroid Biochem Mol Biol* 2013;**137**:124–35.
21. Jia G, Aroor AR, Sowers JR. Estrogen and mitochondria function in cardiorenal metabolic syndrome. *Prog Mol Biol Transl Sci* 2014;**127**:229.
22. Arias-Loza P-A, Muehlfelder M, Pelzer T. Estrogen and estrogen receptors in cardiovascular oxidative stress. *Pflügers Arch Eur J Physiol* 2013;**465**(5):739–46.
23. Levin ER. Rapid signaling by steroid receptors. *Am J Physiol-Regul Integr Comp Physiol* 2008;**295**(5):R1425–30.
24. Gupte AA, Pownall HJ, Hamilton DJ. Estrogen: an emerging regulator of insulin action and mitochondrial function. *J Diabetes Res* 2015;**2015**:916585.
25. Curl C, Wendt I, Kotsanas G. *Effects of gender on intracellular [Ca2^{+}] in rat cardiac myocytes. Pflügers Arch* 2001;**441**(5):709–16.
26. Curl CL, et al. Effects of ovariectomy and 17β-oestradiol replacement on [Ca2^{+}] i in female rat cardiac myocytes. *Clin Exp Pharmacol Physiol* 2003;**30**(7):489–94.
27. Chu SH, et al. Effect of estrogen on calcium-handling proteins, β-adrenergic receptors, and function in rat heart. *Life Sci* 2006;**79**(13):1257–67.
28. Sebag IA, et al. Sex hormone control of left ventricular structure/function: mechanistic insights using echocardiography, expression, and DNA methylation analyses in adult mice. *Am J Physiol-Heart Circul Physiol* 2011;**301**(4):H1706–15.
29. Wittnich C, et al. Sex differences in myocardial metabolism and cardiac function: an emerging concept. *Pflugers Arch* 2013;**465**(5):719–29.
30. Farrell SR, Ross JL, Howlett SE. Sex differences in mechanisms of cardiac excitation-contraction coupling in rat ventricular myocytes. *Am J Physiol-Heart Circul Physiol* 2010;**299**(1):H36–45.
31. Curl CL, Bell JR, Delbridge LM. 'Gain'-ful insight into the cardiomyocyte Ca2^{+} seX factor. *J Mol Cell Cardiol* 2012;**52**(1):7–9.
32. Guo J, et al. 17β-Estradiol prevents cell death and mitochondrial dysfunction by an estrogen receptor-dependent mechanism in astrocytes after oxygen–glucose deprivation/reperfusion. *Free Radic Biol Med* 2012;**52**(11):2151–60.

33. Hsieh Y-C, et al. Inhibition of cardiac PGC-1α expression abolishes ERβ agonist-mediated cardioprotection following trauma-hemorrhage. *FASEB J* 2006;**20**(8):1109–17.
34. Mattingly KA, et al. Estradiol stimulates transcription of nuclear respiratory factor-1 and increases mitochondrial biogenesis. *Mol Endocrinol* 2008;**22**(3):609–22.
35. Vasconsuelo A, Milanesi L, Boland R. Actions of 17β-estradiol and testosterone in the mitochondria and their implications in aging. *Ageing Res Rev* 2013;**12**(4):907–17.
36. Duchen MR. Mitochondria and calcium: from cell signalling to cell death. *J Physiol* 2000;**529**(1):57–68.
37. Roger VL, et al. Gender differences in use of stress testing and coronary heart disease mortality: a population-based study in Olmsted County, Minnesota. *J Am Coll Cardiol* 1998;**32**(2):345–52.
38. Vittinghoff E, et al. Risk factors and secondary prevention in women with heart disease: the Heart and Estrogen/progestin Replacement Study. *Ann Intern Med* 2003;**138**(2):81–9.
39. Bell JR, et al. The intrinsic resistance of female hearts to an ischemic insult is abrogated in primary cardiac hypertrophy. *Am J Physiol-Heart Circul Physiol* 2008;**294**(4):H1514–22.
40. Lagranha CJ, et al. Sex differences in the phosphorylation of mitochondrial proteins result in reduced production of reactive oxygen species and cardioprotection in females. *Circ Res* 2010;**106**(11):1681–91.
41. Sun J, et al. Hypercontractile female hearts exhibit increased S-nitrosylation of the L-type $Ca2^+$ channel α1 subunit and reduced ischemia/reperfusion injury. *Circ Res* 2006;**98**(3):403–11.
42. Pedram A, et al. Estrogen inhibits cardiac hypertrophy: role of estrogen receptor-β to inhibit calcineurin. *Endocrinology* 2008;**149**(7):3361–9.
43. Westphal C, et al. Effects of estrogen, an ERα agonist and raloxifene on pressure overload induced cardiac hypertrophy. *PLoS One* 2012;**7**(12):e50802.
44. Chen C-C, Lin C-C, Lee T-M. 17β-estradiol decreases vulnerability to ventricular arrhythmias by preserving Connexin43 protein in infarcted rats. *Eur J Pharmacol* 2010;**629**(1):73–81.
45. Huss JM, Garbacz WG, Xie W. Constitutive activities of estrogen-related receptors: transcriptional regulation of metabolism by the ERR pathways in health and disease. *Biochim Biophys Acta* 2015;**1852**(9):1912–27.
46. Giguère V, et al. Identification of a new class of steroid hormone receptors. *Nature* 1988;**331**(6151):91–4.
47. Vu EH, Kraus RJ, Mertz JE. Phosphorylation-dependent sumoylation of estrogen-related receptor α1. *Biochemistry* 2007;**46**(34):9795–804.
48. Chen S, et al. Molecular basis for the constitutive activity of estrogen-related receptor α-1. *J Biol Chem* 2001;**276**(30):28465–70.
49. Giguere V. Transcriptional control of energy homeostasis by the estrogen-related receptors. *Endocr Rev* 2008;**29**(6):677–96.
50. Kim MS, et al. Suppression of estrogen-related receptor α and medium-chain acyl-coenzyme A dehydrogenase in the acute-phase response. *J Lipid Res* 2005;**46**(10):2282–8.
51. Dufour CR, et al. Genome-wide orchestration of cardiac functions by the orphan nuclear receptors ERRα and γ. *Cell Metab* 2007;**5**(5):345–56.
52. Schreiber SN, et al. The transcriptional coactivator PGC-1 regulates the expression and activity of the orphan nuclear receptor estrogen-related receptor α (ERRα). *J Biol Chem* 2003;**278**(11):9013–8.
53. Huss JM, et al. Estrogen-related receptor α directs peroxisome proliferator-activated receptor α signaling in the transcriptional control of energy metabolism in cardiac and skeletal muscle. *Mol Cell Biol* 2004;**24**(20):9079–91.
54. Alaynick WA, et al. ERRγ directs and maintains the transition to oxidative metabolism in the postnatal heart. *Cell Metab* 2007;**6**(1):13–24.
55. Vanacker J-M, et al. Activation of the thyroid hormone receptor gene promoter by the orphan nuclear receptor ERR. *Oncogene* 1998;**17**(19):2429–36.
56. Castet A, et al. Receptor-interacting protein 140 differentially regulates estrogen receptor-related receptor transactivation depending on target genes. *Mol Endocrinol* 2006;**20**(5):1035–47.

57. Finck BN, Kelly DP. PGC-1 coactivators: inducible regulators of energy metabolism in health and disease. *J Clin Invest* 2006;**116**(3):615.
58. Seth A, et al. The transcriptional corepressor RIP140 regulates oxidative metabolism in skeletal muscle. *Cell Metab* 2007;**6**(3):236–45.
59. Fritah A, et al. Elevated expression of the metabolic regulator receptor-interacting protein 140 results in cardiac hypertrophy and impaired cardiac function. *Cardiovasc Res* 2010;**86**(3):443–51.
60. Abel ED, Doenst T. Mitochondrial adaptations to physiological vs. pathological cardiac hypertrophy. *Cardiovasc Res* 2011:cvr015.
61. Huss JM, et al. The nuclear receptor ERRα is required for the bioenergetic and functional adaptation to cardiac pressure overload. *Cell Metab* 2007;**6**(1):25–37.
62. Chen Y, et al. Roles of transcriptional corepressor RIP140 and coactivator PGC-1α in energy state of chronically infarcted rat hearts and mitochondrial function of cardiomyocytes. *Mol Cell Endocrinol* 2012;**362**(1):11–18.
63. Gomez-Arroyo J, et al. Metabolic gene remodeling and mitochondrial dysfunction in failing right ventricular hypertrophy secondary to pulmonary arterial hypertension. *Circul Heart Fail* 2013;**6**(1):136–44.
64. Arany Z, et al. Transverse aortic constriction leads to accelerated heart failure in mice lacking PPAR-γ coactivator 1α. *Proc Natl Acad Sci* 2006;**103**(26):10086–91.
65. Sihag S, et al. PGC-1α and ERRα target gene downregulation is a signature of the failing human heart. *J Mol Cell Cardiol* 2009;**46**(2):201–12.
66. Hu X, et al. AMP activated protein kinase-α2 regulates expression of estrogen-related receptor-α, a metabolic transcription factor related to heart failure development. *Hypertension* 2011;**58**(4):696–703.
67. Palomer X, et al. An overview of the crosstalk between inflammatory processes and metabolic dysregulation during diabetic cardiomyopathy. *Int J Cardiol* 2013;**168**(4):3160–72.
68. Oka S-i, et al. Suppression of ERR targets by a PPARα/Sirt1 complex in the failing heart. *Cell Cycle* 2012;**11**(5):856–64.
69. Cain DW, Cidlowski JA. Specificity and sensitivity of glucocorticoid signaling in health and disease. *Best Pract Res Clin Endocrinol Metab* 2015;**29**(4):545–56.
70. Oakley RH, Cidlowski JA. Glucocorticoid signaling in the heart: a cardiomyocyte perspective. *J Steroid Biochem Mol Biol* 2015;**153**:27–34.
71. Grad I, Picard D. The glucocorticoid responses are shaped by molecular chaperones. *Mol Cell Endocrinol* 2007;**275**(1):2–12.
72. Rosenfeld MG, Glass CK. Coregulator codes of transcriptional regulation by nuclear receptors. *J Biol Chem* 2001;**276**(40):36865–8.
73. Meijsing SH, et al. DNA binding site sequence directs glucocorticoid receptor structure and activity. *Science* 2009;**324**(5925):407–10.
74. Kadmiel M, Cidlowski JA. Glucocorticoid receptor signaling in health and disease. *Trends Pharmacol Sci* 2013;**34**(9):518–30.
75. Oakley RH, Cidlowski JA. The biology of the glucocorticoid receptor: new signaling mechanisms in health and disease. *J Allergy Clin Immunol* 2013;**132**(5):1033–44.
76. Rhen T, Cidlowski JA. Antiinflammatory action of glucocorticoids—new mechanisms for old drugs. *New Engl J Med* 2005;**353**(16):1711–23.
77. Sainte-Marie Y, et al. Conditional glucocorticoid receptor expression in the heart induces atrio-ventricular block. *FASEB J* 2007;**21**(12):3133–41.
78. Rog-Zielinska E, et al. Glucocorticoids promote structural and functional maturation of foetal cardiomyocytes: a role for PGC-1α. *Cell Death Differ* 2014;**22**(7):1–11.
79. Oakley RH, et al. Essential role of stress hormone signaling in cardiomyocytes for the prevention of heart disease. *Proc Natl Acad Sci* 2013;**110**(42):17035–40.
80. Pereg D, et al. Cortisol and testosterone in hair as biological markers of systolic heart failure. *Psychoneuroendocrinology* 2013;**38**(12):2875–82.

81. Addison, T., On the constitutional and local effects of disease of the supura-renal capsules. Samuel Highley, London, 1855.
82. Krug JJ. Cardiac arrest secondary to Addison's disease. *Ann Emerg Med* 1986;**15**(6):735–7.
83. Moreira RP, et al. Impact of glucocorticoid receptor gene polymorphisms on the metabolic profile of adult patients with the classical form of 21-hydroxylase deficiency. *PLoS One* 2012;**7**(9):e44893.
84. Debono M, Ross RJ, Newell-Price J. Inadequacies of glucocorticoid replacement and improvements by physiological circadian therapy. *Eur J Endocrinol* 2009;**160**(5):719–29.
85. Mooij CF, et al. Unfavourable trends in cardiovascular and metabolic risk in paediatric and adult patients with congenital adrenal hyperplasia? *Clin Endocrinol (Oxf)* 2010;**73**(2):137–46.
86. Busic Z, Tintor G, Culic V. Cellular mechanisms of cortisol in heart failure. *Psychoneuroendocrinology* 2014;**46**:100–1.
87. Otte C, et al. Glucocorticoid receptor gene, low-grade inflammation, and heart failure: the Heart and Soul study. *J Clin Endocrinol Metab* 2010;**95**(6):2885–91.
88. van den Akker EL, et al. Glucocorticoid receptor gene and risk of cardiovascular disease. *Arch Intern Med* 2008;**168**(1):33–9.
89. Lother A, et al. Mineralocorticoids in the heart and vasculature: new insights for old hormones. *Annu Rev Pharmacol Toxicol* 2015;**55**:289–312.
90. Bauersachs J, Jaisser F, Toto R. Mineralocorticoid receptor activation and mineralocorticoid receptor antagonist treatment in cardiac and renal diseases. *Hypertension* 2015;**65**(2):257–63.
91. Ferrari P. The role of 11β-hydroxysteroid dehydrogenase type 2 in human hypertension. *Biochim Biophys Acta-Mol Basis Dis* 2010;**1802**(12):1178–87.
92. Odermatt A, Kratschmar DV. Tissue-specific modulation of mineralocorticoid receptor function by 11β-hydroxysteroid dehydrogenases: an overview. *Mol Cell Endocrinol* 2012;**350**(2):168–86.
93. Grossmann C, et al. Nuclear shuttling precedes dimerization in mineralocorticoid receptor signaling. *Chem Biol* 2012;**19**(6):742–51.
94. Funder M, John W. Glucocorticoid and mineralocorticoid receptors: biology and clinical relevance. *Annu Rev Med* 1997;**48**(1):231–40.
95. Yang J, Young MJ. The mineralocorticoid receptor and its coregulators. *J Mol Endocrinol* 2009;**43**(2): 53–64.
96. Yang J, Fuller PJ. Interactions of the mineralocorticoid receptor–within and without. *Mol Cell Endocrinol* 2012;**350**(2):196–205.
97. Murai-Takeda A, et al. NF-YC functions as a corepressor of agonist-bound mineralocorticoid receptor. *J Biol Chem* 2010;**285**(11):8084–93.
98. Le Moëllic C, et al. Early nongenomic events in aldosterone action in renal collecting duct cells: PKCα activation, mineralocorticoid receptor phosphorylation, and cross-talk with the genomic response. *J Am Soc Nephrol* 2004;**15**(5):1145–60.
99. Lee H-A, et al. Histone deacetylase inhibition attenuates transcriptional activity of mineralocorticoid receptor through its acetylation and prevents development of hypertension. *Circ Res* 2013;**112**(7):1004–12.
100. Gros R, et al. Aldosterone mediates its rapid effects in vascular endothelial cells through GPER activation. *Am J Physiol-Cell Physiol* 2013;**304**(6):C532–40.
101. Ding Q, et al. Estradiol-mediated ERK phosphorylation and apoptosis in vascular smooth muscle cells requires GPR 30. *Am J Physiol-Cell Physiol* 2009;**297**(5):C1178–87.
102. Vallon V, et al. SGK1-dependent cardiac CTGF formation and fibrosis following DOCA treatment. *J Mol Med* 2006;**84**(5):396–404.
103. Latouche C, et al. Molecular signature of mineralocorticoid receptor signaling in cardiomyocytes: from cultured cells to mouse heart. *Endocrinology* 2010;**151**(9):4467–76.
104. Fejes-Tóth G, Náray-Fejes-Tóth A. Early aldosterone-regulated genes in cardiomyocytes: clues to cardiac remodeling? *Endocrinology* 2007;**148**(4):1502–10.

105. Takeda M, et al. Spironolactone modulates expressions of cardiac mineralocorticoid receptor and 11beta-hydroxysteroid dehydrogenase 2 and prevents ventricular remodeling in post-infarct rat hearts. *Hyper Res* 2007;**30**(5):427.
106. Nagata K, et al. Mineralocorticoid receptor antagonism attenuates cardiac hypertrophy and failure in low-aldosterone hypertensive rats. *Hypertension* 2006;**47**(4):656–64.
107. Lother A, et al. Ablation of mineralocorticoid receptors in myocytes but not in fibroblasts preserves cardiac function. *Hypertension* 2011;**57**(4):746–54.
108. Fraccarollo D, et al. Deletion of cardiomyocyte mineralocorticoid receptor ameliorates adverse remodeling after myocardial infarction. *Circulation* 2011;**123**(4):400–8.
109. Ouvrard-Pascaud A, et al. Conditional mineralocorticoid receptor expression in the heart leads to life-threatening arrhythmias. *Circulation* 2005;**111**(23):3025–33.
110. Rocha R, et al. Aldosterone induces a vascular inflammatory phenotype in the rat heart. *Am J Physiol-Heart Circul Physiol* 2002;**283**(5):H1802–10.
111. López-Andrés N, et al. A role for cardiotrophin-1 in myocardial remodeling induced by aldosterone. *Am J Physiol-Heart Circul Physiol* 2011;**301**(6):H2372–82.
112. Martín-Fernández B, et al. Structural, functional, and molecular alterations produced by aldosterone plus salt in rat heart: association with enhanced serum and glucocorticoid–regulated kinase-1 expression. *J Cardiovasc Pharmacol* 2011;**57**(1):114–21.
113. He BJ, et al. Oxidation of CaMKII determines the cardiotoxic effects of aldosterone. *Nat Med* 2011;**17**(12):1610–8.
114. Ducharme A, et al. Targeted deletion of matrix metalloproteinase-9 attenuates left ventricular enlargement and collagen accumulation after experimental myocardial infarction. *J Clin Invest* 2000;**106**(1):55.
115. Taube A, et al. Inflammation and metabolic dysfunction: links to cardiovascular diseases. *Am J Physiol-Heart Circul Physiol* 2012;**302**(11):H2148–65.
116. Pitt B. The role of mineralocorticoid receptor antagonists (MRAs) in very old patients with heart failure. *Heart Fail Rev* 2012;**17**(4–5):573–9.
117. Shah AM, et al. The prognostic importance of changes in cardiac structure and function in heart failure with preserved ejection fraction and the impact of spironolactone. *Circ Heart Fail* 2015;**8**(6):1052–8.
118. Capuano A, et al. Mineralocorticoid receptor antagonists in heart failure with preserved ejection fraction (HFpEF). *Int J Cardiol* 2015;**200**:15–19.
119. Solomon SD, et al. Influence of ejection fraction on outcomes and efficacy of spironolactone in patients with heart failure with preserved ejection fraction. *Eur Heart J* 2016;**37**(5):455–62.
120. Sanchez-Sanchez C, et al. Spironolactone in patients with heart failure and preserved ejection fraction. *Rev Clin Esp* 2015;**215**(6):301–7.
121. Hamo CE, et al. Baseline distribution of participants with depression and impaired quality of life in the Treatment of Preserved Cardiac Function Heart Failure with an Aldosterone Antagonist Trial. *Circ Heart Fail* 2015;**8**(2):268–77.
122. Edelmann F, et al. Galectin-3 in patients with heart failure with preserved ejection fraction: results from the Aldo-DHF trial. *Eur J Heart Fail* 2015;**17**(2):214–23.
123. Zhang XK, Kahl M. Regulation of retinoid and thyroid hormone action through homodimeric and heterodimeric receptors. *Trends Endocrinol Metab* 1993;**4**(5):156–62.
124. Jepsen K, Rosenfeld MG. Biological roles and mechanistic actions of co-repressor complexes. *J Cell Sci* 2002;**115**(Pt 4):689–98.
125. Casas F, et al. Characterization of a novel thyroid hormone receptor alpha variant involved in the regulation of myoblast differentiation. *Mol Endocrinol* 2006;**20**(4):749–63.
126. Mitsuhashi T, Tennyson GE, Nikodem VM. Alternative splicing generates messages encoding rat c-erbA proteins that do not bind thyroid hormone. *Proc Natl Acad Sci USA* 1988;**85**(16):5804–8.

127. Chassande O, et al. Identification of transcripts initiated from an internal promoter in the c-erbA alpha locus that encode inhibitors of retinoic acid receptor-alpha and triiodothyronine receptor activities. *Mol Endocrinol* 1997;**11**(9):1278–90.
128. Master A, Nauman A. THRB (Thyroid Hormone Receptor, Beta). *Atlas Genet Cytogenet Oncol Haematol* 2014;**18**(6):400–33.
129. Williams GR. Cloning and characterization of two novel thyroid hormone receptor beta isoforms. *Mol Cell Biol* 2000;**20**(22):8329–42.
130. Cheng SY. Multiple mechanisms for regulation of the transcriptional activity of thyroid hormone receptors. *Rev Endocr Metab Disord* 2000;**1**(1–2):9–18.
131. Lazar MA. Thyroid hormone receptors: multiple forms, multiple possibilities. *Endocr Rev* 1993;**14**(2):184–93.
132. Cheng SY, Leonard JL, Davis PJ. Molecular aspects of thyroid hormone actions. *Endocr Rev* 2010;**31**(2):139–70.
133. Cheng SY. Isoform-dependent actions of thyroid hormone nuclear receptors: lessons from knockin mutant mice. *Steroids* 2005;**70**(5–7):450–4.
134. Abel ED, et al. Divergent roles for thyroid hormone receptor beta isoforms in the endocrine axis and auditory system. *J Clin Invest* 1999;**104**(3):291–300.
135. Nunez J, et al. Multigenic control of thyroid hormone functions in the nervous system. *Mol Cell Endocrinol* 2008;**287**(1–2):1–12.
136. Gauthier K, et al. Genetic analysis reveals different functions for the products of the thyroid hormone receptor alpha locus. *Mol Cell Biol* 2001;**21**(14):4748–60.
137. Biondi B, et al. Left ventricular diastolic dysfunction in patients with subclinical hypothyroidism. *J Clin Endocrinol Metab* 1999;**84**(6):2064–7.
138. Monzani F, et al. Effect of levothyroxine on cardiac function and structure in subclinical hypothyroidism: a double blind, placebo-controlled study. *J Clin Endocrinol Metab* 2001;**86**(3):1110–5.
139. Henderson KK, et al. Physiological replacement of T3 improves left ventricular function in an animal model of myocardial infarction-induced congestive heart failure. *Circ Heart Fail* 2009;**2**(3):243–52.
140. Dillmann WH. Editorial: thyroid hormone action and cardiac contractility - a complex affair. *Endocrinology* 1996;**137**(3):799–801.
141. Dillmann WH. Biochemical basis of thyroid hormone action in the heart. *Am J Med* 1990;**88**(6):626–30.
142. Dillmann W. Cardiac hypertrophy and thyroid hormone signaling. *Heart Fail Rev* 2010;**15**(2):125–32.
143. Degens H, et al. Functional and metabolic adaptation of the heart to prolonged thyroid hormone treatment. *Am J Physiol Heart Circ Physiol* 2003;**284**(1):H108–15.
144. Cappola AR, Ladenson PW. Hypothyroidism and atherosclerosis. *J Clin Endocrinol Metab* 2003;**88**(6):2438–44.
145. Duntas LH. Thyroid disease and lipids. *Thyroid* 2002;**12**(4):287–93.
146. Palmieri EA, et al. Subclinical hypothyroidism and cardiovascular risk: a reason to treat? *Treat Endocrinol* 2004;**3**(4):233–44.
147. Shuvy M, et al. Hypothyroidism-induced myocardial damage and heart failure: an overlooked entity. *Cardiovasc Pathol* 2009;**18**(3):183–6.
148. Pazos-Moura C, et al. Cardiac dysfunction caused by myocardium-specific expression of a mutant thyroid hormone receptor. *Circ Res* 2000;**86**(6):700–6.
149. Imperio GE, et al. The impact of a non-functional thyroid receptor beta upon triiodotironine-induced cardiac hypertrophy in mice. *Cell Physiol Biochem* 2015;**37**(2):477–90.
150. Macchia PE, et al. Increased sensitivity to thyroid hormone in mice with complete deficiency of thyroid hormone receptor alpha. *Proc Natl Acad Sci USA* 2001;**98**(1):349–54.
151. Kinugawa K, et al. Regulation of thyroid hormone receptor isoforms in physiological and pathological cardiac hypertrophy. *Circ Res* 2001;**89**(7):591–8.

152. Tylki-Szymanska A, et al. Thyroid hormone resistance syndrome due to mutations in the thyroid hormone receptor alpha gene (THRA). *J Med Genet* 2015;**52**(5):312–6.
153. Moran C, et al. An adult female with resistance to thyroid hormone mediated by defective thyroid hormone receptor alpha. *J Clin Endocrinol Metab* 2013;**98**(11):4254–61.
154. Bochukova E, et al. A mutation in the thyroid hormone receptor alpha gene. *N Engl J Med* 2012;**366**(3):243–9.
155. van Mullem AA, Visser TJ, Peeters RP. Clinical consequences of mutations in thyroid hormone receptor-alpha1. *Eur Thyroid J* 2014;**3**(1):17–24.
156. Amor AJ, et al. Identification of four novel mutations in the thyroid hormone receptor-beta gene in 164 Spanish and 2 Greek patients with resistance to thyroid hormone. *Hormones (Athens)* 2014;**13**(1):74–8.
157. Moran C, Chatterjee K. Resistance to thyroid hormone due to defective thyroid receptor alpha. *Best Pract Res Clin Endocrinol Metab* 2015;**29**(4):647–57.
158. Refetoff S, Dumitrescu AM. Syndromes of reduced sensitivity to thyroid hormone: genetic defects in hormone receptors, cell transporters and deiodination. *Best Pract Res Clin Endocrinol Metab* 2007;**21**(2): 277–305.
159. van Mullem A, et al. Clinical phenotype and mutant TRalpha1. *N Engl J Med* 2012;**366**(15):1451–3.
160. Moran C, et al. Resistance to thyroid hormone caused by a mutation in thyroid hormone receptor (TR) alpha1 and TRalpha2: clinical, biochemical, and genetic analyses of three related patients. *Lancet Diabetes Endocrinol* 2014;**2**(8):619–26.
161. Espiard S, et al. A novel mutation in THRA gene associated with an atypical phenotype of resistance to thyroid hormone. *J Clin Endocrinol Metab* 2015;**100**(8):2841–8.
162. Yuen RK, et al. Whole-genome sequencing of quartet families with autism spectrum disorder. *Nat Med* 2015;**21**(2):185–91.
163. Adams M, et al. Genetic analysis of 29 kindreds with generalized and pituitary resistance to thyroid hormone. Identification of thirteen novel mutations in the thyroid hormone receptor beta gene. *J Clin Invest* 1994;**94**(2):506–15.
164. Collingwood TN, et al. A role for helix 3 of the TRbeta ligand-binding domain in coactivator recruitment identified by characterization of a third cluster of mutations in resistance to thyroid hormone. *EMBO J* 1998;**17**(16):4760–70.
165. Buroker NE, et al. The dominant negative thyroid hormone receptor beta-mutant {Delta}337T alters PPAR{alpha} signaling in heart. *Am J Physiol Endocrinol Metab* 2007;**292**(2):E453–60.
166. Usala SJ, et al. A new point mutation in the 3,5,3′-triiodothyronine-binding domain of the c-erbA beta thyroid hormone receptor is tightly linked to generalized thyroid hormone resistance. *J Clin Endocrinol Metab* 1991;**72**(1):32–8.
167. Kojetin DJ, et al. Structural mechanism for signal transduction in RXR nuclear receptor heterodimers. *Nat Commun* 2015;**6**:8013.
168. Chu R, et al. Thyroid hormone (T3) inhibits ciprofibrate-induced transcription of genes encoding beta-oxidation enzymes: cross talk between peroxisome proliferator and T3 signaling pathways. *Proc Natl Acad Sci USA* 1995;**92**(25):11593–7.
169. Miyamoto T, et al. Inhibition of peroxisome proliferator signaling pathways by thyroid hormone receptor. Competitive binding to the response element. *J Biol Chem* 1997;**272**(12):7752–8.
170. Lin HM, Zhao L, Cheng SY. Cyclin D1 is a ligand-independent co-repressor for thyroid hormone receptors. *J Biol Chem* 2002;**277**(32):28733–41.
171. Bergh JJ, et al. Integrin alphaVbeta3 contains a cell surface receptor site for thyroid hormone that is linked to activation of mitogen-activated protein kinase and induction of angiogenesis. *Endocrinology* 2005;**146**(7):2864–71.
172. Aranda A, et al. Thyroid receptor: roles in cancer. *Trends Endocrinol Metab* 2009;**20**(7):318–24.
173. Furuya F, Hanover JA, Cheng SY. Activation of phosphatidylinositol 3-kinase signaling by a mutant thyroid hormone beta receptor. *Proc Natl Acad Sci USA* 2006;**103**(6):1780–5.

174. Kenessey A, Ojamaa K. Thyroid hormone stimulates protein synthesis in the cardiomyocyte by activating the Akt-mTOR and p70S6K pathways. *J Biol Chem* 2006;**281**(30):20666–72.
175. Kliewer SA, et al. Differential expression and activation of a family of murine peroxisome proliferator-activated receptors. *Proc Natl Acad Sci USA* 1994;**91**(15):7355–9.
176. Kliewer SA, et al. Convergence of 9-cis retinoic acid and peroxisome proliferator signalling pathways through heterodimer formation of their receptors. *Nature* 1992;**358**(6389):771–4.
177. Rosenson RS, et al. Modulating peroxisome proliferator-activated receptors for therapeutic benefit? Biology, clinical experience, and future prospects. *Am Heart J* 2012;**164**(5):672–80.
178. DiRenzo J, et al. Peroxisome proliferator-activated receptors and retinoic acid receptors differentially control the interactions of retinoid X receptor heterodimers with ligands, coactivators, and corepressors. *Mol Cell Biol* 1997;**17**(4):2166–76.
179. Chandra V, et al. Structure of the intact PPAR-gamma-RXR- nuclear receptor complex on DNA. *Nature* 2008;**456**(7220):350–6.
180. Keller H, et al. Fatty acids and retinoids control lipid metabolism through activation of peroxisome proliferator-activated receptor-retinoid X receptor heterodimers. *Proc Natl Acad Sci USA* 1993;**90**(6):2160–4.
181. Gulick T, et al. The peroxisome proliferator-activated receptor regulates mitochondrial fatty acid oxidative enzyme gene expression. *Proc Natl Acad Sci USA* 1994;**91**(23):11012–6.
182. Braissant O, et al. Differential expression of peroxisome proliferator-activated receptors (PPARs): tissue distribution of PPAR-alpha, -beta, and -gamma in the adult rat. *Endocrinology* 1996;**137**(1):354–66.
183. Ziouzenkova O, et al. Peroxisome proliferator-activated receptors. *Curr Atheroscler Rep* 2002;**4**(1):59–64.
184. Inoue I, et al. Expression of peroxisome proliferator-activated receptor alpha (PPAR alpha) in primary cultures of human vascular endothelial cells. *Biochem Biophys Res Commun* 1998;**246**(2):370–4.
185. Marx N, et al. PPARalpha activators inhibit cytokine-induced vascular cell adhesion molecule-1 expression in human endothelial cells. *Circulation* 1999;**99**(24):3125–31.
186. Freitag CM, Miller RJ. Peroxisome proliferator-activated receptor agonists modulate neuropathic pain: a link to chemokines? *Front Cell Neurosci* 2014;**8**:238.
187. Bishop-Bailey D. Peroxisome proliferator-activated receptors in the cardiovascular system. *Br J Pharmacol* 2000;**129**(5):823–34.
188. Guellich A, et al. Role of oxidative stress in cardiac dysfunction of PPARalpha−/− mice. *Am J Physiol Heart Circ Physiol* 2007;**293**(1):H93–H102.
189. Nissen SE, et al. Effects of a potent and selective PPAR-alpha agonist in patients with atherogenic dyslipidemia or hypercholesterolemia: two randomized controlled trials. *JAMA* 2007;**297**(12):1362–73.
190. Wayman NS, et al. Ligands of the peroxisome proliferator-activated receptors (PPAR-gamma and PPAR-alpha) reduce myocardial infarct size. *FASEB J* 2002;**16**(9):1027–40.
191. Ichihara S, et al. Attenuation of cardiac dysfunction by a PPAR-alpha agonist is associated with down-regulation of redox-regulated transcription factors. *J Mol Cell Cardiol* 2006;**41**(2):318–29.
192. Finck BN, et al. The cardiac phenotype induced by PPARalpha overexpression mimics that caused by diabetes mellitus. *J Clin Invest* 2002;**109**(1):121–30.
193. Finck BN, et al. A critical role for PPARalpha-mediated lipotoxicity in the pathogenesis of diabetic cardiomyopathy: modulation by dietary fat content. *Proc Natl Acad Sci USA* 2003;**100**(3):1226–31.
194. Duncan JG, et al. Rescue of cardiomyopathy in peroxisome proliferator-activated receptor-alpha transgenic mice by deletion of lipoprotein lipase identifies sources of cardiac lipids and peroxisome proliferator-activated receptor-alpha activators. *Circulation* 2010;**121**(3):426–35.
195. Fredenrich A, Grimaldi PA. PPAR delta: an uncompletely known nuclear receptor. *Diabetes Metab* 2005;**31**(1):23–7.
196. Ehrenborg E, Krook A. Regulation of skeletal muscle physiology and metabolism by peroxisome proliferator-activated receptor delta. *Pharmacol Rev* 2009;**61**(3):373–93.

197. Chen W, et al. Peroxisome proliferator-activated receptor delta-agonist, GW501516, ameliorates insulin resistance, improves dyslipidaemia in monosodium L-glutamate metabolic syndrome mice. *Basic Clin Pharmacol Toxicol* 2008;**103**(3):240–6.
198. Riserus U, et al. Activation of peroxisome proliferator-activated receptor (PPAR)delta promotes reversal of multiple metabolic abnormalities, reduces oxidative stress, and increases fatty acid oxidation in moderately obese men. *Diabetes* 2008;**57**(2):332–9.
199. Chen ZC, et al. Cardiac peroxisome proliferator-activated receptor delta (PPARdelta) as a new target for increased contractility without altering heart rate. *PLoS One* 2013;**8**(5):e64229.
200. Wagner N, et al. Peroxisome proliferator-activated receptor beta stimulation induces rapid cardiac growth and angiogenesis via direct activation of calcineurin. *Cardiovasc Res* 2009;**83**(1):61–71.
201. Oliver Jr. WR, et al. A selective peroxisome proliferator-activated receptor delta agonist promotes reverse cholesterol transport. *Proc Natl Acad Sci USA* 2001;**98**(9):5306–11.
202. Wallace JM, et al. Effects of peroxisome proliferator-activated receptor alpha/delta agonists on HDL-cholesterol in vervet monkeys. *J Lipid Res* 2005;**46**(5):1009–16.
203. Sprecher DL, et al. Triglyceride:high-density lipoprotein cholesterol effects in healthy subjects administered a peroxisome proliferator activated receptor delta agonist. *Arterioscler Thromb Vasc Biol* 2007;**27**(2):359–65.
204. Cheng L, et al. Cardiomyocyte-restricted peroxisome proliferator-activated receptor-delta deletion perturbs myocardial fatty acid oxidation and leads to cardiomyopathy. *Nat Med* 2004;**10**(11):1245–50.
205. Burkart EM, et al. Nuclear receptors PPARbeta/delta and PPARalpha direct distinct metabolic regulatory programs in the mouse heart. *J Clin Invest* 2007;**117**(12):3930–9.
206. Fajas L, Fruchart JC, Auwerx J. PPARgamma3 mRNA: a distinct PPARgamma mRNA subtype transcribed from an independent promoter. *FEBS Lett* 1998;**438**(1–2):55–60.
207. Tontonoz P, et al. Adipocyte-specific transcription factor ARF6 is a heterodimeric complex of two nuclear hormone receptors, PPAR gamma and RXR alpha. *Nucl Acids Res* 1994;**22**(25):5628–34.
208. Tamori Y, et al. Role of peroxisome proliferator-activated receptor-gamma in maintenance of the characteristics of mature 3T3-L1 adipocytes. *Diabetes* 2002;**51**(7):2045–55.
209. Gray SL, et al. Leptin deficiency unmasks the deleterious effects of impaired peroxisome proliferator-activated receptor gamma function (P465L PPARgamma) in mice. *Diabetes* 2006;**55**(10):2669–77.
210. Sidell RJ, et al. Thiazolidinedione treatment normalizes insulin resistance and ischemic injury in the zucker Fatty rat heart. *Diabetes* 2002;**51**(4):1110–7.
211. Yue TL. Cardioprotective effects of thiazolidinediones, peroxisome proliferator-activated receptor-gamma agonists. *Drugs Today (Barc)* 2003;**39**(12):949–60.
212. Smeets PJ, et al. Peroxisome proliferator-activated receptors and inflammation: take it to heart. *Acta Physiol (Oxf)* 2007;**191**(3):171–88.
213. Yuan Z, et al. Peroxisome proliferation-activated receptor-gamma ligands ameliorate experimental autoimmune myocarditis. *Cardiovasc Res* 2003;**59**(3):685–94.
214. Borchert M, et al. Review of the pleiotropic effects of peroxisome proliferator-activated receptor gamma agonists on platelet function. *Diabetes Technol Ther* 2007;**9**(5):410–20.
215. Ihm SH, et al. Peroxisome proliferator-activated receptor-gamma activation attenuates cardiac fibrosis in type 2 diabetic rats: the effect of rosiglitazone on myocardial expression of receptor for advanced glycation end products and of connective tissue growth factor. *Basic Res Cardiol* 2010;**105**(3):399–407.
216. Wynne AM, Mocanu MM, Yellon DM. Pioglitazone mimics preconditioning in the isolated perfused rat heart: a role for the prosurvival kinases PI3K and P42/44MAPK. *J Cardiovasc Pharmacol* 2005;**46**(6):817–22.
217. Wu L, et al. Beneficial and deleterious effects of rosiglitazone on hypertension development in spontaneously hypertensive rats. *Am J Hypertens* 2004;**17**(9):749–56.
218. Lee TI, et al. Cardiac peroxisome-proliferator-activated receptor expression in hypertension co-existing with diabetes. *Clin Sci (Lond)* 2011;**121**(7):305–12.

219. Duan SZ, et al. Cardiomyocyte-specific knockout and agonist of peroxisome proliferator-activated receptor-gamma both induce cardiac hypertrophy in mice. *Circ Res* 2005;**97**(4):372–9.
220. Ding G, et al. Cardiac peroxisome proliferator-activated receptor gamma is essential in protecting cardiomyocytes from oxidative damage. *Cardiovasc Res* 2007;**76**(2):269–79.
221. Son NH, et al. Cardiomyocyte expression of PPARgamma leads to cardiac dysfunction in mice. *J Clin Invest* 2007;**117**(10):2791–801.
222. Moraes LA, Piqueras L, Bishop-Bailey D. Peroxisome proliferator-activated receptors and inflammation. *Pharmacol Ther* 2006;**110**(3):371–85.
223. Wright MB, et al. Minireview: challenges and opportunities in development of PPAR agonists. *Mol Endocrinol* 2014;**28**(11):1756–68.
224. Forman BM, et al. 15-Deoxy-delta 12, 14-prostaglandin J2 is a ligand for the adipocyte determination factor PPAR gamma. *Cell* 1995;**83**(5):803–12.
225. Chinetti G, et al. PPAR-alpha and PPAR-gamma activators induce cholesterol removal from human macrophage foam cells through stimulation of the ABCA1 pathway. *Nat Med* 2001;**7**(1):53–8.
226. Frick MH, et al. Helsinki Heart Study: primary-prevention trial with gemfibrozil in middle-aged men with dyslipidemia. Safety of treatment, changes in risk factors, and incidence of coronary heart disease. *N Engl J Med* 1987;**317**(20):1237–45.
227. Rubins HB, et al. Gemfibrozil for the secondary prevention of coronary heart disease in men with low levels of high-density lipoprotein cholesterol. Veterans Affairs High-Density Lipoprotein Cholesterol Intervention Trial Study Group. *N Engl J Med* 1999;**341**(6):410–8.
228. Birjmohun RS, et al. Efficacy and safety of high-density lipoprotein cholesterol-increasing compounds: a meta-analysis of randomized controlled trials. *J Am Coll Cardiol* 2005;**45**(2):185–97.
229. Tontonoz P, Spiegelman BM. Fat and beyond: the diverse biology of PPARgamma. *Annu Rev Biochem* 2008;**77**:289–312.
230. Ghazzi MN, et al. Cardiac and glycemic benefits of troglitazone treatment in NIDDM. The Troglitazone Study Group. *Diabetes* 1997;**46**(3):433–9.
231. Graham DJ, et al. Risk of acute myocardial infarction, stroke, heart failure, and death in elderly medicare patients treated with rosiglitazone or pioglitazone. *JAMA* 2010;**304**(4):411–8.
232. Home P. Safety of PPAR agonists. *Diabetes Care* 2011;**34**(Suppl. 2):S215–9.
233. Lu CJ, et al. Risk of stroke with thiazolidinediones: a ten-year nationwide population-based cohort study. *Cerebrovasc Dis* 2013;**36**(2):145–51.
234. Breunig IM, et al. Development of heart failure in Medicaid patients with type 2 diabetes treated with pioglitazone, rosiglitazone, or metformin. *J Manag Care Spec Pharm* 2014;**20**(9):895–903.
235. Varas-Lorenzo C, et al. The risk of heart failure associated with the use of noninsulin blood glucose-lowering drugs: systematic review and meta-analysis of published observational studies. *BMC Cardiovasc Disord* 2014;**14**:129.
236. Lincoff AM, et al. Pioglitazone and risk of cardiovascular events in patients with type 2 diabetes mellitus: a meta-analysis of randomized trials. *JAMA* 2007;**298**(10):1180–8.
237. Starner CI, et al. Rosiglitazone and pioglitazone utilization from January 2007 through May 2008 associated with five risk-warning events. *J Manag Care Pharm* 2008;**14**(6):523–31.
238. Fievet C, Fruchart JC, Staels B. PPARalpha and PPARgamma dual agonists for the treatment of type 2 diabetes and the metabolic syndrome. *Curr Opin Pharmacol* 2006;**6**(6):606–14.
239. Lincoff AM, et al. Effect of aleglitazar on cardiovascular outcomes after acute coronary syndrome in patients with type 2 diabetes mellitus: the AleCardio randomized clinical trial. *JAMA* 2014;**311**(15):1515–25.
240. Rai A, et al. CDK5-induced p-PPARgamma(Ser 112) downregulates GFAP via PPREs in developing rat brain: effect of metal mixture and troglitazone in astrocytes. *Cell Death Dis* 2014;**5**:e1033.
241. Hu E, et al. Inhibition of adipogenesis through MAP kinase-mediated phosphorylation of PPARgamma. *Science* 1996;**274**(5295):2100–3.

242. Compe E, et al. Dysregulation of the peroxisome proliferator-activated receptor target genes by XPD mutations. *Mol Cell Biol* 2005;**25**(14):6065–76.
243. Choi JH, et al. Anti-diabetic drugs inhibit obesity-linked phosphorylation of PPARgamma by Cdk5. *Nature* 2010;**466**(7305):451–6.
244. Choi JH, et al. Thrap3 docks on phosphoserine 273 of PPARgamma and controls diabetic gene programming. *Genes Dev* 2014;**28**(21):2361–9.
245. Lu Y, et al. SUMOylation of PPARgamma by rosiglitazone prevents LPS-induced NCoR degradation mediating down regulation of chemokines expression in renal proximal tubular cells. *PLoS One* 2013;**8**(11):e79815.
246. Wadosky KM, Willis MS. The story so far: post-translational regulation of peroxisome proliferator-activated receptors by ubiquitination and SUMOylation. *Am J Physiol Heart Circ Physiol* 2012;**302**(3):H515–26.
247. Chung SS, et al. Control of adipogenesis by the SUMO-specific protease SENP2. *Mol Cell Biol* 2010;**30**(9):2135–46.
248. Diezko R, Suske G. Ligand binding reduces SUMOylation of the peroxisome proliferator-activated receptor gamma (PPARgamma) activation function 1 (AF1) domain. *PLoS One* 2013;**8**(6):e66947.
249. Rodriguez JE, et al. The ubiquitin ligase MuRF1 regulates PPARalpha activity in the heart by enhancing nuclear export via monoubiquitination. *Mol Cell Endocrinol* 2015;**413**:36–48.
250. He J, et al. MuRF2 regulates PPARgamma1 activity to protect against diabetic cardiomyopathy and enhance weight gain induced by a high fat diet. *Cardiovasc Diabetol* 2015;**14**:97.
251. Ji S, et al. O-GlcNAc modification of PPARgamma reduces its transcriptional activity. *Biochem Biophys Res Commun* 2012;**417**(4):1158–63.
252. Tian L, et al. Acetylation-defective mutant of Ppargamma is associated with decreased lipid synthesis in breast cancer cells. *Oncotarget* 2014;**5**(17):7303–15.
253. Cohen HY, et al. Calorie restriction promotes mammalian cell survival by inducing the SIRT1 deacetylase. *Science* 2004;**305**(5682):390–2.
254. Han L, et al. SIRT1 is regulated by a PPAR{gamma}-SIRT1 negative feedback loop associated with senescence. *Nucl Acids Res* 2010;**38**(21):7458–71.
255. Choi JH, et al. Antidiabetic actions of a non-agonist PPARgamma ligand blocking Cdk5-mediated phosphorylation. *Nature* 2011;**477**(7365):477–81.
256. Norman PE, Powell JT. Vitamin D and cardiovascular disease. *Circul Res* 2014;**114**(2):379–93.

CHAPTER

ADRENERGIC RECEPTORS

11

M. Ciccarelli[1], D. Sorriento[2], E. Coscioni[3], G. Iaccarino[1] and G. Santulli[4]

[1]University of Salerno, Baronissi, SA, Italy [2]Institute of Biostructure and Bioimaging (IBB) of the Italian National Research Council (CNR), Naples, Italy [3]Azienda Ospedaliera Universitaria OO.RR. San Giovanni di Dio Ruggi d'Aragona, Salerno, Italy [4]Columbia University Medical Center, New York, NY, United States

ADRENERGIC SIGNALING: SYSTEMATIC AND UPDATED OVERVIEW

Adrenergic receptors (also known as adrenoceptors, ARs) belong to the guanine nucleotide-binding G protein–coupled receptor (GPCR) superfamily, and are membrane receptors that activate heterotrimeric G proteins following the binding of a ligand. GPCRs consist of one extracellular N-terminal domain, seven membrane-spanning domains, three intra- and three extracellular loops, and one intracellular C-terminal tail (Fig. 11.1). These heptahelical trans-membrane sensors account for approximately 4% of the total protein-coding genome and are considered the most important drug targets in medicine and physiology. G proteins typically stimulate (via G_s protein) or inhibit (via G_i protein) the enzyme adenylyl-cyclase or activate (via G_q protein) phospholipase C (PLC). A detailed and updated overview of the main cardiovascular GPCRs was recently published.[1] GPCR signaling is terminated by phosphorylation of the intracellular domains of the receptor by the family of G protein–coupled receptor kinases (GRKs).[2,3] GRK-mediated phosphorylation increases the affinity of GPCRs for the arrestin class of proteins, which uncouples the phosphorylated receptor from G protein and successively targets the receptor for internalization. Downregulation of GPCRs reduces the functional activity of classical signaling paradigms up to 80%[4,5] (Fig. 11.1).

Two classes of ARs have been identified: αAR and βAR. Phenylephrine is a selective pharmacological agonist of αAR while isoproterenol is considered a nonselective agonist for βAR.[6] The subfamily of α_1AR (G_q coupled receptors) consists of three highly homologous subtypes, including α_1A-, α_1B-, and α_1D-AR.[7] The α_2AR subfamily (coupled to G_i) comprises three subtypes: α_2A-, α_2B-, and α_2C-AR.[8] Some species other than humans express a fourth α_2D-AR as well.[9] In the βAR family there are three receptor subtypes:β_1AR is found at its highest levels in the heart,[10] β_2AR is distributed extensively throughout the body,[11] and β_3AR is mainly expressed in the white and brown adipose tissue.[12] All three βARs couple primarily to $G\alpha_s$ and subsequent cAMP-related pathways, although under certain conditions can also couple to $G\alpha_i$.[13] β_2AR and β_3AR signaling can also occur via G protein independent mechanisms.[14] In particular, cardiac β_3AR causes negative inotropic effects mainly mediated by activation of nitric oxide (NO) synthase, serving thereby as a brake in sympathetic overstimulation. These paradigms of signaling can be observed in the same cell type based on the functional state of the cell. Henceforth, the response to GPCR stimulus can be modified by various conditions, including chronic stimulation, acidosis, cell hypoxia, and aging.[15–17]

Endocrinology of the Heart in Health and Disease. DOI: http://dx.doi.org/10.1016/B978-0-12-803111-7.00011-7

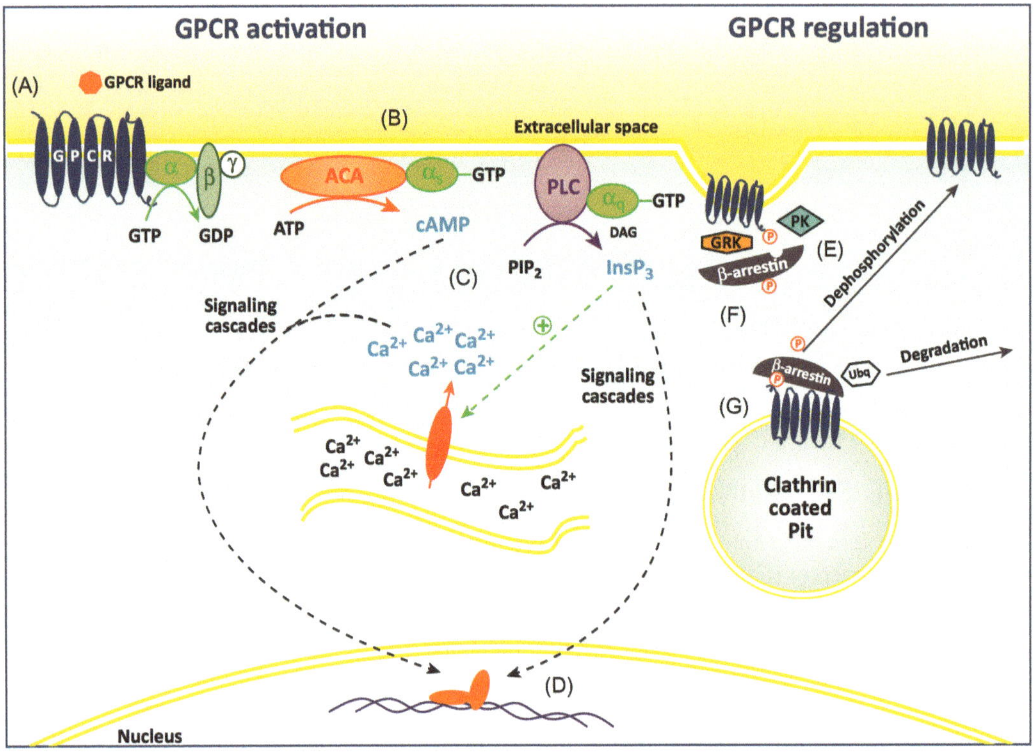

FIGURE 11.1

G protein–coupled receptor (GPCR) activation and regulation. (A) Binding of a GPCR ligand to the extracellular side of the receptor enables the exchange of GDP to GTP by the α subunit of the G protein. (B) The GTP-bound α subunit then acts on a second messenger-releasing enzyme such as adenylate cyclase (*ACA*) (Gαs) or phospholipase C (*PLC*) (Gαq), leading to their activation. (C) Second-messenger molecules such as cAMP and inositol-1,4,5-triphosphate ($InsP_3$) are direct products of enzymatic conversion of ATP and phosphatidylinositol-4,5-bisphosphate (PIP_2) respectively, whereas cytosolic Ca^{2+} is released upon activation of reticular calcium channels. (D) Second-messenger molecules can trigger cascade reactions that will lead to a downstream biological event (frequently gene expression regulation). (E) GPCR responsive elements such as protein kinases (*PKs*) or G protein–coupled receptor kinases (*GRKs*) phosphorylate the intracellular side of the receptor and decouple the G protein by steric exclusion. (F) β-Arrestins can recognize the phosphorylated GPCR and trigger the internalization process. (G) Modifications on the β-arrestin molecule such as dephosphorylation or ubiquitination define the fate of the internalized molecule either to recycling or degradation, respectively.

*Adapted from Martins SA, Trabuco JR, Monteiro GA, Chu V, Conde JP, Prazeres DM. Towards the miniaturization of GPCR-based live-cell screening assays. Trends Biotechnol 2012;**30**(11):566–74. (10.1016/j.tibtech.2012.07.004).*

SYMPATHETIC SYSTEM AND HYPERTENSION

ROLE OF ADRENERGIC SYSTEM IN REGULATION OF VASCULAR HOMEOSTASIS AND OXIDATIVE STRESS

The endothelium is central in the regulation of several vascular functions, including vasculature tone and permeability, thrombosis, hemostasis, and angiogenesis.[18–20] This integrates the overall information originating from the bloodstream and furnishing, in a time- and space-dependent manner, a fine tuning of vascular homeostasis by releasing specific factors including catecholamines, NO, vasoactive peptides, arachidonic acid metabolites, and reactive oxygen species (ROS).[21] The adrenergic system is the major regulator of cardiac and vascular function, and this is accomplished also through the activation of specific receptors localized on endothelial surface by local and systemic release of catecholamines.[22–25]

These receptors actively participate in the release of NO to regulate endothelial function.[26,27] Following its release, NO diffuses to the subjacent vascular smooth muscle where it elicits vasorelaxation through activation of soluble guanylyl-cyclase enzyme, which then catalyzes the formation of cGMP and hence activation of cGMP-dependent protein kinase.[28,29] Classically, NO is released from endothelial cells following activation of the endothelial or type 3 isoform of NO synthase (NOS-3 or eNOS), which is a Ca^{2+} and calmodulin-dependent enzyme; hence, many endothelium-dependent vasodilators cause NO release via an increase in intracellular Ca^{2+}. However, other pathways have also identified to act in Ca^{2+} independent manner and involve phosphorylation of various eNOS serine residues by a number of protein kinases.[30] Such a mechanism is particularly evident for β_2AR signaling where activation of eNOS involves specific kinases such as protein kinase A (PKA) and AKT.[31] The impaired ability of endothelium to appropriately vasodilate is defined as "endothelial dysfunction" and the major cause is decreased NO bioavailability (Fig. 11.2). Endothelial dysfunction has been associated with development of several cardiovascular disorders including hypertension, type 2 diabetes mellitus, and heart failure.[21,32]

However, altered NO production is not the only feature of the endothelial dysfunction. Indeed, increased ROS bioavailability and dysregulated redox signaling (oxidative stress) together with decreased NO production and increased NO consumption by ROS contribute to many of the molecular events underlying endothelial injury. [33,34] These findings have modified the molecular definition of endothelial dysfunction, leading to the concept of "eNOS uncoupling," characterized by the discrepancy between eNOS protein levels and NO production, with a switch in the enzymatic activity of eNOS to generate superoxide (O_2) rather than NO.[35]

ADRENERGIC SIGNALING AND ROS

ROS are products of normal cellular metabolism and derived from many sources in different cellular compartments. Enzymatic sources of ROS in endothelial cells include uncoupled NOS, xanthine oxidoreductase, mitochondrial respiratory enzymes, and NADPH oxidase.[36–38] However, the perceived role of ROS in regulation of cellular physiology has changed in the recent years. Indeed, on the one hand they can be considered detrimental for cell survival; however, they also have important physiological roles and act as part of the intracellular signaling, promoting beneficial cellular process such as mitohormesis (e.g., replacement and organization of the mitochondrial network), induction of host

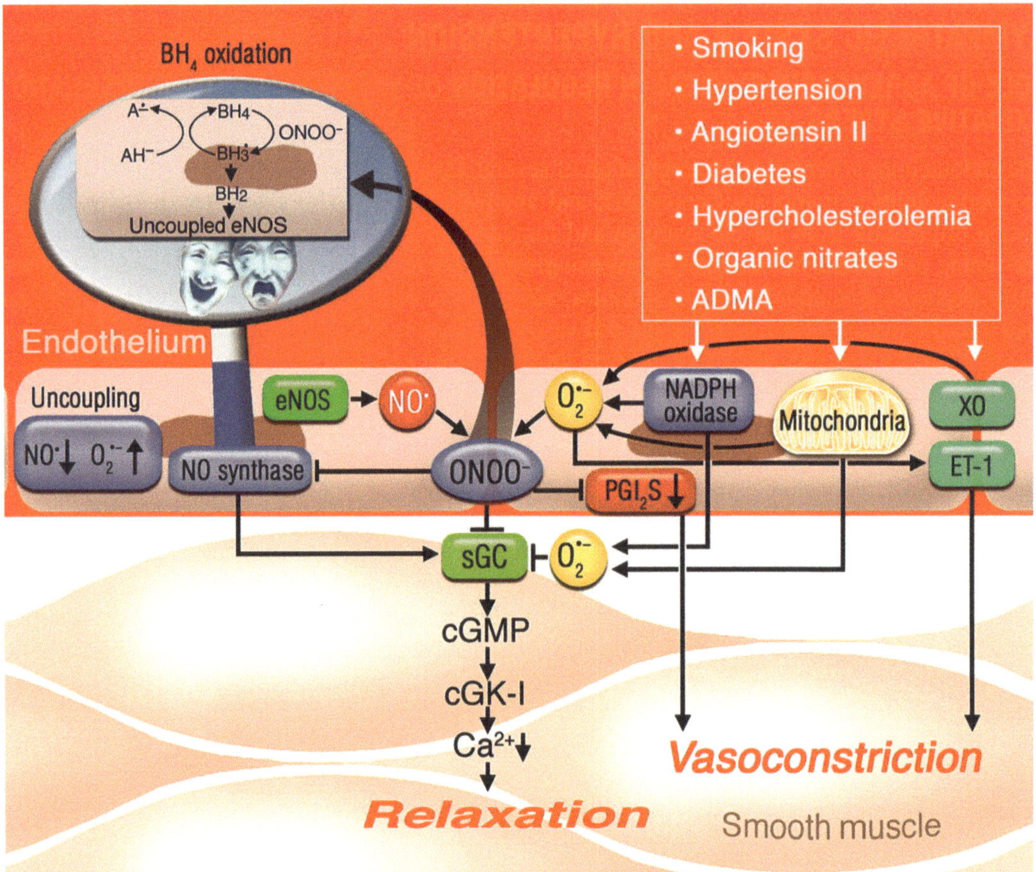

FIGURE 11.2

Mechanisms underlying endothelial (vascular) dysfunction in vascular disease. An unbalanced production of nitric oxide (NO) and superoxide (O_2^-) leads to inappropriate formation of peroxynitrite ($ONOO^-$). Peroxynitrite and superoxide cause vascular dysfunction through several mechanisms (reviewed in Forstermann and Munzel [1]). Peroxynitrite is a strong inhibitor of NO and prostacyclin (PGI_2) signaling, and it may cause eNOS uncoupling, causing this enzyme to produce superoxide instead of NO. *ADMA* = asymmetrical dimethylarginine; *cGMP* = guanosine 3′,5′-cyclic monophosphate; *cGK* = cGMP-dependent kinase; *eNOS* = endothelial nitric oxide synthase; *ET* = endothelin; *sGC* = soluble guanylate cyclase; *TXA* = thromboxane.

*From Münzel T, Gori T. Nebivolol. J Am Coll Cardiol 2009;***54***(16):1491–9. (10.1016/j.jacc.2009.05.066).*

defense genes, activation of transcription factors and stimulation of ion transport systems.[39] In the vascular system, ROS play a physiological role in controlling endothelial function, vascular tone, and vascular integrity but also a pathophysiological role in inflammation, hypertrophy, proliferation, apoptosis, constriction, migration, fibrosis, angiogenesis, and rarefaction, important factors contributing to endothelial dysfunction, vascular contraction, and arterial remodeling in cardiovascular diseases.

These various lines of evidence suggest ROS as a specific cellular messenger able to promote either cellular survival and adaptation or apoptosis, according to the specific characteristics of the stressors. According to this view, the physiological or pathological ROS level is more likely to be associated to the impaired redox signaling and equilibrium rather than the imbalance between pro-oxidants and antioxidants.[40]

The adrenergic system is also implicated in ROS production by the endothelium. Mounting evidence suggest an important roles for catecholamines in vascular cell growth and tissue remodeling following atherosclerosis, hypertension, and vascular injury.[41] Meanwhile, noradrenaline (norepinephrine) is also known to be a potential pro-inflammatory factor, since noradrenaline induces TNF-α, matrix metalloproteinase (MMP)-2, MMP-9, ROS, and toll-like receptor (TLR4) release from cells.[42] Furthermore, data suggest that noradrenaline stimulates the phosphorylation of mitogen-activated protein kinases (MAPK) and ROS synthesis leading to cell proliferation in vitro.[43]

THE ROLE OF G PROTEIN–COUPLED RECEPTOR KINASE 2 IN VASCULAR HOMEOSTASIS

GRKs have a significant role in adrenergic regulation of endothelial function (Figs. 11.1 and 11.2). Of the seven mammalian isoforms of GRKs, G protein-coupled receptor kinase 2 (GRK2) appears to be the most important isoform related to cardiac physiology. GRK2 is found in the striated (heart and skeletal) and smooth muscle in addition to WBCs (bone marrow, lymph nodes, and thymus) and many other organs. Indeed, homozygous GRK2-deficient mice exhibited embryonic lethality whereas gene ablation for the other GRKs resulted in relatively mild phenotypes.[44–46] The physiological relevance of GRK2 was further confirmed by its participation in diverse fundamental cellular processes, including cell cycle progression, migration, and differentiation.[47,48] Notably, GRK-mediated desensitization does not always rely on its catalytic activity but also on protein–protein interactions[49,50] that occur in different cellular compartments.[51] It is likely that both up- and downregulation of GRK2 affect cellular function and survival. Alterations in GRK2 expression and activity were observed in several diseases, such as heart failure,[2] Alzheimer's disease,[52] multiple sclerosis,[53] thyroid gland disorders,[54] opioid addiction,[55] rheumatoid arthritis,[56] ovarian cancer,[57] and cystic fibrosis.[58]

GRK2 participates in the development of experimental portal hypertension, which appears dependent upon the physical interaction between GRK2 and AKT.[59] Since AKT is able to activate eNOS, the GRK2-mediated inhibition of AKT shifts the vascular tone toward constriction in the setting of endothelial dysfunction due to decreased eNOS activity.[59] Given its close relationship to the adrenergic system, GRK2 may represent the specific link between adrenergic system and endothelial ROS production.

The functional role of GRK2 in vascular smooth muscle cells was explored in a transgenic animal model (targeted overexpression of GRK2),[60] where mice exhibited an increase in resting mean arterial pressure accompanied by an attenuated response to β-AR signaling compared with nontransgenic littermates. The increased blood pressure was also accompanied by cardiac hypertrophy and vascular thickening, two hallmarks of hypertensive phenotype.[60]

The endothelium-mediated modulation of the contractile state of vascular smooth muscle is impaired in atherosclerosis and in several conditions associated with the premature development of atherosclerosis.[61] The correlation between GRK2 abundance and hypertension is also present in other conditions characterized by increased blood pressure, such as portal hypertension[59] and preeclampsia.[62] In gestational hypertension, the increase in GRK2 in the placental vasculature seems to be compensatory rather than causative of increased blood pressure. This compensation helps balance the excessive vascular tension as the lack of protective effect of elevated GRK2 expression levels negatively affect the outcome of the hypertensive state.[62] In this case, a potential explanation could rely on the metabolic effect of GRK2, which is able to place the cell in a low energy state that might favor survival in stress conditions.[51,63–65]

GRK2 levels in peripheral blood lymphocytes was reported to mirror changes in kinase expression in other organs under several pathophysiological settings. In particular, GRK2 levels and activity were increased in lymphocytes from hypertensive patients. Impairment of β-adrenergic-mediated vasodilation was reported in both human hypertensive subjects[22,66] and animal models of hypertension[67]; such alterations have been related to the increased GRK2 abundance and activity.[66] Decreased β-adrenergic signaling due to increased GRK2 activity would reduce the vasodilatative response, leading to high blood pressure. This view is supported by the inverse correlation of GRK2 expression with blood pressure.[68] Other data from spontaneously hypertensive rats and Dahl salt-sensitive rats confirmed increased levels of GRK2 in vascular smooth muscle cells, consistent with the observations in peripheral lymphocytes.[69] An subsequent study observed higher GRK2 protein levels in circulating lymphocytes from patients with myocardial infarction; additionally, increased GRK2 levels associated with worse systolic and diastolic function.[70] Importantly, at 2-year follow-up patients with higher GRK2 levels at admission had worse systolic function and cardiac remodeling,[70] suggesting that GRK2 levels may reflect hemodynamic impairment and might have a meaningful prognostic value after myocardial infarction (Fig. 11.3).

Elevated GRK2 levels might imply metabolic alterations and lead to insulin resistance, a common feature of hypertensive state.[14,71,72] In myoblasts, increased GRK2 expression mediated insulin resistance via a mechanism that involves sequestration of G_q and the insulin receptor substrate-1 (IRS-1).[73] In addition, GRK2 was shown to bind and phosphorylate IRS1 and the inhibition of GRK2 action ameliorated insulin sensitivity.[74,75] Also, GRK2 negatively affected cardiac glucose uptake and lowering GRK2 after ischemic injury contributed to restoring cardiac metabolism and prevented the development of subsequent heart failure.[72,74] GRK2 appears to regulate cardiomyocyte function in part by controlling β_1-AR in the regulation of cardiac contractility and chronotropy; interestingly, GRK3 was implicated in the regulation of cardiac growth and hypertrophy by selectively controlling endothelin and α_1-AR (PMID 17573483). Taken together, the control of endothelial homeostasis relies on a complex interaction between adrenergic system and nitroxidative stress; specific molecules such as GRKs may interplay with and modulate the crosstalk across multiple cell types involved in vascular function.

ADRENERGIC SIGNALING IN HEART FAILURE

The sympathetic nervous system (SNS) has pronounced effects on cardiac physiology, including increases in atrioventricular conduction (positive dromotropy), heart rate (positive chronotropy), cardiac contractility (positive inotropy), and cardiac relaxation (positive lusitropy). Likewise, the SNS plays a crucial role in the regulation of vascular tone due by controlling peripheral resistance and cardiac output.[76]

Heart failure is a chronic clinical syndrome in which the heart is incapable of pumping a sufficient supply of blood to meet the metabolic requirements of the body or generating the required elevated ventricular filling pressures to maintain output.[72] Heart failure leads to a debilitating illness characterized by

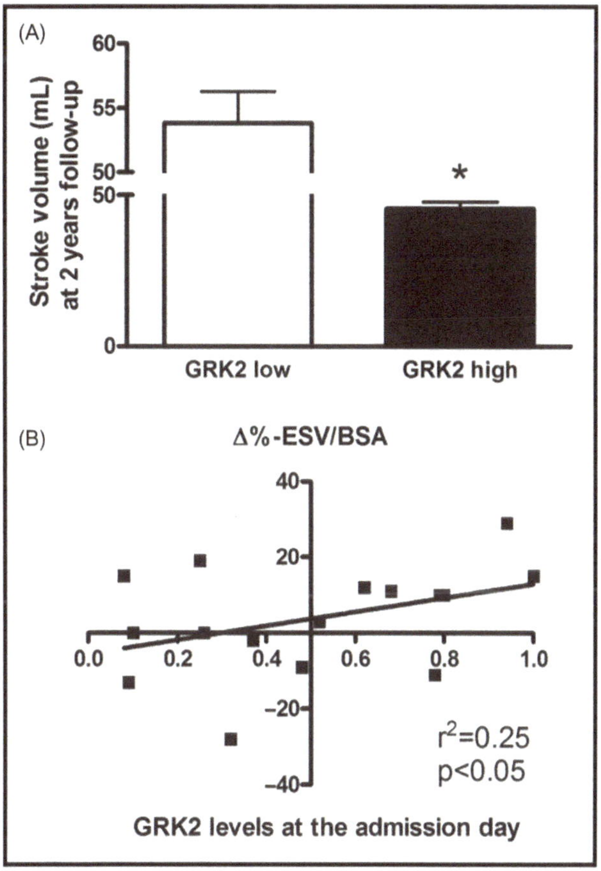

FIGURE 11.3

GRK2 levels and outcomes after myocardial infarction. (A) Two years after myocardial infarction, patients with higher GRK2 levels at admission had worse systolic function, with lower stroke volumes, than those with low GRK2 levels (independent-samples Student's *t*-test). (B) Also, cardiac remodeling, assessed by the change in end-systolic volume (ESV) corrected by body surface area (BSA) after 2 years of follow-up (Δ%-ESV/BSA) was correlated with GRK2 level at admission ($r^2 = 0.25$, $p < 0.05$).

From Santulli G, Campanile A, Spinelli L, et al. G protein-coupled receptor kinase 2 in patients with acute myocardial infarction. Am J Cardiol 2011;107(8):1125–30.

poor exercise tolerance and chronic fatigue, representing one of the most important causes of morbidity and mortality worldwide. Notwithstanding considerable advances in its treatment, heart failure still represents a severe social and clinical burden.[77,78] A complex neurohormonal regulatory system exists between the heart and multiple organ systems, including feedback loops mediated through a variety of vasoactive substances secreted by the adrenals, kidneys, lungs, and endothelium.[79] Perturbations of function in any of these organs affect the others. Accordingly, the cardiovascular system is best viewed as a complex dynamic system, continually adapting to optimize organ perfusion. During heart failure, diverse neurohormonal mechanisms are triggered to maintain cardiac output.[4] Heart failure is indeed a progressive disease that begins long before symptoms or signs become evident. It is initially characterized by a complex adaptive neurohormonal activation, which includes the nervous system (see chapter: Neuronal Hormones and the Sympathetic/Parasympathetic Regulation of the Heart), the renin-angiotensin-aldosterone system (see chapter: Renin Angiotensin Aldosterone System and Heart Function), natriuretic peptides (see chapter: Cardiac Natriuretic Peptides), endothelin (see chapter: Endothelin-1 as a Cardiac-Derived Autocrine, Paracrine and Intracrine Factor in Heart Health and Disease), and vasopressin (see chapter: Renin Angiotensin Aldosterone System and Heart Function). These and other regulatory mechanisms are required to compensate for cardiac dysfunction[80]; however, the process progressively becomes maladaptive when the left ventricular (LV) dysfunction is persistent. This eventually leads to increased mechanical stress on the failing heart, causing detrimental electrical and structural events, further impairment of systolic and diastolic function, and progressive cardiac fibrosis and apoptosis.[81] Thus, β-blockers, angiotensin-converting enzyme inhibitors, Angiotensin II AT_1 receptor blockers and mineralocorticoid receptor antagonists represent cornerstones for the treatment of patients with a failing heart.[82]

The central part of the adrenal gland, called adrenal medulla, is the main source of catecholamines and comprises groups of adrenergic and noradrenergic chromaffin cells and, to a lesser extent, ganglionic neurons.[83] Chromaffin cells secrete roughly 80% adrenaline and 20% noradrenaline whereas this proportion is reversed in the sympathetic nerves, which contain and secrete predominantly noradrenaline.[79] The adrenergic and noradrenergic secretion in different groups of chromaffin cells relies on the different α_2AR subtypes expression.[84] The adrenal gland can be compared to a specialized sympathetic ganglion, receiving inputs from the SNS via preganglionic fibers.[85] However, the adrenal gland directly secretes neurohormones into the bloodstream. Indeed, chromaffin cells are postganglionic sympathetic neurons that have lost part of their characteristics as axons and dendrites and are able to secrete their hormones into the blood by exocytosis. The suggestive link between the adrenal gland and the heart has become quite interesting and stimulating in the last few years, with several studies investigating the molecular mechanisms underlying such a complex relationship, especially in the pathophysiology of heart failure.[79]

Adrenaline and noradrenaline generally have similar effects, although they differ from each other in certain of their actions. In particular, noradrenaline constricts almost all blood vessels, while adrenaline constricts many networks of minute blood vessels but dilates the vessels in the skeletal muscles and the liver.[86] Both sympathomimetic agents increase heart rate and myocardial contractility, thereby augmenting cardiac output and blood pressure.[87] Sympathetic overdrive observed in heart failure correlates with a higher risk of arrhythmias and LV dysfunction.[88] Plasma concentrations of noradrenaline are negatively associated with survival in heart failure patients.[89] Augmented levels of circulating catecholamines can cause myocardial damage via enhanced cardiac oxygen demand and by increasing peroxidative (and lipoperoxidative) metabolism and the ensuing production of free radicals.[90] These reactive species lead to structural alterations in the myocardium, including focal necrosis and inflammation, increased collagen deposition and subsequent interstitial fibrosis.[91] Noradrenaline can also increase cardiac oxygen consumption and cause apoptosis, ultimately leading to dilated cardiomyopathy.[92,93]

At the vascular level, systemically circulating or locally released catecholamines[94] trigger two main classes of ARs: α_1AR and β_2AR, causing vasoconstriction and vasodilatation, respectively.[23,95] With aging, such a fine equilibrium is progressively shifted toward increased vasoconstriction, most likely due to a defective vasodilatation in response to βAR stimulation. Supporting this hypothesis, βAR agonist administration in the human brachial artery induces vasodilatation and this response is attenuated in hypertensive patients.[66] The mechanistic role of β_2AR in the vasculature is also corroborated by the fact that genetic variants of β_2AR cause excessive desensitization and lead to reduced vasodilation, promoting the development of atherosclerosis.[96]

Increased basal levels of circulating catecholamines were observed both in heart failure and with advancing age, mirrored by a decrease in the number of high-affinity βARs, suggesting that these alterations might be due to βAR desensitization rather than actual reduction in βAR density.[11] As mentioned above, βAR affinity for the ligand is mainly dependent upon GPCR phosphorylation, which in turn is in the domain of GRKs.[70] Modulation of sympathetic nervous signaling via GRKs mediated downregulation of βARs in the heart plays a key role in heart failure. In particular, heterozygous GRK2 knockout mice display augmented cardiac contractility and function, whereas transgenic mice overexpressing cardiac GRK2 exhibit decreased myocardial function due to βAR dysfunction.[97]

GRK2 expression and activity increase in vascular tissue with aging.[1] Equally important, an impairment in βAR-mediated vasorelaxation was observed in hypertensive patients[66] and in animal models of hypertension[21,67]: these alterations related to increased GRK2 abundance and activity. Transgenic overexpression of GRK2 in the vasculature impaired βAR signaling and the vasodilatative response, eliciting a hypertensive phenotype in rodents. This aspect was confirmed in humans: GRK2 expression correlated with blood pressure and impaired βAR-mediated adenylyl-cyclase activity.[1] Additionally, genetic variants of the β_2AR that affect its translational efficiency associated with longevity.[11] The decrease in βAR-mediated responses were attributed to different mechanisms, including attenuation of PKA activation, impaired generation of cyclic AMP, decreased receptor density, and less efficient coupling to adenylyl-cyclase.[11] Variations in cyclooxygenase expression and vasoactive prostanoids levels are suggested as potential mechanisms. However, currently there is no single molecular or cellular factor that fully explains the decline in βAR function. Nevertheless, the etiology seems to be most likely associated with alterations in the ability of βAR to respond to agonists at the cellular level.

ADRENERGIC SYSTEM IN THE HEART: BEYOND THE REGULATION OF CONTRACTILITY

The activation of the sympathetic system leads to noteworthy metabolic responses, including increased gluconeogenesis and lipolysis with subsequent elevated plasma levels of free fatty acids (FFAs) and glucose.[98,99] Essentially, the increased availability of glucose and FFAs can be used by the organism as fuel in times of stress or danger, when increased exertion or alertness is required.[100] Different therapeutic approaches targeting myocardial metabolism have been suggested to regulate metabolic pathways in the failing heart, in an attempt to improve cardiac function and metabolic elasticity.[101]

During the flight or fight response, sympathetic activation causes α_1-AR–mediated vasoconstriction in less vital vascular beds, including splanchnic and skin, diverting blood to skeletal muscle. AR activation also mobilizes blood from the capacitance veins, involving α_1 and α_2ARs.[102] These acute physiological responses, typical of the stress conditions, are disadvantageous when they become chronic. Actually, a common feature of many pathological conditions involving sympathetic system hyperactivity is the development of metabolic alterations, including insulin resistance, impaired glucose and lipid metabolism, and mitochondrial dysfunction.[103,104] The myocardium has high metabolic demands, among the highest in the body: with minimal ATP reserves and complete ATP turnover approximately every ten seconds, the heart heavily depends on a continuous energy supply,[105] though the heart possesses a strategic metabolic flexibility that supports its function during stressful conditions. Cardiac muscle generates ATP almost exclusively via oxidative phosphorylation by using different metabolic substrates: in the healthy state cardiac ATP production mainly relies on FFA oxidation, whereas the relative contribution of glucose increases during stress or injury.[106]

Imbalance in adrenergic activation and cardiac energy metabolism represents a risk factor for the development of cardiac disease. Therefore, heart failure represents a classical endpoint in the study of metabolic alterations related to the sympathetic system. Indeed, there are multiple disturbances in various metabolic pathways, including the tricarboxylic acid cycle and β-oxidation in heart under pathological conditions. Metabolic remodeling observed in failing hearts is characterized by a lower oxidative capacity, contractile dysfunction, and insulin resistance.[107,108] Circulating insulin levels are chronically augmented in both type 2 diabetes mellitus and heart failure, leading to persistent stimulation of insulin receptors[109,110] (see chapter: Insulin Signaling in Cardiac Health and Disease). Such an increase in insulin signaling in the heart promotes FFAs uptake and enhances lipotoxicity.[111] Moreover, hyperactive insulin signaling also accelerates adverse LV remodeling.[112,113] Insulin itself can directly impair adrenergic signaling pathways required for contractile function via an insulin receptor/β_2AR signaling complex,[107] providing a potential novel mechanism underlying cardiac dysfunction in heart failure. Of note, insulin resistance highly correlates with neuroadrenergic function,[21] and the onset of type 2 diabetes is associated with increased central sympathetic outflow.[114] In addition, both nutritional sympathetic responsiveness and baseline sympathetic drive are important prognostic biological markers for dietary weight loss outcome in obese subjects with metabolic syndrome.[115,116]

The prevalence of sympathetic over parasympathetic activity might be initially responsible, at least in part, for an increased metabolic state. However, as in different hormone-regulated pathways, such a state is subsequently followed by a decrease in βAR metabolic responsiveness. This compensatory response results in a reduced basal metabolic rate and an increased tendency toward anabolic processes, leading to insulin resistance and reduced ability to dissipate energy, with an overall weight gain, particularly at the visceral level.[117] This complex metabolic network can eventually cause a vicious circle, where insulin resistance further stimulates sympathetic activity, worsening insulin resistance itself. A sustained βAR stimulation is widely known to induce insulin resistance.[118] β_2ARs and β_3ARs seem to play a pivotal, although not exclusive, role in regulating glucose and lipid homeostasis, respectively: whereas β_2AR regulates both pancreatic β-cell hormone secretion and peripheral glucose metabolism,[14] β_3AR is more involved in the modulation of FFAs metabolism.[119] GRKs actively participate in this complex scenario. In fact, GRKs have been proposed as pleiotropic proteins involved in the regulation of countless cellular functions, not exclusively via the classic phosphorylation pathway. Mounting evidence indicates that GRKs exert different effects depending on cell type, localization, stimuli, and pathophysiological context.[120–123] For instance, Iaccarino and colleagues were the first to demonstrate the mitochondrial localization of GRK2,[51] later confirmed by other investigators[124] with imperative functional implications (Fig. 11.4).

Insulin also up-regulates GRK2, which in turn inhibits insulin signaling and glucose uptake.[1,125] Various conditions associated with insulin resistance, including hypertension and diabetes, are characterized by elevated GRK2 levels.[1] In murine failing hearts, GRK2 inhibition was demonstrated to be beneficial, preventing the derangement of insulin signaling and delaying the reduction of glucose uptake, thereby preserving myocardial function.[74] In the clinical setting, lymphocyte GRK2 levels were augmented in patients with end-stage heart failure[126] and in patients with myocardial infarction, correlating with a worse systolic and diastolic function.[70]

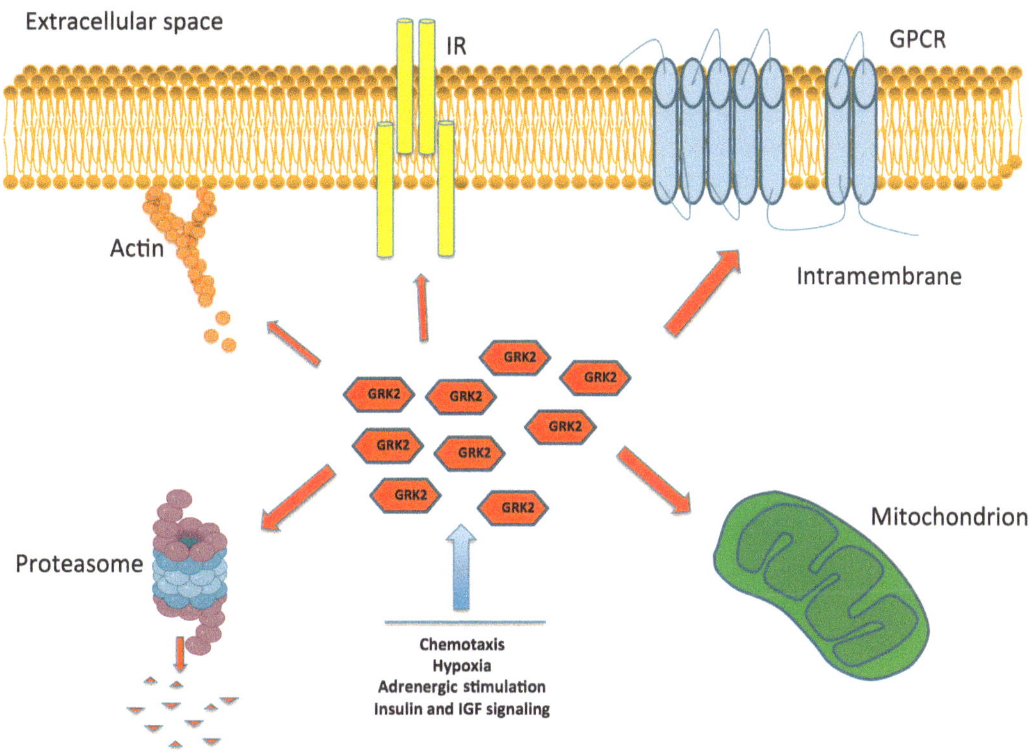

FIGURE 11.4

Intracellular localization of GRK2. GRK2 is localized to the cytosol in resting conditions, but GRK2 translocates in response to a variety of stimuli to different subcellular compartments where GRK2 regulates several cellular functions, including GPCR and IR desensitization at the plasma membrane level, actin polymerization in the cytoskeleton, metabolism, and ROS production in mitochondria. *GPCR*: G protein–coupled receptor; *IR*: insulin receptor.

ADRENERGIC RECEPTORS AND CARDIAC METABOLISM

Cardiac function relies to a great extent on oxidative metabolism. Given its the high mitochondrial content cardiac muscle generates ATP almost exclusively through oxidative phosphorylation.[127] Accordingly, cardiac muscle possesses a metabolic flexibility or plasticity, allowing it to maintain its function during stressful conditions. In the adult heart the major pathway for ATP production is fatty acid oxidation, while the relative contribution of glucose increases during stress or injury, such as exercise or ischemia.[128,129] Thus, it is not surprising that an impairment of cardiac muscle energy metabolism represents an important risk factor for the development of cardiac diseases.[130] The heart exhibits a severe malfunction of different pathways with a metabolic remodeling characterized by a lower oxidative capacity, contractile dysfunction, and cardiac muscle insulin resistance under pathological conditions.[127,130] Different therapeutic strategies have been undertaken to modulate metabolic pathways in the failing heart, though it remains controversial whether targeting glucose versus fatty acid metabolism individually or in combination represents an optimal approach to improve metabolic flexibility and cardiac function.[131]

Activation of the adrenergic system is deeply involved in regulating diverse metabolic pathways. Increased circulating catecholamines and activation of the different adrenergic receptors present in the various organs produce important metabolic responses which include: (1) increased lipolysis and elevated levels of fatty acids in plasma, (2) increased gluconeogenesis by the liver to provide substrate for the brain, and (3) moderate inhibition of insulin release by the pancreas to conserve glucose and to shift fuel metabolism of muscle in the direction of fatty acid oxidation (Fig. 11.5). This physiological

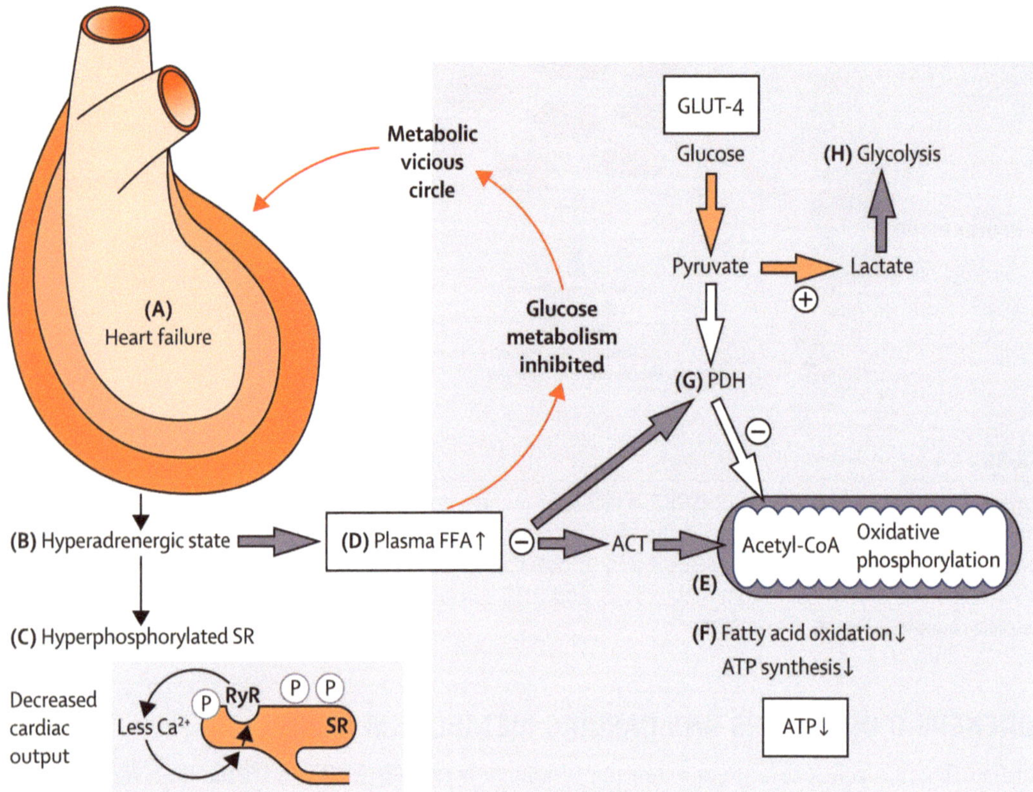

FIGURE 11.5

The metabolic vicious circle in heart failure. Dilation of the myocardium in heart failure (A) leads to adrenergic activation (B) that in turn hyperphosphorylates the SR (C) and increases concentrations of circulating FFA (D). FFA inhibit mitochondrial function at the level of ACT (E), thus inhibiting fatty acid oxidation and synthesis of ATP (F). Plasma FFA also inhibit PDH (G) to promote anaerobic glycolysis (H) rather than oxidative metabolism. SR = sarcoplasmic reticulum. RyR = ryanodine receptor. *FFA* = free fatty acids. *ACT* = acyl carnitine transferase. *PDH* = pyruvate dehydrogenase. *GLUT-4* = glucose uptake transporter 4.

*Adapted from Heusch G, Libby P, Gersh B, Yellon D, Böhm M, Lopaschuk G, Opie L. Cardiovascular remodelling in coronary artery disease and heart failure. Lancet 2014;***383***(9932):1933–43. (10.1016/S0140-6736(14)60107-0).*

response, typical of the stress condition, was demonstrated to be detrimental for the functioning of different organs like the cardiac muscle when it becomes chronic. Indeed, a common feature of many pathological conditions involving over-activation of the adrenergic system is the development of metabolic alterations which can include insulin resistance, altered glucose and lipid metabolism, and mitochondrial dysfunction.[104] These alterations are seen in a number of different pathological conditions; however, they are, in general, highly correlated to the level of activation of the adrenergic system.

The SNS is maladaptively activated in response to a chronic reduction in cardiac output and this response is characterized by an increased adrenal secretion and reduced cardiac reuptake of catecholamines.[132] The effects of the catecholamine secretion on cardiac metabolism are mediated by both central and peripheral mechanisms. For example, increased catecholamines have directly detrimental effects on the heart, which cause marked enzyme loss as an index of diffuse myocardial damage, and substantial oxygen-wastage even in the absence of FFAs in the perfusate.[133,134] Furthermore, noradrenaline promotes both coronary vasoconstriction and increased plasma FFA levels, which further promote oxygen-wastage.[134] In turn, FFAs reciprocally augment sympathetic activity. In human skeletal muscle, a dose-response relationship exists between plasma FFAs[135] and defects in insulin signaling. This may in part be attributable to FFA-mediated activation of PKC, which phosphorylates insulin receptors and results in reduced capillary opening and reduced myocyte glucose uptake.[136]

Locally activated SNS appears to be relevant in altering cardiac metabolism. Using positron emission tomography in conjunction with a noradrenaline analog and 18F-fluorodeoxyglucose, myocardial segments with contractile dysfunction have reduced presynaptic noradrenaline reuptake and myocardial glucose uptake, compared to less impaired myocardial segments in the same patients.[118] Thus, after control for confounding variables, altered metabolism and insulin resistance directly relate to local sympathetic activity. The adverse effects of the SNS on the heart are mediated by ARs; however, extensive research indicates that ARs are differently involved in pathophysiology of heart failure, and so it is likely to be the same for modifications of cardiac metabolism observed during disease. Indeed, β_1- and β_2-adrenoceptors regulate different signal pathways, producing different outcomes on cardiac function. Stimulation of both β_1AR and β_2AR can activate the stimulatory G protein ($G\alpha_s$)/adenylyl-cyclase/cAMP/PKA signaling pathway, which subsequently leads to the phosphorylation of several target proteins within the cardiac myocyte, including intracellular calcium release channels (ryanodine receptors), L-type calcium channels, and phospholamban[16,127,137] (Fig. 11.1). Nonetheless, this signaling pathway is the main mechanism by which β_1AR rather than β_2AR regulates cardiac contractility/relaxation and rate.[138] In contrast, β_2ARregulates an alternative signaling pathway via activation of the inhibitory G protein ($G\alpha_i$) and the heterodimer formed by the β and γ subunits of the G protein ($G\beta\gamma$).[13] Besides the inhibition of adenylyl-cyclase, the main signal pathway regulated by β_2AR through $G\alpha_i$/$G\beta\gamma$ appears to be the phosphatidylinositol-3 kinase (PI3K)–signaling cascade, although other proteins such as the AMP-dependent protein kinase (AMPK), mammalian target of rapamycin, and extracellular signal-regulated kinase 1 and 2 (ERK1/2) have been proposed as novel targets of β_2AR.[139,140]

Regarding the effects of adrenergic system on metabolism, it is known that sustained beta adrenergic stimulation induces insulin resistance and in this context the β_2AR appears to have a major role in overall glucose homeostasis by modulating pancreatic islet hormone secretion as well as liver and muscle glucose homeostasis. For the heart, several studies have raised the possibility of using selective β_2AR agonists as potential modulators of cardiac muscle energy metabolism. Short- and long-term stimulation of the β_2AR has been associated with the modulation of fatty acid and glucose metabolism.[141] Indeed, acute treatment of myocytes in vitro or skeletal muscle ex vivo with β_2AR agonists increases glucose uptake to levels comparable to those seen after insulin stimulation.[142]

A putative mechanism for β_2AR function in insulin resistance involves the activation of PI3K and its downstream signal pathway[143,144] and in particular the phosphorylation and inactivation of TBC1D4 (also known as AKT substrate of 160 kDa, AS160) by AKT.[145] TBC1D4 inhibits the translocation of the glucose transporter type4 (GLUT4) from intracellular vesicles to the plasma membrane, hence an increase in TBC1D4 phosphorylation enhances glucose uptake.[145] Moreover, TBC1D4 is also targeted by AMPK, which represents a key mechanism in the regulation of insulin-independent glucose uptake.[145,146] Consistent with the potential role of β_2AR in glucose metabolism, higher levels of AMPK phosphorylation, and activity was seen in response to βAR stimulation[109,147] as a result of changes in the AMP/ATP ratio or activation of upstream AMPK kinases.[148] Therefore, it is tempting to speculate that β_2AR-agonists would induce GLUT4 translocation in this situation in an insulin-independent manner. Moreover in vivo studies show a greater efficiency of carvedilol, a nonselective beta AR antagonist, in ameliorating myocardial insulin sensitivity and glucose extraction in an animal model of heart failure, compared to the selective β1AR antagonist metoprolol.[149] These conflicting results may be due to differences in preclinical models but are more likely due to differences in response to acute and chronic stimulation of the β_2AR. While acute activation of the receptor can favor glucose uptake by increasing GLUT4 translocation to the plasma membrane, chronic adrenergic stimulation, as seen during heart failure, would be detrimental by mechanisms involving other molecular mechanisms, such as JNK, β-arrestins, and GRKs.[4,150]

ROLE OF ADRENERGIC RECEPTORS IN THE PATHOPHYSIOLOGY OF CARDIAC HYPERTROPHY

Cardiac hypertrophy can be observed in both physiological and pathological conditions where the increased hemodynamic or metabolic stress produces a remodeling of cardiac geometry.[151,152] However, under pathological conditions the hypertrophy is not compensatory, rather it reflects activation of maladaptive cellular processes that promote disease progression. In this sense, myocardial hypertrophy might serve as diagnostic and prognostic marker of cardiac remodeling (Fig. 11.6), and underlies several biochemical and molecular changes involved in metabolic and contractile regulatory pathways.[153,154]

The pathways attributed to pathological hypertrophy promoted the identification of specific pharmacological targets able to counteract adverse remodeling and foster prognosis improvement. Common triggers of cardiac remodeling include hypertension, myocardial infarction, chronic ischemia, inflammation, valvular disease, prolonged tachycardia or bradycardia, and genetic predisposition.[113] Cardiac remodeling represents the result of increased cell death (apoptosis and/or necrosis) and hypertrophy of the surviving cardiomyocytes. A resulting increase in LV mass is defined by LV wall thickness and LV diameter as concentric or eccentric hypertrophy.[155] In LV concentric hypertrophy cardiomyocytes grow thicker but retain normal length, while dilation of the LV in eccentric hypertrophy is associated with cardiomyocyte elongation through sequential addition of sarcomeres.[156] The type of hypertrophic remodeling depends on the trigger and concomitant progression of contractile dysfunction, such that concentric hypertrophy is a common response to increased afterload (valve stenosis, hypertensive heart disease), whereas eccentric hypertrophy is often observed in conditions of LV volume overload (e.g., valve regurgitation or shunt) or after myocardial infarction (as a late response).[157] Overall, cardiac hypertrophy can be considered a general term that indicates both concentric hypertrophy, with prevalent diastolic dysfunction, and eccentric hypertrophy with prevalent systolic dysfunction. These two patterns of cardiac remodeling represent the two extremes of a continuum.[158] Clinical echocardiography defines four distinct geometric

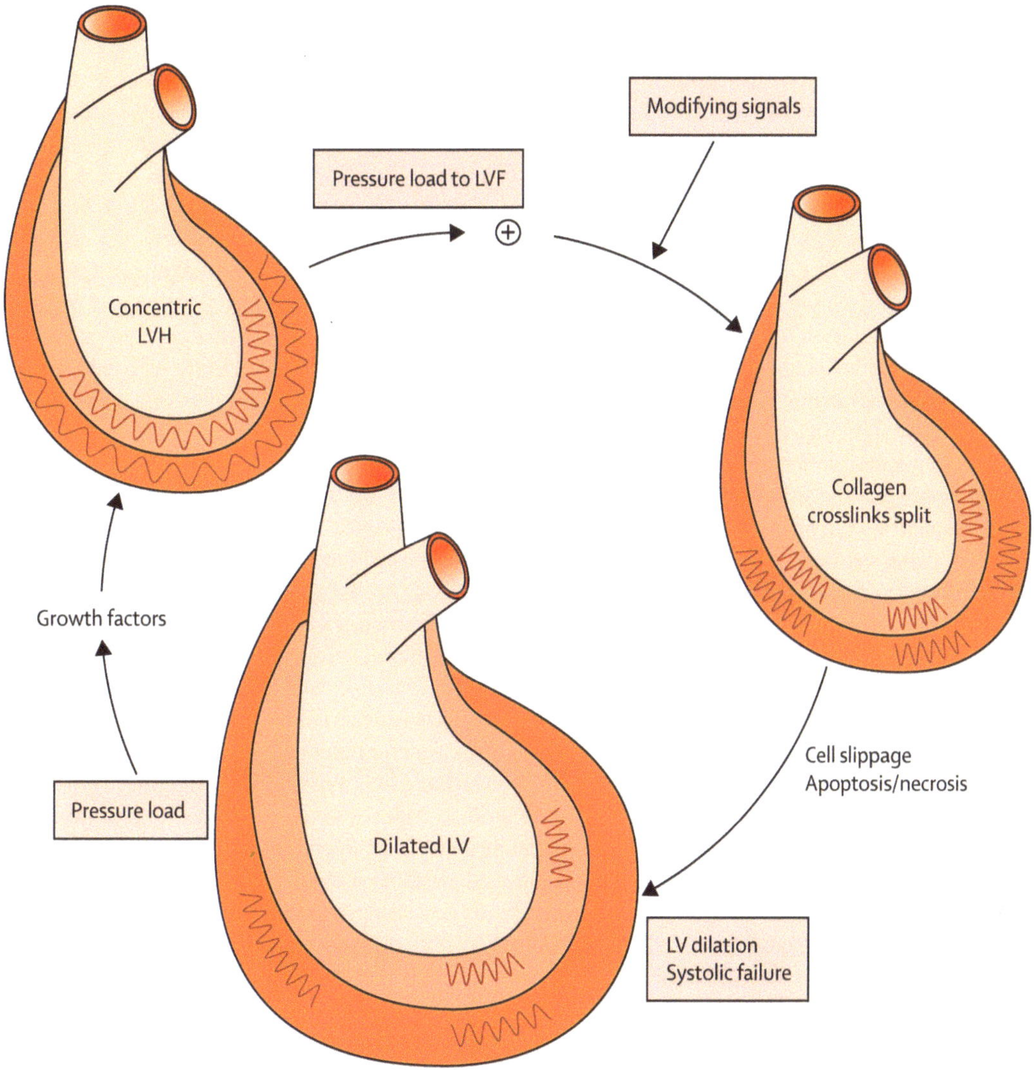

FIGURE 11.6

Myocardial remodeling in response to pressure load. Proposed transition from pressure load to concentric hypertrophy to dilated failing left ventricle (LV). Concentric remodeled myocardium undergoes splitting of the collagen crosslinks in response to modifying molecular signals such as metalloproteinases and other signals that disrupt collagen crosslinks to promote LV dilation and systolic heart failure. *LVF* = left ventricular failure. *LVH* = left ventricular hypertrophy.

*Adapted from Heusch G, Libby P, Gersh B, Yellon D, Böhm M, Lopaschuk G, Opie L. Cardiovascular remodelling in coronary artery disease and heart failure. Lancet 2014;***383***(9932):1933–43. (10.1016/S0140-6736(14)60107-0).*

patterns: (1) normal geometry, (2) concentric remodeling, (3) concentric hypertrophy, and (4) eccentric hypertrophy.[159] Additionally, nine intermediate phenotypes have been recently identified.[160]

Activation of the SNS in response to normal or disease-related stimuli is essential to maintain homeostasis and for the body to adapt in a constantly changing environment. The physiological and metabolic responses to sympathetic activation are mediated through the action of the endogenous catecholamines on adrenergic receptors. Regulation of cardiac function in response to catecholamine stimulation is controlled primarily through activation of βARs. As mentioned above, both β_1 and β_2AR subtypes couple to G_s and activate adenylyl-cyclase, thereby increasing cAMP levels and activating PKA.[161] In addition to G_s, β_2ARs also possess a nonclassic pathway through which are coupled to G_i (pertussis-toxin sensitive pathway).[162] Studies in neonatal cardiomyocytes of β_2AR knockout mice showed that stimulation of β_2AR is characterized by a biphasic effect on contraction rate with an initial PKA-independent increase in rate, followed by a PTX-sensitive decrease in rate of contraction.[163] Switching of β_2AR from G_s to G_i-coupling was found not only to inhibit adenylyl-cyclase activity but also to initiate signaling of MAPK by the Gβγ subunits of G_i in a process that is regulated by PKA-mediated phosphorylation of the receptor. βAR/G_i coupling can also activate the cytosolic effector molecule phospholipase A2 (cPLA2) in the heart in a cascade that triggers positive enhancement of calcium signaling and contraction, and which is independent of cAMP production.[164] In contrast with β_1-β_2ARs, β_3ARs are expressed at very low levels in the unstressed heart and are upregulated in various conditions with adrenergic overstimulation. Moreover, β_3ARs are typically activated by high concentrations of catecholamines (e.g., noradrenaline), are resistant to homologous desensitization, and their activation has potential negative inotropic effects since genetic deletion of β_3ARs results in enhancement of cardiac myocyte contractility.[165]

Transgenic overexpression of β_3ARs in the mouse heart was described as a neutral phenotype, with no deterioration of LV function at baseline.[166] However, systemic deletion of β_3ARs in mice subjected to transverse aortic constriction produced an adverse cardiac phenotype, thus arguing in favor of protection conferred by β_3ARs.[167] Nonetheless, mouse models with cardiac-specific overexpression of the human β_3ARs subjected to various neurohormonal stresses appear protected from hypertrophic and fibrotic remodeling. Dissection of signaling in isolated cardiomyocytes identifies β_3AR coupling to NOS/cGMP and downstream protein kinase G (PKG) as key components for this protection.[12]

Cardiac hypertrophy and heart failure are typically characterized by derangement of βARs signaling and a reduction of the adrenergic reserve of the heart.[168] This is primarily due to the selective reduction (downregulation) of β_1AR density at the plasma membrane and by the uncoupling of the remaining β_1ARs and β_2ARs from G proteins (functional desensitization). Moreover β_2AR signaling in the failing heart is different from that seen in the normal heart, switching from a compartmentalized to a diffuse pro-apoptotic cAMP signaling pattern, similar to that seen for the β_1AR.[169] These modifications are strictly connected to myocardial levels and activities of the most important, versatile, and ubiquitous GRKs, GRK2, and GRK5, which were elevated both in humans and in animal models of heart failure.[2] Excessive catecholamines stimulation of cardiac βARs triggered the GRK2 upregulation in cardiomyocytes, thus leading to a reduction in cardiac βAR density and responsiveness, ultimately resulting in cardiac inotropic reserve depletion.[4,170] Such GRK2 elevation is a homeostatic protective mechanism aimed at defending the heart against excessive catecholaminergic toxicity.[151] Thus, elevated sympathetic activity in chronic heart failure cause enhanced GRK2-mediated cardiac β_1AR and β_2AR desensitization and β_1ARs downregulation, eventually leading to the progressive loss of the adrenergic and inotropic reserves of the heart.

GRK2 SUBCELLULAR LOCALIZATION: A MOLECULAR LINK BETWEEN MYOCARDIAL CONTRACTILITY AND CARDIAC METABOLISM

Activation of the adrenergic system has a profound effect on cell function and metabolism regulating several metabolic responses. The over-activation in stress conditions becomes detrimental for the correct functioning of organs leading to the development of metabolic alterations (insulin resistance, altered glucose, and lipid metabolism and mitochondrial dysfunction). Among adrenergic receptors, it was demonstrated that the activation of βARs subtypes induces insulin resistance[75] and, in particular the βARs regulates overall glucose homeostasis.[14,73] At the cardiac level, β_2AR stimulation associated with the modulation of fatty acid and glucose metabolism.[141] In particular, acute treatment of myocytes in vitro or skeletal muscle ex vivo with β_2AR agonists increased glucose uptake, comparable to the increase produced by insulin stimulation.[171] Recent discoveries have suggested that GRK2 is a potential molecular link between chronic adrenergic stimulation and development of altered myocardial metabolism observed during heart failure.[74,127] The failing heart is characterized by an upregulation of GRK2 levels,[2] which is involved in the inhibition of βARs signaling and cardiac inotropism[5,172] (Fig. 11.7).

In addition to the effects on heart function, GRK2 upregulation also affects cardiac metabolism, and in particular, myocardial glucose uptake, at the early stages of the disease, when cardiac dilation and reduced function are not yet evident, indicating that metabolic modifications are involved in the progression of heart failure. These findings suggest that GRK2 is the molecular link between the over-activation of the adrenergic system and the altered glucose uptake during heart failure.[5,74] The connection between GRK2 and insulin signaling derives from the proof of concept that insulin increases the cellular content of GRK2.[75] Several reports suggest that GRK2 is a crucial modulator of insulin resistance, both systemically and in the heart.[173] GRK2 can directly induce insulin resistance and reduce glucose metabolism in cardiomyocytes through its catalytic activity. When GRK2 is overexpressed in myocytes, there was a decrease in myocardial glucose uptake and impaired insulin signaling and fatty acid metabolism.[74,174] GRK2 directly phosphorylates IRS1 at the inhibitory Ser^{307} residue, inducing the dissociation of the insulin receptor signaling complex and attenuating signaling to downstream effectors such as AKT and GLUT4.[74,150] Moreover, elevated myocardial GRK2 levels exacerbated defects in cardiac glucose metabolism after ischemic injury, before inducing ventricular contractile dysfunction,[173] demonstrating a proposed link between GRK2 and adrenergic control of contractility and metabolism. To further support this concept, myocardial glucose uptake is elevated in cardiac-specific GRK2 knockout mice, compared to wild-type mice, and glucose uptake is maintained even after ischemia. Moreover, insulin signaling is modified as evidenced by decreased phosphorylation of IRS1. Overall, glucose metabolism was improved, which prevents heart failure because cardiac contractility is not adversely affected.

The interaction between GRK2 and IRS1 is dependent on an intact C terminus of GRK2 as demonstrated in studies using the βARKct peptide, which reproduces the C-terminal sequence, inhibits insulin-mediated GRK2-dependent IRS1 phosphorylation, and improves AKT activation and GLUT4 translocation in response to insulin. Moreover, βARKct gene delivery to the hearts of rats through adeno-associated virus serotype 6 before ischemic injury prevented insulin resistance and myocardial glucose uptake remained high. These results could suggest that the direct interaction between GRK2 and IRS1 occurs within the C-terminal tail of GRK2 or that activation of the insulin receptor stimulates a pool of G proteins that recruit GRK2 to the membrane through Gβγ where it can interact with IRS1.

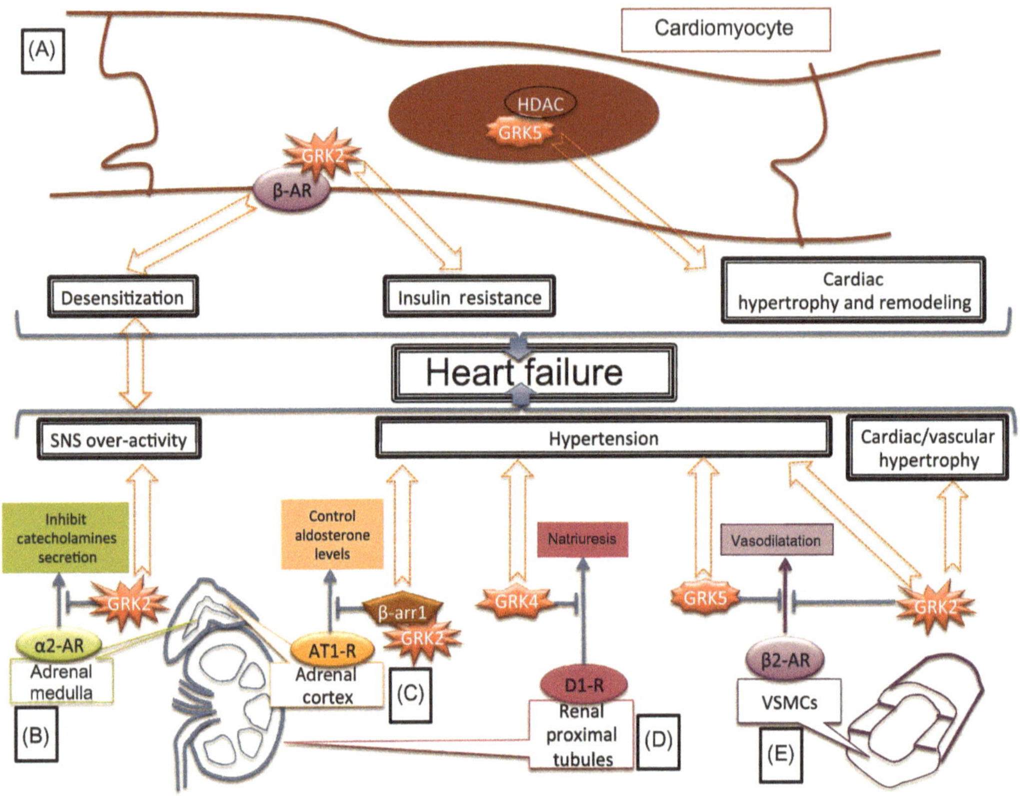

FIGURE 11.7

GRKs and cardiovascular disease. Persistent sympathetic stimulation of the cardiomyocyte triggers GRK2 upregulation that aggravates β-AR desensitization and impairs adrenergic signaling. GRK2 upregulation due to sympathetic nervous system overdrive has also been shown to be involved in the development of insulin resistance. (A) In the nucleus, GRK5 mediates cardiac hypertrophy by phosphorylating HDAC. (B) The adrenal gland was recently recognized as an attractive target for HF therapy because adrenal medullary chromaffin cells are the sites of catecholamine synthesis. GRK2 upregulation has been correlated with elevated catecholamine synthesis and secretion, primarily due to desensitization of the inhibitory α2-AR receptors. (C) In the adrenal cortex, angiotensin regulates aldosterone synthesis, where GRK2-β-arrestin 1–mediated signaling interferes with this regulatory pathway and elevated aldosterone secretion. (D) In the kidneys, dopamine 1-R–mediated natriuresis is dampened by GRK4; water and sodium retention are key factors of hypertension. (E) In the vasculature, β2-AR–mediated vasodilation is impaired by GRK2, leading to hypertension and cardiac and vascular hypertrophy. GRK5 hyperactivity in the vasculature precipitates hypertension.

*Adapted from Kamal FA, Travers JG, Blaxall BC. G protein–coupled receptor kinases in cardiovascular disease: why "where" matters. Trends Cardiovasc Med 2012;***22***(8):213–19.*

Overall, given the higher efficiency of glucose in ATP production and the lower effect in oxidative stress with respect to other substrates, these data argue that the role of GRK2 in the pathogenesis of heart failure is due, at least in part, to negative alterations in cardiac metabolism.[74,174] Since GRK2 upregulation causes insulin resistance, its inhibition has positive effects on cellular metabolism. Indeed, peptide inhibitors of GRK2 have been designed that prevent its binding to the substrate[175] and correct glucose levels in diabetic gerbils. In spontaneously hypertensive rats, chronic treatment with a similar inhibitor of GRK2 kinase activity, Ant-124, ameliorates the glucose dyshomeostasis and reduction of the blood pressure levels.[75] Moreover, the inhibition of GRK2 delays the reduction of glucose uptake and protects insulin signaling in the heart, preserving cardiac dimension and function.[74] This nurtures a novel scenario in which GRK2 inhibition might correct impaired metabolism in those conditions characterized by poor energy utilization by the cell, such as heart failure. In particular, it is known that GRK2 inhibition obtained through means of βARKct transgenic expression of the truncated mutant which prevents GRK2 localization on membranes or deletion of GRK2 gene is beneficial for the failing heart. Nevertheless, this benefit is thought to be dependent upon inhibition of βARs in the heart.

GRK2 inhibition may lead to an improved cardiac energy utilization. Indeed, as described above, during the development of heart failure impaired glucose metabolism precedes depressed cardiac contractility in mice with myocardial infarction.[13] These findings support the idea that the inhibition of GRK2 kinase activity could be a potential therapeutic target and that excessive elevation of GRK2 is deleterious for the cell. However, recent evidence challenges this view, since GRK2 exerts different effects within the cell depending on its localization, cell type, stimuli, and the pathophysiological context (Fig. 11.4). Beside the known localization of GRK2 in plasma membrane and cytosol, recently it has been demonstrated that GRK2 is also able to localize in mitochondria under specific experimental conditions.[51] Such mitochondrial localization suggests a potential role of GRK2 in the regulation of energy metabolism but to date there are only few and apparently contradictory reports on this topic. In the basal condition, GRK2 is in mitochondria and stressors can induce further accumulation. In macrophages, GRK2 levels in mitochondria increase during inflammation or endotoxin stimulation, facilitating biogenesis, and restoring mitochondrial function.[176] In the early pathogenesis of Alzheimer's disease and in models of ischemia/reperfusion brain injury, GRK2 accumulates in damaged mitochondria.[177] Furthermore, both in hearts in vivo and in cultured myocytes, GRK2 localizes into mitochondria after ischemia/reperfusion[124]. As to the role of GRK2 in mitochondria, in HEK-293 cells the kinase enhances mitochondrial biogenesis, leading to an increase of ATP cellular content.[51] The removal of GRK2 from the skeletal muscle in vivo leads to reduced ATP production and impaired tolerance to ischemia.[51] These findings support a positive regulatory role of GRK2 for mitochondrial biogenesis and ATP generation.[176]

In conclusion, GRK2 is involved in the regulation of cell metabolism, and its effects are strictly dependent on its subcellular localization. Collectively, the literature demonstrates this kinase is an important adaptive mechanism to stress, such as receptor dependent and independent stimuli. As for all adaptive mechanisms, the effect is beneficial in the beginning but then becomes detrimental. Indeed, increased levels of GRK2 have a deleterious effect in the development of heart failure and insulin resistance when it is increased on plasma membranes,[74,75] whereas it is advantageous for energy metabolism when it is localized in mitochondria.[51,176] Subcellular localization of GRK2 might in the future pose the strategy for selective inhibition of the kinase, and the possibility to modulate GRK2 accumulation within cellular compartments could be a useful approach to regulate its negative or positive effects on cell metabolism.

PHARMACOLOGY OF ADRENERGIC RECEPTOR BLOCKADE

α-ADRENERGIC RECEPTOR BLOCKADE

As powerful vasodilators, α_1AR blockers were initially considered as promising drugs to treat heart failure. Nevertheless, chronic administration of the α_1AR blocker prazosin led to increased catecholamine levels. Two clinical trials failed to support the use of α_1AR blockers to treat heart failure: in the Veterans Administration Cooperative Study (aka Vasodilator Heart Failure Trial or V-HeFT)) patients receiving prazosin experienced worse outcomes than those receiving the combined vasodilator therapy of isosorbide dinitrate and hydralazine;[178] and in the ALLHAT (Antihypertensive and Lipid-Lowering Treatment to prevent Heart Attack Trial) study, the doxazosin arm was terminated early because of higher incidence of heart failure.[179] Growing evidence indicates that the central nervous system plays a determinant role in the sympathetic excitation observed in heart failure.[83] Moreover, the association between the degree of sympathetic activation and mortality raised the possibility that a more complete adrenergic blockade might produce better outcome. Since the excitation of central α_2AR inhibits the activation of the SNS, such a receptor has been considered a possible target in the treatment of heart failure.[180] Clonidine is a centrally acting drug with α_2AR agonist action that at modest doses can markedly attenuates cardiac and renal sympathetic tone in patients with failing hearts enrolled in a small and short-term clinical study. However, a trial investigating the centrally acting sympatholytic agent moxonidine, had to be terminated early,[181] despite a significant dose-related reduction in plasma noradrenaline, because the drug was associated with increased mortality and hospitalizations for heart failure and myocardial infarction. These findings indicate that peripheral receptor inhibition may be better tolerated than central suppression of the SNS. A marked sympatholytic effect has also been associated with adverse outcomes in the Beta Blocker Evaluation of Survival Trial, where patients receiving bucindolol showed a decrease in noradrenaline levels and exhibited a 169% increase in mortality.[182] Notably, one of the oldest drugs used to treat heart failure, digoxin, which mainly acts by indirectly increasing intracellular Ca^{2+} available in the sarcoplasmic reticulum, has been also shown to modulate the adrenergic nervous system by improving baroreceptor function and decreasing sympathetic tone.[183]

β-ADRENERGIC RECEPTOR BLOCKADE

Based on receptor-level activity, β-blockers can be classified into three generations (Fig. 11.8): (1) first generation—nonselective drugs that block both β_1AR and β_2AR; (2) second generation—cardioselective agents, with higher affinity for β_1AR; and (3) third generation—β-blockers with vasodilative properties, mediated by α_1AR blockade, β_2AR agonism, or NO synthesis. Both selective and nonselective β-blockers have negative inotropic and chronotropic effects. The reduced inhibitory effect on β_2ARs makes the selective β-blockers less likely to cause peripheral vasoconstriction.[184] Hence, exercise performance may be impaired to a lesser extent by β_1AR selective drugs, at least in part because β_2AR blockade tends to blunt the exercise-induced increase in skeletal muscle blood flow.[103] Exercise training can improve βAR signaling and function, augmenting peak oxygen uptake, increasing cardiac inotropic reserves, and restoring normal sympathetic outflow and circulating catecholamine levels.[103]

β-blockers differ in their physicochemical properties. For instance, lipophilic compounds, including metoprolol, carvedilol, nebivolol, and bucindolol are rapidly adsorbed in the gastrointestinal tract and are extensively metabolized in the liver (first-pass metabolism), resulting in a shorter half-life when

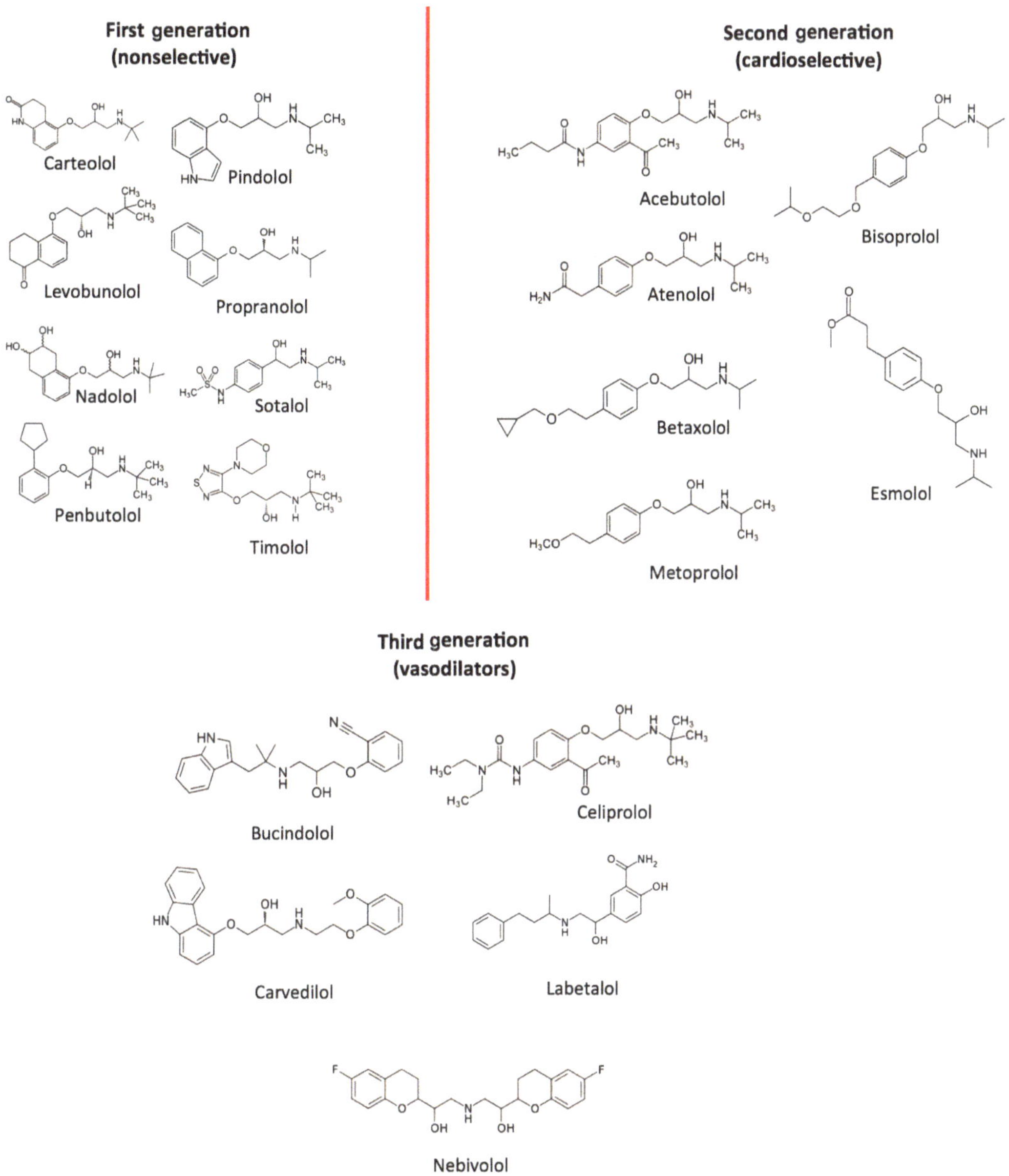

FIGURE 11.8

Graphic representation of the molecular structures of the three generations of β-blockers.

compared to other β-blockers. Additionally, the high lipophilicity leads to an enhanced penetration across the blood-brain barrier, which may justify the increased number of central effects as well as the membrane-stabilizing properties of antiarrhythmic molecules.[185]

The most common adverse events of β-blockers are attributable to the blockade of sympathetic stimulation, resulting in acute or chronic consequences at cardiovascular, metabolic, and respiratory levels.[186] In the heart, acute blockade of catecholamine effects worsens myocardial contractility and induces bradycardia. Starting with low doses and slowly titrating up is a commonly used approach to reduce these risks, patients may experience worsening of their symptoms during β-blocker titration, often requiring increased diuretic doses. Since a prolonged β-blocker treatment can enhance the sensitivity to catecholamines, an abrupt withdrawal should be avoided. As a result of antagonizing β_2ARs, β-blockers can cause bronchoconstriction, therefore β-blockers, especially nonselective agents, are contraindicated in patients suffering from asthma or chronic obstructive pulmonary disease. A risk/benefit assessment should be performed in each patient to avoid under treatment of heart failure.

The variability in the response to β-blockers has been at least in part ascribed to polymorphisms in the cytochrome P450 (CYP) gene CYP2D6, which is highly polymorphic in humans.[187] Indeed, many β-blockers are partially or totally metabolized by CYP2D6, and opportune dose modifications should be accurately considered in patients treated with drugs processed by the same cytochrome P450 isoforms, including antipsychotics and antidepressants.[188] Equally important, half-life and peak plasma concentration are influenced by the formulation of the molecule.[189] For instance, metoprolol is available in two different formulations: metoprolol-succinate, with a long-lasting action (Metoprolol CR/XL Randomized Intervention Trial in Congestive Heart Failure—MERIT-HF), and metoprolol-tartrate, which has a short half-life and demonstrated a reduced efficacy when compared to carvedilol (Carvedilol or Metoprolol European Trial—COMET study). The FDA has approved metoprolol-succinate for the treatment of patients with heart failure.[189]

Counteracting adrenergic overdrive via βAR antagonists reduces cardiac workload and increases O_2 sparing in patients with failing heart.[189] However, β-blockers have also noteworthy metabolic implications, including alterations in the lipoprotein profile, namely, a reduction in high-density lipoprotein cholesterol and an increase in triglycerides, and a deranged glucose homeostasis, which can be partially attributed to the blockade of β_2AR-dependent insulin release from the pancreatic islets of Langerhans.[14,190] Thus, β_1AR selective antagonists are generally preferred in patients with diabetes and heart failure.[110,186]

REFERENCES

1. Santulli G, Trimarco B, Iaccarino G. G-protein-coupled receptor kinase 2 and hypertension: molecular insights and pathophysiological mechanisms. *High Blood Press Cardiovasc Prev Off J Italian Soc Hypertens* 2013;**20**(1):5–12.
2. Iaccarino G, Barbato E, Cipolletta E, et al. Elevated myocardial and lymphocyte GRK2 expression and activity in human heart failure. *Eur Heart J* 2005;**26**(17):1752–8.
3. Penela P, Ribas C, Mayor Jr. F. Mechanisms of regulation of the expression and function of G protein-coupled receptor kinases. *Cell Signal* 2003;**15**(11):973–81.
4. Hatton R, Cvjeticanin A, Lymperopoulos A. The adrenergic system of the adrenal glands as a remote control of cardiac function. *JCvD* 2015;**5**(3):394–7.

5. Kamal FA, Travers JG, Blaxall BC. G protein-coupled receptor kinases in cardiovascular disease: why “where” matters. *Trends Cardiovasc Med* 2012;**22**(8):213–9.
6. Mei Y, Yin N, Jin X, He J, Yin Z. The regulatory role of the adrenergic agonists phenylephrine and isoproterenol on fetal hemoglobin expression and erythroid differentiation. *Endocrinology* 2013;**154**(12):4640–9.
7. Lampri E, Ioachim E.. In: Santulli G, editor. *Angiogenesis: something old, something new. Angiogenesis: insight from a systematic overview*. New York, NY: Nova Science Publishers; 2013. p. 1–30.
8. O’Connell TD, Jensen BC, Baker AJ, Simpson PC. Cardiac alpha1-adrenergic receptors: novel aspects of expression, signaling mechanisms, physiologic function, and clinical importance. *Pharmacol Rev* 2014;**66**(1):308–33.
9. Ruuskanen JO, Laurila J, Xhaard H, et al. Conserved structural, pharmacological and functional properties among the three human and five zebrafish alpha 2-adrenoceptors. *Br J Pharmacol* 2005;**144**(2): 165–77.
10. Vicco MH, Pujato N, Bontempi I, Rodeles L, Marcipar I, Bottasso OA. beta1-Selective adrenoceptor antagonists increase plasma levels of Anti-p2beta antibodies and decrease cardiac involvement in chronic progressive chagas heart disease. *Can J Cardiol* 2014;**30**(3):332–7.
11. Santulli G, Iaccarino G. Pinpointing beta adrenergic receptor in ageing pathophysiology: victim or executioner? Evidence from crime scenes. *Immun Ageing* 2013;**10**(1):10.
12. Belge C, Hammond J, Dubois-Deruy E, et al. Enhanced expression of beta3-adrenoceptors in cardiac myocytes attenuates neurohormone-induced hypertrophic remodeling through nitric oxide synthase. *Circulation* 2014;**129**(4):451–62.
13. Xiao RP. Beta-adrenergic signaling in the heart: dual coupling of the beta2-adrenergic receptor to G(s) and G(i) proteins. *Sci STKE* 2001;**2001**(104):re15.
14. Santulli G, Lombardi A, Sorriento D, et al. Age-related impairment in insulin release: the essential role of beta(2)-adrenergic receptor. *Diabetes* 2012;**61**(3):692–701.
15. Kaya AI, Onaran HO, Ozcan G, et al. Cell contact-dependent functional selectivity of beta2-adrenergic receptor ligands in stimulating cAMP accumulation and extracellular signal-regulated kinase phosphorylation. *J Biol Chem* 2012;**287**(9):6362–74.
16. Santulli G, Marks AR. Essential roles of intracellular calcium release channels in muscle, brain, metabolism, and aging. *Curr Mol Pharmacol* 2015;**8**(2):206–22.
17. Yuan Q, Chen Z, Santulli G, et al. Functional role of Calstabin2 in age-related cardiac alterations. *Sci Rep* 2014;**4**:7425.
18. Santulli G, Wronska A, Uryu K, et al. A selective microRNA-based strategy inhibits restenosis while preserving endothelial function. *J Clin Invest* 2014;**124**(9):4102–14.
19. Santulli G, Basilicata MF, De Simone M, et al. Evaluation of the anti-angiogenic properties of the new selective alphaVbeta3 integrin antagonist RGDechiHCit. *J Transl Med* 2011;**9**:7.
20. Santulli G, Ciccarelli M, Palumbo G, et al. In vivo properties of the proangiogenic peptide QK. *J Transl Med* 2009;**7**:41.
21. Iaccarino G, Ciccarelli M, Sorriento D, et al. AKT participates in endothelial dysfunction in hypertension. *Circulation* 2004;**109**(21):2587–93.
22. Iaccarino G, Cipolletta E, Fiorillo A, et al. Beta(2)-adrenergic receptor gene delivery to the endothelium corrects impaired adrenergic vasorelaxation in hypertension. *Circulation* 2002;**106**(3):349–55.
23. Iaccarino G, Ciccarelli M, Sorriento D, et al. Ischemic neoangiogenesis enhanced by beta2-adrenergic receptor overexpression: a novel role for the endothelial adrenergic system. *Circul Res* 2005;**97**(11):1182–9.
24. Ciccarelli M, Sorriento D, Cipolletta E, et al. Impaired neoangiogenesis in beta-adrenoceptor gene-deficient mice: restoration by intravascular human beta-adrenoceptor gene transfer and role of NFkappaB and CREB transcription factors. *Br J Pharmacol* 2011;**162**(3):712–21.
25. Santulli G. Angiopoietin-like proteins: a comprehensive look. *Front Endocrinol* 2014;**5**:4.

26. Boer C, Scheffer GJ, de Lange JJ, Westerhof N, Sipkema P. Alpha-1-adrenoceptor stimulation induces nitric oxide release in rat pulmonary arteries. *J Vasc Res* 1999;**36**(1):79–81.
27. Guimaraes S, Moura D. Vascular adrenoceptors: an update. *Pharmacol Rev* 2001;**53**(2):319–56.
28. Ignarro LJ, Buga GM, Wood KS, Byrns RE, Chaudhuri G. Endothelium-derived relaxing factor produced and released from artery and vein is nitric oxide. *Proc Natl Acad Sci USA* 1987;**84**(24):9265–9.
29. Palmer RM, Ferrige AG, Moncada S. Nitric oxide release accounts for the biological activity of endothelium-derived relaxing factor. *Nature* 1987;**327**(6122):524–6.
30. Bockman CS, Gonzalez-Cabrera I, Abel PW. Alpha-2 adrenoceptor subtype causing nitric oxide-mediated vascular relaxation in rats. *J Pharmacol Exp Ther* 1996;**278**(3):1235–43.
31. Queen LR, Ji Y, Xu B, et al. Mechanisms underlying beta2-adrenoceptor-mediated nitric oxide generation by human umbilical vein endothelial cells. *J Physiol* 2006;**576**(Pt 2):585–94.
32. Lembo G, Iaccarino G, Vecchione C, et al. Insulin modulation of an endothelial nitric oxide component present in the alpha2- and beta-adrenergic responses in human forearm. *J Clin Invest* 1997;**100**(8):2007–14.
33. Ozaki M, Kawashima S, Yamashita T, et al. Overexpression of endothelial nitric oxide synthase accelerates atherosclerotic lesion formation in apoE-deficient mice. *J Clin Invest* 2002;**110**(3):331–40.
34. Endemann DH, Schiffrin EL. Endothelial dysfunction. *J Am Soc Nephrol* 2004;**15**(8):1983–92.
35. Bouloumie A, Bauersachs J, Linz W, et al. Endothelial dysfunction coincides with an enhanced nitric oxide synthase expression and superoxide anion production. *Hypertension* 1997;**30**(4):934–41.
36. Forstermann U. Oxidative stress in vascular disease: causes, defense mechanisms and potential therapies. *Nat Clin Pract* 2008;**5**(6):338–49.
37. Lambeth JD. NOX enzymes and the biology of reactive oxygen. *Nat Rev Immunol* 2004;**4**(3):181–9.
38. Theccanat T, Philip JL, Razzaque AM, et al. Regulation of cellular oxidative stress and apoptosis by G protein-coupled receptor kinase-2; The role of NADPH oxidase 4. *Cell Signal* 2016;**28**(3):190–203.
39. Droge W. Free radicals in the physiological control of cell function. *Physiol Rev* 2002;**82**(1):47–95.
40. Gutierrez J, Ballinger SW, Darley-Usmar VM, Landar A. Free radicals, mitochondria, and oxidized lipids: the emerging role in signal transduction in vascular cells. *Circul Res* 2006;**99**(9):924–32.
41. Fu YC, Yin SC, Chi CS, Hwang B, Hsu SL. Norepinephrine induces apoptosis in neonatal rat endothelial cells via a ROS-dependent JNK activation pathway. *Apoptosis* 2006;**11**(11):2053–63.
42. Lopez Farre A, Casado S. Heart failure, redox alterations, and endothelial dysfunction. *Hypertension* 2001;**38**(6):1400–5.
43. Finkel T. Reactive oxygen species and signal transduction. *IUBMB Life* 2001;**52**(1–2):3–6.
44. Gainetdinov RR, Bohn LM, Sotnikova TD, et al. Dopaminergic supersensitivity in G protein-coupled receptor kinase 6-deficient mice. *Neuron* 2003;**38**(2):291–303.
45. Lyubarsky AL, Chen C, Simon MI, Pugh Jr. EN. Mice lacking G-protein receptor kinase 1 have profoundly slowed recovery of cone-driven retinal responses. *J Neurosci* 2000;**20**(6):2209–17.
46. Walker JK, Gainetdinov RR, Feldman DS, et al. G protein-coupled receptor kinase 5 regulates airway responses induced by muscarinic receptor activation. *Am J Physiol Lung Cell Mol Physiol* 2004;**286**(2):L312–9.
47. Kahsai AW, Zhu S, Fenteany G. G protein-coupled receptor kinase 2 activates radixin, regulating membrane protrusion and motility in epithelial cells. *Biochim Biophys Acta* 2010;**1803**(2):300–10.
48. Chen Y, Sasai N, Ma G, et al. Sonic Hedgehog dependent phosphorylation by CK1alpha and GRK2 is required for ciliary accumulation and activation of smoothened. *PLoS Biol* 2011;**9**(6):e1001083.
49. Lodowski DT, Pitcher JA, Capel WD, Lefkowitz RJ, Tesmer JJ. Keeping G proteins at bay: a complex between G protein-coupled receptor kinase 2 and Gbetagamma. *Science* 2003;**300**(5623):1256–62.
50. Tesmer VM, Kawano T, Shankaranarayanan A, Kozasa T, Tesmer JJ. Snapshot of activated G proteins at the membrane: the Galphaq-GRK2-Gbetagamma complex. *Science* 2005;**310**(5754):1686–90.
51. Fusco A, Santulli G, Sorriento D, et al. Mitochondrial localization unveils a novel role for GRK2 in organelle biogenesis. *Cell Signal* 2011;**24**(2):468–75.

52. Obrenovich ME, Morales LA, Cobb CJ, et al. Insights into cerebrovascular complications and Alzheimer disease through the selective loss of GRK2 regulation. *J Cell Mol Med* 2009;**13**(5):853–65.
53. Vroon A, Kavelaars A, Limmroth V, et al. G protein-coupled receptor kinase 2 in multiple sclerosis and experimental autoimmune encephalomyelitis. *J Immunol* 2005;**174**(7):4400–6.
54. Iacovelli L, Franchetti R, Masini M, De Blasi A. GRK2 and beta-arrestin 1 as negative regulators of thyrotropin receptor-stimulated response. *Mol Endocrinol* 1996;**10**(9):1138–46.
55. Ferrer-Alcon M, La Harpe R, Garcia-Sevilla JA. Decreased immunodensities of micro-opioid receptors, receptor kinases GRK 2/6 and beta-arrestin-2 in postmortem brains of opiate addicts. *Brain Res Mol Brain Res* 2004;**121**(1–2):114–22.
56. Lombardi MS, Kavelaars A, Cobelens PM, Schmidt RE, Schedlowski M, Heijnen CJ. Adjuvant arthritis induces down-regulation of G protein-coupled receptor kinases in the immune system. *J Immunol* 2001;**166**(3):1635–40.
57. King DW, Steinmetz R, Wagoner HA, et al. Differential expression of GRK isoforms in nonmalignant and malignant human granulosa cells. *Endocrine* 2003;**22**(2):135–42.
58. Mak JC, Chuang TT, Harris CA, Barnes PJ. Increased expression of G protein-coupled receptor kinases in cystic fibrosis lung. *Eur J Pharmacol* 2002;**436**(3):165–72.
59. Liu S, Premont RT, Kontos CD, Zhu S, Rockey DC. A crucial role for GRK2 in regulation of endothelial cell nitric oxide synthase function in portal hypertension. *Nat Med* 2005;**11**(9):952–8.
60. Eckhart AD, Ozaki T, Tevaearai H, Rockman HA, Koch WJ. Vascular-targeted overexpression of G protein-coupled receptor kinase-2 in transgenic mice attenuates beta-adrenergic receptor signaling and increases resting blood pressure. *Mol Pharmacol* 2002;**61**(4):749–58.
61. Santulli G. microRNAs distinctively regulate vascular smooth muscle and endothelial cells: functional implications in angiogenesis, atherosclerosis, and in-stent restenosis. *Adv Exp Med Biol* 2015;**887**:53–77.
62. Napolitano R, Campanile A, Sarno L, et al. GRK2 levels in umbilical arteries of pregnancies complicated by gestational hypertension and preeclampsia. *Am J Hypertens* 2012;**25**(3):366–71.
63. Maynard SE, Min JY, Merchan J, et al. Excess placental soluble fms-like tyrosine kinase 1 (sFlt1) may contribute to endothelial dysfunction, hypertension, and proteinuria in preeclampsia. *J Clin Invest* 2003;**111**(5):649–58.
64. Rana S, Powe CE, Salahuddin S, et al. Angiogenic factors and the risk of adverse outcomes in women with suspected preeclampsia. *Circulation* 2012;**125**(7):911–9.
65. Abd Alla J, Graemer M, Fu X, Quitterer U. Inhibition of G-protein-coupled receptor kinase 2 prevents the dysfunctional cardiac substrate metabolism in fatty acid synthase-transgenic mice. *J Biol Chem* 2015;**291**(6):2583–600.
66. Izzo R, Cipolletta E, Ciccarelli M, et al. Enhanced GRK2 expression and desensitization of betaAR vasodilatation in hypertensive patients. *Clin Transl Sci* 2008;**1**(3):215–20.
67. Borkowski KR, Gros R, Schneider H. Vascular beta-adrenoceptor-mediated responses in hypertension and ageing in rats. *J Auton Pharmacol* 1992;**12**(6):389–401.
68. Gros R, Benovic JL, Tan CM, Feldman RD. G-protein-coupled receptor kinase activity is increased in hypertension. *J Clin Invest* 1997;**99**(9):2087–93.
69. Gros R, Chorazyczewski J, Meek MD, Benovic JL, Ferguson SS, Feldman RD. G-Protein-coupled receptor kinase activity in hypertension: increased vascular and lymphocyte G-protein receptor kinase-2 protein expression. *Hypertension* 2000;**35**(1 Pt 1):38–42.
70. Santulli G, Campanile A, Spinelli L, et al. G protein-coupled receptor kinase 2 in patients with acute myocardial infarction. *Am J Cardiol* 2011;**107**(8):1125–30.
71. De Boer MP, Meijer RI, Wijnstok NJ, et al. Microvascular dysfunction: a potential mechanism in the pathogenesis of obesity-associated insulin resistance and hypertension. *Microcirculation* 2012;**19**(1):5–18.

72. Santulli G. The adrenergic system in cardiovascular metabolism and aging.. In: Lymperopoulos A, editor. *The cardiovascular adrenergic system*. New York, NY: Springer; 2015. p. 97–116.
73. Usui I, Imamura T, Babendure JL, et al. G protein-coupled receptor kinase 2 mediates endothelin-1-induced insulin resistance via the inhibition of both Galphaq/11 and insulin receptor substrate-1 pathways in 3T3-L1 adipocytes. *Mol Endocrinol* 2005;**19**(11):2760–8.
74. Ciccarelli M, Chuprun JK, Rengo G, et al. G protein-coupled receptor kinase 2 activity impairs cardiac glucose uptake and promotes insulin resistance after myocardial ischemia. *Circulation* 2011;**123**(18): 1953–62.
75. Cipolletta E, Campanile A, Santulli G, et al. The G protein coupled receptor kinase 2 plays an essential role in beta-adrenergic receptor-induced insulin resistance. *Cardiovasc Res* 2009;**84**(3):407–15.
76. Heinonen I, Wendelin-Saarenhovi M, Kaskinoro K, Knuuti J, Scheinin M, Kalliokoski KK. Inhibition of alpha-adrenergic tone disturbs the distribution of blood flow in the exercising human limb. *Am J Physiol Heart Circul Physiol* 2013;**305**(2):H163–72.
77. Wu L, Liu L. Systematic review and meta-analysis evaluating the impact of vitamin D on the risk of heart failure: new evidence from population-based studies. *J Cardiovasc Dis* 2014;**2**(3):159–73.
78. Al Maluli H, DeStephan C. Hemodynamic monitoring in the intensive care unit. *J Cardiovas Dis* 2014;**2**(2):101–15.
79. Santulli G. Adrenal signaling in heart failure: something more than a distant ship's smoke on the horizon. *Hypertension* 2014;**63**(2):215–6.
80. Latini R, Masson S, Staszewsky L, Barlera S. Neurohormonal modulation in heart failure of ischemic etiology: correlates with left ventricular remodeling. *Curr Heart Fail Rep* 2006;**3**(4):157–63.
81. Sardu C, Marfella R, Santulli G, Paolisso G. Functional role of miRNA in cardiac resynchronization therapy. *Pharmacogenomics* 2014;**15**(8):1159–68.
82. Senni M, Paulus WJ, Gavazzi A, et al. New strategies for heart failure with preserved ejection fraction: the importance of targeted therapies for heart failure phenotypes. *Eur Heart J* 2014;**35**(40):2797–815.
83. Lymperopoulos A, Chowdhary S, Sankar K, Simon I. Regulation of catecholamine production from the adrenal medulla. In: Santulli G, editor. *Adrenal glands: from pathophysiology to clinical evidence*. New York, NY: Nova Science Publisher; 2015.
84. Perez-Alvarez A, Hernandez-Vivanco A, Albillos A. Past, present and future of human chromaffin cells: role in physiology and therapeutics. *Cell Mol Neurobiol* 2010;**30**(8):1407–15.
85. Chung M, Song J. Imaging of adrenal gland. In: Santulli G, editor. *Adrenal glands: from pathophysiology to clinical evidence*. New York, NY: Nova Science Publisher; 2015.
86. Deo SH, Jenkins NT, Padilla J, Parrish AR, Fadel PJ. Norepinephrine increases NADPH oxidase-derived superoxide in human peripheral blood mononuclear cells via alpha-adrenergic receptors. *Am J Physiol Regul Integr Comp Physiol* 2013;**305**(10):R1124–32.
87. Ma Y, Krueger JJ, Redmon SN, et al. Extracellular norepinephrine clearance by the norepinephrine transporter is required for skeletal homeostasis. *J Biol Chem* 2013;**288**(42):30105–13.
88. Thireau J, Karam S, Roberge S, et al. Beta-adrenergic blockade combined with subcutaneous B-type natriuretic peptide: a promising approach to reduce ventricular arrhythmia in heart failure? *Heart* 2014;**100**(11):833–41.
89. Staroukine M, Devriendt J, Decoodt P, Verniory A. Relationships between plasma epinephrine, norepinephrine, dopamine and angiotensin II concentrations, renin activity, hemodynamic state and prognosis in acute heart failure. *Acta Cardiol* 1984;**39**(2):131–8.
90. Shiny KS, Kumar SH, Farvin KH, Anandan R, Devadasan K. Protective effect of taurine on myocardial antioxidant status in isoprenaline-induced myocardial infarction in rats. *J Pharm Pharmacol* 2005;**57**(10): 1313–7.
91. Huang CJ, Webb HE, Zourdos MC, Acevedo EO. Cardiovascular reactivity, stress, and physical activity. *Front Physiol* 2013;**4**:314.

92. Weng TP, Fu TC, Wang CH, Hsu CC, Wang JS. Activation of lymphocyte autophagy/apoptosis reflects haemodynamic inefficiency and functional aerobic impairment in patients with heart failure. *Clin Sci* 2014;**127**(10):589–602.
93. Berezin A, Kremzer A, Samura T, Martovitskaya Y. Apoptotic microparticles to progenitor mononuclear cells ratio in heart failure: relevance of clinical status and outcomes. *J Cardiovasc Dis* 2014;**2**(2):50–7.
94. Sorriento D, Santulli G, Del Giudice C, Anastasio A, Trimarco B, Iaccarino G. Endothelial cells are able to synthesize and release catecholamines both in vitro and in vivo. *Hypertension* 2012;**60**(1):129–36.
95. Ciccarelli M, Santulli G, Campanile A, et al. Endothelial alpha1-adrenoceptors regulate neo-angiogenesis. *Br J Pharmacol* 2008;**153**(5):936–46.
96. Gao W, Li J. Femoral artery occlusion increases muscle pressor reflex and expression of hypoxia-inducible factor-1α in sensory neurons. *J Cardiovascu Dis* 2014;**1**(2):34–40.
97. Buroker N. ADRBK1 (GRK2) rSNPs, transcriptional factor binding sites and cardiovascular disease in the black population. *J Cardiovasc Dis* 2014;**2**(2):62–7.
98. Santulli G. Coronary heart disease risk factors and mortality. *JAMA J Am Med Assoc* 2012;**307**(11):1137.
99. Szepietowska B, Zhu W, Czyzyk J, Eid T, Sherwin RS. EphA5-EphrinA5 interactions within the ventromedial hypothalamus influence counterregulatory hormone release and local glutamine/glutamate balance during hypoglycemia. *Diabetes* 2013;**62**(4):1282–8.
100. Neglia D, De Caterina A, Marraccini P, et al. Impaired myocardial metabolic reserve and substrate selection flexibility during stress in patients with idiopathic dilated cardiomyopathy. *Am J Physiol Heart Circul Physiol* 2007;**293**(6):H3270–8.
101. Dias P, Terracciano CM. Hyperpolarization-activated cyclic nucleotide-gated channels and ventricular arrhythmias in heart failure: a novel target for therapy? *J Am Heart Assoc* 2013;**2**(3):e000287.
102. Li YF, Shi ST. Age-dependent differential crosstalk between alpha(1)-adrenergic and angiotensin receptors. *Can J Cardiol* 2009;**25**(8):481–5.
103. Santulli G, Ciccarelli M, Trimarco B, Iaccarino G. Physical activity ameliorates cardiovascular health in elderly subjects: the functional role of the beta adrenergic system. *Front Physiol* 2013;**4**:209.
104. Ciccarelli M, Santulli G, Pascale V, Trimarco B, Iaccarino G. Adrenergic receptors and metabolism: role in development of cardiovascular disease. *Front Physiol* 2013;**4**:265.
105. Chakraborty M, Phillips A, Macdonald J, Windsor J, Hickey A. Mitochondrial respiration in mononuclear cells and heart fibers in spontaneously hypertensive rats. *J Cardiovascu Dis* 2014;**2**(1):7–14.
106. Leone TC, Kelly DP. Transcriptional control of cardiac fuel metabolism and mitochondrial function. *Cold Spring Harbor Symp Quant Biol* 2011;**76**:175–82.
107. Fu Q, Xu B, Liu Y, et al. Insulin inhibits cardiac contractility by inducing a Gi-biased beta2 adrenergic signaling in hearts. *Diabetes* 2014;**63**(8):2676–89.
108. Msolly A, Miled A, Kassab A. Hydrogen peroxide: an oxidant stress indicator in type 2 diabetes mellitus. *J Cardiovasc Dis* 2014;**1**(2):48–52.
109. Oriente F, Iovino S, Cassese A, et al. Overproduction of phosphoprotein enriched in diabetes (PED) induces mesangial expansion and upregulates protein kinase C-beta activity and TGF-beta1 expression. *Diabetologia* 2009;**52**(12):2642–52.
110. Sardu C, Marfella R, Santulli G. Impact of diabetes mellitus on the clinical response to cardiac resynchronization therapy in elderly people. *J Cardiovasc Transl Res* 2014;**7**(3):362–8.
111. Azevedo PS, Minicucci MF, Santos PP, Paiva SA, Zornoff LA. Energy metabolism in cardiac remodeling and heart failure. *Cardiol Rev* 2013;**21**(3):135–40.
112. Shimizu I, Minamino T, Toko H, et al. Excessive cardiac insulin signaling exacerbates systolic dysfunction induced by pressure overload in rodents. *J Clin Invest* 2010;**120**(5):1506–14.
113. Sorriento D, Santulli G, Fusco A, Anastasio A, Trimarco B, Iaccarino G. Intracardiac injection of AdGRK5-NT reduces left ventricular hypertrophy by inhibiting NF-kappaB-dependent hypertrophic gene expression. *Hypertension* 2010;**56**(4):696–704.

114. Badimon L, Hernandez Vera R, Vilahur G. Determinants of cardiovascular risk in diabetes beyond hyperglycemia. *J Cardiovasc Dis* 2014;**1**(2):53–62.
115. Masuo K, Rakugi H, Ogihara T, Lambert GW. Different mechanisms in weight loss-induced blood pressure reduction between a calorie-restricted diet and exercise. *Hypertens Res Off J Jpn Soc Hypertens* 2012;**35**(1):41–7.
116. Santulli G. Effects of low-carbohydrate and low-fat diets. *Ann Int Med* 2015;**162**(5):392.
117. Quinones MJ, Nicholas SB, Lyon CJ. Insulin resistance and the endothelium. *Curr Diabetes Rep* 2005;**5**(4):246–53.
118. Mongillo M, John AS, Leccisotti L, Pennell DJ, Camici PG. Myocardial pre-synaptic sympathetic function correlates with glucose uptake in the failing human heart. *Eur J Nucl Med Mol Imaging* 2007;**34**(8):1172–7.
119. Larsen TM, Toubro S, van Baak MA, et al. Effect of a 28-d treatment with L-796568, a novel beta(3)-adrenergic receptor agonist, on energy expenditure and body composition in obese men. *Am J Clin Nutr* 2002;**76**(4):780–8.
120. Sorriento D, Ciccarelli M, Santulli G, Illario M, Trimarco B, Iaccarino G. Trafficking GRK2: cellular and metabolic consequences of GRK2 subcellular localization. *Transl Med UniSa* 2014;**10**:3–7.
121. Horinouchi T, Hoshi A, Harada T, et al. Endothelin-1 suppresses insulin-stimulated Akt phosphorylation and glucose uptake via G protein-coupled receptor kinase 2 in skeletal muscle cells. *Br J Pharmacol* 2016;**173**(6):1018–32.
122. Lucas E, Cruces-Sande M, Briones AM, et al. Molecular physiopathology of obesity-related diseases: multi-organ integration by GRK2. *Arch Physiol Biochem* 2015;**121**(5):163–77.
123. Mehta N, Cheng AH, Chiang CK, et al. GRK2 fine-tunes circadian clock speed and entrainment via transcriptional and post-translational control of PERIOD proteins. *Cell Rep* 2015;**12**(8):1272–88.
124. Chen M, Sato PY, Chuprun JK, et al. Prodeath signaling of G protein-coupled receptor kinase 2 in cardiac myocytes after ischemic stress occurs via extracellular signal-regulated kinase-dependent heat shock protein 90-mediated mitochondrial targeting. *Circul Res* 2013;**112**(8):1121–34.
125. Taguchi K, Sakata K, Ohashi W, Imaizumi T, Imura J, Hattori Y. Tonic inhibition by G protein-coupled receptor kinase 2 of Akt/endothelial nitric-oxide synthase signaling in human vascular endothelial cells under conditions of hyperglycemia with high insulin levels. *J Pharmacol Exp Ther* 2014;**349**(2):199–208.
126. Hata JA, Williams ML, Koch WJ. Genetic manipulation of myocardial beta-adrenergic receptor activation and desensitization. *J Mol Cell Cardiol* 2004;**37**(1):11–21.
127. Santulli G, Xie W, Reiken SR, Marks AR. Mitochondrial calcium overload is a key determinant in heart failure. *Proc Natl Acad Sci USA* 2015;**112**(36):11389–94.
128. Wisneski JA, Gertz EW, Neese RA, Mayr M. Myocardial metabolism of free fatty acids. Studies with 14C-labeled substrates in humans. *J Clin Invest* 1987;**79**(2):359–66.
129. Bing RJ, Siegel A, Ungar I, Gilbert M. Metabolism of the human heart. II. Studies on fat, ketone and amino acid metabolism. *Am J Med* 1954;**16**(4):504–15.
130. Neubauer S. The failing heart—an engine out of fuel. *New Engl J Med* 2007;**356**(11):1140–51.
131. Kolwicz Jr. SC, Tian R. Metabolic therapy at the crossroad: how to optimize myocardial substrate utilization? *Trends Cardiovasc Med* 2009;**19**(6):201–7.
132. Eisenhofer G, Friberg P, Rundqvist B, et al. Cardiac sympathetic nerve function in congestive heart failure. *Circulation* 1996;**93**(9):1667–76.
133. Opie LH, Thandroyen FT, Muller C, Bricknell OL. Adrenaline-induced "oxygen-wastage" and enzyme release from working rat heart. Effects of calcium antagonism, beta-blockade, nicotinic acid and coronary artery ligation. *J Mol Cell Cardiol* 1979;**11**(10):1073–94.
134. Sasaoka T, Wada T, Tsuneki H. Lipid phosphatases as a possible therapeutic target in cases of type 2 diabetes and obesity. *Pharmacol Ther* 2006;**112**(3):799–809.
135. Banerjee S, Peterson LR. Myocardial metabolism and cardiac performance in obesity and insulin resistance. *Curr Cardiol Rep* 2007;**9**(2):143–9.

136. Wagenmakers AJ, van Riel NA, Frenneaux MP, Stewart PM. Integration of the metabolic and cardiovascular effects of exercise. *Essays Biochem* 2006;**42**:193–210.
137. Xiao RP, Cheng H, Zhou YY, Kuschel M, Lakatta EG. Recent advances in cardiac beta(2)-adrenergic signal transduction. *Circul Res* 1999;**85**(11):1092–100.
138. Baruscotti M, Barbuti A, Bucchi A. The cardiac pacemaker current. *J Mol Cell Cardiol* 2010;**48**(1):55–64.
139. Santulli G, Totary-Jain H. Tailoring mTOR-based therapy: molecular evidence and clinical challenges. *Pharmacogenomics* 2013;**14**(12):1517–26.
140. Perino A, Ghigo A, Ferrero E, et al. Integrating cardiac PIP(3) and cAMP signaling through a PKA anchoring function of p110gamma. *Mol Cell* 2011;**42**(1):84–95.
141. Philipson LH. beta-Agonists and metabolism. *J Allergy Clin Immunol* 2002;**110**(6 Suppl.):S313–7.
142. Ngala RA, O'Dowd J, Wang SJ, et al. Metabolic responses to BRL37344 and clenbuterol in soleus muscle and C2C12 cells via different atypical pharmacologies and beta2-adrenoceptor mechanisms. *Br J Pharmacol* 2008;**155**(3):395–406.
143. Jo SH, Leblais V, Wang PH, Crow MT, Xiao RP. Phosphatidylinositol 3-kinase functionally compartmentalizes the concurrent G(s) signaling during beta2-adrenergic stimulation. *Circul Res* 2002;**91**(1):46–53.
144. Zhu WZ, Zheng M, Koch WJ, Lefkowitz RJ, Kobilka BK, Xiao RP. Dual modulation of cell survival and cell death by beta(2)-adrenergic signaling in adult mouse cardiac myocytes. *Proc Natl Acad Sci USA* 2001;**98**(4):1607–12.
145. Sakamoto K, Holman GD. Emerging role for AS160/TBC1D4 and TBC1D1 in the regulation of GLUT4 traffic. *Am J Physiol* 2008;**295**(1):E29–37.
146. Maarbjerg SJ, Sylow L, Richter EA. Current understanding of increased insulin sensitivity after exercise - emerging candidates. *Acta Physiol (Oxford, England)* 2011;**202**(3):323–35.
147. Perez-Schindler J, Philp A, Baar K, Hernandez-Cascales J. Regulation of contractility and metabolic signaling by the beta2-adrenergic receptor in rat ventricular muscle. *Life Sci* 2011;**88**(19–20):892–7.
148. Hardie DG, Ross FA, Hawley SA. AMPK: a nutrient and energy sensor that maintains energy homeostasis. *Nat Rev* 2012;**13**(4):251–62.
149. Nikolaidis LA, Poornima I, Parikh P, Magovern M, Shen YT, Shannon RP. The effects of combined versus selective adrenergic blockade on left ventricular and systemic hemodynamics, myocardial substrate preference, and regional perfusion in conscious dogs with dilated cardiomyopathy. *J Am College Cardiol* 2006;**47**(9):1871–81.
150. Shahid G, Hussain T. GRK2 negatively regulates glycogen synthesis in mouse liver FL83B cells. *J Biol Chem* 2007;**282**(28):20612–20.
151. Sorriento D, Santulli G, Franco A, et al. Integrating GRK2 and NFkappaB in the pathophysiology of cardiac hypertrophy. *J Cardiovasc Transl Res* 2015;**8**(8):493–502.
152. Santulli G, Cipolletta E, Sorriento D, et al. CaMK4 gene deletion induces hypertension. *J Am Heart Assoc* 2012;**1**(4):e001081.
153. Opie LH, Commerford PJ, Gersh BJ, Pfeffer MA. Controversies in ventricular remodelling. *Lancet (London, England)* 2006;**367**(9507):356–67.
154. Heusch G, Libby P, Gersh B, et al. Cardiovascular remodelling in coronary artery disease and heart failure. *Lancet* 2014;**383**(9932):1933–43.
155. Ganau A, Devereux RB, Roman MJ, et al. Patterns of left ventricular hypertrophy and geometric remodeling in essential hypertension. *J Am College Cardiol* 1992;**19**(7):1550–8.
156. Gerdes AM, Kellerman SE, Moore JA, et al. Structural remodeling of cardiac myocytes in patients with ischemic cardiomyopathy. *Circulation* 1992;**86**(2):426–30.
157. Pfeffer MA, Braunwald E. Ventricular remodeling after myocardial infarction. Experimental observations and clinical implications. *Circulation* 1990;**81**(4):1161–72.
158. Lorell BH, Carabello BA. Left ventricular hypertrophy: pathogenesis, detection, and prognosis. *Circulation* 2000;**102**(4):470–9.

159. Foppa M, Duncan BB, Rohde LE. Echocardiography-based left ventricular mass estimation. How should we define hypertrophy? *Cardiovasc Ultrasound* 2005;**3**:17.
160. Tarone G, Balligand JL, Bauersachs J, et al. Targeting myocardial remodelling to develop novel therapies for heart failure: a position paper from the Working Group on Myocardial Function of the European Society of Cardiology. *Eur J Heart Fail* 2014;**16**(5):494–508.
161. Brodde OE, Michel MC, Zerkowski HR. Signal transduction mechanisms controlling cardiac contractility and their alterations in chronic heart failure. *Cardiovasc Res* 1995;**30**(4):570–84.
162. Xiao RP, Avdonin P, Zhou YY, et al. Coupling of beta2-adrenoceptor to Gi proteins and its physiological relevance in murine cardiac myocytes. *Circul Res* 1999;**84**(1):43–52.
163. Devic E, Xiang Y, Gould D, Kobilka B. Beta-adrenergic receptor subtype-specific signaling in cardiac myocytes from beta(1) and beta(2) adrenoceptor knockout mice. *Mol Pharmacol* 2001;**60**(3):577–83.
164. Pavoine C, Behforouz N, Gauthier C, et al. beta2-adrenergic signaling in human heart: shift from the cyclic AMP to the arachidonic acid pathway. *Mol Pharmacol* 2003;**64**(5):1117–25.
165. Moniotte S, Kobzik L, Feron O, Trochu JN, Gauthier C, Balligand JL. Upregulation of beta(3)-adrenoceptors and altered contractile response to inotropic amines in human failing myocardium. *Circulation* 2001;**103**(12):1649–55.
166. Kohout TA, Takaoka H, McDonald PH, et al. Augmentation of cardiac contractility mediated by the human beta(3)-adrenergic receptor overexpressed in the hearts of transgenic mice. *Circulation* 2001;**104**(20):2485–91.
167. Moens AL, Leyton-Mange JS, Niu X, et al. Adverse ventricular remodeling and exacerbated NOS uncoupling from pressure-overload in mice lacking the beta3-adrenoreceptor. *J Mol Cell Cardiol* 2009;**47**(5):576–85.
168. Port JD, Bristow MR. Altered beta-adrenergic receptor gene regulation and signaling in chronic heart failure. *J Mol Cell Cardiol* 2001;**33**(5):887–905.
169. Nikolaev VO, Moshkov A, Lyon AR, et al. Beta2-adrenergic receptor redistribution in heart failure changes cAMP compartmentation. *Science New York, NY* 2010;**327**(5973):1653–7.
170. Sorriento D, Ciccarelli M, Santulli G, et al. The G-protein-coupled receptor kinase 5 inhibits NFkappaB transcriptional activity by inducing nuclear accumulation of IkappaB alpha. *Proc Natl Acad Sci USA* 2008;**105**(46):17818–23.
171. Nevzorova J, Evans BA, Bengtsson T, Summers RJ. Multiple signalling pathways involved in beta2-adrenoceptor-mediated glucose uptake in rat skeletal muscle cells. *Br J Pharmacol* 2006;**147**(4):446–54.
172. Koch WJ, Rockman HA, Samama P, et al. Cardiac function in mice overexpressing the beta-adrenergic receptor kinase or a beta ARK inhibitor. *Science New York, NY* 1995;**268**(5215):1350–3.
173. Ciccarelli M, Cipolletta E, Iaccarino G. GRK2 at the control shaft of cellular metabolism. *Curr Pharm Des* 2012;**18**(2):121–7.
174. Sato PY, Chuprun JK, Ibetti J, et al. GRK2 compromises cardiomyocyte mitochondrial function by diminishing fatty acid-mediated oxygen consumption and increasing superoxide levels. *J Mol Cell Cardiol* 2015;**89**(Pt B):360–4.
175. Anis Y, Leshem O, Reuveni H, et al. Antidiabetic effect of novel modulating peptides of G-protein-coupled kinase in experimental models of diabetes. *Diabetologia* 2004;**47**(7):1232–44.
176. Sorriento D, Fusco A, Ciccarelli M, et al. Mitochondrial G protein coupled receptor kinase 2 regulates proinflammatory responses in macrophages. *FEBS Lett* 2013;**587**(21):3487–94.
177. Obrenovich ME, Smith MA, Siedlak SL, et al. Overexpression of GRK2 in Alzheimer disease and in a chronic hypoperfusion rat model is an early marker of brain mitochondrial lesions. *Neurotox Res* 2006;**10**(1):43–56.
178. Cheng JW. A review of isosorbide dinitrate and hydralazine in the management of heart failure in black patients, with a focus on a new fixed-dose combination. *Clin Ther* 2006;**28**(5):666–78.
179. Oparil S, Davis BR, Cushman WC, et al. Mortality and morbidity during and after Antihypertensive and Lipid-Lowering Treatment to Prevent Heart Attack Trial: results by sex. *Hypertension* 2013;**61**(5):977–86.

180. Gavras I, Manolis AJ, Gavras H. The alpha2 -adrenergic receptors in hypertension and heart failure: experimental and clinical studies. *J Hypertens* 2001;**19**(12):2115–24.
181. Pocock S, Wilhelmsen L, Dickstein K, Francis G, Wittes J. The data monitoring experience in the MOXCON trial. *Eur Heart J* 2004;**25**(22):1974–8.
182. Frantz RP, Lowes BD, Grayburn PA, et al. Baseline and serial neurohormones in patients with congestive heart failure treated with and without bucindolol: results of the neurohumoral substudy of the Beta-Blocker Evaluation of Survival Study (BEST). *J Card Fail* 2007;**13**(6):437–44.
183. Deneer VH, van Hemel NM. Is antiarrhythmic treatment in the elderly different? a review of the specific changes. *Drugs Aging* 2011;**28**(8):617–33.
184. Wong GW, Laugerotte A, Wright JM. Blood pressure lowering efficacy of dual alpha and beta blockers for primary hypertension. *Cochrane Database Syst Rev* 2015;**8**:CD007449.
185. Ellison KE, Gandhi G. Optimising the use of beta-adrenoceptor antagonists in coronary artery disease. *Drugs* 2005;**65**(6):787–97.
186. Santulli G. beta-Blockers in diabetic patients with heart failure. *JAMA Intern Med* 2015;**175**(4):657.
187. Lazalde-Ramos BP, Martinez-Fierro Mde L, Galaviz-Hernandez C, et al. CYP2D6 gene polymorphisms and predicted phenotypes in eight indigenous groups from northwestern Mexico. *Pharmacogenomics* 2014;**15**(3):339–48.
188. Rossello X, Pocock SJ, Julian DG. Long-term use of cardiovascular drugs: challenges for research and for patient care. *J Am Coll Cardiol* 2015;**66**(11):1273–85.
189. Santulli G. Sympathetic nervous system signaling in heart failure and cardiac aging. In: Jagadeesh G, editor. *Pathophysiology and pharmacotherapy of cardiovascular disease*. New York, NY: Springer; 2015. p. 83–105.
190. Santulli G, Pagano G, Sardu C, et al. Calcium release channel RyR2 regulates insulin release and glucose homeostasis. *J Clin Invest* 2015;**125**(5):1968–78.

CHAPTER

12

INSULIN SIGNALING IN CARDIAC HEALTH AND DISEASE*

J. Bartlett, P. Trivedi and T. Pulinilkunnil

Dalhousie Medicine New Brunswick (DMNB), Saint John, NB, Canada

ABBREVIATIONS

4E-BP1	eIF4E-binding protein1
ACC	acetyl-CoA carboxylase
ACSL1	acyl-CoA synthase long-chain family member 1
AFX/FOXO4	forkhead box protein O4
AMPK	AMP-activated protein kinase
AS160	Akt substrate of 160 kDa, also known as TBC1D4
ATGL	adipose triglyceride lipase, produces DAG
ATP	adenosine triphosphate
β2AR	β2-adrenergic receptor
cAMP	cyclic adenosine monophosphate
CD36	cluster of differentiation 36
CIRKO	cardiac insulin receptor knockout
CPT-1	carnitine palmitoyl-transferase 1
DAG	diacylglycerol
eEF2	eukaryotic elongation factor 2
eEF2K	eEF2 kinase
eIF4E	eukaryotic initiation factor 4E
eNOS	endothelial nitric oxide synthase
F-2,6-BP	fructose-2,6-bisphophate
FA	fatty acid
FFA	free fatty acids
FKHR/FOXO1	forkhead in rhabdomyosarcoma, also known as forkhead box protein O1
FKHRL-1/FOXO3	forkhead box protein O3
FOXO	forkhead box O proteins
G4H-/-	cardiac-specific deletion of GLUT4
G-6-P	glucose-6-phosphate
GDP	guanosine diphosphate
GFAT	glutamine: fructose-6-phosphate aminotransferase, a rate-limiting enzyme in HBP

* Bartlett et al. Biology and Pathology of Cardiac Insulin Signaling

Endocrinology of the Heart in Health and Disease. DOI: http://dx.doi.org/10.1016/B978-0-12-803111-7.00012-9

GH	growth hormone
G_i	inhibitory G-protein
GLUT-1(-4)	glucose transporter-1(-4)
Grb2	growth-factor receptor-bound protein 2
GRK2	G-protein receptor kinase 2
GS	glycogen synthase
GSK3 (α/β)	glycogen synthase kinase 3 (α/β)
GTP	guanosine triphosphate
HBP	hexosamine biosynthetic pathway
HF	heart failure
HSL	hormone sensitive lipase, produces MG
HW/BW	ratio of heart weight/body weight
IGF-1	insulin growth-like factor-1
IL-6	interleukin-6
I/R	ischemia/reperfusion
InsR	insulin receptor
IRS-1(-2,-3,-4)	insulin-receptor substrate-1(-2,-3,-4)
JNK	c-Jun NH2-terminal kinase
LCFA	long-chain fatty acid
LDH	lactate dehydrogenase
LPL	lipoprotein lipase
MAPK	mitogen-activated kinase, (p38, 38 kDa MAPK protein)
MCD	malonyl-CoA decarboxylase
MG	monoacylglycerol
MGL	monoacylglycerol lipase, produces FA
mTOR	mammalian/mechanistic target of rapamycin
mTORC1/2	mTOR complex ½
Nck	non-catalytic region of tyrosine kinase adaptor protein
nFAT	nuclear factor of activated T-cells
p110	110kDa subunit of PI3K
p70S6K	S6K of 70 kDa
p85	85 kDa subunit of PI3K
PDH	pyruvate dehydrogenase
PDK-1(-4)	phosphoinositide-dependent kinase-1(-4)
PFK-1(-2)	phosphofructo-1(-2)-kinase
PI3K	phosphoinositol-3-kinase
PIP2	phosphatidylinositol-4,5-diphosphate
PIP3	phosphatidylinositol-3,4,5-triphosphate
PKA	protein kinase A
PKB	protein kinase B, a serine-threonine protein kinase, also known as Akt
PKC-ζ	protein kinase C, ζ-isoform
PLN	phospholamban
PPAR-α	peroxisome proliferator-activated receptor, α-isoform
PTEN	phosphatase and tensin homolog deleted from chromosome 10
PTP1B	protein-tyrosine phosphatase 1B
Rab GAP	GTPase-activating protein of Ras superfamily G-protein
Rheb	Ras homolog enriched in brain
RYD	ryanodine

RyR2	ryanodine receptor 2
S6K	ribosomal protein S6 kinase
SERCA	sarcoplasmic reticulum calcium uptake pump
SH2	Src-homology domain 2
Shc	adaptor protein with homologies to Src and collagen
SPT	serine palmitoyltransferase
SR	sarcoplasmic reticulum
T1/2DM	type 1/2 diabetes mellitus
TAG	triacylglycerol
TBC1D1	TBC1 domain family member 1
TBC1D4	TBC1 domain family member 4, also known as AS160
TCA	tricarboxylic acid cycle
TNF-α	tumor necrosis factor-α
TSC2	tuberous sclerosis factor 2

INTRODUCTION

Insulin is the primary hormone regulating glucose utilization in the muscle, adipose tissue, and liver by virtue of a complex signaling program.[1,2] Systemic action of insulin exerts a tight control over metabolic processes within insulin-responsive tissues to maintain metabolic homeostasis.[3] Cardiac muscle is an insulin-responsive organ that expresses insulin receptors[2,4] and harbors an insulin signal transduction network of proteins. Within the myocardium, insulin promotes glucose utilization and prevents fatty acid (FA) oxidation. Furthermore, by sparing utilization of amino acids, insulin's mitogenic abilities govern the structural and functional development of the heart.[5] In addition to the key effect on cardiomyocytes, insulin also regulates vascular metabolism and function to maintain functional homeostasis in the myocardium. Insulin's effect on cardiac metabolism is a prerequisite for optimal cardiac function.[2,4] However, a lack of insulin or a disruption in the insulin signaling program precipitates detrimental cardiac outcomes.[6] In the present chapter, we first describe the fundamental insulin signaling mechanism(s) mediating the vast majority of biological effects in cardiac development, energy maintenance, and function. In the second part, we discuss how aberrant insulin signaling affects these normal physiological processes to cause serious detrimental effects on cardiac health. Loss of insulin signaling in Types 1 and 2 diabetes mellitus (T1/2DM) engender structural and functional abnormalities in the heart, which render the heart susceptible to dysfunction and failure. These abnormalities are indisputably related to insulin's loss of control over myocardial glucose metabolism that subsequently affects growth and survival pathways.[6] Randle's cycle explains the allosteric mechanisms by which deficits in glucose-derived energy propels over-usage and over-activation of FA utilization pathways in the heart resulting in metabolic inflexibility. Excessive use of FA results in accumulation of lipotoxic metabolites, rendering the heart more susceptible to increased pathogenesis and further exacerbating malfunction of the insulin signaling program. In addition, FA also behave as signaling molecules that activate peroxisome proliferator-activated receptors (PPARs), transcriptional regulators of myocardial energy metabolism. In the last 15 years of insulin-signaling research, molecular effectors of the insulin signaling program were directly targeted in the cardiomyocyte to ascertain their physiological importance in the heart and to decipher their contribution to whole body metabolism and function.[7,8]

FUNCTIONAL IMPORTANCE OF INSULIN RECEPTOR SIGNALING IN THE HEART

Elevated blood glucose triggers pancreatic islets (β cells) to secrete insulin into the systemic circulation, which then facilitates glucose uptake and metabolism in insulin-responsive tissues. Circulating insulin binds to the insulin receptor (InsR) in the heart, which acts as a "gatekeeper" of insulin-glucose communication between extra- and intra-cellular environments. The InsR is a hetero-tetrameric structure consisting of two extracellular α-subunits and two transmembrane β-subunits[9] (Fig. 12.1(A)). The

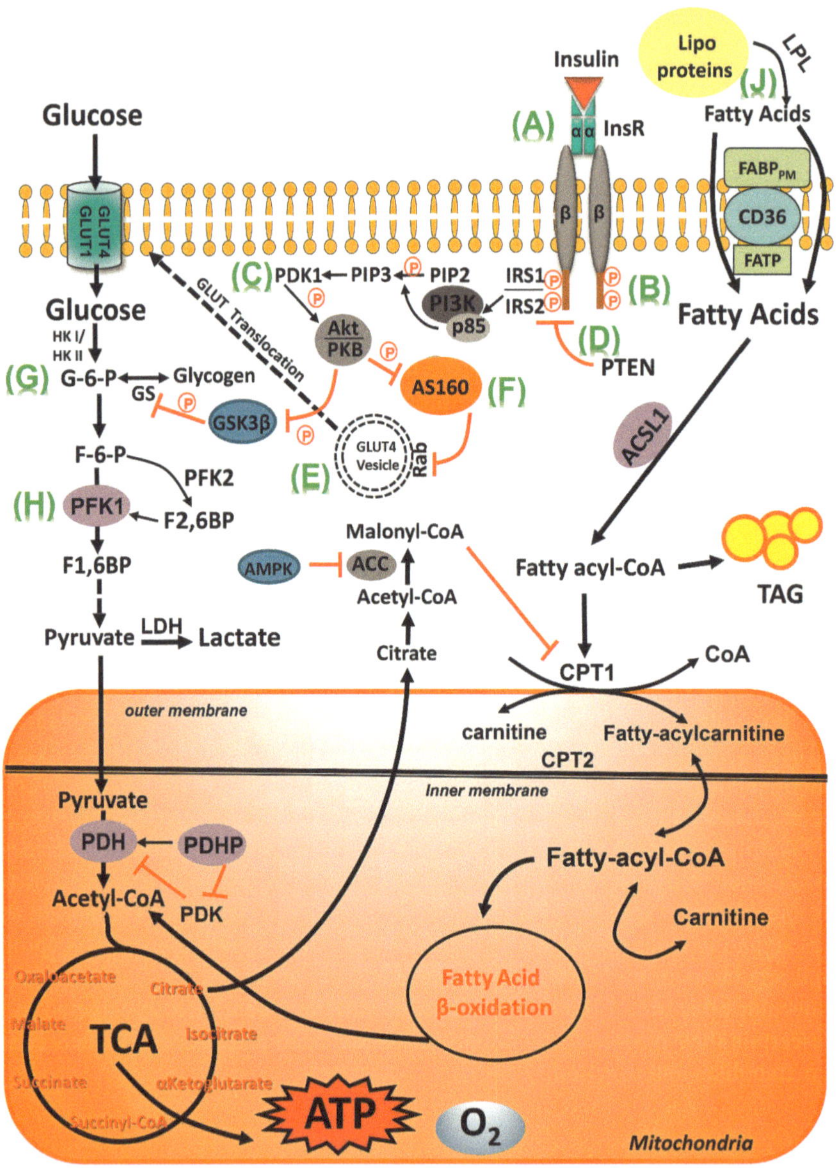

two β-subunits have tyrosine-kinase catalytic activity and facilitate an autophosphorylation cascade upon insulin binding on α-subunits.[9] The β-subunit autophosphorylation results in phosphorylation of several tyrosine residues on one of the β-subunits.[9] The insulin signaling cascade is negatively regulated by protein tyrosine phosphatases (PTP) that dephosphorylates the InsR. Notably, genetic deletion of PTP1B was found to be protective against septic shock-induced cardiomyopathy, and this was due to heightened insulin-stimulated reduction in inflammation,[10] signifying the benefits of enhanced insulin signaling in the myocardium.

The physiological importance of cardiomyocyte insulin signaling was established when cardiac-specific insulin receptor knockout (CIRKO) mice were generated. CIRKO mice exhibited a significant reduction in myocyte size and displayed metabolic features similar to the fetal heart signifying the importance of insulin signaling in cardiac tissue.[11] The control of insulin over myocardial metabolism is evident from the fact that CIRKO hearts persistently express immature fetal myosin gene programs resulting in augmented glycolysis and attenuated FA oxidation. Apart from the InsR, downstream insulin-signaling effectors also play an equally important role in governing cardiac metabolism and function. InsR activation following autophosphorylation leads to InsR–mediated phosphorylation of two indispensable molecular targets: insulin receptor substrate-1 & -2 (IRS-1/2) and Shc.[9] IRS-1 phosphorylation at several tyrosine residues induce IRS-1 activation (Fig. 12.1(B)). IRS activation leads to the association of a subset of cellular proteins containing an SH2-domain including Grb2, Nck, and lipid kinase phosphoinositol-3-kinase (PI3K).[12] Tyrosine phosphorylated residues on InsR and IRS-1 directly

FIGURE 12.1

Insulin regulation of cardiac energy metabolism in the healthy heart. Insulin regulates cardiac energy metabolism by activating metabolic pathways involving glucose and fatty acid utilization. Insulin's binding to its transmembrane receptor (A) initiates an intracellular autophosphorylation cascade that activates IRS-1 (B) and promotes PI3K-phosphorylation of PIP2 to increase intracellular PIP3 concentrations. Increased PIP3 concentrations facilitate recruitment of PDK1 and Akt to the cardiomyocyte membrane whereby PDK1 phosphorylates Akt at Ser473 (C). PTEN, a protein phosphatase, negatively regulates insulin signaling by dephosphorylating PI3K (D). Activating phosphorylation of Akt induces inhibitory phosphorylation of AS160, relieving inhibition on GLUT-4 translocation (F). GLUT-4 allows facilitated transport of glucose through the cardiomyocyte sarcolemma. Insulin-induced GLUT-4 translocation (E) facilitates cellular glucose uptake and utilization. Intracellularly, glucose is processed to G-6-P (G) that is either shunted into glycogen storage via glycogen synthase or processed further via glycolytic pathway. Insulin promotes myocyte glycolytic flux through the activation of PFK-2 (H), facilitating the feed-forward action of glycolysis. The glycolytic end-product pyruvate is transported into the mitochondrial matrix and converted by PDH to form acetyl-CoA, which is processed via the TCA cycle to generate ATP. Within the mitochondria, citrate generated during the TCA cycle translocates into the cytosol to form acetyl-CoA that is further converted to malonyl-CoA by ACC action. The pumping ability of the heart requires uninterrupted ATP production that is garnered via reliance on fatty acid oxidation. LPL-derived FA enter into the myocardium via the concerted action of fatty acid translocase CD36 and FABP/FATP (I), a mechanism similar to GLUT-4 translocation. Insulin inhibits fatty acid oxidation and directs the incorporation of fatty acids into TAG. Insulin increases malonyl-CoA levels, which inhibits CPT-1 and the ensuing mitochondrial β-oxidation of FAs. Insulin limits the heart's reliance on fatty acid oxidation by augmenting glucose utilization rendering energetic homeostasis within the heart. *Solid black arrow: indicate reaction is proceeding forward in a single step; Dashed black arrow: indicate reaction is proceeding forward in multiple steps; Solid red line: indicate reaction is inhibited.*

associate with PI3K's p85 subunit through its SH2-domain to mediate a wide array of cellular functions. Notably, mice with a double knockout of IRS-1 & -2 proteins exhibited a reduction in ventricular mass and a defect in metabolic gene expression resulting in impaired ATP production, cardiac cell death, and fibrosis,[13] all of which attest to the critical role of IRS proteins in maintaining functional homeostasis in the heart. Similarly, class-IA PI3K regulates myocardial growth and hypertrophy independent of changes in contractile function,[14,15] whereas class-IB PI3K does not affect heart growth at baseline but negatively regulates cardiac contractility. Furthermore, the gamma isoform of PI3K inhibits cardiac contractility by decreasing intracellular concentrations of cyclic adenosine monophosphate (cAMP).[16] Recruitment of PI3K to the plasma membrane stimulates its catalytic phosphorylation of phosphatidylinositol (4,5)-diphosphate (PIP2) to phosphatidylinositol (3,4,5)-trisphosphate (PIP3).[12] Increases in PIP3 levels at the plasma membrane mediate further recruitment of protein kinase B (PKB)/Akt along with phosphoinositide-dependent kinase 1 (PDK1)[12] (Fig. 12.1(C)). At the plasma membrane, PDK1 phosphorylates and activates Akt isoforms to further relay insulin's signal to downstream targets. Importantly, heart muscle-specific PDK1 knockout (KO) mice display thinner ventricular walls, enlarged atria and right ventricles with marked reduction in cardiomyocyte size.[17] PDK1 KO mice also exhibit sensitivity to hypoxia and increases in markers of heart failure (HF) and mortality by 11 weeks of age,[17] which was associated with decreased Akt signaling. Indeed, PDK1-mediated phosphorylation of Akt, particularly phosphorylation of the Akt2 cardiac isoform, is thought to be essential for insulin's metabolic effects on the heart since loss of Akt2 gene leads to abnormal glucose metabolism and mild growth deficiency.[18] In agreement with this phenotypic data, interestingly, loss of Akt1 gene leads to general growth retardation[19,20] and Akt3 deletion in mice results in stunted brain development[21,22] signifying the critical role of Akt2 in regulating cardiac metabolism and function. Walsh and colleagues elegantly demonstrated the critical role of Akt in regulating myocardial capillary growth with an inducible model of active Akt overexpression.[23] Short-term Akt activation preserves contractile function, as the induced hypertrophy is reversible.[23] However, long-term Akt induction remodels the myocardium to cause pathological hypertrophy and extensive growth associated with interstitial fibrosis, fetal gene expression, dilation of the left ventricle (LV), and dysfunction of contractility mechanisms.[24] Endogenous inhibition of Akt signaling is executed by phosphatase and tensin homolog deleted from chromosome 10 (PTEN), which dephosphorylates PIP3, inactivates Akt and subsequently terminates insulin signaling (Fig. 12.1(D)). Indeed, cardiomyocyte-specific PTEN knockout elicited cardiac hypertrophy and contractile dysfunction associated with interrupted autophagy and autophagic flux[25,26], a phenotype that was associated with chronic Akt activation. Abnormalities in PTEN deletion phenotypes are secondary to PI3K over-activation, since the loss of PTEN-induced hypertrophy is corrected upon the introduction of dominant negative p110α and induced pathological contractility is normalized upon the additional deletion of p110γ of PI3K subunits.[27] Phenotypic characterization of mouse models with genetic modification of key insulin signaling proteins point to the fine balance in insulin receptor signaling that is essential to maintain functional homeostasis in the heart.

METABOLIC EFFECTS OF INSULIN SIGNALING IN THE MYOCARDIUM

EFFECTS OF INSULIN ON GLUCOSE TRANSPORT

FAs are the preferred energy substrate for the heart and accounts for more than 60% of ATP production under most physiological conditions.[9,28,29] Despite glucose not being the dominant fuel in the heart, cardiac tissue exhibits extreme dependence on this substrate and glucose consumption amounts to 25–50 g in a 24-hour period in humans. Due to glucose's hydrophilic nature, transmembrane delivery is impeded, thus necessitating a protein transporter that can circumvent the hydrophobic cellular cardiomyocyte membrane. A specific class of transmembrane transporters, known as glucose transporters (GLUT), is used to facilitate glucose uptake into the cardiomyocyte[30] (Fig. 12.1(E)). Two GLUT transporters are particularly predominant within cardiac tissue: GLUT-1 and GLUT-4. Cardiac GLUT-4 is insulin-dependent and outnumbers cardiac GLUT-1 3-to-1.[31] Heart muscle expresses the highest levels of the "insulin sensitive" GLUT-4 isoform. GLUT-1 isoform is an insulin-independent GLUT present in high abundance in erythrocytes and at lesser amounts within the heart, allowing the heart to uptake glucose in the absence of insulin.[30] Activation of myocardial glucose transport by insulin involves membrane translocation of both GLUT isoforms. The expression of GLUT-1 but not GLUT-4 is known to decline within the rat heart following starvation for two days.[32] These studies found that basal glucose transport was diminished, but maximal stimulation by insulin remained unaltered. GLUT-1 and GLUT-4 reside within two populations in the cardiomyocyte: one at the plasma membrane and the other in an intracellular "reservoir" that can be accessed in times of insulin stimulation.[33] Plasma membrane targeting of GLUT requires insulin-mediated signaling. Indeed, an important substrate of activated PKB/Akt kinase activity is the Rab GAP, Akt substrate of 160 kDa (AS160), or TBC1D4[33] (Fig. 12.1(F)). At basal state, AS160 inhibits GLUT translocation to the plasma membrane. However, upon phosphorylation of AS160 by Akt, AS160 becomes inactivated, releasing its inhibitory control over GLUT exocytosis. After AS160 inhibition, the resultant GLUT membrane translocation seems to play a predominant role in glucose uptake in muscle and adipose tissue but to a lesser extent in the myocardium. Another substrate that is important in GLUT exocytosis includes the Rab GAP, TBC1D1[9]. TBC1D1 is a substrate of Akt present only at low levels in cardiac tissue[9,33] and seems to play a role similar to AS160. The Rab-GTPase-activating proteins TBC1D1 and TBC1D4 (AS160) regulate GLUT-4 translocation in response to activation of Akt and AMP-dependent kinase.[33–35] Mice with combined inactivation of TBC1D1 and AS160 displayed normal fasting glucose concentrations; however, insulin-stimulated glucose uptake in muscle and adipose tissue was almost completely abolished. In skeletal muscle and white adipose tissue, the abundance of GLUT-4 protein, but not GLUT-4 mRNA, was substantially reduced.[34] Cell surface labeling of GLUTs indicated that Rab GAP deficiency impairs retention of GLUT-4 in intracellular vesicles in the basal state.[34] Taken together, these observations suggest that in the contracting heart GLUT-4 translocation and recycling is under the direct control of insulin and that AS160 is a key regulator of insulin-dependent cardiac glucose uptake in vivo (Fig. 12.1).

EFFECTS OF INSULIN ON GLUCOSE UTILIZATION

Within cardiomyocytes, glucose is processed for storage as glycogen or is subjected to glycolysis and glucose oxidation for ATP generation. Intracellular glucose is phosphorylated by hexokinase to glucose-6-phosphate (G-6-P) (Fig. 12.1(G)). Hexokinase I is the abundant isoform in the fetal heart, and hexokinase II is the dominant isoform in the adult heart[36–38] (Fig. 12.1(G)). G-6-P is metabolized through the glycolytic pathway and contributes to less than 10% of the total ATP generated within the heart.[39] The excess G-6-P is mobilized towards glycogen storage. Glycogen synthesis is dependent on the activity of the enzyme glycogen synthase (GS), which is inactivated by glycogen synthase kinase α/β (GSK3α/β) via inhibitory phosphorylation of GS.[40] Insulin activates Akt which phosphorylates and inactivates GSK3α/β,[41] allowing GS to remain in an active dephosphorylated state, resulting in increased glycogen synthesis. In addition to insulin's control over cardiac glycogen stores, insulin-dependent glucose utilization is also secondary to insulin's promotion of cardiac glycolysis. Insulin-dependent glycolysis results from PI3K/PDK-mediated activating phosphorylation of 6-phosphofructo-2-kinase (PFK-2) that induces production of fructose-2-6-bisphosphate (F-2,6-BP), a potent activator of glycolysis.[42] Furthermore, F-2,6-BP activates 6-phosphofructo-1-kinase (PFK-1), a central regulator of glycolysis[42] (Fig. 12.1(H)). Notably, PFK-2 activation is obligatory for cardiac glycolysis[43,44] since insulin-mediated augmentation of cardiac glycolysis is abolished in mouse heart expressing kinase-dead PFK-2, resulting in decreased glycolytic flux, hypertrophy, fibrosis, and reduced cardiomyocyte function.[45] Conversely, chronically elevated glycolysis is observed in heart from mice overexpressing phosphatase-deficient PFK-2[46] leading to constitutive activation of PFK-2 and threefold elevation of F-2,6-BP.[46] In oxygen-rich conditions, G-6-P is catabolized to pyruvate and in hypoxic conditions, G-6-P is converted to lactate by the enzyme lactate dehydrogenase (LDH). Pyruvate and lactate flux into the mitochondria is governed by putative monocarboxylate transporters.[47–49] In an insulin-dependent manner, pyruvate generated by glycolysis is transformed via three sets of reactions (Fig. 12.1(I)): (1) conversion to oxaloacetate or malate via a carboxylation reaction, (2) conversion to lactate, and/or (3) decarboxylation to acetyl-CoA through the multienzyme complex pyruvate dehydrogenase (PDH).[50,51] Insulin augments PDH activity by activating its corresponding phosphatase which dephosphorylates PDH and inhibits the actions of pyruvate dehydrogenase kinase (PDK) 2 and 4 isoforms.[52,53] Negative feedback from high matrix acetyl-CoA concentrations stimulates PDK and reduces PDH activity. Notably, in conditions where insulin levels are low such as during starvation, disinhibition of FA utilization activates PDK, which inactivates PDH and inhibits glucose oxidation,[52] signifying the impact of insulin on substrate competition within the heart.

EFFECTS OF INSULIN ON FATTY ACID UTILIZATION

The heart is an energy-intensive machine, requiring a continuous and uninterrupted supply of 3.5–5 KG of ATP per day to maintain adequate pumping action.[54–57] To achieve a high level of ATP consumption, the heart relies on glucose and FA metabolism. In the healthy heart, oxidation of long-chain fatty acids (LCFA) accounts for approximately 65–80% of ATP production.[54–57] LCFAs are the preferred energy substrate for the heart, but nonetheless glucose and lactate oxidation account for considerable ATP production, representing 15–25% and 5–10%, respectively.[54–57] Serum FAs increase during starvation;[58] however, during fed conditions, secretion of insulin inhibits lipolysis leading to a decrease in serum FA levels. Serum FAs exist in triacylglycerol (TAG)-containing lipoproteins and are also present in the albumin-bound form.[59] Exogenous FA importation is necessary to maintain optimal β-oxidative function, which is accomplished by the concerted action of lipoprotein lipase (LPL) and myocyte FA transporters.[60] Insulin facilitates the "selectivity and usage" of substrates within the heart by inhibiting LPL activation and promoting glucose utilization.[61–63] Notably, cardiac-specific knockout of LPL switches the cardiac substrate selection preference to glucose[59,64], signifying competing traits of different substrates. During physiological states, FA uptake into the cardiomyocyte occurs via passive diffusion or via FA transporters such as the FA translocase, CD36, or FA transport proteins (Fig. 12.1(J)), a process that is insulin sensitive.[65–67] A recent study demonstrated that insulin and AMP-activated protein kinase (AMPK) regulate CD36 plasma membrane recruitment in cardiomyocytes via AS160 and Rab8α, a Rab-GTPase.[35] FAs are targeted to either storage as TAG or mitochondrial FA β-oxidation for energy production.[68,69] Long-chain fatty acyl-CoA synthase (ACSL1) converts FAs into fatty acyl-CoA esters in an ATP-dependent manner.[68,70] Carnitine palmitoyl-transferase 1 (CPT-1) is the rate-limiting enzyme for mitochondrial FA uptake and subsequent FA β-oxidation.[68] CPT-1 resides on the outer mitochondrial membrane and converts fatty acyl-CoA esters into their corresponding fatty acylcarnitine moieties.[68,71] Fatty acyl-CoA esters are sequentially oxidized within the mitochondria. In cardiac muscle, insulin can inhibit CPT-1 and subsequent FA β-oxidation rates by increasing expression of malonyl-CoA, a potent endogenous inhibitor of CPT-1.[68,72,73] Insulin activates acetyl-CoA carboxylase (ACC), which is required for the formation of malonyl-CoA,[31,74] a process that is inhibited by stress kinase AMPK.[75,76] Glucose-derived acetyl-CoA is exported to cytosol where it serves as a substrate for ACC.[77] Furthermore, ACC converts acetyl-CoA to malonyl-CoA which inhibits the rate-limiting step prior to FA import into the mitochondria.[68,78] In isolated working heart perfusions, citrate's positive effect on ACC activity is blunted in the absence of insulin.[79] Randle and his coworkers demonstrated that FA impairs basal and insulin-stimulated glucose uptake and oxidation, a pathway known as Randle cycle.[55] Augmented intracellular FA derivatives, such as fatty acyl-CoA, diacylglycerols (DAG) and ceramides impair insulin-mediated glucose uptake through inhibition of IRS and Akt.[80] Increased intracellular FAs also activate PPAR-α (Fig. 12.3) that promote the expression of genes involved in FA oxidation, such as PDK4, which inhibits PDH and pyruvate flux.[81,82] Moreover, increased acetyl-CoA/free CoA and NADH/NAD^+ratios caused by high rates of FA oxidation also activate PDK4, leading to inactivation of PDH.[83] Augmented acetyl-CoA/free CoA also causes accumulation of citrate in the cytosol, which subsequently inhibits PFK and glycolysis. FA-derived acetyl-CoA increases FA substrate selection through inhibition of PDH. Furthermore, in the absence of insulin or insulin function, FAs regulate cardiac function by transcriptional regulation of PPAR-α, which is associated with increased FA uptake, mitochondrial transport, and β-oxidation.[84] Overexpression of PPAR-α in mouse models have demonstrated an increase in FA uptake and oxidation, TAG storage, and a reduction in glucose substrate preference, producing a cardiac phenotype similar to a diabetic or an insulin-resistant heart.[85] FAs derived from TAG hydrolysis are important cardiac energy substrates and are also utilized for formation of complex lipids and construction of membranes.[86] TAG hydrolysis represents a tightly regulated process and involves the concerted action of ATGL (adipose triglyceride lipase producing DAG), HSL (hormone sensitive lipase producing monoacylglycerol (MG)), and MGL (monoacylglycerol lipase producing FA).[69] Insulin inhibition of cardiac lipolysis occurs via the inhibitory effect of insulin on ATGL and HSL.[87,88] Therefore, insulin plays a central role in achieving metabolic outcomes of Randle cycle by promoting substrate competition (Fig. 12.1(K)).

EFFECTS OF INSULIN ON PROTEIN SYNTHESIS

Insulin is a mitogenic hormone that prevents amino acid mobilization, enabling the storage of amino acids into proteins. Biosynthesis of proteins involves a complex interplay between signal transduction proteins and machinery involving translation and ribosomal biogenesis (summarized in Fig. 12.2). Insulin mediates its effect on protein synthesis via its downstream effector, the mammalian or mechanistic target of rapamycin (mTOR).[83,89–91] Insulin signaling activates Akt which inactivates tuberous sclerosis factor 2 (TSC2) by inhibitory phosphorylation.[92] Active TSC2 enables addition of GDP to G protein Rheb leading to Rheb inactivation[93] (Fig. 12.2(A)). By inactivating TSC2, Akt activates Rheb, which phosphorylates and activates mTOR.[93] mTOR exists in two distinct complexes: mTOR complex 1 (mTORC1) and mTOR complex 2 (mTORC2).[89] mTORC1 regulates the function of proteins involved in the initiation

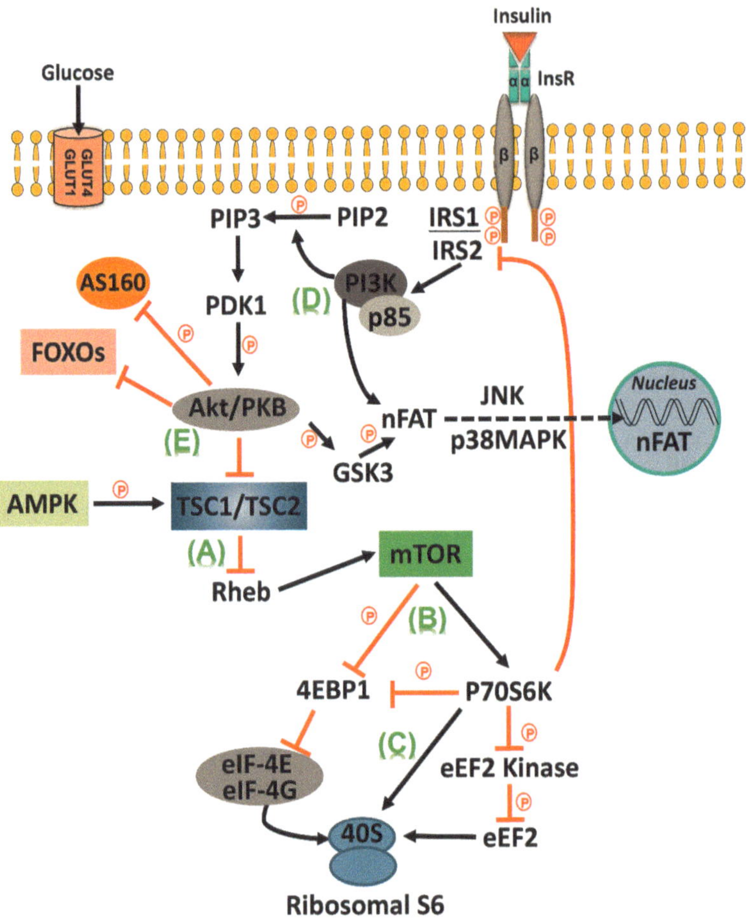

FIGURE 12.2

Insulin coordinates protein synthesis with energy metabolism in the healthy heart: insulin not only facilitates the heart's uptake and metabolism of energy substrates to generate ATP but also promotes the use of derived energy to initiate mitogenic program to synthesize proteins in the heart. Upon insulin-pathway stimulation, activated Akt initiate protein synthesis signaling cascades by inhibiting TSC1/2 activity, relieving inhibition on mTOR (A). Activated mTOR inhibits 4E-BP1, allowing eIF4E and eIF4G to promote initiation of protein translation (B). Additionally, active mTOR increases kinase activity of p70S6K, further promoting protein synthesis mechanisms by p70S6K-mediated inhibition of 4E-BP1 and activation of eukaryotic elongation factors, thereby facilitating protein translational elongation (C). p70S6K also regulates insulin signaling via a negative feedback mechanism by inhibiting IRS-1, a mechanism contributing to insulin resistance. *Solid black arrow: indicate reaction is proceeding forward in a single step; Dashed black arrow: indicate reaction is proceeding forward in multiple steps; Solid red line: indicate reaction is inhibited.*

and elongation stages of mRNA translation such as the eukaryotic initiation factor 4E (eIF4E), eIF4E-binding proteins (4E-BP), ribosomal protein S6 kinase (S6Ks) and eukaryotic elongation factor 2 (eEF2)[90,91,94–96] (Fig. 12.2(B)). Initiation of protein translation occurs upon binding of the ribosomal 40 S subunit to the 5′-cap structure of the mRNA, a process that is facilitated by eIF4E with its binding partner eIF4G, with the former being tightly bound to 4E-BP1. The above step in protein synthesis is insulin dependent.[97,98] Following insulin-receptor activation, mTOR performs inhibitory phosphorylation of 4E-BP1 at either Thr37, Thr46, Thr70, or Ser65, thereby relieving its inhibition of eIF4E and facilitating protein translation.[94,99] mTOR also activates p70S6K which further phosphorylates the S6 ribosomal protein to regulate expression of translation factors and ribosomal proteins (Fig. 12.2(C)) and thereby augment translational capacity and ribosomal biogenesis.[100,101] Another activator of protein translation is eEF2, whose phosphorylation and activity is coordinately regulated by mTOR and eEF2 kinases (eEF2K).[94,102] eEF2K is a calcium- and calmodulin-dependent kinase and a bona fide substrate of p70S6K.[103,104] eEF2 is dephosphorylated and activated by insulin-induced mTOR activation, whereas a lack of insulin or insulin function augments phosphorylation by eEF2K, rendering eEF2 inactive.[105–108] Similarly, insulin also regulates the function of 4E-BP1 in the cardiac cell by inducing mTOR-mediated inhibitory phosphorylation of 4E-BP1 and thus preventing it from binding to (eIF), allowing eIF4E to bind the mRNA cap and initiate protein synthesis.[105–108] Besides insulin signaling, glucose utilization per se is also a prerequisite for mTOR activation. Indeed, it was demonstrated that glucose phosphorylation is required for insulin-dependent mTOR signaling in the heart.[109]

CARDIAC INSULIN SIGNALING DURING OBESITY AND TYPE 2 DIABETES

Insulin resistance develops as a result of obesity, which is an outcome of a combination of excessive calorie intake and lack of physical activity. Uncontrolled and untreated insulin resistance culminates into T2DM, a clinical condition that increases susceptibility to cardio-metabolic inflexibility and ensuing HF.[2,6,56,57,68] Hallmark symptoms of diabetes such as hyperinsulinemia, hyperglycemia, and hyperlipidemia result in secondary aberrant cardiac energy metabolism, disrupting cardiac insulin signaling by the attenuation of insulin-induced phosphorylation of IRS-1/2 and Akt in cardiomyocytes.[2,6,56,57,68] During obesity and diabetes, GLUT-4 protein expression is reduced resulting in impairment in glucose uptake and utilization and leading to impaired insulin signaling.[110,111] Insulin resistance causes impairment in insulin-mediated increases in IRS leading to PI3K inactivation and decreases in PDK1 activation (Figs. 12.2(D), 12.3(A)); as a consequence, PDK1-mediated translocation of GLUT-4 to the sarcolemmal membrane is decreased.[112] Akt is also a downstream target of PI3K signaling (Fig. 12.2(E)), which appears to regulate glucose uptake by phosphorylating and inhibiting the Rab-GTPase–activating protein AS160. Notably, skeletal muscle from T2DM patients exhibited impairment in insulin-mediated phosphorylation of AS160 and TBC1D1, which is associated with defects in glucose uptake as a consequence of reduced GLUT-4 translocation.[7,113] However, the direct effect of substrates and insulin on AS160 regulation in the cardiac muscle is yet to be investigated. Germline deletion of GLUT-4 (*GLUT4*-null) causes cardiac hypertrophy in mice that are 2 to 4 months old.[114–116] Furthermore, *GLUT4*-null mice hearts demonstrated increases in glucose uptake, resulting from increases in insulin-independent GLUT-1 expression.[114–116] On the other hand, cardiac-specific deletion of GLUT-4 (G4H-/-) caused cardiac hypertrophy with preserved cardiac contractile function and systemic metabolism.[114,117–119] Interestingly, G4H-/- mice heart exhibited normal glucose uptake, which was found to

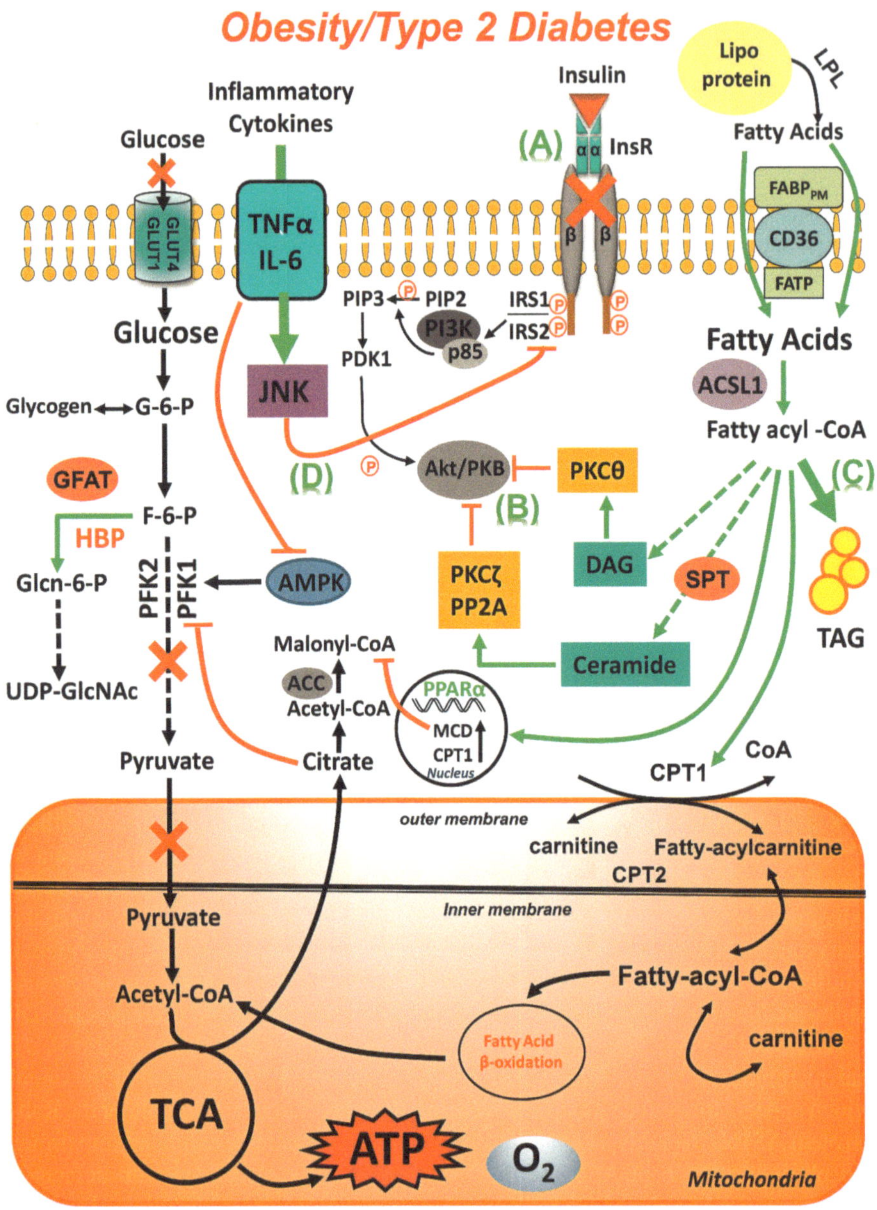

FIGURE 12.3

Altered cardiac energy metabolism and utilization in the insulin-resistant/diabetic heart. During cardiac insulin resistance, impaired insulin signaling halts glycolytic flux redirecting glucose intermediates into the HBP. Decreased reliance on glucose is compensated by enhanced cardiac dependence on fatty acid oxidation via the Randle cycle (A). Intracellular FA is processed by ACSL1 (A), generating intermediate fatty acyl-CoA that is be associated with upregulation of cardiac GLUT-1 expression.[114,117–119] Insulin stimulates glucose uptake and oxidation in the heart and accounts for a total of ~20% of cardiac energy generation. Intracellularly, excess glucose is diverted into hexosamine biosynthetic pathway (HBP), polyol pathway and glycolysis, which accounts for 20% of total myocardial energy production. Indeed, mice overexpressing GFAT (Glutamine: fructose-6-phosphate aminotransferase, a rate-limiting enzyme in HBP pathway), developed muscle insulin resistance, which was associated with a decreased level of muscle GLUT-4 transporter.[120] In an aerobic state, the heart utilizes both glucose (25–30%) and FAs (65–70%) for its energy requirements.[68,121–123] During obesity T2DM, impaired insulin response compels the heart to switch almost exclusively towards FA oxidation for energy.[68,121–123] Though insulin promotes increases in FA uptake in the heart, it also inhibits FA utilization for ATP synthesis. Indeed, insulin signaling plays an important role in regulating glucose and LCFA metabolism. During obesity and T2DM, loss of insulin function (Fig. 12.3(A)) diminishes insulin's inhibitory control on adipose tissue lipolysis.[29,124] Systemic increases in lipolysis elevates circulating plasma FFA, which are known to inhibit glucose utilization (glucose uptake, glycolysis, and pyruvate oxidation) in the heart[6] by inducing a reduction in cardiac GLUT-4 expression.[6] Furthermore, intramyocellular increases in FA and FA metabolites such as fatty acyl-CoA also impair cardiac-insulin signaling.[6] FAs are shown to inhibit insulin signaling in the heart (Fig. 12.3) by multiple mechanisms.[125,126] FAs cause ceramide accumulation that induces activation of atypical protein kinase C, which inactivates Akt. Ceramide-dependent inhibition of Akt/PKB is mediated by two distinct mechanisms.[127–129] First, ceramide blocks translocation of Akt/PKB to the plasma membrane and second, it dephosphorylates Akt/PKB by protein phosphatase 2A (PP2A).[129] Ceramides interfere with insulin signaling by activating protein kinase C-ζ (PKC- ζ) which inhibits Akt phosphorylation at Ser473 and Thr308[6,130] (Fig. 12.3(B)). Indeed, when C2C12 (mouse muscle myoblast) and 3T3L1 pre-adipocytes (mouse embryonic fibroblast) are exposed to a ceramide load, activation of Akt/PKB becomes attenuated.[131] FAs also induce DAG accumulation which activates typical and novel protein kinase C to promote the inhibitory Akt signaling,[80]

FIGURE 12.3

further processed via the mitochondrial β-oxidation pathway via rate-limiting CPT-1 and CPT-2 to generate ATP through TCA cycle. Citrate derived from the TCA cycle is exported to the cytosol to inhibit PFK-2, which inhibits glycolysis. A part of the fatty acyl-CoA is stored as TAG (C) and the remaining as lipotoxic intermediates; DAGs and SPT-generated ceramides. Following diabetes or diet-induced obesity, increased FA load within the cardiomyocyte activates PPAR-α, which provokes further maladaptive use of β-oxidation pathway by increasing expression of CPT-1 and malonyl-CoA decarboxylase, which depletes malonyl-CoA and releases its inhibition on FA oxidation. Additionally, the lipotoxic DAGs and ceramides activate PKCθ and PKCζ and PP2A (B) which further inhibit Akt function. Furthermore, during obesity and diabetes serum concentrations of inflammatory cytokines TNF-α and IL-6 increase and also result in the inhibition and suppression of glycolysis and the insulin signaling program via inactivation of AMPK- and JNK-mediated inhibitory Serine phosphorylation of IRS-1/2 (D), respectively. Thus, when cardiac insulin signaling is dysfunctional, glucose oxidation is attenuated and fatty acid oxidation is augmented, leading to metabolic inflexibility within the cardiomyocyte and ensuing accumulation of lipotoxic intermediates. *Solid black arrow: indicate reaction is proceeding forward in a single step; Solid green arrow: indicate reaction is pathologically increased; Solid red line: indicate reaction is inhibited. Solid red X: indicates reaction is halted.*

Furthermore, FAs augment negative feedback loop in which the insulin-dependent activation of mTOR/p70S6K induces serine phosphorylation and inhibition of IRS-1.[132,133] Increases in FAs also drives activation of PPAR-α, which induces the gene expression of various enzymes involved in FA oxidation (e.g., malonyl-CoA decarboxylase and CPT-1). Cardiac-specific overexpression of PPAR-α results in excess fat oxidation, lipid deposition, oxidative stress, and cardiomyopathy.[85,134–136] Using a perfused heart model, it was demonstrated that the negative effect of FA oxidation in the obese and diabetic heart could be attenuated by inhibition of serine palmitoyltransferase, a rate-limiting enzyme in ceramide biosynthesis resulting in increases in glucose oxidation.[137,138] In *db/db* mice, a model of T2DM, there are increases in FA oxidation with subsequent increases in citrate synthesis from tricarboxylic acid cycle.[110,139,140] Higher citrate levels inhibit PFK-1, the rate-limiting enzyme in glycolysis.[141,142] In addition, hyper-activation of Akt during insulin resistance increases the translocation of CD36 to plasma membrane and upregulates β- oxidation.[143] This results in the increased production of acetyl-CoA, NADH, and FADH2 and citrate, which further inhibits PDH and phosphofructokinase and exacerbates the lipotoxicity in the heart.[6] Conversely, according to Randle, glucose and FA metabolism do not occur independently. Indeed, it has been demonstrated that FAs decrease glucose utilization by impairing insulin-stimulated glucose uptake and oxidation, an event known as the Randle cycle.[28,54,55,144] Studies in rodent heart and diaphragm by Randle and colleagues demonstrated that FAs impaired insulin-dependent glucose uptake resulting in decreased glucose oxidation and increased accumulation of glycolytic intermediates, which is further suggested to be mediated by inhibition of PDH.[55,125] During obesity and/or insulin resistance, following saturation of FA oxidation, excessive FFA is channeled towards storage in the form of TAGs resulting in cardiac steatosis (Fig. 12.3(C)), which can also precipitate cardiac contractile impairment.[69,145] Chronic TAG accumulation leads to cytosolic accumulation of lipid metabolites such as ceramides, DAG, long-chain acyl-CoA and acylcarnitines.[146–148] Increases in glucose, FA or TAG not only cause insulin resistance but also generate free radicals that can cause mitochondrial dysfunction, cell death, and cardiomyocyte failure in the setting of obesity and diabetes.[149–154] Mitochondrial pathology in the setting of insulin resistance, obesity, and diabetes will not be discussed in this chapter. Insulin resistance is also associated with systemic and intramyocellular inflammatory pathways.[155] During obesity and diabetes, there is an elevation of circulating levels of proinflammatory cytokines such as tumor necrosis factor-α and interleukin-6 (IL-6), which promote insulin resistance in multiple tissue including the heart.[156] In the obese and diabetic heart, inflammation causes cardiac tissue to become dependent on TAG and FFA to generate energy. Mice fed high-fat diet displayed increased cardiac infiltration of inflammatory cytokines such as IL-6. It is postulated that inflammation in the heart likely impairs insulin signaling and contributes to myocardial insulin resistance by activating intracellular signaling kinases such as Jun N-terminal kinase (JNK) (Fig. 12.3(D)), which then further increases the serine phosphorylation of IRS-mediated by IL-6.[157] Additionally, IL-6 causes insulin resistance by inhibiting AMPK and IRS-1 and suppressing myocardial glucose metabolism, highlighting the role of inflammation in the pathogenesis of obese and diabetic heart.[6,157]

INSULIN SIGNALING AND CARDIAC HYPERTROPHY

Insulin couples growth pathway signaling to energy metabolism for effective cardiac functioning.[158] Insulin's impact on cardiac growth and size correlates with serum insulin level, since in response to a hyperinsulinemic environment, hearts respond by increasing in size. This is attributed to insulin's anabolic effects following an increased flux of glucose and FAs into growth activating molecular programs. However, insulin's effects on cardiac growth can become maladaptive, particularly during pathologies such as obesity and T2DM.[159,160] In fact, risk of heart disease in the form of diabetic cardiomyopathy is elevated in patients with T2DM.[161,162] A hallmark symptom of diabetic cardiomyopathy is cardiac hypertrophy, particularly of the LV.[161,162] Mouse models of acute insulin infusion display enhanced cardiac protein synthesis,[163,164] whereas mice exposed to chronic insulin infusion display an increase in LV mass and relative wall thickness and reduced stroke volume and cardiac output, similar to diabetic cardiomyopathy.[28,56,161,162] Insulin's unprecedented effect on cardiac growth and size is exemplified in animal models of insulin signaling pathway substrate knockouts. Models of CIRKO mice display significant reductions in cardiomyocyte size and overall cardiac weight.[11] This reduction in cardiac weight was associated with reduction in phosphorylation of Akt, p70S6K, and 4E-BP1, targets of master regulator of growth signaling, mTOR.[11] This reduction in cardiac weight and myofibril diameter were reversed upon forced cardiac expression of myristoylated Akt in vivo, revealing that Akt signaling is an important mediator of cardiac growth induction. Furthermore, models employing targeted deletion of the IRS-1 gene display significant reductions in heart weight/body weight ratio.[5] IRS-1 appears to be the key regulator of cardiac growth programs in this context as models of IRS-2, IRS-3, and IRS-4–deficient mice did not display gross abnormalities in cardiac phenotype.[165–167] Models utilizing dominant negative PI3K transgenes also exhibited reduced cardiac size, similar to CIRKO mice, further testifying to insulin's potent stimulation of cardiac growth.[168] In addition, rodents with overexpression of constitutively active PI3K or Akt by muscle-specific inactivation of PTEN, a phosphatase regulating phosphorylation status of PI3K, displayed severe cardiac hypertrophy.[19,20,23,25–27] Taken together, these models continually recapitulate the growth-stimulating effect of insulin on cardiac tissue notably during both physiological and pathological processes. In addition to insulin's anabolic effects through PI3K-Akt–signaling pathways, insulin induces cardiomyocyte growth by augmenting GSK3, which is reported to activate nuclear factors of translation, particularly the nuclear factor of activated T-cells (nFAT) transcription factors, which are indispensable for cardiac hypertrophic signaling[169] (Fig. 12.4). nFAT plays a pivotal role in cardiac development by regulating gene expression for maintenance of an adult-differentiated cardiac phenotype, and also by activating remodeling processes in hypertrophy and HF.[170–172] Studies using rabbit ventricular myocytes demonstrated that nFAT regulation was mediated by a PI3K and Akt signaling involving activation of GSK3β, JNK, p38 mitogen-activated kinase (p38MAPK), resulting in phosphorylation, deactivation, and nuclear export of nFAT[171] (Fig. 12.4(A)). In addition to nFAT, the forkhead transcription factors (FOXO) family of proteins contribute to a plethora of diverse cellular functions including differentiation, metabolism, proliferation, and survival.[173] This subfamily consists of three members present in cardiomyocytes, FOXO1 (FKHR), FOXO3a (FKHRL-1), and FOXO4 (AFX), all of which are inactivated by Akt.[174–177] Inhibitory phosphorylation by Akt leads to nuclear export and deactivation of FOXOs. FOXO1-dependent IRS-1 downregulation lead to blunted Akt signaling and resistance to insulin function.[178] Akt activation following pro-hypertrophic stimuli, such as growth factors, stretch, angiotensin II, and pressure overload, inactivates FOXO via Akt-mediated phosphorylation.[173–175,177] Conversely, states of nutrient restriction inactivate PI3K/Akt signaling, relieving inhibition on FOXO, and promoting FOXO translocation to the nucleus[179] to activate genes that are associated with "atrophy" also termed as atrogenes[175] (Fig. 12.4(B)). Specifically, FOXO3a is a putative negative regulator of cardiomyocyte size that regulates gene expression of atrophy program.[177] In addition to atrophy, FOXO proteins are

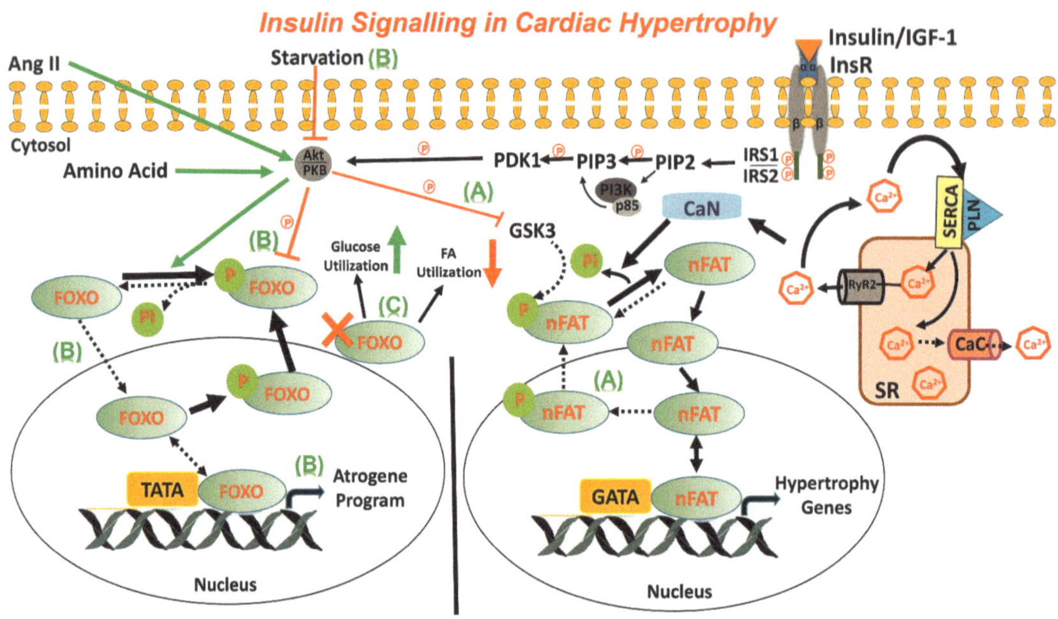

FIGURE 12.4

Defects in insulin signaling in the pathological hypertrophy heart. Growth signals, such as angiotensin and insulin promote cardiac growth and protein synthesis via transcriptional activation of nFAT and FOXO proteins. Insulin activates Akt which phosphorylates FOXO (B). Inhibitory phosphorylation of FOXO results in the nuclear exclusion of FOXO preventing it from transcribing atrogenic markers. Furthermore, deletion of cardiac FOXO compels the heart to utilize glucose over fatty acids to generate ATP (C). In addition, GSK3, a downstream target of Akt, is a bona fide nFAT kinase (A). Inhibitory phosphorylation of nFAT results in the nuclear exclusion of nFAT preventing it from transcribing hypertrophic markers. Following insulin stimulation, activation of Akt and inhibition of GSK3, leads to nFAT dephosphorylation and entry into nucleus for cellular proliferation and growth programming (A). Insulin governs energy metabolic programs and promotes mitogenic signaling resulting in cardiomyocyte protein synthesis, initiating activation of downstream substrates of initiation and elongation of protein translation at the ribosome, and facilitating synthesis of proteins indispensable for cardiac functioning. *Solid black arrow: indicate reaction is proceeding forward in a single step; Dashed black arrow: indicate reaction is proceeding forward in multiple steps; Solid red line: indicate reaction is inhibited.*

strongly associated with the development of metabolic cardiomyopathy.[178] Notably in hearts of diet-induced obese and diabetic mice, loss of insulin signaling prevents Akt activation, relieving inhibition on FOXO and rendering FOXO constitutively active.[178] Furthermore, cardiomyocyte-specific deletion of FOXO1 rescued hearts from high-fat diet-induced dysfunction by preserving cardiomyocyte insulin responsiveness.[178] Mechanistically, FOXO1 deletion switched metabolic preference of heart to favor glucose and not FA utilization as evident from decreased accumulation of lipids in the heart following obesity and diabetes[178] (Fig. 12.4(C)). Together, these data evidences point to FOXOs being a bona fide transcriptional effector of insulin and hypertrophic signals in the myocardium.[174] FOXO proteins not only regulate insulin signaling but also regulate insulin growth-like factor (IGF-1) signaling, which is a critical node in growth hormone signaling.[5,176] IGF-1 is a peptide hormone produced primarily in the liver, muscle, and heart, and is similar to insulin in structure. Models employing double deletion of FOXO1 and FOXO3, exhibited increased cell cycle processes and augmented IGF-1 expression within cardiomyocytes, signifying FOXO1 and FOXO3's important role in hypertrophic and IGF-1 regulation in the heart.[176] These lines of evidences suggest that insulin and IGF-1 signaling axes contributes to cardiac growth and metabolism and disruptions in this pathway remodel hypertrophy phenotype of the cardiomyocyte (Fig. 12.4).

CARDIO-PROTECTIVE ROLE OF INSULIN SIGNALING IN ISCHEMIA REPERFUSION AND CONTRACTILE FAILURE

Vasoconstriction of the coronary vasculature triggers myocardial ischemia limiting oxygen and substrate supply to the heart. Reduction in glucose and FA oxidation during ischemia suppresses ATP generation.[68,180] To maintain adequate ATP for contractile function, glycolysis is increased during ischemia.[181] However, glycolytic end-product pyruvate is subsequently converted to lactate since pyruvate is unable to enter the mitochondria.[182,183] Increasing accumulation of lactate compromises proton gradient in the cardiomyocyte, augmenting proton load and declining intracellular pH.[183,184] Acidic pH within the myocardium impairs the functioning of sarco-endoplasmic reticulum calcium ATPase (SERCA) & phospholamban (PLN) and inhibits Akt and eNOS activity.[185,186] While long-term ischemia irreversibly damages the myocardium, timely reperfusion of ischemic tissue salvages the myocardium. Insulin signaling mediated regulation of substrate energy metabolism is the key determinant of the functional recovery of the reperfused myocardium.[187] During ischemia-reperfusion, formation of superoxides and peroxynitrite trigger oxidative/nitrative stress causing mitochondrial demise and cell death, a process that is inhibited by insulin-activated cell survival pathways.[188] Insulin exerts a cardioprotective effect against ischemia-reperfusion (I/R) injury by blocking ONOO(–) formation, increasing eNOS activity to generate nitric oxide and augment cellular antioxidant status with concomitant reduction in superoxide, all of which are secondary to activation of PI3K and Akt.[189] Insulin decreases inflammatory cytokine expression and apoptosis via PI3K/Akt-mediated inhibition of p38MAPK[190] and prevents activation of the cardiac mitochondrial-dependent apoptotic pathway. Glucose-insulin-potassium administration at the onset of the reperfusion period functions to protect cardiac tissue by activating cell-survival programs.[187,191,192]

Although the heart is a “fat-loving” organ due to high levels of ATP production from FA oxidation, it is actually beneficial for the heart to utilize glucose since the use of glucose expends 12% less O_2 than FA oxidation to generate the same amount of ATP[4,68,123,193] (Fig. 12.5). Insulin promotes cardiomyocyte function and efficiency by stimulating contractile and relaxation processes and by reducing myocardial O_2 demand[4,68,123,193] (Fig. 12.5(A)). Insulin augments efficiency of energy utilization within the cardiomyocyte to improve contractile function. Cardiomyocyte functioning depends on proper contractility and relaxation mechanisms which ultimately rely on adequate functioning of ion pumps. Sodium pumps (Na^+/K^+-ATPase) and sarco-endoplasmic reticulum calcium ATPase uptake pumps (SERCA) are both important ion pumps in cardiomyocyte functioning[194–196] (Fig. 12.5B). Upon cardiomyocyte depolarization, Ca^{2+} enters into the sarcoplasm through reverse Na^+/Ca^{2+} exchangers and Ca^{2+}

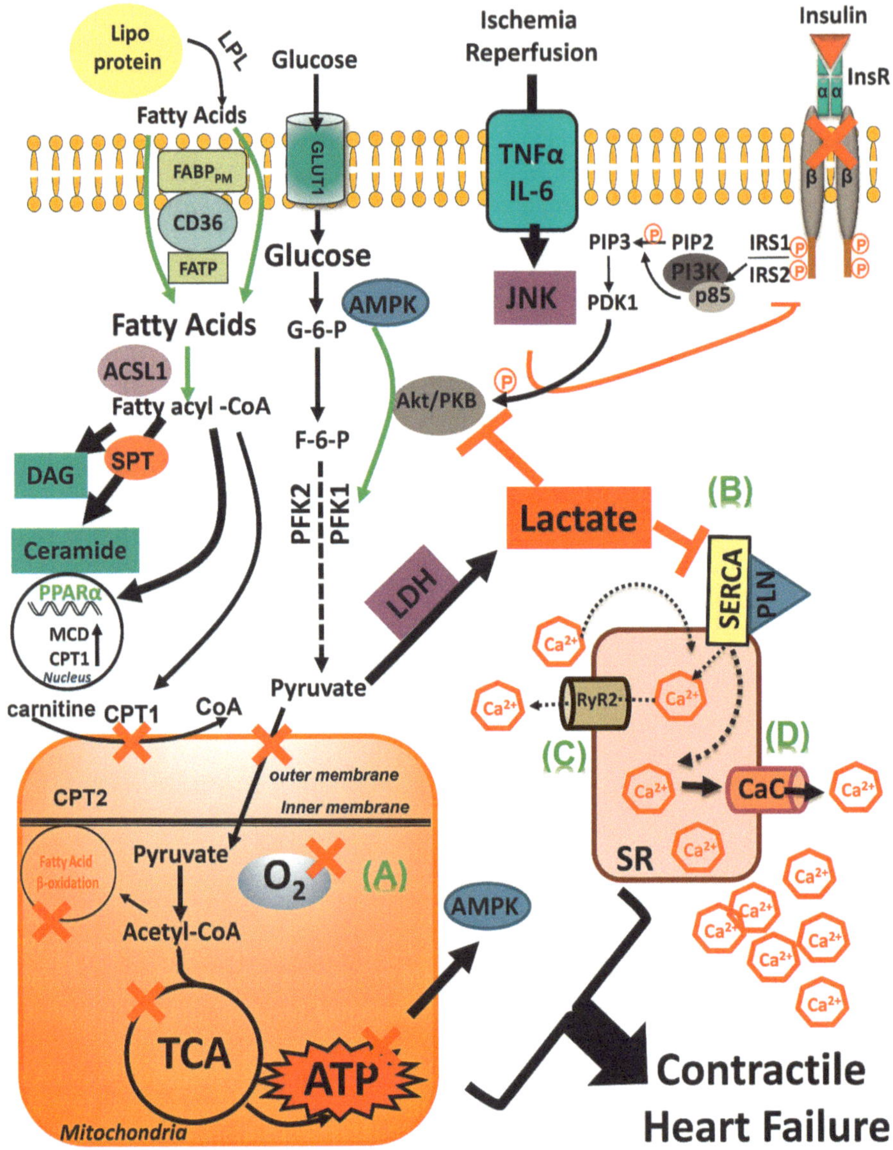

FIGURE 12.5

Metabolic maladaptation in insulin signaling in the heart post-ischemia-reperfusion injury. Following occlusion of coronary arteries during ischemia, lack of molecular oxygen prevents oxidation phosphorylation of glucose and FA in the mitochondria (A), leading to accumulation of pyruvate and fatty acyl-CoA in the cardiomyocyte. Since a substantial portion of the fatty acyl-CoA remains unoxidized, they are converted into lipotoxic intermediates; DAGs and SPT-generated ceramides which exacerbate mitochondrial dysfunction and endoplasmic reticulum stress. Deficits in substrate-derived cellular ATP activates AMPK which activates

L-channels.[194,197,198] Entrance of Ca^{2+} within the cardiomyocyte activates ryanodine (RYD) receptors, which further facilitates Ca^{2+} release from the sarcoplasmic reticulum (SR) resulting in a positive feedback mechanism.[196,199,200] Free-released Ca^{2+} within the sarcoplasm binds to cardiac troponin C, resulting in sliding of actin and myosin filaments and overall shortening and contraction of cardiomyocytes. Upon cardiomyocyte repolarization, free Ca^{2+} within the sarcoplasm is "recycled" back to the SR by uptake via SERCA or discarded by transference to extracellular regions via utilization of Na^{+}/Ca^{2+} exchanger pumps, all of which ultimately result in cardiomyocyte relaxation.[194–196] Insulin stimulation increases Ca^{2+} release to the sarcoplasm by acting on Ca^{2+} L-channels and by facilitating uptake of Ca^{2+} by reverse Na^{+}/Ca^{2+} exchanger pumps (Fig. 12.5(C,D)). Insulin not only acts to increase functioning of the aforementioned pumps, it also acts to increase mRNA expression of RYD receptors and SERCA calcium pumps, further promoting cardiomyocyte contraction and relaxation processes.[201–203] Energy required for proper ion pump functioning also depends substantially on insulin signaling processes; specifically, functioning of Na^{+}/Ca^{2+} and SERCA rely heavily on ATP derived from glycolytic processes that are upregulated upon insulin stimulation. Notably, mice with cardiac-specific GLUT-4 deletion display significant cardiac enlargement due to increased cardiomyocyte volume and fibrosis.[117] Furthermore, in GLUT-4 KO myocytes maximal rates of shortening and relaxation were decreased with associated decreases in myocyte contractility.[117] Contractile changes were associated with a decline in SERCA2 and RyR2 expression in GLUT-4 KO myocytes signifying that GLUT-4 deficiency per se profoundly impacts calcium mechanics in cardiomyocyte. In insulin-dependent T1DM, depressed contractile performance is associated with diminished SERCA2 and decreased L-type voltage calcium channel activity.[204] This contractility defect in diabetic mice was secondary to reduced PI3K signaling in the heart,[205] which was reversed by insulin treatment or by intracellular infusion of PIP3. Notably, genetic deletion and pharmacological inhibition of PI3K regulatory subunit p110α blocked insulin signaling and decreased calcium currents in myocytes.[206] Similarly, dysregulation in calcium mechanics in the heart was also observed in PTEN(-/-)/DN-p110α double mutant mice, an effect that was reversed by activation of Akt or inactivation of PTEN which results in PI3Kα-dependent increase in PKB activation.[207] Interestingly, Sprague–Dawley rats administered adenovirus overexpressing Akt exhibited increased systolic Ca^{2+} levels, augmented myofilament responsiveness, and increased SERCA protein levels.[208] Not only T1DM but also T2DM models exhibit impaired cardiac contractility.[202,203] The *db/db* insulin-resistant mouse hearts showed decreased diastolic and systolic levels of Ca^{2+} and pointed toward a reduced ability to clear cytosolic calcium due to increased leakage of calcium from SR.[140] In agreement with findings observed in *db/db* mice,

FIGURE 12.5

glycolysis, augmenting pyruvate levels. Glucose-derived pyruvate is converted into lactate via the enzyme LDH, leading to decreases in intramyocellular pH. Increased serum concentrations of inflammatory cytokines TNF-α and IL-6 with concomitant increases in lactate impairs insulin signaling and subsequent activation of AKT. Acidic pH also directly counter-regulates the SR-calcium transport machinery by inactivating SERCA and PLN (B). Calcium sequestration in the SR is impaired leading to elevation of cytosolic calcium and contractile failure of the myocardium. Metabolic maladaptation in the ischemic and reperfused myocardium impairs insulin signaling, triggering contractile failure of the myocardium. *Solid black arrow: indicate reaction is proceeding forward in a single step; Solid green arrow: indicate reaction is pathologically increased; Solid red line: indicate reaction is inhibited. Solid red X: indicates reaction is halted.*

mice that ate a high-fat diet exhibited decreases in myofilament sensitivity to Ca^{2+} that was suggested to be responsible for impaired contractility in an hyperinsulinemic, insulin-resistant state.;[209] Although physiological insulin levels promote beneficial cellular phenomena to improve cardiac contractility and relaxation, there are also recent reports that augmented insulin signaling during hyperinsulinemic conditions such as T2DM, impairs cardiac contractility mechanisms.[210] Insulin-dependent impairment in cardiac contractility results from alterations in β2-adrenergic receptor (β2AR) signaling. Specifically, upon insulin stimulation IRS-1 and IRS-2 mediate protein kinase A (PKA) and G-protein receptor kinase 2 (GRK2) induced phosphorylation of β2AR, which upon phosphorylation, becomes coupled to an inhibitory Gi subtype of G-protein.[210] Impaired cardiac insulin sensitivity and metabolic dysregulation in the obese and diabetic heart have emerged as the primary contributor to contractile impairment (Fig. 12.5) in obesity- and diabetes-related cardiomyopathy.

SCOPE AND FUTURE PERSPECTIVES

This chapter has presented emerging molecular mechanisms in cardiac insulin signaling and how they are altered in disease states, including diabetes/insulin resistance, cardiac hypertrophy, and ischemic injuries. These findings highlight the critical role of insulin signaling in regulating calcium sensing and contractility, as well as growth and energy generation via glucose and FA metabolism during various disease states. While insulin signaling appears to be primarily responsible for regulating cellular metabolism and energetics, insulin also influences ion channel activity, glycogen storage, ischemia/reperfusion injury, autophagy, cytoskeletal assembly, and endoplasmic reticulum and nucleus remodeling through a myriad of signaling pathways which are beyond the scope of this book chapter. While not discussed completely, the mechanisms by which mitochondria play an effector role for insulin signaling is an important aspect of insulin signaling given that recent evidence demonstrates that insulin can govern mitochondrial fusion–fission dynamics, biogenesis, mitophagy, and mitochondrial membrane potential. Moreover, the role that insulin plays in the endothelium, fibroblasts, and macrophages during disease has not been addressed herein, but this regulation likely plays a major role in regulating cardiac function.[211–213] Indeed, numerous studies have now established that insulin's effect on vasculature is impaired if endothelium is damaged. Insulin signaling in the vasculature maintains vessel tone, attenuates oxidative stress, improves nitric oxide signaling related function, and exerts an anti-inflammatory effect. Additionally, the transcriptional effectors of insulin signaling in noncardiomyocyte cell types are largely understudied and require further research. Consistent with this, increasing our knowledge of the role that insulin signaling plays in the heart may allow us to design novel and effective strategies that modulate insulin signaling to treat prevalent disorders in clinical cardiology such as cardiac hypertrophy, ischemia/reperfusion injury, glycogen-storage cardiomyopathy and obesity, and diabetes-associated lipotoxic complications.

REFERENCES

1. Ijuin T, Takenawa T. Regulation of insulin signaling and glucose transporter 4 (GLUT4) exocytosis by phosphatidylinositol 3,4,5-trisphosphate (PIP3) phosphatase, skeletal muscle, and kidney enriched inositol polyphosphate phosphatase (SKIP). *J Biol Chem* 2012;**287**(10):6991–9.

2. Rask-Madsen C, Kahn CR. Tissue-specific insulin signaling, metabolic syndrome, and cardiovascular disease. *Arterioscler Thromb Vasc Biol* 2012;**32**(9):2052–9.
3. Bedinger DH, Adams SH. Metabolic, anabolic, and mitogenic insulin responses: a tissue-specific perspective for insulin receptor activators. *Mol Cell Endocrinol* 2015;**415**:143–56.
4. Iliadis F, Kadoglou N, Didangelos T. Insulin and the heart. *Diabetes Res Clin Pract* 2011;**93**(1):S86–91.
5. DeBosch BJ, Muslin AJ. Insulin signaling pathways and cardiac growth. *J Mol Cell Cardiol* 2008;**44**(5):855–64.
6. Abel ED, O'Shea KM, Ramasamy R. Insulin resistance: metabolic mechanisms and consequences in the heart. *Arterioscler Thromb Vasc Biol* 2012;**32**(9):2068–76.
7. Abel ED. Insulin signaling in heart muscle: lessons from genetically engineered mouse models. *Curr Hypertens Rep* 2004;**6**(6):416–23.
8. Velez M, Kohli S, Sabbah HN. Animal models of insulin resistance and heart failure. *Heart Fail Rev* 2014;**19**(1):1–13.
9. Bertrand L, Horman S, Beauloye C, Vanoverschelde JL. Insulin signalling in the heart. *Cardiovasc Res* 2008;**79**(2):238–48.
10. Coquerel D, Neviere R, Delile E, et al. Gene deletion of protein tyrosine phosphatase 1B protects against sepsis-induced cardiovascular dysfunction and mortality. *Arterioscler Thromb Vasc Biol* 2014;**34**(5):1032–44.
11. Belke DD, Betuing S, Tuttle MJ, et al. Insulin signaling coordinately regulates cardiac size, metabolism, and contractile protein isoform expression. *J Clin Invest* 2002;**109**(5):629–39.
12. Frojdo S, Vidal H, Pirola L. Alterations of insulin signaling in type 2 diabetes: a review of the current evidence from humans. *Biochim Biophys Acta* 2009;**1792**(2):83–92.
13. Qi Y, Xu Z, Zhu Q, et al. Myocardial loss of IRS1 and IRS2 causes heart failure and is controlled by p38alpha MAPK during insulin resistance. *Diabetes* 2013;**62**(11):3887–900.
14. Luo J, McMullen JR, Sobkiw CL, et al. Class IA phosphoinositide 3-kinase regulates heart size and physiological cardiac hypertrophy. *Mol Cell Biol* 2005;**25**(21):9491–502.
15. McMullen JR, Shioi T, Zhang L, et al. Phosphoinositide 3-kinase(p110alpha) plays a critical role for the induction of physiological, but not pathological, cardiac hypertrophy. *Proc Natl Acad Sci USA* 2003;**100**(21):12355–60.
16. Patrucco E, Notte A, Barberis L, et al. PI3Kgamma modulates the cardiac response to chronic pressure overload by distinct kinase-dependent and -independent effects. *Cell* 2004;**118**(3):375–87.
17. Mora A, Davies AM, Bertrand L, et al. Deficiency of PDK1 in cardiac muscle results in heart failure and increased sensitivity to hypoxia. *EMBO J* 2003;**22**(18):4666–76.
18. Garofalo RS, Orena SJ, Rafidi K, et al. Severe diabetes, age-dependent loss of adipose tissue, and mild growth deficiency in mice lacking Akt2/PKB beta. *J Clin Invest* 2003;**112**(2):197–208.
19. Chen WS, Xu PZ, Gottlob K, et al. Growth retardation and increased apoptosis in mice with homozygous disruption of the Akt1 gene. *Genes Dev* 2001;**15**(17):2203–8.
20. Cho H, Thorvaldsen JL, Chu Q, Feng F, Birnbaum MJ. Akt1/PKBalpha is required for normal growth but dispensable for maintenance of glucose homeostasis in mice. *J Biol Chem* 2001;**276**(42):38349–52.
21. Easton RM, Cho H, Roovers K, et al. Role for Akt3/protein kinase Bgamma in attainment of normal brain size. *Mol Cell Biol* 2005;**25**(5):1869–78.
22. Tschopp O, Yang ZZ, Brodbeck D, et al. Essential role of protein kinase B gamma (PKB gamma/Akt3) in postnatal brain development but not in glucose homeostasis. *Development* 2005;**132**(13):2943–54.
23. Shiojima I, Schiekofer S, Schneider JG, et al. Short-term akt activation in cardiac muscle cells improves contractile function in failing hearts. *Am J Pathol* 2012;**181**(6):1969–76.
24. Shiojima I, Sato K, Izumiya Y, et al. Disruption of coordinated cardiac hypertrophy and angiogenesis contributes to the transition to heart failure. *J Clin Invest* 2005;**115**(8):2108–18.
25. Roe ND, Xu X, Kandadi MR, et al. Targeted deletion of PTEN in cardiomyocytes renders cardiac contractile dysfunction through interruption of Pink1-AMPK signaling and autophagy. *Biochim Biophys Acta* 2015;**1852**(2):290–8.

26. Xu X, Roe ND, Weiser-Evans MC, Ren J. Inhibition of mammalian target of rapamycin with rapamycin reverses hypertrophic cardiomyopathy in mice with cardiomyocyte-specific knockout of PTEN. *Hypertension* 2014;**63**(4):729–39.
27. Crackower MA, Oudit GY, Kozieradzki I, et al. Regulation of myocardial contractility and cell size by distinct PI3K-PTEN signaling pathways. *Cell* 2002;**110**(6):737–49.
28. An D, Rodrigues B. Role of changes in cardiac metabolism in development of diabetic cardiomyopathy. *Am J Physiol Heart Circ Physiol* 2006;**291**(4):H1489–506.
29. Pulinilkunnil T, Rodrigues B. Cardiac lipoprotein lipase: metabolic basis for diabetic heart disease. *Cardiovasc Res* 2006;**69**(2):329–40.
30. Thorens B, Mueckler M. Glucose transporters in the 21st century. *Am J Physiol Endocrinol Metab* 2010;**298**(2):E141–5.
31. Brownsey RW, Boone AN, Allard MF. Actions of insulin on the mammalian heart: metabolism, pathology and biochemical mechanisms. *Cardiovasc Res* 1997;**34**(1):3–24.
32. Kraegen EW, Sowden JA, Halstead MB, et al. Glucose transporters and in vivo glucose uptake in skeletal and cardiac muscle: fasting, insulin stimulation and immunoisolation studies of GLUT1 and GLUT4. *Biochem J* 1993;**295**(Pt 1):287–93.
33. Montessuit C, Lerch R. Regulation and dysregulation of glucose transport in cardiomyocytes. *Biochim Biophys Acta* 2013;**1833**(4):848–56.
34. Chadt A, Immisch A, de Wendt C, et al. Deletion of both Rab-GTPase-activating proteins TBC1D1 and TBC1D4 in mice eliminates insulin- and AICAR-stimulated glucose transport [corrected]. *Diabetes* 2015;**64**(3):746–59.
35. Samovski D, Su X, Xu Y, Abumrad NA, Stahl PD. Insulin and AMPK regulate FA translocase/CD36 plasma membrane recruitment in cardiomyocytes via Rab GAP AS160 and Rab8a Rab GTPase. *J Lipid Res* 2012;**53**(4):709–17.
36. McCommis KS, Douglas DL, Krenz M, Baines CP. Cardiac-specific hexokinase 2 overexpression attenuates hypertrophy by increasing pentose phosphate pathway flux. *J Am Heart Assoc* 2013;**2**(6):e000355.
37. Wu R, Smeele KM, Wyatt E, et al. Reduction in hexokinase II levels results in decreased cardiac function and altered remodeling after ischemia/reperfusion injury. *Circ Res* 2011;**108**(1):60–9.
38. Wu R, Wyatt E, Chawla K, et al. Hexokinase II knockdown results in exaggerated cardiac hypertrophy via increased ROS production. *EMBO Mol Med* 2012;**4**(7):633–46.
39. Hue L, Depre C, Lefebvre V, Rider MH, Veitch K. Regulation of glucose metabolism in cardiac muscle. *Biochem Soc Trans* 1995;**23**(2):311–4.
40. Shulman RG, Bloch G, Rothman DL. In vivo regulation of muscle glycogen synthase and the control of glycogen synthesis. *Proc Natl Acad Sci USA* 1995;**92**(19):8535–42.
41. Markou T, Cullingford TE, Giraldo A, et al. Glycogen synthase kinases 3alpha and 3beta in cardiac myocytes: regulation and consequences of their inhibition. *Cell Signal* 2008;**20**(1):206–18.
42. Hue L, Beauloye C, Marsin AS, Bertrand L, Horman S, Rider MH. Insulin and ischemia stimulate glycolysis by acting on the same targets through different and opposing signaling pathways. *J Mol Cell Cardiol* 2002;**34**(9):1091–7.
43. Bertrand L, Alessi DR, Deprez J, et al. Heart 6-phosphofructo-2-kinase activation by insulin results from Ser-466 and Ser-483 phosphorylation and requires 3-phosphoinositide-dependent kinase-1, but not protein kinase B. *J Biol Chem* 1999;**274**(43):30927–33.
44. Deprez J, Vertommen D, Alessi DR, Hue L, Rider MH. Phosphorylation and activation of heart 6-phosphofructo-2-kinase by protein kinase B and other protein kinases of the insulin signaling cascades. *J Biol Chem* 1997;**272**(28):17269–75.
45. Donthi RV, Ye G, Wu C, McClain DA, Lange AJ, Epstein PN. Cardiac expression of kinase-deficient 6-phosphofructo-2-kinase/fructose-2,6-bisphosphatase inhibits glycolysis, promotes hypertrophy, impairs myocyte function, and reduces insulin sensitivity. *J Biol Chem* 2004;**279**(46):48085–90.

46. Wang Q, Donthi RV, Wang J, et al. Cardiac phosphatase-deficient 6-phosphofructo-2-kinase/fructose-2,6-bisphosphatase increases glycolysis, hypertrophy, and myocyte resistance to hypoxia. *Am J Physiol Heart Circ Physiol* 2008;**294**(6):H2889–97.
47. Evans RK, Schwartz DD, Gladden LB. Effect of myocardial volume overload and heart failure on lactate transport into isolated cardiac myocytes. *J Appl Physiol (1985)* 2003;**94**(3):1169–76.
48. Valenti D, de Bari L, Atlante A, Passarella S. L-Lactate transport into rat heart mitochondria and reconstruction of the L-lactate/pyruvate shuttle. *Biochem J* 2002;**364**(Pt 1):101–4.
49. Halestrap A, Price N. The proton-linked monocarboxylate transporter (MCT) family: structure, function and regulation. *Biochem J* 1999;**343**:281–99.
50. Depre C, Vanoverschelde JL, Taegtmeyer H. Glucose for the heart. *Circulation* 1999;**99**(4):578–88.
51. Watanabe T, Smith MM, Robinson FW, Kono T. Insulin action on glucose transport in cardiac muscle. *J Biol Chem* 1984;**259**(21):13117–22.
52. Lee FN, Zhang L, Zheng D, Choi WS, Youn JH. Insulin suppresses PDK-4 expression in skeletal muscle independently of plasma FFA. *Am J Physiol Endocrinol Metab* 2004;**287**(1):E69–74.
53. Kim YI, Lee FN, Choi WS, Lee S, Youn JH. Insulin regulation of skeletal muscle PDK4 mRNA expression is impaired in acute insulin-resistant states. *Diabetes* 2006;**55**(8):2311–7.
54. Randle PJ. The biochemical basis of the relation between glucose and fatty acid metabolism. *Acta Chir Scand Suppl* 1980;**498**:111–4.
55. Randle PJ, Garland PB, Hales CN, Newsholme EA. The glucose fatty-acid cycle. Its role in insulin sensitivity and the metabolic disturbances of diabetes mellitus. *Lancet* 1963;**1**(7285):785–9.
56. Rodrigues B, Cam MC, McNeill JH. Myocardial substrate metabolism: implications for diabetic cardiomyopathy. *J Mol Cell Cardiol* 1995;**27**(1):169–79.
57. Rodrigues B, McNeill JH. The diabetic heart: metabolic causes for the development of a cardiomyopathy. *Cardiovasc Res* 1992;**26**(10):913–22.
58. Brumby PE, Anderson M, Tuckley B, Storry JE, Hibbit KG. Lipid metabolism in the cow during starvation-induced ketosis. *Biochem J* 1975;**146**(3):609–15.
59. Khan RS, Lin Y, Hu Y, et al. Rescue of heart lipoprotein lipase-knockout mice confirms a role for triglyceride in optimal heart metabolism and function. *Am J Physiol Endocrinol Metab* 2013;**305**(11):E1339–47.
60. Yagyu H, Chen G, Yokoyama M, et al. Lipoprotein lipase (LpL) on the surface of cardiomyocytes increases lipid uptake and produces a cardiomyopathy. *J Clin Invest* 2003;**111**(3):419–26.
61. Pulinilkunnil T, An D, Yip P, et al. Palmitoyl lysophosphatidylcholine mediated mobilization of LPL to the coronary luminal surface requires PKC activation. *J Mol Cell Cardiol* 2004;**37**(5):931–8.
62. Qi D, Pulinilkunnil T, An D, et al. Single-dose dexamethasone induces whole-body insulin resistance and alters both cardiac fatty acid and carbohydrate metabolism. *Diabetes* 2004;**53**(7):1790–7.
63. Lloyd S, Brocks C, Chatham JC. Differential modulation of glucose, lactate, and pyruvate oxidation by insulin and dichloroacetate in the rat heart. *Am J Physiol Heart Circ Physiol* 2003;**285**(1):H163–72.
64. Augustus A, Yagyu H, Haemmerle G, et al. Cardiac-specific knock-out of lipoprotein lipase alters plasma lipoprotein triglyceride metabolism and cardiac gene expression. *J Biol Chem* 2004;**279**(24):25050–7.
65. Luiken JJ, Coort SL, Willems J, et al. Contraction-induced fatty acid translocase/CD36 translocation in rat cardiac myocytes is mediated through AMP-activated protein kinase signaling. *Diabetes* 2003;**52**(7):1627–34.
66. Luiken JJ, Schaap FG, van Nieuwenhoven FA, van der Vusse GJ, Bonen A, Glatz JF. Cellular fatty acid transport in heart and skeletal muscle as facilitated by proteins. *Lipids* 1999(34 Suppl):S169–75.
67. Luiken JJ, Turcotte LP, Bonen A. Protein-mediated palmitate uptake and expression of fatty acid transport proteins in heart giant vesicles. *J Lipid Res* 1999;**40**(6):1007–16.
68. Lopaschuk GD, Ussher JR, Folmes CD, Jaswal JS, Stanley WC. Myocardial fatty acid metabolism in health and disease. *Physiol Rev* 2010;**90**(1):207–58.
69. Kienesberger PC, Pulinilkunnil T, Nagendran J, Dyck JR. Myocardial triacylglycerol metabolism. *J Mol Cell Cardiol* 2013;**55**:101–10.

70. Knudsen J, Neergaard TB, Gaigg B, Jensen MV, Hansen JK. Role of acyl-CoA binding protein in acyl-CoA metabolism and acyl-CoA–mediated cell signaling. *J Nutr* 2000;**130**(2):294S–298SS.
71. McCoin CS, Knotts TA, Adams SH. Acylcarnitines–old actors auditioning for new roles in metabolic physiology. *Nat Rev Endocrinol* 2015;**11**(10):617–25.
72. McGarry JD, Brown NF. The mitochondrial carnitine palmitoyltransferase system—from concept to molecular analysis. *Eur J Biochem* 1997;**244**(1):1–14.
73. McGarry JD, Woeltje KF, Kuwajima M, Foster DW. Regulation of ketogenesis and the renaissance of carnitine palmitoyltransferase. *Diabetes Metab Rev* 1989;**5**(3):271–84.
74. Brownsey RW, Boone AN, Elliott JE, Kulpa JE, Lee WM. Regulation of acetyl-CoA carboxylase. *Biochem Soc Trans* 2006;**34**(Pt 2):223–7.
75. Steinberg GR, Kemp BE. AMPK in Health and Disease. *Physiol Rev* 2009;**89**(3):1025–78.
76. Zordoky BN, Nagendran J, Pulinilkunnil T, et al. AMPK-dependent inhibitory phosphorylation of ACC is not essential for maintaining myocardial fatty acid oxidation. *Circ Res* 2014;**115**(5):518–24.
77. Louis NA, Witters LA. Glucose regulation of acetyl-CoA carboxylase in hepatoma and islet cells. *J Biol Chem* 1992;**267**(4):2287–93.
78. Mazumder PK, O'Neill BT, Roberts MW, et al. Impaired cardiac efficiency and increased fatty acid oxidation in insulin-resistant ob/ob mouse hearts. *Diabetes* 2004;**53**(9):2366–74.
79. Vincent G, Bouchard B, Khairallah M, Des Rosiers C. Differential modulation of citrate synthesis and release by fatty acids in perfused working rat hearts. *Am J Physiol Heart Circ Physiol* 2004;**286**(1):H257–66.
80. Yu C, Chen Y, Cline GW, et al. Mechanism by which fatty acids inhibit insulin activation of insulin receptor substrate-1 (IRS-1)-associated phosphatidylinositol 3-kinase activity in muscle. *J Biol Chem* 2002;**277**(52):50230–6.
81. Djouadi F, Brandt J, Weinheimer C, Leone T, Gonzalez F, Kelly D. The role of the peroxisome proliferator-activated receptor α (PPARα) in the control of cardiac lipid metabolism. *Prostaglandins Leukot Essent Fatty Acids* 1999;**60**(5):339–43.
82. Wu P, Peters JM, Harris RA. Adaptive increase in pyruvate dehydrogenase kinase 4 during starvation is mediated by peroxisome proliferator-activated receptor alpha. *Biochem Biophys Res Commun* 2001;**287**(2):391–6.
83. Huang B, Wu P, Bowker-Kinley MM, Harris RA. Regulation of pyruvate dehydrogenase kinase expression by peroxisome proliferator-activated receptor-alpha ligands, glucocorticoids, and insulin. *Diabetes* 2002;**51**(2):276–83.
84. Varga T, Czimmerer Z, Nagy L. PPARs are a unique set of fatty acid regulated transcription factors controlling both lipid metabolism and inflammation. *Biochim Biophys Acta* 2011;**1812**(8):1007–22.
85. Finck BN, Lehman JJ, Leone TC, et al. The cardiac phenotype induced by PPARalpha overexpression mimics that caused by diabetes mellitus. *J Clin Invest* 2002;**109**(1):121–30.
86. Aon MA, Bhatt N, Cortassa SC. Mitochondrial and cellular mechanisms for managing lipid excess. *Front Physiol* 2014;**5**:282.
87. Chakrabarti P, Kandror KV. Adipose triglyceride lipase: a new target in the regulation of lipolysis by insulin. *Curr Diabetes Rev* 2011;**7**(4):270–7.
88. Stralfors P, Honnor RC. Insulin-induced dephosphorylation of hormone-sensitive lipase. Correlation with lipolysis and cAMP-dependent protein kinase activity. *Eur J Biochem/FEBS* 1989;**182**(2):379–85.
89. Sengupta S, Peterson TR, Sabatini DM. Regulation of the mTOR complex 1 pathway by nutrients, growth factors, and stress. *Mol Cell* 2010;**40**(2):310–22.
90. Wang X, Proud CG. The mTOR pathway in the control of protein synthesis. *Physiology (Bethesda)* 2006;**21**:362–9.
91. Wang X, Proud CG. mTORC1 signaling: what we still don't know. *J Mol Cell Biol* 2010;**4**:206–20.
92. Rolfe M, McLeod LE, Pratt PF, Proud CG. Activation of protein synthesis in cardiomyocytes by the hypertrophic agent phenylephrine requires the activation of ERK and involves phosphorylation of tuberous sclerosis complex 2 (TSC2). *Biochem J* 2005;**388**(Pt 3):973–84.

93. Inoki K, Zhu T, Guan KL. TSC2 mediates cellular energy response to control cell growth and survival. *Cell* 2003;**115**(5):577–90.
94. Wang X, Beugnet A, Murakami M, Yamanaka S, Proud CG. Distinct signaling events downstream of mTOR cooperate to mediate the effects of amino acids and insulin on initiation factor 4E-binding proteins. *Mol Cell Biol* 2005;**25**(7):2558–72.
95. Wang X, Li W, Williams M, Terada N, Alessi DR, Proud CG. Regulation of elongation factor 2 kinase by p90(RSK1) and p70 S6 kinase. *EMBO J* 2001;**20**(16):4370–9.
96. Wullschleger S, Loewith R, Hall MN. TOR signaling in growth and metabolism. *Cell* 2006;**124**(3):471–84.
97. Maillet M, van Berlo JH, Molkentin JD. Molecular basis of physiological heart growth: fundamental concepts and new players. *Nat Rev Mol Cell Biol* 2013;**14**(1):38–48.
98. Yang Z, Ming XF. mTOR signalling: the molecular interface connecting metabolic stress, aging and cardiovascular diseases. *Obes Rev Off J Int Assoc Study Obes* 2012(13 Suppl 2):58–68.
99. Beugnet A, Wang X, Proud CG. Target of rapamycin (TOR)-signaling and RAIP motifs play distinct roles in the mammalian TOR-dependent phosphorylation of initiation factor 4E-binding protein 1. *J Biol Chem* 2003;**278**(42):40717–22.
100. Demeulder B, Zarrinpashneh E, Ginion A, et al. Differential regulation of eEF2 and p70S6K by AMPKalpha2 in heart. *Biochim Biophys Acta* 2013;**1832**(6):780–90.
101. Wang L, Wang X, Proud CG. Activation of mRNA translation in rat cardiac myocytes by insulin involves multiple rapamycin-sensitive steps. *Am J Physiol Heart Circ Physiol* 2000;**278**(4):H1056–68.
102. Ryazanov AG, Pavur KS, Dorovkov MV. Alpha-kinases: a new class of protein kinases with a novel catalytic domain. *Curr Biol* 1999;**9**(2):R43–5.
103. Browne GJ, Finn SG, Proud CG. Stimulation of the AMP-activated protein kinase leads to activation of eukaryotic elongation factor 2 kinase and to its phosphorylation at a novel site, serine 398. *J Biol Chem* 2004;**279**(13):12220–31.
104. Chan AY, Soltys CL, Young ME, Proud CG, Dyck JR. Activation of AMP-activated protein kinase inhibits protein synthesis associated with hypertrophy in the cardiac myocyte. *J Biol Chem* 2004;**279**(31):32771–9.
105. Proud CG. mTOR-mediated regulation of translation factors by amino acids. *Biochem Biophys Res Commun* 2004;**313**(2):429–36.
106. Proud CG. Regulation of protein synthesis by insulin. *Biochem Soc Trans* 2006;**34**(Pt 2):213–6.
107. Proud CG, Denton RM. Molecular mechanisms for the control of translation by insulin. *Biochem J* 1997;**328**(Pt 2):329–41.
108. Proud CG, Wang X, Patel JV, et al. Interplay between insulin and nutrients in the regulation of translation factors. *Biochem Soc Trans* 2001;**29**(Pt 4):541–7.
109. Sharma S, Guthrie PH, Chan SS, Haq S, Taegtmeyer H. Glucose phosphorylation is required for insulin-dependent mTOR signalling in the heart. *Cardiovasc Res* 2007;**76**(1):71–80.
110. Carroll R, Carley AN, Dyck JR, Severson DL. Metabolic effects of insulin on cardiomyocytes from control and diabetic db/db mouse hearts. *Am J Physiol Endocrinol Metab* 2005;**288**(5):E900–6.
111. Young ME, Guthrie PH, Razeghi P, et al. Impaired long-chain fatty acid oxidation and contractile dysfunction in the obese Zucker rat heart. *Diabetes* 2002;**51**(8):2587–95.
112. Leguisamo NM, Lehnen AM, Machado UF, et al. GLUT4 content decreases along with insulin resistance and high levels of inflammatory markers in rats with metabolic syndrome. *Cardiovasc Diabetol* 2012;**11**:100.
113. Middelbeek RJ, Chambers MA, Tantiwong P, et al. Insulin stimulation regulates AS160 and TBC1D1 phosphorylation sites in human skeletal muscle. *Nutr Diabetes* 2013;**3**:e74.
114. Abel ED, Kaulbach HC, Tian R, et al. Cardiac hypertrophy with preserved contractile function after selective deletion of GLUT4 from the heart. *J Clin Invest* 1999;**104**(12):1703–14.
115. Stenbit AE, Katz EB, Chatham JC, et al. Preservation of glucose metabolism in hypertrophic GLUT4-null hearts. *Am J Physiol Heart Circ Physiol* 2000;**279**(1):H313–8.
116. Weiss RG, Chatham JC, Georgakopolous D, et al. An increase in the myocardial PCr/ATP ratio in GLUT4 null mice. *Faseb J* 2002;**16**(6):613–5.

117. Domenighetti AA, Danes VR, Curl CL, Favaloro JM, Proietto J, Delbridge LM. Targeted GLUT-4 deficiency in the heart induces cardiomyocyte hypertrophy and impaired contractility linked with Ca(2+) and proton flux dysregulation. *J Mol Cell Cardiol* 2010;**48**(4):663–72.
118. Li Y, Wende AR, Nunthakungwan O, et al. Cytosolic, but not mitochondrial, oxidative stress is a likely contributor to cardiac hypertrophy resulting from cardiac specific GLUT4 deletion in mice. *FEBS J* 2012;**279**(4):599–611.
119. Zisman A, Peroni OD, Abel ED, et al. Targeted disruption of the glucose transporter 4 selectively in muscle causes insulin resistance and glucose intolerance. *Nat Med* 2000;**6**(8):924–8.
120. Hebert Jr. LF, Daniels MC, Zhou J, et al. Overexpression of glutamine:fructose-6-phosphate amidotransferase in transgenic mice leads to insulin resistance. *J Clin Invest* 1996;**98**(4):930–6.
121. Lopaschuk GD, Belke DD, Gamble J, Itoi T, Schonekess BO. Regulation of fatty acid oxidation in the mammalian heart in health and disease. *Biochim Biophys Acta* 1994;**1213**(3):263–76.
122. Stanley WC, Lopaschuk GD, Hall JL, McCormack JG. Regulation of myocardial carbohydrate metabolism under normal and ischaemic conditions. Potential for pharmacological interventions. *Cardiovasc Res* 1997;**33**(2):243–57.
123. Stanley WC, Recchia FA, Lopaschuk GD. Myocardial substrate metabolism in the normal and failing heart. *Physiol Rev* 2005;**85**(3):1093–129.
124. Pulinilkunnil T, Qi D, Ghosh S, et al. Circulating triglyceride lipolysis facilitates lipoprotein lipase translocation from cardiomyocyte to myocardial endothelial lining. *Cardiovasc Res* 2003;**59**(3):788–97.
125. Samuel VT, Shulman GI. Mechanisms for insulin resistance: common threads and missing links. *Cell* 2012;**148**(5):852–71.
126. Savage DB, Petersen KF, Shulman GI. Disordered lipid metabolism and the pathogenesis of insulin resistance. *Physiol Rev* 2007;**87**(2):507–20.
127. Hsieh CT, Chuang JH, Yang WC, Yin Y, Lin Y. Ceramide inhibits insulin-stimulated Akt phosphorylation through activation of Rheb/mTORC1/S6K signaling in skeletal muscle. *Cell Signal* 2014;**26**(7):1400–8.
128. Ritter O, Jelenik T, Roden M. Lipid-mediated muscle insulin resistance: different fat, different pathways? *J Mol Med* 2015;**93**(8):831–43.
129. Stratford S, Hoehn KL, Liu F, Summers SA. Regulation of insulin action by ceramide: dual mechanisms linking ceramide accumulation to the inhibition of Akt/protein kinase B. *J Biol Chem* 2004;**279**(35):36608–15.
130. JeBailey L, Wanono O, Niu W, Roessler J, Rudich A, Klip A. Ceramide- and oxidant-induced insulin resistance involve loss of insulin-dependent Rac-activation and actin remodeling in muscle cells. *Diabetes* 2007;**56**(2):394–403.
131. Mahfouz R, Khoury R, Blachnio-Zabielska A, et al. Characterising the inhibitory actions of ceramide upon insulin signaling in different skeletal muscle cell models: a mechanistic insight. *PloS One* 2014;**9**(7):e101865.
132. Mothe I, Van Obberghen E. Phosphorylation of insulin receptor substrate-1 on multiple serine residues, 612, 632, 662, and 731, modulates insulin action. *J Biol Chem* 1996;**271**(19):11222–7.
133. Shah OJ, Wang Z, Hunter T. Inappropriate activation of the TSC/Rheb/mTOR/S6K cassette induces IRS1/2 depletion, insulin resistance, and cell survival deficiencies. *Curr Biol* 2004;**14**(18):1650–6.
134. Finck BN, Han X, Courtois M, et al. A critical role for PPARalpha-mediated lipotoxicity in the pathogenesis of diabetic cardiomyopathy: modulation by dietary fat content. *Proc Natl Acad Sci USA* 2003;**100**(3):1226–31.
135. Park SY, Cho YR, Finck BN, et al. Cardiac-specific overexpression of peroxisome proliferator-activated receptor-alpha causes insulin resistance in heart and liver. *Diabetes* 2005;**54**(9):2514–24.
136. Son NH, Yu S, Tuinei J, et al. PPARgamma-induced cardiolipotoxicity in mice is ameliorated by PPARalpha deficiency despite increases in fatty acid oxidation. *J Clin Invest* 2010;**120**(10):3443–54.
137. Chavez JA, Summers SA. A ceramide-centric view of insulin resistance. *Cell Metab* 2012;**15**(5):585–94.
138. Park TS, Hu Y, Noh HL, et al. Ceramide is a cardiotoxin in lipotoxic cardiomyopathy. *J Lipid Res* 2008;**49**(10):2101–12.
139. Belke DD, Larsen TS, Gibbs EM, Severson DL. Altered metabolism causes cardiac dysfunction in perfused hearts from diabetic (db/db) mice. *Am J Physiol-Endocrinolo Metabol* 2000;**279**(5):E1104–13.

140. Belke DD, Swanson EA, Dillmann WH. Decreased sarcoplasmic reticulum activity and contractility in diabetic db/db mouse heart. *Diabetes* 2004;**53**(12):3201–8.
141. Newsholme EA, Sugden PH, Williams T. Effect of citrate on the activities of 6-phosphofructokinase from nervous and muscle tissues from different animals and its relationships to the regulation of glycolysis. *Biochem J* 1977;**166**(1):123–9.
142. Usenik A, Legisa M. Evolution of allosteric citrate binding sites on 6-phosphofructo-1-kinase. *PloS One* 2010;**5**(11):e15447.
143. Jain SS, Luiken JJ, Snook LA, et al. Fatty acid transport and transporters in muscle are critically regulated by Akt2. *FEBS Lett* 2015;**589**(19 Pt B):2769–75.
144. Randle PJ. Regulatory interactions between lipids and carbohydrates: the glucose fatty acid cycle after 35 years. *Diabetes Metab Rev* 1998;**14**(4):263–83.
145. Kienesberger PC, Lee D, Pulinilkunnil T, et al. Adipose triglyceride lipase deficiency causes tissue-specific changes in insulin signaling. *J Biol Chem* 2009;**284**(44):30218–29.
146. Glenn DJ, Wang F, Nishimoto M, et al. A murine model of isolated cardiac steatosis leads to cardiomyopathy. *Hypertension* 2011;**57**(2):216–22.
147. Pulinilkunnil T, Kienesberger PC, Nagendran J, Sharma N, Young ME, Dyck JR. Cardiac-specific adipose triglyceride lipase overexpression protects from cardiac steatosis and dilated cardiomyopathy following diet-induced obesity. *Int J Obes (Lond)* 2014;**38**(2):205–15.
148. Newgard CB. Interplay between lipids and branched-chain amino acids in development of insulin resistance. *Cell Metab* 2012;**15**(5):606–14.
149. Ghosh S, An D, Pulinilkunnil T, et al. Role of dietary fatty acids and acute hyperglycemia in modulating cardiac cell death. *Nutrition* 2004;**20**(10):916–23.
150. Ghosh S, Kewalramani G, Yuen G, et al. Induction of mitochondrial nitrative damage and cardiac dysfunction by chronic provision of dietary omega-6 polyunsaturated fatty acids. *Free Radic Biol Med* 2006;**41**(9):1413–24.
151. Ghosh S, Pulinilkunnil T, Yuen G, et al. Cardiomyocyte apoptosis induced by short-term diabetes requires mitochondrial GSH depletion. *Am J Physiol Heart Circ Physiol* 2005;**289**(2):H768–76.
152. Ghosh S, Qi D, An D, et al. Brief episode of STZ-induced hyperglycemia produces cardiac abnormalities in rats fed a diet rich in n-6 PUFA. *Am J Physiol Heart Circ Physiol* 2004;**287**(6):H2518–27.
153. Ghosh S, Rodrigues B. Cardiac cell death in early diabetes and its modulation by dietary fatty acids. *Biochim Biophys Acta* 2006;**1761**(10):1148–62.
154. Ghosh S, Ting S, Lau H, et al. Increased efflux of glutathione conjugate in acutely diabetic cardiomyocytes. *Can J Physiol Pharmacol* 2004;**82**(10):879–87.
155. Eguchi K, Manabe I. Toll-like receptor, lipotoxicity and chronic inflammation: the pathological link between obesity and cardiometabolic disease. *J Atheroscler Thromb* 2014;**21**(7):629–39.
156. Rana JS, Nieuwdorp M, Jukema JW, Kastelein JJ. Cardiovascular metabolic syndrome-an interplay of, obesity, inflammation, diabetes and coronary heart disease. *Diabetes Obes Metab* 2007;**9**(3):218–32.
157. Ko HJ, Zhang Z, Jung DY, et al. Nutrient stress activates inflammation and reduces glucose metabolism by suppressing AMP-activated protein kinase in the heart. *Diabetes* 2009;**58**(11):2536–46.
158. Kolwicz Jr. SC, Purohit S, Tian R. Cardiac metabolism and its interactions with contraction, growth, and survival of cardiomyocytes. *Circ Res* 2013;**113**(5):603–16.
159. de Simone G, Izzo R, De Luca N, Gerdts E. Left ventricular geometry in obesity: Is it what we expect? *Nutr Metabol Cardiovasc Dis NMCD* 2013;**23**(10):905–12.
160. Murdolo G, Angeli F, Reboldi G, et al. Left ventricular hypertrophy and obesity: only a matter of fat? *High Blood Press Cardiovascr Prevention Off J Italian Soc Hypertension* 2015;**22**(1):29–41.
161. Jia G, DeMarco VG, Sowers JR. Insulin resistance and hyperinsulinaemia in diabetic cardiomyopathy. *Nat Rev Endocrinol* 2015;**12**(3):144–53.
162. Ussher JR. The role of cardiac lipotoxicity in the pathogenesis of diabetic cardiomyopathy. *Expert Rev Cardiovasc Ther* 2014;**12**(3):345–58.

163. Bark TH, McNurlan MA, Lang CH, Garlick PJ. Increased protein synthesis after acute IGF-I or insulin infusion is localized to muscle in mice. *Am J Physiol* 1998;**275**(1 Pt 1):E118–23.
164. McNulty PH, Louard RJ, Deckelbaum LI, Zaret BL, Young LH. Hyperinsulinemia inhibits myocardial protein degradation in patients with cardiovascular disease and insulin resistance. *Circulation* 1995;**92**(8):2151–6.
165. Kido Y, Burks DJ, Withers D, et al. Tissue-specific insulin resistance in mice with mutations in the insulin receptor, IRS-1, and IRS-2. *J Clin Invest* 2000;**105**(2):199–205.
166. Laustsen PG, Michael MD, Crute BE, et al. Lipoatrophic diabetes in Irs1(-/-)/Irs3(-/-) double knockout mice. *Genes Dev* 2002;**16**(24):3213–22.
167. Long YC, Cheng Z, Copps KD, White MF. Insulin receptor substrates Irs1 and Irs2 coordinate skeletal muscle growth and metabolism via the Akt and AMPK pathways. *Mol Cell Biol* 2011;**31**(3):430–41.
168. Lin RC, Weeks KL, Gao XM, et al. PI3K(p110 alpha) protects against myocardial infarction-induced heart failure: identification of PI3K-regulated miRNA and mRNA. *Arterioscler Thromb Vasc Biol* 2010;**30**(4):724–32.
169. Heineke J, Molkentin JD. Regulation of cardiac hypertrophy by intracellular signalling pathways. *Nat Rev Mol Cell Biol* 2006;**7**(8):589–600.
170. Molkentin JD. Calcineurin-NFAT signaling regulates the cardiac hypertrophic response in coordination with the MAPKs. *Cardiovasc Res* 2004;**63**(3):467–75.
171. Walther S, Awad S, Lonchyna VA, Blatter LA. NFAT transcription factor regulation by urocortin II in cardiac myocytes and heart failure. *Am J Physiol Heart Circ Physiol* 2014;**306**(6):H856–66.
172. Yang TT, Suk HY, Yang X, et al. Role of transcription factor NFAT in glucose and insulin homeostasis. *Mol Cell Biol* 2006;**26**(20):7372–87.
173. Zhang X, Tang N, Hadden TJ, Rishi AK. Akt, FoxO and regulation of apoptosis. *Biochim Biophys Acta* 2011;**1813**(11):1978–86.
174. Evans-Anderson HJ, Alfieri CM, Yutzey KE. Regulation of cardiomyocyte proliferation and myocardial growth during development by FOXO transcription factors. *Circ Res* 2008;**102**(6):686–94.
175. Ni YG, Wang N, Cao DJ, et al. FoxO transcription factors activate Akt and attenuate insulin signaling in heart by inhibiting protein phosphatases. *Proc Natl Acad Sci USA* 2007;**104**(51):20517–22.
176. Sengupta A, Kalinichenko VV, Yutzey KE. FoxO1 and FoxM1 transcription factors have antagonistic functions in neonatal cardiomyocyte cell-cycle withdrawal and IGF1 gene regulation. *Circ Res* 2013;**112**(2):267–77.
177. Skurk C, Izumiya Y, Maatz H, et al. The FOXO3a transcription factor regulates cardiac myocyte size downstream of AKT signaling. *J Biol Chem* 2005;**280**(21):20814–23.
178. Battiprolu PK, Hojayev B, Jiang N, et al. Metabolic stress-induced activation of FoxO1 triggers diabetic cardiomyopathy in mice. *J Clin Invest* 2012;**122**(3):1109–18.
179. Paula-Gomes S, Goncalves DA, Baviera AM, Zanon NM, Navegantes LC, Kettelhut IC. Insulin suppresses atrophy- and autophagy-related genes in heart tissue and cardiomyocytes through AKT/FOXO signaling. *Horm Metab Res* 2013;**45**(12):849–55.
180. Lopaschuk GD. Alterations in fatty acid oxidation during reperfusion of the heart after myocardial ischemia. *Am J Cardiol* 1997;**80**(3A):11A–16AA.
181. Oliver MF, Opie LH. Effects of glucose and fatty acids on myocardial ischaemia and arrhythmias. *Lancet* 1994;**343**(8890):155–8.
182. Kloner RA, Jennings RB. Consequences of brief ischemia: stunning, preconditioning, and their clinical implications: part 1. *Circulation* 2001;**104**(24):2981–9.
183. Liu Q, Docherty JC, Rendell JC, Clanachan AS, Lopaschuk GD. High levels of fatty acids delay the recovery of intracellular pH and cardiac efficiency in post-ischemic hearts by inhibiting glucose oxidation. *J Am Coll Cardiol* 2002;**39**(4):718–25.

184. Ponticos M, Lu QL, Morgan JE, Hardie DG, Partridge TA, Carling D. Dual regulation of the AMP-activated protein kinase provides a novel mechanism for the control of creatine kinase in skeletal muscle. *EMBO J* 1998;**17**(6):1688–99.
185. Dennis SC, Gevers W, Opie LH. Protons in ischemia: where do they come from; where do they go to? *J Mol Cell Cardiol* 1991;**23**(9):1077–86.
186. Opie LH. Myocardial ischemia--metabolic pathways and implications of increased glycolysis. *Cardiovasc Drugs Ther* 1990(4 Suppl 4):777–90.
187. Sack MN, Yellon DM. Insulin therapy as an adjunct to reperfusion after acute coronary ischemia: a proposed direct myocardial cell survival effect independent of metabolic modulation. *J Am Coll Cardiol* 2003;**41**(8):1404–7.
188. Yao H, Han X, Han X. The cardioprotection of the insulin-mediated PI3K/Akt/mTOR signaling pathway. *Am J Cardiovasc Drugs* 2014;**14**(6):433–42.
189. Teshima Y, Takahashi N, Thuc LC, et al. High-glucose condition reduces cardioprotective effects of insulin against mechanical stress-induced cell injury. *Life Sci* 2010;**87**(5–6):154–61.
190. Lv GF, Dong ML, Hu DH, et al. Insulin-mediated inhibition of p38 mitogen-activated protein kinase protects cardiomyocytes in severe burns. *J Burn Care Res Off Publ Am Burn Assoc* 2011;**32**(6):591–9.
191. Zuurbier CJ, Van Wezel HB. Glucose-insulin therapy, plasma substrate levels and cardiac recovery after cardiac ischemic events. *Cardiovasc Drugs Ther* 2008;**22**(2):125–31.
192. Jonassen AK, Aasum E, Riemersma RA, Mjos OD, Larsen TS. Glucose-insulin-potassium reduces infarct size when administered during reperfusion. *Cardiovasc Drugs Ther* 2000;**14**(6):615–23.
193. Taegtmeyer H, Lubrano G. Rethinking cardiac metabolism: metabolic cycles to refuel and rebuild the failing heart. *F1000Prime Rep* 2014;**6**:90.
194. Allen DG, Xiao X-H. Role of the cardiac Na+/H+ exchanger during ischemia and reperfusion. *Cardiovasc Res* 2003;**57**(4):934–41.
195. Azevedo PS, Minicucci MF, Santos PP, Paiva SA, Zornoff LA. Energy metabolism in cardiac remodeling and heart failure. *Cardiol Rev* 2013;**21**(3):135–40.
196. Dhalla NS, Liu X, Panagia V, Takeda N. Subcellular remodeling and heart dysfunction in chronic diabetes. *Cardiovasc Res* 1998;**40**(2):239–47.
197. Piper H, Garcña-Dorado D, Ovize M. A fresh look at reperfusion injury. *Cardiovasc Res* 1998;**38**(2):291–300.
198. Piper HM, García-Dorado D. Prime causes of rapid cardiomyocyte death during reperfusion. *Ann Thorac Surg* 1999;**68**(5):1913–9.
199. Dhalla NS, Saini HK, Tappia PS, Sethi R, Mengi SA, Gupta SK. Potential role and mechanisms of subcellular remodeling in cardiac dysfunction due to ischemic heart disease. *J Cardiovasc Med* 2007;**8**(4):238–50.
200. Temsah RM, Netticadan T, Chapman D, Takeda S, Mochizuki S, Dhalla NS. Alterations in sarcoplasmic reticulum function and gene expression in ischemic-reperfused rat heart. *Am J Physiol* 1999;**277**(2 Pt 2):H584–94.
201. Abdallah Y, Gkatzoflia A, Gligorievski D, et al. Insulin protects cardiomyocytes against reoxygenation-induced hypercontracture by a survival pathway targeting SR Ca2+ storage. *Cardiovasc Res* 2006;**70**(2):346–53.
202. Fredersdorf S, Thumann C, Zimmermann WH, et al. Increased myocardial SERCA expression in early type 2 diabetes mellitus is insulin dependent: In vivo and in vitro data. *Cardiovasc Diabetol* 2012;**11**:57.
203. Wold LE, Dutta K, Mason MM, et al. Impaired SERCA function contributes to cardiomyocyte dysfunction in insulin resistant rats. *J Mol Cell Cardiol* 2005;**39**(2):297–307.
204. Zarain-Herzberg A, Garcia-Rivas G, Estrada-Aviles R. Regulation of SERCA pumps expression in diabetes. *Cell Calcium* 2014;**56**(5):302–10.

205. Lu Z, Jiang YP, Xu XH, Ballou LM, Cohen IS, Lin RZ. Decreased L-type Ca2+ current in cardiac myocytes of type 1 diabetic Akita mice due to reduced phosphatidylinositol 3-kinase signaling. *Diabetes* 2007;**56**(11):2780–9.
206. Lu Z, Jiang YP, Wang W, et al. Loss of cardiac phosphoinositide 3-kinase p110 alpha results in contractile dysfunction. *Circulation* 2009;**120**(4):318–25.
207. Sun H, Kerfant BG, Zhao D, et al. Insulin-like growth factor-1 and PTEN deletion enhance cardiac L-type Ca2+ currents via increased PI3Kalpha/PKB signaling. *Circ Res* 2006;**98**(11):1390–7.
208. Cittadini A, Monti MG, Iaccarino G, et al. Adenoviral gene transfer of Akt enhances myocardial contractility and intracellular calcium handling. *Gene Ther* 2006;**13**(1):8–19.
209. Howarth FC, Qureshi MA, Gbewonyo AJ, Tariq S, Adeghate E. The progressive effects of a fat enriched diet on ventricular myocyte contraction and intracellular Ca2+ in the C57BL/6J mouse. *Mol Cell Biochem* 2005;**273**(1–2):87–95.
210. Limitations of resuscitation. *Lancet* 1972;**1**(7761):1169–70.
211. Kolluru GK, Bir SC, Kevil CG. Endothelial dysfunction and diabetes: effects on angiogenesis, vascular remodeling, and wound healing. *Int J Vasc Med* 2012;**2012**:918267.
212. Frantz S, Nahrendorf M. Cardiac macrophages and their role in ischaemic heart disease. *Cardiovasc Res* 2014;**102**(2):240–8.
213. Takeda N, Manabe I. Cellular Interplay between Cardiomyocytes and Nonmyocytes in Cardiac Remodeling. *Int J Inflam* 2011;**2011**:535241.

Index

Note: Page numbers followed by "*f*" and "*t*" refer to figures and tables, respectively.

B

Kolibri 360 GmbH
Ferdinand-Jühlke-Straße 7
99095 Erfurt, Deutschland
produktsicherheit@kolibri360.de